# Tumors in
# Domestic Animals

# Tumors in Domestic Animals

Third Edition,
Revised and Expanded

**Edited by Jack E. Moulton**

University of California Press
Berkeley · Los Angeles · London

to Sally Moulton Borges, D.V.M.

University of California Press
Berkeley and Los Angeles, California

University of California Press, Ltd.
London, England

Copyright © 1961, 1978, 1990 by The Regents of the University of California
First edition 1961   Second Edition 1978   Third Edition, revised and expanded 1990

LIBRARY OF CONGRESS CATALOGING-IN-PUBLICATION DATA
Tumors in domestic animals / edited by Jack E. Moulton.—3rd ed.,
   rev. and expanded.
      p.   cm.
   Includes bibliographies.
   ISBN 0-520-05818-6 (alk. paper)
   1. Tumors in animals.   2. Veterinary oncology.   I. Moulton, Jack E.
   [DNLM: 1. Animals, Domestic.   2. Neoplasms—veterinary. SF910.T8 T295]
SF910.T8M6   1990
636.089′6992—dc19
DNLM/DLC
for Library of Congress          87-30248

Printed in the United States of America
1 2 3 4 5 6 7 8 9

# Contents

## 12. Tumors of the Mammary Gland    518

by Jack E. Moulton

## 13. Tumors of the Endocrine Glands    553

by Charles C. Capen

## 14. Tumors of the Nervous System and Eye    640

by Donald R. Cordy

# Contributing Authors

Charles C. Capen, D.V.M., Ph.D.
Professor and Chairman, Department of Veterinary Pathobiology, College of Veterinary Medicine; Professor of Endocrinology and Metabolism, Department of Medicine, College of Medicine, Ohio State University, Columbus, Ohio.

Donald R. Cordy, D.V.M., Ph.D.
Professor Emeritus, Department of Pathology, School of Veterinary Medicine, University of California, Davis, California.

John W. Harvey, D.V.M., Ph.D.
Professor, Department of Physiological Sciences, and Chief, Clinical Pathology Service, College of Veterinary Medicine, University of Florida, Gainesville, Florida.

Kenneth W. Head, BSc., M.R.C.V.S.
Senior Lecturer, Department of Pathology, Royal (Dick) School of Veterinary Studies, Edinburgh, Scotland, U.K.

Thomas J. Hulland, D.V.M., Ph.D.
Professor, Department of Pathology, and Associate Dean, Academic, Ontario Veterinary College, University of Guelph, Guelph, Ontario, Canada.

Peter C. Kennedy, D.V.M., Ph.D.
Professor, Department of Pathology, School of Veterinary Medicine, University of California, Davis, California.

Wim Misdorp, D.V.M., Ph.D.
Member of the Staff, Netherlands Cancer Institute, Amsterdam, The Netherlands, and Professor, Veterinary Oncology, Veterinary Faculty, State University, Utrecht, The Netherlands.

Jack E. Moulton, D.V.M., Ph.D.
Professor Emeritus, Department of Pathology, School of Veterinary Medicine, University of California, Davis, California.

Svend W. Nielson, D.V.M., Ph.D.
Professor of Pathobiology and Director, Northeastern Research Center for Wildlife Diseases, University of Connecticut, Storrs, Connecticut.

Roy R. Pool, D.V.M., Ph.D.
Professor, Department of Pathology, and Research Pathologist, Laboratory for Energy-Related Health Research, School of Veterinary Medicine, University of California, Davis, California.

James A. Popp, D.V.M., Ph.D.
Head, Experimental Pathology and Toxicology, CIIT, Research Triangle Park, North Carolina.

L. Thomas Pulley, D.V.M., Ph.D.
Department Head, Clinical Pathology, Syntex Research, Palo Alto, California.

Anthony A. Stannard, D.V.M., Ph.D.
Professor, Department of Medicine, School of Veterinary Medicine, University of California, Davis, California.

# Preface to the Third Edition

The third edition of *Tumors in Domestic Animals* is considerably enlarged from the previous edition because of the great expansion of published data in veterinary oncology. There has been some attempt to balance the chapter subject matter based on importance in veterinary practice today, but this has not always been possible. I feel that everything significant is included, although some unevenness will be apparent.

The number of chapters has increased from 13 to 14 because of the need of adding a chapter on proliferative lesions of the joints.

A number of new authors have been added. These include Drs. Head and Misdorp from Europe and Drs. Kennedy, Nielsen, Popp, and Harvey from the United States.

The book, as before, is directed mainly toward students and graduate veterinarians, but I hope it will also be of value to individuals in comparative oncology, including those interested in human and experimental pathology.

We have been unable to include neoplasms of domestic and pet avian species and those of captive wild species. Neoplasms of laboratory animals have also been excluded.

I wish to acknowledge the patience and consideration of my university colleagues. Finally, I would like to thank the University Press, especially my editors, Shirley Warren and Kathy Walker, and Ellen Herman; and my proofreader, Jess Bell of Kachergis Book Design.

JACK E. MOULTON

*February 15, 1989*

# Tumors in
# Domestic Animals

**1**

*Wim Misdorp*
# General Considerations

Tumours are space filling lesions
For the cell growth we don't know the reasons
     They expand and can spread
     From the toe to the head
They're the host's own parts guilty of treason.
(After Sobin, 1978)

## The Pathologist's Task in Veterinary Oncology

The primary task of the veterinary pathologist working in the field of clinical oncology is to determine the nature and type of a given tumor, to assess the completeness of surgery, and if possible, to indicate the prognosis.

Good cooperation between pathologist and clinician is indispensable to this task. The clinician has to provide data concerning the stage of the disease and the patient's condition. The pathologist can then give valuable information regarding further treatment.

Unfortunately, the pathologist's involvement in the study of tumors often begins at a relatively late stage, and his observations tend to be both fragmentary and static. Microscopical observations are necessarily limited to some selected centimeters of what may be a very extensive battlefield between tumor cells and the host and one that is fixed at a particular moment in time.

Nevertheless, veterinary pathologists have contributed much to the classification and further characterization of tumor diseases in animals. With the growing interest in tumor therapy studies in animals, the veterinary pathologist has an important role in determining whether a given tumor patient is to be included in a trial or not and, at the end of such a patient's life, in determining the cause of death and the effect of the treatment. There are many aspects of veterinary oncology, such as epi-demiological, etiological, tumor kinetic, and cyto-photometric studies, which benefit from the participation of a pathologist.

Once a diagnosis of neoplasia is established, the nature of the tumor, that is, whether it is malignant or benign, has to be determined (table 1.1). Post-mortem examination and other retrospective studies are valuable for this. In recent years, however, prospective "follow-up" studies have been found to be of particular assistance in determining the true nature of several tumor types in domestic animals. Some tumors occupy the borderland between malignant and benign: for example, those tumors that metastasize only rarely, those that may lead to euthanasia due to ingrowth into vital structures, and those that produce excessive amounts of hormones or other products.

Neoplasms are usually of epithelial or mesenchymal (connective tissue) type. The former usually have an organoid organization of neoplastic epithelium and of stromal tissue, which consists of connective tissue with newly formed blood vessels. Thus, carcinomas (malignant epithelial neoplasms) can be categorized according to the relative amount of stroma: scirrhous (much stroma), simplex (moderate amount), or medullary (little stroma). Sarcomas (malignant connective tissue neoplasms) lack the organoid type of structure shown by carcinomas. As shown in table 1.2, tumors can be diagnosed according to their tissue of origin.

In poorly differentiated tumors, the diagnosis in some cases can be established by the application of

**TABLE 1.1. Criteria for Distinguishing Between Benign and Malignant Tumors**

| Cytologic features | Benign | Malignant |
|---|---|---|
| Cell size | Uniform | Pleomorphic |
| Nucleoli | Normal | Large, usually multiple |
| Chromatin, DNA | Usually normal amount | Hyperchromatic, often polyploid |
| Mitoses | Few | Usually numerous, including pathologic ones |
| Nuclear:cytoplasmic ratio | Rather low | Rather high |
| Structure | Well-differentiated | Imperfectly differentiated (anaplastic) |
| Mode of growth | Usually expansive and a capsule formed | Infiltrative as well as expansive, not encapsulated |
| Rate of growth[a] | Usually slow | May be rapid |
| Course of growth | May come to a standstill | Rarely ceases growing |
| Effect on host | Usually not dangerous, metastasis absent | Dangerous because of destructive infiltrative growth; prone to recurrence and metastasis |

[a] Little is known of the rate of growth of untreated primary tumors in domestic animals.

**TABLE 1.2. Most Common Types of Benign and Malignant Tumors in Domestic Animals**

| Benign tumor | Malignant tumor (with metastatic potential) |
|---|---|
| A. Connective tissue and its derivatives | |
| Fibroma (fibropapilloma) | Fibrosarcoma |
| Chondroma (and osteochondroma) | Chondrosarcoma |
| Osteoma (and osteoblastoma) | Osteosarcoma (osteogenic sarcoma) |
| Lipoma | Liposarcoma |
| Giant cell tumor (osteoclastoma) | Malignant giant cell tumor |
| Synovioma (fibroxanthoma) | Synovial sarcoma |
| Mastocytoma | Mast cell sarcoma |
| Histiocytoma | Histiocytic sarcoma |
| B. Endothelial tissue and its derivatives | |
| Hemangioma | Hemangiosarcoma |
| Lymphangioma | Lymphangiosarcoma |
| C. Hematopoietic tissue and its derivatives | |
| Solitary plasmacytoma | Myeloma (and primary macroglobulinemia) |
| Mastocytoma | Malignant mastocytoma |
| Thymoma | Malignant thymoma |
| | Lymphoma (lymphosarcoma) |
| | Lymphoid leukemia |
| | Miscellaneous myeloid neoplasms (erythremia and polycythemia vera) |
| D. Muscle | |
| Leiomyoma | Leiomyosarcoma |
| Rhabdomyoma | Rhabdomyosarcoma |

**TABLE 1.2 (continued)**

| Benign tumor | Malignant tumor (with metastatic potential) |
|---|---|
| **E. Nervous system** | |
| Schwannoma (neurinoma, neurofibroma) | Malignant Schwannoma (neurofibrosarcoma) |
| Astrocytoma | |
| Gangliocytoma | |
| | Medulloblastoma |
| Ganglioneuroma | Neuroblastoma |
| **F. Epithelium** | |
| Papilloma | Squamous cell carcinoma (epidermoid carcinoma) |
| Adenoma | Adenocarcinoma |
| Basal cell tumor | Transitional cell carcinoma |
| **G. Mixed (derived from more than one germ layer or more than one derivative of a single germ layer)** | |
| Teratoma, benign | Teratoma, malignant |
| Mixed tumor, benign (mammary gland) (epithelial and myoepithelial and/or mesenchymal tumor cells) | Mixed tumor, malignant (carcinosarcoma) |
| **H. Miscellaneous tumors and tumors of special organs** | |
| Melanoma, benign | Melanoma, malignant |
| Myoepithelioma, benign | Myoepithelioma, malignant |
| Chemoreceptor tumor, benign (chemodectoma, nonchromaffin paraganglioma) | Chemoreceptor tumor, malignant |
| Epulis | |
| Odontoma | |
| Sertoli cell tumor, benign | Sertoli cell tumor, malignant |
| | Seminoma[a] |
| Interstitial cell tumor (testis) | |
| Granulosa cell tumor, benign | Granulosa cell tumor, malignant |
| | Mesothelioma |
| | Embryonal nephroma |
| | Transmissible venereal tumor |
| Pheochromocytoma | Malignant pheochromocytoma |
| **I. Locally aggressive but rarely metastasizing tumors** | |
| Canine hemangiopericytoma (soft tissues) | |
| Equine sarcoid (soft tissues) | |
| Ependymoma (brain) | |
| Plexus papilloma (brain) | |
| Oligodendroglioma (brain) | |
| Meningioma (meninges) | |
| Ameloblastoma, or adamantinoma (gingiva) | |

[a] Metastasizes rarely in the dog in spite of malignant histological features.

special stains. These can accentuate either the epithelial or mesenchymal structure (e.g., reticulum fiber stain) or special cellular products (e.g., melanin, mucin, or metachromatic mast cell granules).

Cytology can be a useful diagnostic tool in the hands of a well-skilled cytologist familiar with the histologic and cytologic appearance of tumors and normal tissues. The diagnosis of processes in locations not easily accessible for incisional or excisional biopsy (e.g., body cavities) can be facilitated by cytology.

Needle biopsy can be of practical importance in the differentiation between "carcinomatous mastitis" (treatment contraindicated) and true mastitis (treatable) in dogs. Also, differentiation between tumorous (lymphomatous or carcinomatous) and nontumorous enlarged lymph nodes can be facilitated by cytology. Impression smears can be used for the cytologic diagnosis of superficial processes or as a complementary tool to histology in the detailed diagnosis of lymphoma.

This chapter is meant to help the student in veterinary oncologic pathology to become familiar with various branches of the subject, in particular with morphology. In general, emphasis is laid on the veterinary literature, but where information is lacking, relevant data from studies on human and experimental cancer have been used to explain current concepts of special importance.

Our knowledge of the naturally occurring tumors of domestic animals and our understanding of the important role that the veterinary pathologist can play in comparative pathology owes much to the work of Professor Ernest Cotchin of the Royal Veterinary College, London. Some of his many contributions to the literature are cited below (Cotchin, 1956, 1959, 1966).

## Diagnosis

A neoplasm can be defined as a disturbance of growth characterized by excessive, uncontrolled proliferation of cells. The term *cancer* has been used as a synonym for malignant tumor. Neoplasms usually appear as swellings, but inflammatory and hyperplastic lesions may also cause swellings. Reliable differentiation among these categories is often only possible by histological or cytological examination.

This also holds true for the differentiation between malignant and benign neoplasms.

Tumors and hyperplasias usually consist of one or two main cell types arranged in a way that resembles an organ or tissue. In contrast, inflammatory lesions are generally built up of a mixture of inflammatory cells often intermingled with newly formed blood vessels, collagen, and reticulum fibers.

Some tumors, for example, canine cutaneous histiocytoma, mastocytoma, and equine sarcoid, are sometimes difficult to differentiate from inflammatory lesions, especially when ulcerated. Necrotic and infected sarcomas can mimic abscesses. Hemangiomas and hemangiosarcomas of the spleen can mimic hematomas. The difference between neoplasms, especially benign neoplasms, and hyperplasias is sometimes debatable, although the latter generally show resemblance to the structure of the organ from which they stem and tend to be small and nonencapsulated.

Cytology permits a better identification of cellular characteristics, but is inferior to histopathology with respect to information about the architecture of tumors. The various applications of cytology in veterinary oncology were reviewed by Roszel (1981). The morphology of malignant tumor cells in the dog as determined by cytology was reported by Saar (1967).

Lymphoma can be characterized by using cytological, cytoenzymological, and immunochemical methods. In cattle and dogs the majority of lymphoma cases are derived from B lymphocytes (Parodi *et al.*, 1982). Also, in the dog it appears that most of the lymphomas are of B-cell type (Holmberg *et al.*, 1977).

Hematology is a valuable method for the diagnosis of leukemic diseases. Electron microscopy can help in diagnosing badly differentiated tumors (e.g., mast cell tumors). The ultrastructure of several types of tumors in domestic animals was depicted by Cheville (1976), whose contribution includes many references.

Monoclonal and polyclonal antibodies against cytoskeletal proteins and cell surface antigens are of potential value in the differential diagnosis of tumors (epithelial–mesenchymal and fibrous tissue–muscle melanomas).

## Classification

A classification of tumors in domestic animals, based on defined histological criteria, is necessary for avoiding misunderstanding in the exchange of information and for comparative epidemiologic and therapeutic studies. Most classifications are based on combinations of histogenetic (organs or tissues of origin), histological (descriptive), and biological (benign or malignant) criteria (Misdorp, 1976).

The process of classification includes the following steps: (1) identification and description of types, (2) categorization in a logical scheme, and (3) adoption of the most suitable nomenclature.

For teaching purposes the classification used must be simple. The names of each group of tumors should reflect as much as possible what the student sees under the microscope. The classification of tumors into many small groups ("splitting") has the advantage that all the histological details of the tumor are reflected in the classification. The disadvantages are that the subdivision is often arbitrary because many tumors have a variegated structure, and statistical evaluation can be difficult because of the limited numbers of cases per group. Other pathologists prefer the "lumping" approach where the tumors are classified into a small number of groups. This procedure facilitates statistical evaluation, but the disadvantage is that certain features that later might prove to be important (e.g., for prognosis) are not listed in a statistically acceptable way. Probably the best procedure is to start with splitting into many subgroups that can then be compressed, if necessary, into a few main groups of tumors having different biologic behavior. This method was adopted in a detailed study of canine mammary cancer (Misdorp and Hart, 1976).

The World Health Organization (WHO) Comparative Oncology Group developed an international histologic classification of tumors of domestic animals in parallel with a similar project for the classification of human tumors. The main purpose of the project was to provide a sound basis for research in comparative oncology and to help advance veterinary pathology. This classification, like any other, is arbitrary and temporary. Revision will be indicated as soon as newer data, especially concerning the biologic behavior of different tumor types, can be included. The classification has been published (WHO, 1974, 1976), and study sets of representative color transparencies (diapositives) are available at the WHO Collaboration Center of Worldwide Reference on Comparative Oncology, which is located at the Armed Forces Institute of Pathology in Washington, D.C.

## Structure and Composition

The microscopic structure of tumors varies from the relatively simple to the very complex. Developmental tumors such as teratomas and nephroblastomas are well known for their complex and variegated structures. The multipotential embryonal cells of which they are composed are capable of differentiating into various cell types and tissues. Canine mammary mixed tumors are also good examples of structurally complex tumors. Their complexity is probably due to the great metaplastic capacity of the myoepithelial cells surrounding the acini of the mammary gland or to the presence of multipotential precursor (stem) cells. Synoviomas and mesotheliomas, although basically derived from one cell type, show a bimodal (biphasic) epithelial-mesenchymal structure. Melanomas may structurally resemble epithelial or mesenchymal tissue or both. Tumors often show a wide range in growth pattern, degree of differentiation, and cellular pleomorphism. Therefore, the study of several histological sections of the same tumor may be required to characterize a tumor properly. Tumors can show not only structural complexity, but also a severe heteroploidy (an abnormal number of chromosomes), as indicated by Johnson *et al.* (1981). These authors found heteroploidy in 80% of canine tumors studied (60 to 80% heteroploidy in human tumors). In the group of canine mammary carcinomas and skeletal osteosarcomas, bimodal stemlines have been observed, and in feline mammary carcinomas studied in Amsterdam (T. Erich *et al.*, personal communication, 1982), heteroploidy was also found to be a common phenomenon.

The complexity of tumors seems to be more readily explainable by the multiclonal or field theory of carcinogenesis than by the monoclonal (one-cell origin) theory. Although little is known about the genesis of tumors of domestic animals, studies of human tumors (Fialkow, 1976) suggest a monoclonal origin for most human tumors. Complexity in tumors of monoclonal origin could be caused by stepwise progression of a number of tumor cells.

## Cell Kinetics

The population of tumor cells observed by the pathologist under the microscope is a mixture of cycling and dividing cells, resting and nondividing cells, and dying cells (cell loss). The relative proportion of these three components is associated with the speed of growth of the tumor and the response to chemotherapy and radiotherapy.

The cycling cell population undergoes a sequence of events occurring during the interval from one cell division to the next. Mitosis is followed by a period during which RNA and protein synthesis occur prior to DNA synthesis. New DNA synthesis (S) and finally RNA and protein synthesis precede mitosis. The length of each phase can be calculated, as has been demonstrated in the study of transmissible venereal tumor of the dog (Cohen and Steel, 1972). This calculation was done by determining the percentage of labeled mitoses on repeated biopsies after injection of radioactive thymidine, which is incorporated into the S phase of dividing cells.

The potential value of the dog as a model for the study of cell kinetics was demonstrated by Owen and Steel (1969) who compared the cell cycles of primary and secondary tumors and tumor doubling times. It appears from this study that in canine tumors, as in human tumors, extensive cell loss takes place. The volume doubling time of pulmonary metastases, determined by radiography in dogs, ranges from 8 to 150 days (Bech-Nielsen *et al.,* 1976; Owen and Steel, 1969; van Peperzeel, 1972) with a median of 25 days. This is much shorter than the amount of 66 days calculated for human tumors.

The number of mitotic figures as an indicator of cellular proliferation has often been determined by examination of a number of high power fields. However, use of the mitotic index (number of mitoses per 1000 cells determined in multiple foci of viable tumor tissue) provides a more objective and reliable method. The number of mitoses was found to be an important parameter in distinguishing ma-

lignant from benign melanomas (Bostock, 1979).

In some tumors, the mitotic rate is a parameter that has proved useful as a guide to prognosis.

## Metastasis

Metastasis is a multistep mechanism, involving (1) the release of tumor cells from the primary tumor; (2) invasion of lymphatics, blood vessels, or celomic cavities; and (3) dissemination to distant organs where secondary tumors develop. The morphologic aspects of metastasis were reviewed by Willis (1952), and the fundamental and functional aspects more recently by Liotta and Hart (1982).

Cancers (i.e., malignant tumors) consist of subpopulations of cells with different metastatic potential. The clonal (one-cell) origin of at least a proportion of spontaneous metastases became evident in a study of radiation-induced chromosomal mosaicism of malignant melanoma in mice (Talmadge *et al.,* 1982). The same study showed that although metastasis is a highly selective process, different metastases originate from different progenitor cells.

When tumor cells are released into lymphatics, they may be trapped in the subcapsular sinuses of the regional lymph node. There, the tumor cells can either be destroyed, remain in a stationary state, or "grow out." By growing out, tumor cells gradually occupy the whole node and release new emboli that can reach the next node in the chain. Lymph node involvement is more frequent with carcinomas than with sarcomas.

The bypassing of regional lymph nodes by tumor cells was found to be a rare event, at least in the case of canine mammary carcinoma (Misdorp and Hart, 1979b). With the slow stream of lymph, tumor cells can reach venous tributaries, causing secondary hematogenous metastasis in the lungs. Primary blood-borne metastasis arises when tumor cells, after penetrating blood vessels, are arrested in the first capillary bed encountered where they adhere to the endothelium and penetrate either between (in the lungs) or through endothelial cells (in the liver).

Depending on the site of the primary tumor, the lungs (reached by the vena cava pathway) or the liver (via the portal vein) are the first filter organs

## TABLE 1.3. Prognostic Factors

| Characteristics | Canine mammary cancer | | | Feline mammary cancer | Canine mastocytoma | Canine melanoma | | | Canine osteosarcoma | |
|---|---|---|---|---|---|---|---|---|---|---|
| | Bostock (1975) | Misdorp and Hart (1976) | Else and Hannant (1979) | Weijer et al. (1972) | Bostock (1973) | skin/oral | | oral | Brodey and Abt (1976) | Misdorp and Hart (1979a) |
| | | | | | | Bostock (1979) | Frese (1978) | Harvey et al. (1981) | | |
| Breed | | | | | + | | | | | |
| Sex | | | | | | − | | | − | − |
| Age | + | | | | | | | | − | − |
| Location | | − | − | − | | + | + | − | − | + |
| Clinical stage[a] | | + | | | | | | | | |
| Size and volume | + | + | − | + | + | − | + | − | | + |
| Histological subtype | + | + | + | | | | − | | | + |
| Mode of growth[b] | + | + | + | | + | − | + | | | + |
| Mitosis | | − | | + | | + | − | | | − |
| Pleomorphism | | − | | + | | | | | | |
| Differentiation | | − | | + | + | − | | − | | |
| Histological grade of malignancy[c] | | + | | + | + | − | | | | − |
| Peritumorous lymphocytes[d] | | + | | − | | | | | | − |
| Type of surgery | − [e] | | | | | | | + [f] | | |

[a] Only with complex carcinoma; the clinical stage was determined by the size of the tumor and the involvement of skin and underlying tissue.

[b] Severely infiltrating tumors had a worse prognosis than moderately infiltrating or expansive growing tumors.

[c] The histological grade of malignancy is the sum of the degrees of anaplasia and pleomorphism and the number of mitoses.

[d] Larger amounts of peritumorous lymphocytes were associated with a favorable prognosis only with complex carcinomas.

[e] Radical (*en bloc*) mastectomy was associated with a more favorable prognosis only with complex carcinoma.

[f] Surgery was found to be superior to cryosurgery, possible because of selection of unfavorable cases.

from which tumor cells can disseminate to other distant organs. Large-scale studies in man and mice have led to two theories that attempt to explain the observed organ distribution of metastasis (Weiss *et al.,* 1981). The first, the "seed and soil" theory, emphasizes some affinity between tumor cells and specific organs (e.g., prostatic carcinoma and the vertebral column in humans). The second, the "hemodynamic" theory, stresses the correlation of metastasis rate and target organ blood flow. In veterinary oncology the latter theory seems to be applicable for most cancers with the lungs as the organ having the highest incidence of metastasis (first filter).

Except for one observation in canine osteosarcoma, little is known with certainty about the total "metastatic tumor load" in animals at the moment of first treatment. In dogs killed immediately after the diagnosis osteosarcoma was made, slight to moderate involvement of lungs was found in 35% of cases (Misdorp and Hart, 1979*c*). Additional study of selected giant sections of grossly uninvolved lungs showed micrometastasis in 6 out of 13 lungs examined. These findings indicate that, as could be expected from the follow-up studies of dogs after amputation of a limb for osteosarcoma, metastasis was present in a fair number of untreated dogs at the time of first presentation of the primary tumor. The metastatic tumor load did not seem to be excessive, however, and gives rise to the expectation that, at least in this model, early systemic treatment might prove to be effective in a number of affected dogs.

Pulmonary metastasis can be nodular ("cannon-balls"), diffuse (pneumonia carcinomatosa), or radiating in a linear fashion (lymphangitic). Pleuritic carcinosis in dogs and cats with mammary cancer is, in our experience, invariably associated with pulmonary involvement (Misdorp and Hart, 1979*b*; Weijer *et al.,* 1972).

The skeleton, one of the most frequently involved organs for metastasis in the human, was for a long time considered to be involved only exceptionally in domestic animals. Examination of the cross section of vertebrae yielded 8.8% of bone metastasis (mostly a single focus) in canine mammary cancer (Misdorp and den Herder, 1966). Accurate screening of the whole axial skeleton resulted in 17% bone metastasis in dogs with all types of malignancies (Goedegebuure, 1979).

## Prognosis

The course of a tumor disease in any patient, treated or untreated, may be different from that in other patients. This is due to the influence of a large number of tumor and host characteristics (table 1.3). Among these are the clinical stage and histological grade of malignancy, studies of which have been recently introduced in veterinary oncology. These characteristics are widely used in human oncology and are of veterinary as well as of comparative significance.

Clinical staging is the division of cases into groups by degree of apparent extent of disease (Madewell, 1979; Misdorp, 1976). The TNM system of clinical staging is based on the assessment of the extent of the primary tumor (T), the condition of the regional lymph nodes (N), and the absence or presence of distant metastasis (M). On the basis of this principle, tumor diseases in domestic animals have been classified clinically by cooperation between WHO and the Veterinary Cancer Society. The histological grade is expressed as the sum of degrees of differentiation and pleomorphism and mitotic index (Misdorp, 1976). It is probable that cell kinetics and cellular and serological immunologic factors also influence the course of tumors, but their precise role is still difficult to evaluate.

Too little is known about the natural course of untreated cancers in domestic animals (and humans). Retrospective studies viewed from the standpoint of prognosis can help to identify characteristics of tumor and host that potentially affect biological behavior. Only well-designed prospective studies, however, can provide the controls and stratification needed to allow for the many interacting characteristics inherent in any clinical population.

The prognosis of tumor diseases in domestic animals is often expressed as the percentage of animals surviving 1 or 2 years after treatment. Comparison between overall survival time in humans and animals is somewhat difficult because of the differences in the causes of death (e.g., natural death versus euthanasia) and in the interpretation of survival time. For example, can 2 years survival for dogs be compared with 10 years for humans? Another difficulty can be that death in a proportion of cancer-treated animals is not caused by tumor but by intercurrent diseases, which sometimes can be determined only by careful postmortem examination. Therefore, tumor-free (recurrence- and metastasis-free) survival seems to be a better prognostic parameter than overall survival, provided that the diagnosis of recurrence and/or metastasis can be accurately established.

Statistical analysis is a prerequisite for reliable prognostic studies. These studies are mostly based on unifactorial analysis in which each characteristic is associated with prognosis. In multifactorial analysis, which is superior to unifactorial analysis, the association among characteristics as well as that between characteristics and prognosis is determined. The latter is subsequently corrected for intercharacteristic dependency.

Although one should be cautious in comparing the results of prognostic studies that differ in the composition of patient populations, some tentative findings have been published and are summarized in terms of diagnostic criteria and statistical procedures (table 1.3). Histologic type, mode of growth (figs. 1.1 and 1.2) and, to a lesser extent, tumor size seem to be the most prominent prognostic factors.

Most dogs surgically treated for skeletal osteosarcoma, oral malignant melanoma, and mammary cancer and most cats surgically treated for mammary carcinoma die within 1 year after first treatment. Death in most cases results from pulmonary metastasis, which at the moment of first treatment must have been present as micrometastases. Therefore, surgical excision must be combined with a systemic approach using adjuvant chemotherapy and/or immunotherapy. Another cause of death is recurrence due to incomplete removal of the primary tumor. Metastasis and local recurrence alone or in combination as the major causes of failure of surgical treatment have been specified for the various tumor types by Brodey (1979).

The biological behavior of many tumor diseases in domestic animals shows striking similarities to that of human cancers. New therapy modalities can be tested on spontaneous animal systems, providing valuable data relatively quickly, which may prove to be important for both animals and humans. The course, prognosis, and management of tumors in domestic animals are extensively treated in Theilen and Madewell's (1979) textbook entitled *Veterinary Cancer Medicine*.

## Hormone Production by Tumors

Tumors can produce hormones in an eutopic or ectopic way. Hyperadrenocorticism, hypoglycemia (insulinoma), and hyperthyroidism (thyroid carcinoma) are typical examples of eutopic secretion. Feminization and alopecia are associated with testicular Sertoli cell tumor. Pyometra and endometrial hyperplasia are often found in bitches with ovarian tumors.

Ectopic hormone production can cause paraneoplastic syndromes. A great variety of these syndromes such as anemia, anorexia, cachexia, fever, hemostatic abnormalities, and neuropathy are reported in the medical literature and can involve complex mechanisms (Madewell, 1979).

The hypercalcemia associated with lymphoma,

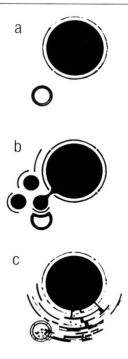

**FIGURE 1.1.** Types of growth. A. Expansive type of growth. B. Moderately invasive, compressing the vessel wall. C. Highly invasive tumor, showing vascular involvement.

**FIGURE 1.2.** Example of prognostic importance of type of growth in a tumor system. Survival curves (survival expressed in 0.5, 1, 1.5, and 2 years) for canine mammary cancer: expansive (———), moderately infiltrating (– – –), and severely infiltrating (–·–·–) type of growth. Numbers along curves indicate numbers of patients alive at beginning of the interval.

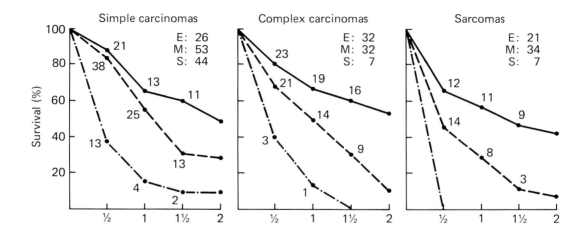

perirectal tumors, and plasmacytoma should be distinguished from primary and secondary parathyroidism.

Extreme emaciation, part of the cachexia complex, is sometimes encountered at autopsy of animal cancer patients, but less frequently than in human patients. Other animals with metastatic disease can be in a surprisingly good state of nutrition. It is not yet clear whether the observed differences in emaciation between domestic animals and humans are only because most animals are killed in earlier stages of the metastatic disease whereas many human cancer patients ultimately die after a long time of extensive treatment.

Pulmonary hypertrophic osteoarthropathy, associated with tumors in the thoracic cavity, perhaps can also be classified as a paraneoplastic syndrome.

## Origin, Pathogenesis, and Further Course of Cancer

### Origin

Normal cells can be transformed *in vitro* and *in vivo* to cancer cells by many agents. Studies on tumors from human patients with (enzyme or immunoglobin) mosaicism as markers provide important clues to the number and nature of cells from which the neoplasms arise (Fialkow, 1976). Most tumors tested appear to have a monoclonal (one-cell) origin. This finding is compatible with somatic mutation theories of carcinogenesis, including the multistep mutation (multihit) theories. Clonal origin of the putative virus-associated Burkitt tumor and endocrine-influenced thyroid tumors seems to exclude the field theory that suggests that a large number of cells undergo neoplastic alteration as a result of a potent carcinogen. The clonal origin of chronic leukemia seems to exclude the possibility that these neoplasms result from continuous recruitment of normal cells. Hare *et al.* (1967) observed that, while enzootic lymphoma in cattle is not characterized by a consistent chromosomal change, neoplastic cells from different tumor sites in each individual case showed the same abnormal karyotype. This observation suggests that the disease is unicentric.

The functional abnormalities of neoplastic cells may be divided into those that concern the control of position, proliferation, or differentiation. We do not know the relative importance of intrinsic genetic programs and immunological factors.

Common cellular changes occurring with malignancy include chromosome abnormalities, (e.g., in canine transmissible venereal tumor [Makino, 1963]), canine osteosarcoma (Pool and Wolf, 1974), ploidy state, and increased proliferative activity (Johnson *et al.*, 1981).

A cancer can either arise *ab initio* as an infiltrating destructive lesion, as a noninfiltrating cancer (intraductal carcinoma) eventually followed by an infiltrating phase, or as the endpoint of successive steps of progression from benign to malignant. Premalignant lesions are those from which cancers arise with a selectively high frequency. Viral-induced papillomas of the skin and alimentary tract can progress to carcinomas. In Scotland, progression of intestinal lesions to carcinomas in cattle was exclusively found in bracken fern areas, leading to the supposition of a possible interaction between virus and bracken fern associated carcinogen (Jarrett *et al.*, 1978). Not all premalignant lesions progress to cancer; some remain stationary or regress. Cameron and Faulkin (1971) carefully screened healthy, middle-aged beagles and studied several hundred proliferative lesions, but the role of these lesions in premalignancy seems difficult to establish. In dogs benign and malignant tumor development were found to be associated, and the occurrence of a benign neoplasm was considered to be an indicator of a parallel predisposition to malignancy (Bender *et al.*, 1982). Lymphocytosis associated with persistent bovine leukemia virus precedes enzootic lymphomas in many but not all cattle.

In domestic animals, some conditions are known as premalignant conditions because they are associated with a higher than normal subsequent occurrence of cancer. Lack of pigmentation at the corneal–scleral junction in cows is associated with ocular carcinoma, white hair in cats and goats is associated with skin carcinoma, and the loss of pigmentation of hairs in older gray horses is associated with equine melanotic disease. Cryptorchidism is associated with a higher than normal rate of testicular tumors in dogs and humans.

## Pathogenesis

The pathogenesis of some neoplasms in animals has been studied in particular detail. Equine melanotic disease (see review by Levene, 1971), which is associated with vitiligo (loss of pigment of hair), was considered to be a special multifocal manifestation of the blue nevus phenomenon. The pathogenesis of benign cutaneous melanoma in swine shows similarities with that in gray horses (Flatt *et al.*, 1968). Using experimental and natural cases, Mackey and Jarrett (1972) studied the phases of development of feline lymphoma. The sites of multiplication and routes of migration through the primary and secondary lymphoid organs were distinct in any of four separate morbid anatomical types of the disease. A parallel was found between the distribution of cells in each form of neoplasia and in different compartments of the immunocyte-producing systems.

## Further Course

The further course of an established neoplasm depends on the tumor (cell kinetics and proteolytic enzymes) as well as the host (vascular and immunologic factors). Necrosis is a relatively frequent regressive sign, but complete regression, with the exception of papillomas and histiocytomas, is uncommon. Little is known of the progression of established tumors in domestic animals. Much knowledge about tumor progression has been acquired from experimental oncology. According to the rules formulated by Foulds (1969), progression occurs independently in different cellular units in the same tumor and may be continuous or discontinuous, by gradual change or by abrupt steps. Progression does not always reach an endpoint within the lifespan of the host, which in domestic animals is often shortened by euthanasia or slaughtering. Treatment also interferes with the course of the disease.

## Cultivation and Transplantation

Both cultivation and transplantation techniques are useful for the preservation and accumulation of living tumor material for various studies. Transplantation is superior to cultivation if large quantities of tumor tissue are required. The following *in vitro* methods are in use.

1. Short-term cultures, in combination with cytophotometry (DNA measurement), are currently used in Amsterdam for testing of cytostatic drugs on feline mammary carcinoma cultures.

2. Long-term tissue cultures and cell lines of various canine malignant tumors (mammary carcinoma, malignant melanoma, osteosarcoma, and fibrosarcoma) and equine sarcoid have been prepared, characterized, and maintained at the WHO Center for Comparative Oncology at Cambridge, United Kingdom (Owen *et al.*, 1981). An important aspect of the Cambridge study is the observation that morphological and biological (e.g., transplantation and metastasis) features are well maintained in most cultured tumors.

3. Organ culture of canine mammary dysplasia promises to be a useful technique for testing hormone responsiveness, a characteristic that can be important for exploring the progression from the normal to neoplasia (Warner, 1977).

## Transplantation

Because of their large size and the common occurrence of spontaneous metastasizing tumors in them, domestic animals are better suited for research on surgical, irradiation, and perfusion techniques in cancer therapy than smaller laboratory animals. Transplantation can provide a sufficient number of tumor-bearing animals for testing of therapy methods. Transplantation in allogeneic animals, with the exception of canine transmissible venereal tumor, is only possible when rejection by the immune system can be suppressed. Transplantation of canine tumors was reviewed by Owen (1980).

### Methods of Transplantation

**Autotransplantation.** Autografting bovine ocular squamous cell carcinoma was in most cases (11 out of 17) successful with pieces of tumor, but not with autologous cultured cells (Hoffmann *et al.*, 1981).

**Whole Body Irradiation.** Transplantation of canine lymphoma (Moldovanu *et al.*, 1966) and carcinoma of the thyroid (Allam *et al.*, 1956) was successful after irradiation of neonatal puppies.

**Intrafetal Injection.** Canine lymphoma (Owen and Nielsen, 1968), lymphatic leukemia (Owen, 1971), and canine osteosarcoma (Owen, 1969) have been successfully transplanted by injection into the fetus *in utero*. The tumors, examined subsequently, had the histological appearance of the original tumors, and the growth rate was found to be faster in the transplanted tumors than in the original tumors.

**Antilymphocyte Serum.** Continued immunosuppression with antilymphocyte serum enabled transplantation of canine melanoma (Betton and Owen, 1976) and of mammary carcinoma into newborn puppies (Owen *et al.*, 1977). Intravenous inoculation of canine osteosarcoma cells resulted in widespread development of tumors in many organs, including the skeleton (Owen, 1980).

*Nude* **Mice.** These mice are characterized by defective development of hair and thymus and are good recipients of tumor transplants. Canine osteosarcoma, mammary carcinoma, transmissible venereal tumor, and melanoma have been successfully transplanted, and, in most cases, give a histological appearance similar to the original tumor. Transplantation of bovine lymphoma and canine lymphoma (Owen, 1980), however, was successful only after whole body irradiation of the *nude* mice.

## Tumor Immunology

There is no general agreement concerning the relationship between transformed cells and the immune system. Malignant change, according to Burnett's theory of immune surveillance, is an unavoidable event associated with the formation of new components (antigens). These components will stimulate an immune response because the host has had no prior experience to develop tolerance; in other words, they are "nonself." Neoplasms will develop cases of insufficient immune response. The validity of the theory of immune surveillance and many other important topics of tumor immunology were discussed by Grant (1979).

In most virally and chemically induced tumors, strongly acting antigens are produced. In cats a truly tumor-specific antigen is associated with feline leukemia virus infection. Tumor-associated antigens have also been demonstrated in a number of spontaneous tumors, including mammary carcinoma (Hannant *et al.*, 1978). In a number of spontaneous tumors, however, antigens are either absent or only weakly active.

It can be assumed that during tumor growth, the immune system becomes sensitized to tumor antigens, but *in vivo* the reaction that occurs is not sufficient to contain tumor growth. Immune response *in vivo* is a spectrum of partly cooperating, partly adverse cellular and humoral reactions in which several classes of lymphocytes and macrophages are involved.

*In vitro* techniques have revealed different types of immune responses in dogs with mammary tumors (Ulvund, 1975), osteosarcoma (Bech-Nielsen *et al.*, 1978), and a variety of other spontaneous tumors (Fidler *et al.*, 1974; Tsoi *et al.*, 1974; Weiden 1974). Dogs that developed metastasis after amputation for osteosarcoma showed a significantly higher cell-mediated and serum-blocking activity than dogs without metastasis or control dogs. Following surgical intervention, serum-blocking activity was detectable a few months before metastasis appeared (Bech-Nielsen *et al.*, 1978). Blocking activity, which may explain the ability of many tumors to escape from immune surveillance, may be caused by the presence of a complex of antibody and tumor antigens protecting the tumor cells against cytotoxic T lymphocytes. Circulating immune complexes have been found in sera of dogs that have benign and malignant mammary tumors. Dogs with a persistent presence of immune complexes are at greater risk of developing metastasis (Gordon et al., 1980). Infiltration of lymphocytes and plasma cells is found around tumors of various types, especially in the cat. Orbital squamous carcinoma in cattle, cutaneous histiocytoma in dogs, and mammary carcinoma in cats are notable for lymphocyte and plasma cell infiltration. The amount of cellular infiltration proved not to be of prognostic importance in dogs with osteosarcoma (Misdorp and Hart, 1979c) or in cats with mammary carcinoma (Weijer *et al.*, 1972). Spontaneous regression has been noted especially with canine histiocytoma and with papillomas in various species. Lymphoma of the skin in cattle, dogs, and horses may also regress, but relapses occur in most cases.

Naturally occurring neoplasms in domestic animals present a closer parallel to those in humans than do experimentally induced neoplasms in inbred laboratory animals. For this reason, a WHO group recommended that more immunological studies of tumors in domestic animals should be carried out, and they selected a series of suitable ones as models for research (WHO, 1973a, b).

## Epidemiology

### Sources of Data

Considerable progress has been made in epidemiological studies of tumors in domestic animals during the past few decades. In California, and later in Oklahoma, for example, a tumor registry concerned mainly with pet animals was established. The incidences of tumors in veterinary practices are compared with populations in the area. In one area a registry of tumors in people was established enabling comparative studies to be made (Schneider, 1976).

The Veterinary Medical Data Program (VMDP) was established through cooperation between the National Cancer Institute and Colleges of Veterinary Medicine in the United States and Canada. The hospital population served as a reference. The results were summarized in a monograph (Priester and McKay, 1980). Epidemiological studies have also been carried out in the School of Veterinary Medicine, University of Pennsylvania, and in some European countries (Germany, United Kingdom, The Netherlands, and Switzerland).

### Age Distribution

In the dog and cat, the frequency of benign and malignant tumors increases with age. In the bovine and equine, malignant but not benign tumors increase with age (Priester, 1979). Sheep and swine, usually slaughtered before middle age, have a lesser chance to develop tumors. In the American (VMDP) study as well as in the European (WHO) study, hematopoietic malignancies are as frequent in young animals as they are in children. Embryonal tumors are more frequent in children than in young animals. Nephroblastoma occurs mainly in young but also in older swine. Histiocytoma of the skin is especially common in young dogs. Viral papilloma in the dog, ox, and horse often occurs before 2 years of age.

### Multiplicity

The majority of multiple primary tumor cases (as with single primaries) were found in dogs when compared with cats, cattle, and horses. The total number of multiple tumors closely approximated a theoretical model of random distribution, but several site pairs seem to occur excessively. One pair (mammary tumors and tumors of internal female organs) might parallel a similar excessive occurrence in humans. Another pair (testes and perianal glands) can be explained by the androgen dependency of the latter type of tumor (Priester, 1977).

## Distribution and Etiology of Spontaneous Tumors

### Skin and Soft Tissues

Tumors of skin and subcutis, including virus-associated papillomas, are frequent in a wide range of animal species. In contrast to the situation with humans, no association between the incidence of canine skin tumors and exposure to sunlight was found by Priester (1973).

Squamous cell carcinomas of the skin of cats and sheep and those of the orbit and vulva in cattle are associated with exposure to ultraviolet light. Orbital carcinomas in the United States and Australia are frequently found in Hereford cattle. These carcinomas are mainly located in the bulbar conjunctiva and are associated with lack of corneoscleral pigment. In the Netherlands, orbital carcinomas in cows are usually located in the membrana nictitans.

Malignant melanomas occur in the skin (and mouth), especially of heavily pigmented dogs. Melanotic disease in gray and white horses, associated with vitiligo of hair, is a very peculiar disease in between benign and malignant tumor neoplasia and storage disease. Multiple cases of a cutaneous melanotic disease in Hormel miniature swine, showing similarity to that in the horse, were reported (Flatt *et al.*, 1968). Malignant melanomas have also been reported in young porcine Duroc–Jersey littermates (Hjerpe and Theilen, 1964).

Hemangiopericytoma, histiocytoma, and perianal gland tumors are almost exclusively found in dog skin. Fibrosarcomas in older cats are usually solitary and probably not virus associated. Fibrosarcomas in young cats are mostly multicentric and associated with feline sarcoma virus (FeSV). Mastocytoma of the skin, very common in the dog, is not rare in the cat. "Sarcoids" are common, locally invasive but not metastasizing tumors in the skin of horses.

### Skeleton

In the dog, in which a great variety of bone tumors occur, osteosarcoma is the most prominent tumor, especially in large and giant breeds (Tjalma, 1966). The reported association of canine osteosarcoma on one hand and pinned fractures and bone infarcts on the other is probably based upon the strong proliferative activity of osteoblasts in both conditions.

### Lymphoid and Hematopoietic System

Lymphoma (lymphosarcoma) is defined here in accordance with the WHO classification (Jarrett and Mackey, 1974) as a malignancy of cells of the lymphoid series involving solid tissues. In lymphoid leukemia, malignant lymphoid cells are present in blood and bone marrow. The term *leukosis* is often used in Europe to label lymphoid malignancies, either localized in solid tissues, in blood, or in both. Lymphoma is a common disease in many species. In cats, feline leukemia virus (FeLV) causes degenerative as well as neoplastic changes in the cell types that it infects, for example, thymus atrophy, erythroleukemia–anemia, and myeloid leukemia–myeloblastopenia. Immunological and epidemiological evidence indicates that leukemic cats that are negative to tests for FeLV still have some association with the virus (Hardy, 1981*a*). In addition, it has proven to be possible to reactivate latent FeLV infection by cultivation or immunomodulation *in vivo* (Rojko *et al.*, 1982). These observations are of importance for those species in which a great degree of viral genomic latency predominates.

In cattle in many countries, an enzootic multicentric type of lymphoma occurs that is associated with bovine leukemia virus. The calf form, the thymus adolescent form, and the skin form are sporadic types and have not yet been associated with a known oncogenic virus.

Porcine lymphoma occurs sporadically in most countries, but in Scotland a multiple case herd was detected. It is suggested that an autosomal recessive gene may play an important role (McTaggart *et al.*, 1971).

### Respiratory System

Endemic ethmoturbinate tumors were reported in sheep in Germany and in Montana, United States; in goats in France; and in cows in Sweden, South Africa, India, and Brazil. Carcinomas were found in most species. Transmission by tumor suspension or bacteria-free filtrates was successful in sheep.

Primary pulmonary tumors are rare in domestic animals. The dog is the only animal in which squamous cell and plastic small cell carcinomas (associated with smoking in humans) occur, although rarely (Stünzi, 1971). There is no association of lung tumors in dogs of urban versus rural environment (Reif and Cohen, 1971).

In sheep in many countries, a multicentric pulmonary tumor (jaagsiekte or pulmonary adenomatosis) occurs, which is transmissible and probably of viral origin. Contrary to its name, pulmonary adenomatosis resembles a malignant neoplasm showing metastasis to local lymph nodes.

### Alimentary System

Tonsillar carcinomas in the dog (London and Philadelphia) and tonsillar, tongue, and esophageal cancer in the cat (London) may be associated with urban environmental pollution. The high incidence of esophageal and stomach cancer in cattle in Brazil, Turkey, and Scotland is associated with the ingestion of bracken fern. A relationship between canine esophageal sarcoma and the parasite *Spirocerca lupi* has been established.

## Urogenital System

Ovarian tumors of epithelial and granulosa cell type are mainly found in the bitch, cow, and mare. Testicular tumors (seminoma, Sertoli cell tumor, and interstitial cell tumor) are common in older dogs, and benign testicular teratoma is almost exclusively found in the horse. Many Sertoli cell tumors produce estrogens causing feminization. Transmissible venereal tumor, transmitted by coitus, is an exclusively canine disease and is primarily located on the penis, sheath, vulva, and vagina. Carcinomas of the corpus uteri are almost exclusively found in cows, but often only after careful postmortem inspection. Leiomyomas of the uterus and vagina are rather frequent in the bitch. Kidney tumors are uncommon in domestic animals with the exception of nephroblastomas in swine. Bladder tumors of different types are frequent in cattle in bracken fern areas. Bladder carcinomas of transitional cell types are not rare in dogs.

## Mammary Gland

Mammary tumors are frequent in the dog (malignant:benign ratio is 1:3), less frequent in the cat (malignant:benign ratio is 8:1), and astonishingly rare in other species, including the cow. The protective effect of ovariectomy at early ages (Schneider *et al.*, 1969) and at later ages, the demonstrated presence of hormone receptors in mammary tumors, and experimental results with progestational compounds all indicate that canine mammary tumors are associated with hormones. In about 30% of feline mammary carcinomas, C-type virus (FeLV or an antigenetically related virus) was demonstrated, but transmission experiments failed (Weijer *et al.*, 1974).

## Nervous System

Nervous tissue tumors are not common in domestic animals with the exception of Schwannoma in cattle and brain tumors in boxer dogs.

## Experimentally Induced Tumors

Most experiments with induced tumors have been conducted with dogs, particularly of the beagle breed.

### Irradiation

External X-radiation was reported not to cause excessive tumors, but those that occurred appeared earlier in life of treated beagle dogs (Andersen and Rosenblatt, 1969). Internal radiation, however, has been associated with tumorigenesis in various organs in dogs. Bronchiolar–alveolar carcinomas (the most common type of natural lung tumor in dogs) were induced by inhalation of plutonium particles (Clarke *et al.*, 1964; Howard, 1970). Inhalation of radioactive cesium resulted in a variety of malignant lung tumors (Hahn *et al.*, 1973). Inhalation of various radionuclides, including strontium, caused a high proportion of hemangiosarcomas in various organs associated with hemolytic anemia (Rebar *et al.*, 1980). Skeletal osteosarcomas were induced by intravenous application of radium, thorium, plutonium, or strontium in dogs (Mays *et al.*, 1966).

### Chemical Carcinogens

Bladder tumor in dogs has been produced by several aromatic amines (see review by Jabara, 1963). Methylcholanthrene induced fibrosarcomas and gliomas in dogs (Mulligan, 1944; Mulligan *et al.*, 1946). Smoking experiments (through tracheostomy) with smoke from nonfiltered cigarettes resulted in frequent development of invasive adenocarcinomas (bronchiolar–alveolar carcinomas). There were no carcinomas in dogs smoking filtered cigarettes or in nonsmoking dogs (Auerbach *et al.*, 1970). Biliary tract carcinomas were produced in dogs fed *o*-aminoazotoluene (Nelson and Woodard, 1953) and aramite (Sternberg *et al.*, 1960). Oral administration of *N*-ethyl-*N*-nitro-*N*-nitrosoguanidine is associated with development of widespread gastric adenocarcinomas in dogs (Kurihara *et al.*, 1974).

## Hormones

Metastasizing ovarian carcinomas, some of which are hormone-dependent, were induced in bitches by the administration of diethylstilbestrol (Jabara, 1962). Progestins alone or in combination with estrogens (Giles *et al.*, 1978) are associated with development of benign tumors and, in high doses, malignant mammary tumors in dogs. The fact that mammary tumor induction by progestins was not affected by prior ovariectomy but was reduced by prior hypophysectomy suggests involvement of pituitary secretion, especially of growth hormone (Concannon *et al.*, 1981).

## Viruses

Extensive studies including transmission experiments have been performed with FeLV and FeSV. This subject was extensively reviewed by Hardy (1981*a,b,c,d*). Some FeLV subgroups can replicate in cells of species other than the cat (e.g., dog and human). Natural or artificial infection with FeLV causes lymphoma in cats and also in newborn puppies after inoculation. The FeSV is a rarely occurring, highly oncogenic virus that can transform human cells in culture and can induce progressing or regressing fibrosarcomas in numerous species, including cats, dogs, and primates. Although the experimental induction of persistent lymphocytosis in cattle has been well documented, conclusive evidence for the induction of lymphoma in cattle inoculated with cell-free bovine leukemia virus (BLV) preparations or BLV-infected cells is still lacking. Lymphoma in sheep was induced by administration of blood from leukemic cows, of BLV producing lymphocytes, and of cell-free supernatant. The induction of malignant melanomas in the skin and eyes of FeSV-inoculated cats shows that, in addition to mesenchymal tumors, ectodermal tumors can also be induced. Cutaneous papillomas in many species are produced by papova viruses (see chap. 2, this volume). The causal viruses are quite host specific with the exception of the bovine papilloma virus. Depending on the site of inoculation, this virus will cause papillomas of the skin, genital mucosa, or bladder or will cause meningiomas.

## Heredity

Tumors were found to be relatively more common in purebred dogs than in crossbred ones (Dorn *et al.*, 1968). Inbreeding was associated with a relatively high frequency of mammary tumors in dogs (Dorn and Schneider, 1976). High risk for particular types of tumors was noted for 14 canine, 1 bovine, and 2 equine breeds (Priester and Mantel, 1971). From table 1.4 it appears that the boxer dog is at high risk for a large variety of tumors, especially those of mesenchymal type. A common ancestral configuration in boxers, Boston terriers, and bull terriers explains their demonstrated increased relative risk to one tumor type: mastocytoma of skin (Peters, 1969). A hereditary factor was established for porcine lymphoma in Scotland (McTaggart *et al.*, 1971) and likely to be associated with congenital melanocytomas in Hormel (Flatt *et al.*, 1968) and Duroc–Jersey (Hjerpe and Theilen, 1964) swine.

## Comparative Aspects

Age-adjusted comparisons of tumor incidence in domestic animals and of humans in the same geographic area (CANR study by Schneider, 1976) showed interesting data. The tumor rate per 100,000 individuals per year does not differ very much between humans (300), dogs (213), and cats (264). Tumors of soft tissues in dogs (27) were more frequent than in cats (13) and much more frequent than in humans (2). Carcinoma of the breast was about equally frequent in dogs (51) and humans (43) and less frequent in cats (14). But in cats, lymphomas and leukemias (180) outnumbered those in dogs (25) and humans (21).

For six major tumor sites human rates were at least three times greater than dog and cat rates, and some tumors (lung, bladder, and intestine) appeared related to environmental effects. Apparently the dog and cat do not share these effects with humans. Cancer rates of gum and testis were threefold greater in the dog. Lymphomas are three times more frequent in the cat than in the human, but the cat has sex and age expressions similar to the human.

Owen, L. N., and Steel, G. G. (1969) The Growth and Cell Population Kinetics of Spontaneous Tumours in Domestic Animals. *Br. J. Cancer* 23, 493–509.

Owen, L. N., Doyle, A., and Littlewood, T. D. (1981) Long-Term Tissue Cultures and Cell Lines of Neoplasms in Domesticated Animals. *J. Comp. Pathol.* 91, 159–163.

Owen, L. N., Morgan, D. R., Bostock, D. E., and Flemans, R. J. (1977) Tissue Culture and Transplantation Studies on Canine Mammary Carcinoma. *Eur. J. Cancer* 13, 1445–1449.

Parodi, A.-L., Mialot, M., Crespeau, F., Lévy, D., Salmon, H., Noguès, G., and Gérard-Marchand, R. (1982) Attempt for a New Cytological and Cytoimmunological Classification of Bovine Malignant Lymphoma (BML) (Lymphosarcoma). In: Straub, O. E., ed., *Proceedings of the Fourth International Symposium on Bovine Leukosis.* Martinus Nijhoff (The Hague), pp. 561–572.

Peters, J. A. (1969) Canine Mastocytoma: Excess Risk as Related to Ancestry. *J. Natl. Cancer Inst.* 42, 435–443.

Pool, R. R., and Wolf, H. G. (1974) An Unusual Case of Canine Osteosarcoma. *Cancer* 34, 771–779.

Priester, W. A. (1967) Canine Lymphoma: Relative Risk in the Boxer Breed. *J. Natl. Cancer Inst.* 39, 833–845.

——. (1973) Skin Tumors in Domestic Animals: Data from 12 United States and Canadian Colleges of Veterinary Medicine. *J. Natl. Cancer Inst.* 50, 457–466.

——. (1974a) Data from Eleven United States and Canadian Colleges of Veterinary Medicine on Pancreatic Carcinoma in Domestic Animals. *Cancer Res.* 34, 1372–1375.

——. (1974b) Pancreatic Islet Cell Tumors in Domestic Animals: Data from 11 Colleges of Veterinary Medicine in the United States and Canada. *J. Natl. Cancer Inst.* 53, 227–229.

——. (1975) Esophageal Cancer in North China; High Rates in Human and Poultry Populations in the Same Areas. *Avian Dis.* 19, 213–215.

——. (1977) Multiple Primary Tumors in Domestic Animals: A Preliminary View with Particular Emphasis on Tumors in Dogs. *Cancer* 40, 1845–1848.

——. (1979) Epidemiology. In: *Veterinary Cancer Medicine.* Lea and Febiger (Philadelphia), 14–32.

Priester, W. A., and Mantel, N. (1971) Occurrence of Tumors in Domestic Animals: Data from 12 United States and Canadian Colleges of Veterinary Medicine. *J. Natl. Cancer Inst.* 47, 1333–1344.

Priester, W. A., and McKay, F. W. (1980) The Occurrence of Tumors in Domestic Animals. *Natl. Cancer Inst. Monogr.* no. 54, Washington, D.C., 210 p.

Priester, W. A., Oleinick, A., and Conner, G. H. (1970) Bovine Leukosis and Human Cancer. *Lancet* 1, 367.

Rebar, A. H., Hahn, F. F., Halliwell, W. H., de Nicola, D. B., and Benjamin, S. A. (1980) Micro Angiopathic Hemolytic Anemia Associated with Radiation-Induced Hemangiosarcomas. *Vet. Path.* 17, 443–454.

Reif, J. S., and Cohen, D. (1971) The Environmental Distribution of Canine Respiratory Tract Neoplasms. *Arch. Environ. Hlth.* 22, 136–140.

Ringertz, N. (1967) Possible Interrelationships between Bovine and Human Leukemia. *Int. Path.* 8, 30–32.

Rojko, J. L., Hoover, E. A., Quackenbusch, S. L., and Olsen, R. G. (1982) Reactivation of Latent Feline Leukemia Virus Infection. *Nature* 298, 385–388.

Roszel, J. F. (1981) Cytologic Procedures. *J. Am. Anim. Hosp. Assoc.* 17, 903–910.

Saar, C. (1967) Die Morphologie der malignen Tumorzelle im Ausstrich. *Zbl. Vet. Med.* A14, 302–314.

Schneider, R. (1976) *Epidemiologic Studies of Cancer in Man and Animals Sharing the Same Environment.* Third Quadrennial Conference on Cancer Epidemiology (San Francisco), 1377–1387.

Schneider, R., and Riggs, J. L. (1973) A Serologic Survey of Veterinarians for Antibody to Feline Leukemia Virus. *J. Am. Vet. Med. Assoc.* 162, 217–219.

Schneider, R., Dorn, C. R., and Taylor, D. O. N. (1969). Factors Influencing Canine Mammary Cancer Development and Postsurgical Survival. *J. Natl. Cancer Inst.* 43, 1249–1261.

Sobin, L. H. (1978) *A Pathology Primer in Verse.* H. K. Lewis & Co., Ltd. (London), 11.

Sternberg, S. S., Popper, H., Oser, B. L., and Oser, M. (1960) Gallbladder and Bile Duct Adenocarcinomas in Dogs after Long Term Feeding of Aramite. *Cancer* 13, 780–789.

Stünzi, H. (1971) Das epidermoide Lungenkarzinom des Hundes als Vergleichsobjekt für das Raucherkarzinom des Menschen. *Schweiz. Arch. Tierheilk.* 113, 311–319.

Talmadge, J. E., Wolman, S. R., and Fidler, I. J. (1982) Evidence for the Clonal Origin of Spontaneous Metastasis. *Science* 217, 361–362.

Theilen, G. H., and Madewell, B. R. (1979) *Veterinary Cancer Medicine.* Lea and Febiger (Philadelphia).

Tjalma, R. A. (1966) Canine Bone Sarcoma: Estimation of Relative Risk as a Function of Body Size. *J. Natl. Cancer Inst.* 36, 1137–1150.

Tsoi, M. S., Weiden, P. L., and Storb, R. (1974) Lymphocyte Reactivity to Autochthonous Tumor Cells in Dogs with Spontaneous Malignancies. *Cell. Immunol.* 13, 431–439.

Ulvund, M. J. (1975) Cellular Immunity to Canine Mammary Tumor Cells Demonstrated by the Leucocyte Migration Technique. *Acta Vet. Scand.* 16, 95–114.

van Peperzeel, H. A. (1972) Effects of Simple Doses of Radiation on Lung Metastases in Man and Experimental Animals. *Eur. J. Cancer* 8, 665–675.

Viola, M. W. (1968) Haematological Malignancy in Patients and Their Pets. *JAMA* 205, 95–97.

von Bomhard, D., and Dreiack, J. (1977) Statistische Erhebungen über Mammatumoren bei Hündinnen. *Kleintier-Praxis* 22, 205–209.

Warner, M. R. (1977) Response of Beagle Mammary

Dysplasias to Various Hormone Supplements *in Vitro*. *Cancer Res.* 37, 2062–2067.

Weiden, P. L. (1974) Immune Reactivity in Dogs Spontaneous Malignancy. *J. Natl. Cancer Inst.* 53, 1049–1056.

Weijer, K., Calafat, J., Daams, J. H., Hageman, P. C., and Misdorp, W. (1974) Feline Malignant Mammary Tumors. II. Immunologic and Electron Microscopic Investigations into a Possible Viral Etiology. *J. Natl. Cancer Inst.* 52, 673–679.

Weijer, K., Head, K. W., Misdorp, W., and Hampe, J. F. (1972). Feline Malignant Mammary Tumors. I. Morphology and Biology: Some Comparisons with Human and Canine Mammary Carcinomas. *J. Natl. Cancer Inst.* 49, 1697–1704.

Weiss, L., Bronk, J., Pickren, J. W., and Lane, W. W. (1981) Metastatic Patterns and Target Organ Arterial Blood Flow. *Invasian Metastasis* 1, 126–135.

Willis, R. A. (1952) *The Spread of Tumours in the Human Body*. Butterworth & Co. (London).

Wolska, A. (1968) Human and Bovine Leukaemias. *Lancet* 1, 1155.

World Health Organization (WHO) (1973a) Immunity to Cancer. Naturally Occurring Tumours in Domestic Animals as Models for Research: 1. *Bull. Wld. Hlth. Org.* 49, 81–91.

———. (1973b) Immunity to Cancer. Naturally Occurring Tumours in Domestic Animals as Models for Research: 2. *Bull. Wld. Hlth. Org.* 49, 205–213.

———. (1974) International Histological Classification of Tumours of Domestic Animals. *Bull. Wld. Hlth. Org.* 50, 1–2, 1–142.

———. (1976) International Histological Classification of Tumours of Domestic Animals. *Bull. Wld. Hlth. Org.* 53, 2–3, 137–304.

## 2

*L. Thomas Pulley and Anthony A. Stannard*

# Tumors of the Skin and Soft Tissues

Tumors of the skin and soft tissues are the most frequently encountered neoplasms in domestic animals. This is to be expected since skin is the largest and most easily observed organ in the body and since the skin and subcutis are composed of a great variety of cell types capable of developing into neoplasms. In addition, the skin is exposed not only to genetic and other internal factors involved in tumor production, but also to many external factors such as infectious agents, sunlight, chronic irritation, and environmental pollutants that may initiate or promote tumor development.

It is not the intent of this chapter to present all of the possible tumor types, variations, or subclassifications that have been described for skin and soft tissues. Rather, the purpose is to present the most commonly occurring or unique tumors and the currently accepted classifications.

## Fibroma

**General Considerations and Classification.** The term *fibroma* is often loosely applied to include any benign fibrous growth whether it is a real neoplasm, reparative tissue, or congenital malformation. Usage of the term *fibroma* should be restricted to a true neoplastic lesion.

**Incidence, Age, Breed, and Sex.** Fibromas occur in all domestic animals, but are most common in the horse (see section on equine sarcoid below).

They usually develop in adult and aged animals. There is no breed or sex prevalence.

**Sites and Gross Morphology.** Fibromas are most common in the dermis or subcutis, but may be present wherever there is fibrous connective tissue.

Fibromas are well-circumscribed neoplasms, usually firm or rubbery, although some are soft. The tumors are round or ovoid and often dome-shaped in the skin, although some are pedunculated. The surface may be ulcerated and secondarily infected. The cut surface is usually homogeneous grayish white.

**Histological Features.** Fibromas have a characteristic structure consisting of whorls and interlacing bundles of fibroblasts and collagen fibers (fig. 2.1). The tumor cells are usually fusiform, but may be stellate in shape, and have large, pale, ovoid to elongated nuclei and multiple nucleoli. Mitotic figures are rare. The collagen fibers are dense or loose as though separated by edema or mucinous ground substance. These tumors show variable degrees of vascularization. The epidermis overlying the fibroma may be hyperplastic.

Fibroma must be differentiated from granulation tissue, which generally has parallel bundles of fibroblasts and collagen fibers with proliferating capillaries running at right angles. Inflammatory polyps, nodular dermal fibrosis, so-called dermal nevi, and skin tags are also confused with this tumor.

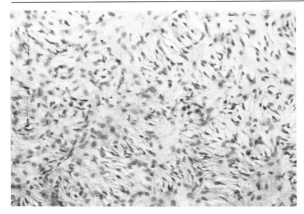

**FIGURE 2.1.** Fibroma of the skin of a dog showing loosely arranged cells and fibers.

## Nodular Fasciitis

**General Considerations.** *Nodular fasciitis* and its synonyms *aggressive fibromatosis* and *pseudosarcomatous fibromatosis* are terms used to describe a nonneoplastic lesion having many features of inflammation, yet clinically exhibiting aggressive behavior suggestive of a locally invasive neoplasm (Konwaler *et al.*, 1955; Price *et al.*, 1961).

**Incidence, Age, Breed, and Sex.** Nodular fasciitis has been recognized in the dog and cat, and the only published reports concern the dog (Belhorn and Henkind, 1967; Lavignette and Carlton, 1974). The actual incidence is not known since it is probable that nodular fasciitis has been diagnosed in the past as inflammation, granulation tissue, fibrosarcoma, and hemangiopericytoma. There is no known age, breed, or sex predisposition.

**Sites and Gross Morphology.** Nodular fasciitis occurs in the subcutis in any location on the body and has occurred with some frequency in deeper fascia and muscles of the head, face, and eyelid. Corneal, scleral, and retrobulbar locations also occur. A similar condition referred to as proliferative episcleritis has been reported by Peiffer *et al.* (1976).

The gross appearance of nodular fasciitis is not distinctive and the lesion can resemble neoplastic or inflammatory tissue. It is usually a firm, poorly circumscribed, nodular mass that can vary greatly in size, from 0.2 to 5.0 cm in diameter or larger. The

cut surface is gray with foci of red and brown discoloration.

**Histological Features.** Nodular fasciitis is composed of large plump or spindle-shaped fibroblasts in a stromal network of variable amounts of collagen and reticulum fibers. Several patterns can exist, with fibroblasts arranged in a haphazard pattern, in short to long fasciculi, or in whorls around well-formed capillaries (fig. 2.2). Parts of the mass may be sparsely cellular, consisting of dense collagen, while other areas may be highly cellular. A few mitotic figures may be present, and some nuclei are hyperchromatic, but in general the fibroblasts are well-differentiated.

Scattered foci of inflammatory cells consisting of lymphocytes, plasma cells, and macrophages are characteristic. Multinucleated giant cells are occasionally seen, usually in or near the inflammatory foci. The periphery is nonencapsulated and often merges with the surrounding connective tissue and muscle.

Although there is apparent infiltrative growth with nodular fasciitis, the cellular morphology of the fibroblasts lacks such characteristic features as anaplasia and numerous mitotic figures found in a malignant neoplasm.

**Growth and Metastasis.** Most cases of nodular fasciitis are slow growing, but a few exhibit rapid growth. Lesions occurring in the subcutis are often diagnosed as fibrosarcoma of low-grade malignancy

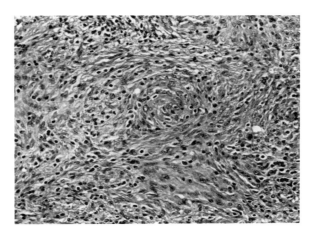

**FIGURE 2.2.** Nodular fasciitis from the skin of a dog. Fibroblasts are in bundles and whorls intermixed with inflammatory cells.

and, as expected, do not recur after complete surgical excision. Some cases of nodular fasciitis associated with the eye or eyelid have been invasive and have recurred multiple times.

## Fibrosarcoma

**General Considerations and Classification.** The category of fibrosarcoma probably represents a heterogeneous group consisting not only of malignant tumors of fibroblasts but also unclassifiable and mixed mesenchymal cell neoplasms capable of collagen production. Undifferentiated leiomyosarcoma, liposarcoma, malignant melanoma, and malignant Schwannoma can be difficult to distinguish from one another, and often the tendency is to classify them as fibrosarcomas. Undifferentiated sarcoma or undifferentiated spindle cell sarcoma may be more appropriate designations.

Special stains are usually of little help in differentiating anaplastic sarcomas and do little more than give the pathologist more time to study the hematoxylin and eosin-stained section. The mere presence of a few fat vacuoles, detected with oil red-O stain, is not conclusive evidence of liposarcoma since other mesenchymal and epithelial cells can contain fat. Masson's trichrome and van Gieson's stains will help to define the stroma, and phosphotungstic acid–hematoxylin will aid in detection of cytoplasmic cross striations and filaments. However, these distinctions can usually be made on thin, well-stained hematoxylin and eosin sections.

**Incidence, Age, Breed, and Sex.** Fibrosarcomas are found most often in the dog and cat, although they do occur in all species. Most of these neoplasms develop in adult and aged animals, but occasionally they are found in dogs and cats as young as 6 months or even younger. No breed predisposition or sex prevalence has been found in domestic animals.

**Sites.** The most common sites for fibrosarcoma in the dog are the skin and subcutis of the trunk and extremities, the oral cavity, and nasal cavity. In cats the tumors occur most often in the dermis and subcutis of the trunk and extremities (Brown *et al.,* 1978). The neoplasms can be found in any location in the body, although internal sites are uncommon.

No particular predilection sites are known in other domestic animals.

**Gross Morphology.** Fibrosacromas are of variable size, and some are very large. They are usually irregular and nodular in shape, poorly demarcated, and nonencapsulated. The consistency is firm or fleshy with soft, friable areas. When they involve the skin and mucous membranes, the surfaces are often ulcerated and secondarily infected. On the cut surface, the neoplasm is lobulated, homogeneous, opaque, and reddish white, and it may exhibit striations. Reddish brown areas of hemorrhage and yellow areas of necrosis are common.

**Histological Features.** The basic pattern of fibrosarcoma consists of interwoven bundles of immature fibroblasts and variable amounts of collagenous fibers (figs. 2.3A–D). The tumor is more cellular than fibroma, and fiber formation is generally minimal, particularly in highly anaplastic fibrosarcoma. Some fibrosarcomas have variable amounts of mucinous ground substance.

The tumor cells are usually fusiform, but may be ovoid or stellate in shape. Undifferentiated tumors may have multinucleated giant cells and cells with bizarre shapes. The nuclei are elongated or oval and hyperchromatic. Nucleoli range from two to five in number and are generally prominent; mitotic figures are common. The amount of cytoplasm varies, and cytoplasmic borders are sometimes difficult to distinguish from stroma. Fibrosarcoma is highly vascular, but the blood vessels are poorly formed and hemorrhage is common. Ischemic necrosis of tumor tissue, inflammation, and edema are also common.

**Growth and Metastasis.** Most fibrosarcomas demonstrate rapid, infiltrative growth. They often recur after surgical removal, but metastasis occurs in less than one-fourth of the cases. Metastasis usually develops via the blood stream with secondary tumors found first in the lungs. Metastasis may be generalized; spread to local lymph nodes occurs less often.

At present, definite criteria for grading fibrosarcomas have not been established. It is possible to estimate the degree of malignancy by infiltration, anaplasia, and number of mitotic figures. According to Bostock (1980) the mitotic index is the most important criterion for predicting behavior of

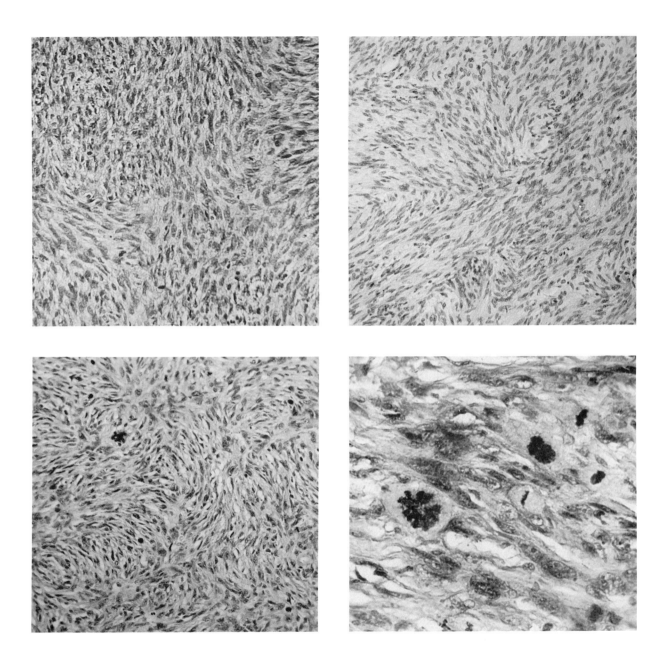

A|B    **FIGURE 2.3.** Fibrosarcoma. A. Fibrosarcoma of the
C|D    skin of a cat showing bundles of anaplastic fibro-
blasts. B. Skin growth in a cow with typical criss-crossing
pattern of cells and fibers. C. Fibrosarcoma of the skin in
a dog with interlocking arrangement of cells and fibers.
D. Mitotic figures in a fibrosarcoma metastasis in the lungs
of a dog.

canine fibrous connective tissue sarcomas. Fibrosarcomas with many mitotic figures and marked nuclear pleomorphism can be designated as "highly malignant," while those with few mitotic figures and abundant collagen production can be referred to as "fibrosarcoma of low-grade malignancy." The problem is that an occasional fibrosarcoma that appears to be of low-grade malignancy will readily recur and metastasize.

## Malignant Fibrous Histiocytoma

**General Considerations.** The use of the term *malignant fibrous histiocytoma* has evolved out of the reevaluation and reclassification of neoplasms in humans having a varied morphological appearance believed to be of histiocytic origin (Fu *et al.,* 1975). Malignant fibrous histiocytoma is thought to arise from a pluripotential mesenchymal cell that differentiates into histiocytelike cells, fibroblastlike cells, and cells with intermediate morphology (Lattes, 1982; Weiss and Enzinger, 1978).

Malignant fibrous histiocytoma has been reported in the dog and cat (Confer *et al.,* 1981; Gleiser *et al.,* 1979*b*; Seiler and Wilkinson, 1980), and there are earlier reports of neoplasms in the dog, cat, and horse having similar morphology (Alexander *et al.,* 1975; Ford *et al.,* 1975; Nielsen, 1952*a*).

**Incidence, Age, Breed, and Sex.** At this time malignant fibrous histiocytoma appears to be a rarely occurring tumor, but it is probable that more cases will be recognized now that it has become a diagnostic entity. Most malignant fibrous histiocytomas have been reported in the cat. The average age is 9 years with a range of 2 to 12 years. Males and females are equally affected. Too few cases have been reported in other species to make meaningful conclusions.

**Sites.** The dorsal thoracic and scapular areas are the most common sites for malignant fibrous histiocytomas in the cat. These locations are also common sites for feline fibrosarcomas. The limbs and pelvic region are other reported locations for malignant fibrous histiocytoma. The tumor has not been reported to occur in internal sites. Most malignant fibrous histiocytomas appear to arise in the subcutis with extension into underlying skeletal muscle. They also develop deep within skeletal muscle or adjacent to bone and can cause bone destruction and proliferation.

**Gross Morphology.** The surface may be smooth or nodular and the skin is occasionally ulcerated. The cut surface is gray, often lobulated, and has foci of red and tan discoloration representing hemorrhage and necrosis. Margins are usually poorly delineated because of the infiltrative nature of the tumor.

**Histological Features.** Malignant fibrous histiocytoma is characterized by cells resembling histiocytes and fibroblasts. Other characteristic features are fibroplasia, storiform pattern, bizarre tumor giant cells, foam cells, inflammatory cells (which are usually lymphocytes), and atypical mitotic figures (figs. 2.4A–C). There can be marked variability within and between tumors, even to the absence of some of these features (Seiler and Wilkinson, 1980). Because of this variability in morphology, malignant fibrous histiocytoma can resemble pleomorphic forms of rhabdomyosarcoma, liposarcoma, chondrosarcoma, fibrosarcoma, and osteosarcoma. Also, because of this great variability in tumor morphology, it is possible that malignant fibrous histiocytoma may become the diagnostic "catch-all" that has generally been referred to as undifferentiated sarcoma.

**Growth and Metastasis.** Malignant fibrous histiocytoma is a rapidly growing neoplasm that infiltrates extensively into surrounding tissues. These tumors recur in a high percentage of cases after surgical removal. Distant metastasis has not been reported.

## Equine Sarcoid

**General Considerations and Incidence.** Equine sarcoid was first described by Jackson (1936) in South Africa. The term was used to refer to a unique, locally aggressive, fibroblastic skin tumor and to distinguish it from papilloma, fibroma, and fibrosarcoma. Horses, donkeys, and mules are susceptible. It should be stressed that equine sarcoid is not related to sarcoids and sarcoidosis of humans.

Equine sarcoid is the most common skin tumor

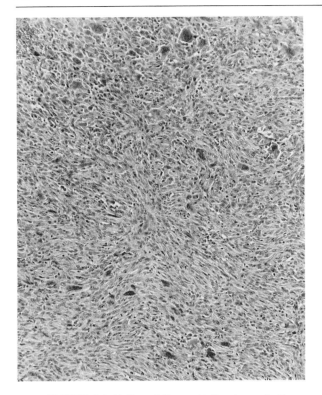

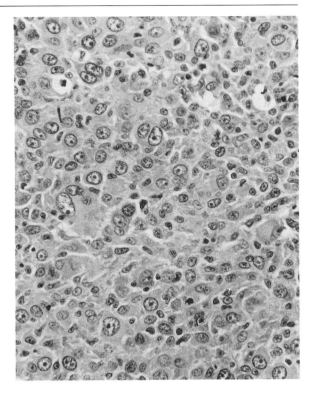

A|B  **FIGURE 2.4.** Malignant fibrous histiocytoma. A. Fi-
—|C  broblastic area with arrangement in short fascicles.
B. An area composed of histiocytic cells. C. Tumor giant
cells mixed with histiocytic and fibroblastic cells. (Photographs courtesy of R. J. Seiler and *Vet. Path.*).

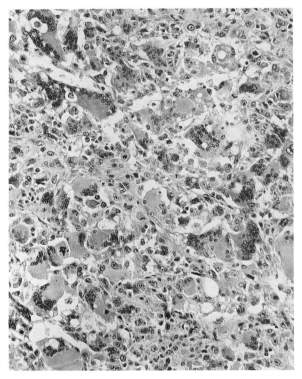

of horses (Jackson, 1936; Ragland *et al.*, 1970*a*).
It is worldwide in distribution.

**Sites, Age, Breed, and Sex.** There apparently is
no predilection for age, breed, sex, or color coat in
equine sarcoid.

The most frequent site for equine sarcoid is the
skin of the legs, ventral trunk, and the head, especially the ears and commissures of the mouth.
About one-third of the affected horses have multiple lesions (Ragland *et al.*, 1970*a*).

**Gross Morphology.** On the basis of gross appearance, it is usually possible to classify the growth
as either the verrucous (warty) type or the fibroblastic ("proud-flesh") type (Ragland *et al.*,
1970*a*). A few tumors are of a mixed type sharing
features of both the verrucous and fibroblastic
types (figs. 2.5A and B).

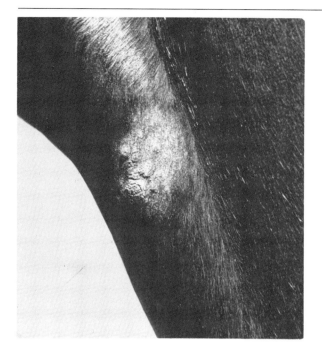

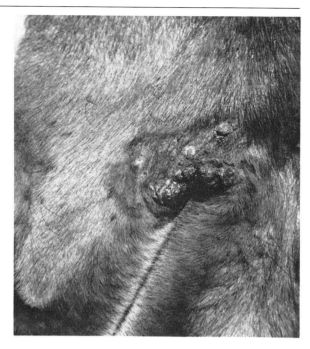

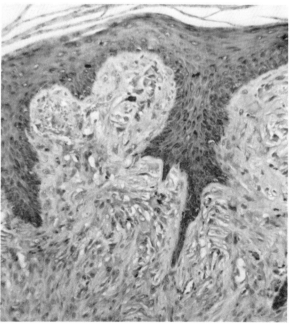

The verrucous type is usually small, rarely larger than 6 cm in diameter. It may be sessile or pedunculated. The surface is dry, horny, and frequently cauliflowerlike in appearance. Some of the very sessile lesions appear as sharply demarcated, thickened areas of skin that are partially or completely devoid of hair and with a slightly roughened surface.

The fibroblastic type has considerable variation in appearance. Some are fairly discrete fibrous nodules situated within the dermis and subcutis, with the overlying epidermis remaining intact. Others are large sessile masses sometimes exceeding 25 cm in diameter, with an ulcerated surface that bleeds easily. In those sarcoids progressing from verrucous to fibroblastic types, features of both types will be present.

**Histological Features.** Almost all equine sarcoids have an epidermal and a dermal component (fig. 2.5C). If the epidermis is intact, it will be acanthotic and hyperkeratotic. Pseudoepitheliomatous hyperplasia, with epithelial pegs extending deep into the underlying tissue, is a characteristic finding. Occasionally small epithelial inclusion cysts are present.

A|B
—
C|

**FIGURE 2.5.** Equine sarcoid. A. Verrucous type sarcoid in the ventral neck of a horse. B. Verrucous type sarcoid at commissures of the lips of a horse. The tumor is undergoing transition to the fibroblastic type. C. Equine sarcoid showing proliferating fibroblasts and pseudoepitheliomatous hyperplasia.

The dermal component of sarcoid consists of fibroblasts and varying amounts of collagen fibers arranged in a whorled or tangled pattern. Occasionally a herringbone pattern is observed. The tumor cells are usually spindle shaped with elongated nuclei. Mitotic figures are numerous in the more rapidly growing tumors. Ragland *et al.* (1970*a*) stressed that the fibroblasts at the epidermal–dermal junction are frequently oriented perpendicularly to the basement membrane in a "picket fence" pattern.

In some fibroblastic sarcoids, especially those that have ulcerated, the epidermal component may be minimal or nonexistent. Likewise, in some of the sessile verrucous sarcoids the epidermal component predominates, and the dermal component is limited to a narrow band of active fibroblasts hugging the epidermis.

**Etiology and Transmission.** In the original description of equine sarcoids, it was reported that they frequently occurred in areas subject to trauma, such as the head and legs, and it was suggested that the neoplasm might spread from one animal to another (Jackson, 1936). Development of equine sarcoids in areas of prior injury to the skin has been documented several times (Ragland *et al.*, 1970*a*).

Cadéac (1901) and Montpellier *et al.* (1939) were the first to successfully autotransplant what were probably equine sarcoids. Olson (1948) was also successful in autotransplanting equine sarcoid, but was unsuccessful with cell-free material. Later, Olson and Cook (1951) demonstrated that the supernatant fluid of ground bovine papilloma tissue could, when inoculated into the skin of the horse, produce fibromas. This suggested a possible relationship between bovine papilloma virus (BPV) and equine sarcoid. Recent findings, however, indicate that BPV and equine sarcoid are unrelated. Horses with equine sarcoid apparently do not have serum-neutralizing antibodies against BPV (Ragland and Spencer, 1968), while horses with BPV-induced lesions do have antibodies against BPV (Segre *et al.*, 1955). Attempts to produce papillomas in calves with equine sarcoid extracts have not been successful (Ragland *et al.*, 1970*b*). The fibroblastic growth produced in the horse's skin with the BPV differs from equine sarcoid in that it lacks an epidermal component and there is no active fibroblastic proliferation at the epidermal–dermal junction (Ragland and Spencer, 1969). When inoculated into equine fibroblasts cultured *in vitro* the BPV will cause neoplasticlike transformation of the cells. The BPV-induced growth in the horse is usually characterized by a short incubation period (10 to 14 days) and a rather rapid regression, which is not typical of naturally occurring equine sarcoids (Ragland and Spencer, 1969).

Despite the negative findings regarding BPV, most available evidence still supports an infectious and presumably viral etiology for equine sarcoid. Ragland *et al.* (1966) reported an epizootic of equine sarcoids in a herd of horses in Washington State. Voss (1969) was successful in transferring, by both autologous and homologous routes, equine sarcoid using whole sarcoid tissue, minced sarcoid material, and more importantly, what was presumed to be cell-free extracts of the tumor. The incubation period with the cell-free extracts averaged 94 days, with a range of 49 to 128 days. Attempts by Ragland *et al.* (1970*b*) to produce equine sarcoid in horses with cell-free extracts of the neoplasm were unsuccessful.

Intracytoplasmic viruslike particles resembling certain retroviruses have been observed in electron microscopic studies of cell lines derived from equine sarcoids (Cheeves *et al.*, 1982; England *et al.*, 1973). Identical viruslike particles were seen in the tumors themselves. The demonstration by Watson and Larson (1974) of tumor-specific antigens in an equine sarcoid cell line is further evidence for a possible rival etiology of equine sarcoid. Consideration must also be given, however, to the possibility that the virus of equine sarcoid is in a "masked" state in the tumor cells, similar to the situation of BPV being in a masked state in the more undifferentiated cells of bovine papilloma.

On two occasions, a possible familial tendency to develop equine sarcoid has been reported (James, 1968; Ragland *et al.*, 1966).

**Growth and Metastasis.** Initially, an equine sarcoid can be of the verrucous or fibroblastic type. Verrucous sarcoid may remain static for years or progress to the usually more aggressive fibroblastic type. Although many sarcoids are locally invasive, they do not metastasize. A characteristic feature of equine sarcoid is its recurrence following surgical removal. A large percentage of equine sarcoids spontaneously regress, but this may take several years.

## Lipoma and Liposarcoma

**General Considerations.** Lipoma and liposarcoma are neoplasms of well-differentiated lipocytes and lipoblasts. Most of the tumors that we refer to as lipomas are so well-differentiated that clinical history indicating that the specimen represents a fatty mass may be necessary to make the diagnosis. It is possible that these growths represent nodular hyperplasia or some type of alteration in fat metabolism rather than true neoplasms.

**Incidence, Age, Breed, and Sex.** Lipomas are most common in the dog. They are seen less frequently in the horse and ox and are rare in the cat, sheep, and pig. Liposarcomas are rare in all animals.

These tumors occur predominantly in adult and aged animals of all species. The average age in the dog is 8 years and the incidence increases with age. There is no known breed predisposition, but the tumors tend to be more common in overweight females than in male dogs.

**Sites.** The growths are single or multiple, and in dogs they are found most often in the subcutis of the lateral and ventral thorax, abdomen, and upper hindlimbs and forelimbs. In the horse, pedunculated lipomas develop in the mesentery, occasionally resulting in strangulation of the intestine. Multiple lipomas (lipomatosis) are occasionally observed in the abdominal cavity of cattle (Papp and Williams, 1970). Lipomas occur in the liver of the cat, which, when combined with myeloid elements, are called myelolipomas (Gourley *et al.*, 1971; Ikede and Downey, 1972).

**Gross Morphology.** Lipomas are usually round, ovoid, or discoid and commonly multilobulated. Most are well-circumscribed, lightly encapsulated, and soft or flabby. Some are more solid due to the presence of fibrous connective tissue, necrosis, or inflammation. When located in the subcutis, the skin is freely movable over the tumor and the tumor is usually not attached to the underlying fascia and muscle. Needle aspiration will reveal oily material with few intact fat cells. The usual color of the lipoma is white or slightly yellow, but the tumor may have areas of red or yellow discoloration. Areas of fat necrosis are chalky white. The tumor will float in formalin fixative.

Liposarcomas are not as well-circumscribed as the benign growths, are gray to white in color, and are firmer than lipomas.

**Histological Features.** Lipomas are often indistinguishable from normal adipose tissue unless there is a fibrous component or capsule (fig. 2.6A). The fat cells are usually well-differentiated and have a full complement of fat. Fibrous septa may divide the neoplasm into lobules, or in some lipomas, the fibrous connective tissue component can make up a large portion of the tumor. These tumors are sometimes referred to as fibrolipomas. The pedunculated lipomas of the horse frequently become infarcted and histologically consist of encapsulated necrotic fat cells with granulation tissue, blood pigment, mononuclear inflammatory cells, and mineralization.

Liposarcomas are more cellular than lipomas (figs. 2.6B and C). Most of the cells are round, but some may be polygonal, stellate, or elongate. There is usually abundant acidophilic, finely vacuolated cytoplasm. A few cells may contain large lipid vacuoles. The nuclei are round or ovoid and, unlike the benign tumor, are not flattened. The cells usually have single large nucleoli. Giant nuclei and multinucleated cells are frequently found. Mitotic figures may be numerous and sometimes atypical in the liposarcoma.

**Growth and Metastasis.** Lipomas are generally characterized by slow growth, usually over a long period, but some tumors have a history of rapid growth. Lipomas do not recur after complete surgical removal. Liposarcomas are locally invasive and have moderate potential for widespread metastasis. The lung is the most common site for metastasis.

## Infiltrative Lipoma

**General Considerations.** Infiltrative lipomas are considered as a separate category since they are distinct both clinically and pathologically from lipomas and liposarcomas. They have been reported in

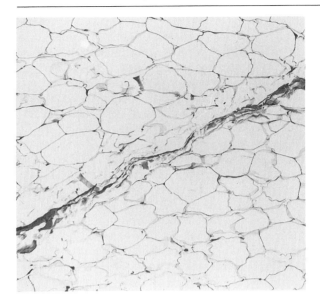

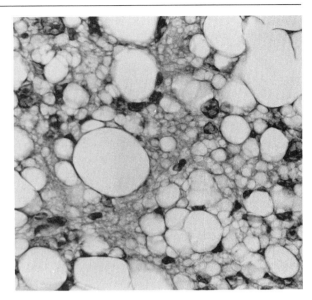

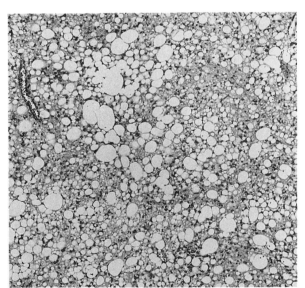

A | B
C |
**FIGURE 2.6.** Lipoma and liposarcoma. A. Lipoma of the skin showing adipose cells with large fat vacuoles. B. Liposarcoma of the skin with cells containing variably sized cytoplasmic vacuoles. C. Liposarcoma of the skin with large, round cells containing round or ovoid nuclei and variably sized cytoplasmic vacuoles.

the dog (Gleiser *et al.*, 1979*a*; McChesney *et al.*, 1980), the horse (Blackwell, 1972), and the cat. The entity is well documented in humans (Dionne and Seemayer, 1974).

**Incidence, Age, Breed, and Sex.** Infiltrative lipoma occurs much less frequently than lipoma. The incidence is not known since their classification has been inconsistent in the past. These tumors have been referred to as atypical lipoma, noncircumscribed lipoma, liposarcoma, accumulation of fat resembling lipoma, lipoma arborescens, or extensive fatty infiltration (marbling) of muscle (McChesney *et al.*, 1980). In the dog the infiltrative lipoma develops more frequently in females, as does the more commonly occuring lipoma, but is not associated with generalized increase in body fat. They tend to occur most frequently in middle-aged dogs, but have been observed in dogs from 1 to 12 years of age. There is no known breed predisposition. In the horse they have been first observed in animals as young as 2 days of age (Blackwell, 1972).

**Sites.** Infiltrative lipomas occur most frequently in muscles of the pelvis, thigh, shoulder, and lateral cervical area. Lower extremities and the abdominal wall are less frequently occurring sites. They are generally single, although bilaterally symmetrical infiltrative lipomas have been observed in the horse.

**Gross Morphology.** These neoplasms are usually soft, poorly circumscribed masses that clinically may appear as localized muscle swelling. Their color and consistency are grossly similar to normal adipose tissue. Some appear to arise in the subcutis and infiltrate into adjacent muscle bundles, while others have no apparent connection to the subcutaneous fat. Depending on their location they can surround tendons, nerves, blood vessels, and lymph nodes. Their margins are often impossible to delineate, making it difficult for complete excision by the surgeon.

**Histological Features.** Infiltrative lipoma, like the more common lipoma, is composed of well-differentiated fat cells that are indistinguishable from normal adipose tissue. The distinctive feature is their infiltration into and between muscle bundles. The neoplastic fat cells in the areas of infiltration will often be arranged in single rows between or separating atrophic muscle fibers (fig. 2.7). Fibrous connective tissue stroma is minimal and there is no encapsulation.

**Growth and Metastasis.** Infiltrative lipoma is generally slow growing but some exhibit periods of rapid growth. Because of its infiltrative nature, complete surgical excision is difficult and the recurrence rate is high. Since it is slow growing, tumor recurrence may not become clinically apparent for several years. Metastasis has not been reported.

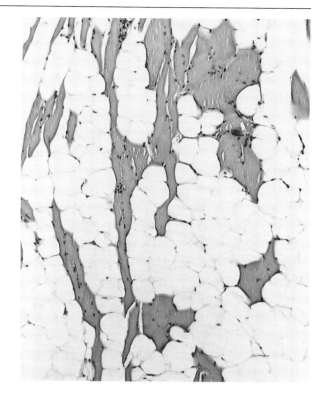

FIGURE 2.7. Infiltrative lipoma showing fat cells infiltrating between and replacing skeletal muscle fibers.

## Myxoma and Myxosarcoma

**General Considerations.** Myxoma and myxosarcoma are considered to be neoplasms of fibroblast origin, but since their histology is distinct from that of the usual fibroma and fibrosarcoma, they have been included in a separate category. Mucin in the intercellular matrix is the chief feature that distinguishes myxoma and myxosarcoma from fibroma and fibrosarcoma.

**Incidence and Sites.** These neoplasms occur in all domestic animals but their incidence is rare. Affected animals are usually adult or aged. There is no breed or sex prevalence.

Myxoma and myxosarcoma, like fibroma and fibrosarcoma, can occur at any site where there is connective tissue. In the dog the skin is the most common site. They have been seen in such unusual locations as the heart, liver, and spinal canal.

**Gross Morphology.** Myxoma and myxosarcoma are generally infiltrative growths that have no definite shape. They are soft, slimy, and nonencapsulated. The color is grayish white with clear, viscid, honeylike areas visible on the cut surface.

**Histological Features, Growth, and Metastasis.** It is difficult to distinguish the benign from the malignant neoplasm because the cells are similar in both (figs. 2.8A and B). Each form of the neoplasm usually displays scattered cells that appear singly or in small clusters. In some areas the cells are more numerous and are in whorls, lobules, or sheets.

The tumor cells are distributed in a vacuolated, basophilic, mucinous stroma that may be partitioned by collagenous connective tissue septa. Loose, wavy collagen fibers are sometimes present in the stroma. The individual tumor cell is usually

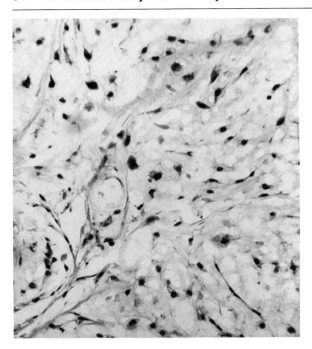

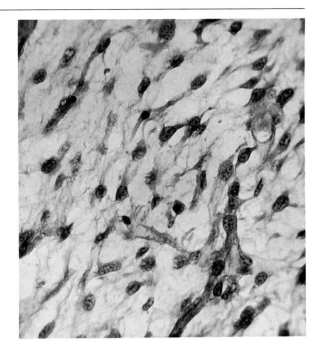

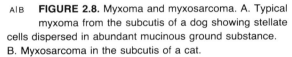

A|B  **FIGURE 2.8.** Myxoma and myxosarcoma. A. Typical myxoma from the subcutis of a dog showing stellate cells dispersed in abundant mucinous ground substance. B. Myxosarcoma in the subcutis of a cat.

stellate in shape but may be fusiform. The cell nuclei are round, ovoid, or elongated, with multiple nucleoli. The cells in myxosarcoma exhibit moderate numbers of mitotic figures, and the nuclei are more hyperchromatic than in the benign tumor.

Since myxosarcoma is infiltrative and difficult to remove completely at surgery, recurrence is common. Metastasis, usually first to the lungs, is uncommon.

## Canine Cutaneous Histiocytoma

**General Considerations.** Canine cutaneous histiocytoma (CCH) is a benign skin growth found only in the dog. Some pathologists doubt that it is a neoplasm, and consider it to be a peculiar focal proliferative inflammatory lesion. Contrary to previous reports (Mulligan, 1948), CCH is not an extragenital form of transmissible venereal tumor. Cytogenetic studies have shown that cells of histiocytoma have chromosomal makeup identical to

that of the normal dog (Smith and Jones, 1966), while those of transmissible venereal tumor show a consistent chromosomal abnormality (Makino, 1963; Smith and Jones, 1966; Weber *et al.*, 1965). The two tumors also exhibit different biological and epidemiological characteristics. The CCH and the histiocytoma of humans are not comparable entities.

**Incidence.** The canine cutaneous histiocytoma is a relatively common tumor of dogs. In an extensive study of these neoplasms, Taylor *et al.* (1969) found the average annual incidence rate during a 3-year period to be 117 per 100,000 dogs.

**Age, Breed, and Sex.** Canine cutaneous histiocytoma characteristically affects young dogs, and approximately 50% of the cases occur in dogs less than 2 years of age (Howard and Nielsen, 1969; Taylor *et al.*, 1969). After 2 years of age the prevalence drops considerably.

Purebred dogs in general, and boxer and dachshund breeds particularly, are predisposed to the de-

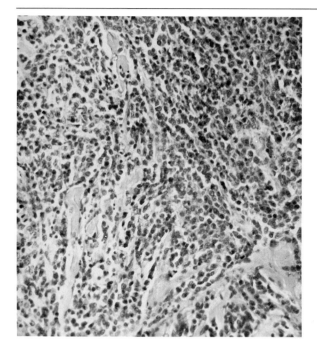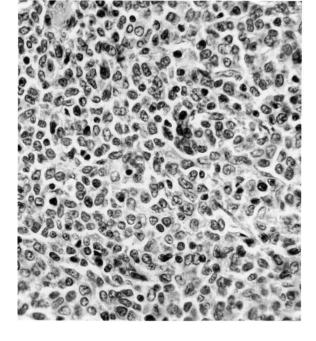

AIB **FIGURE 2.9.** Canine cutaneous histiocytoma. A. Typical histiocytoma with tumor cells infiltrating the dermis. B. Higher magnification of neoplastic cells.

velopment of histiocytoma (Taylor *et al.*, 1969). There is no sex predisposition for the tumor.

**Sites.** Canine cutaneous histiocytoma is usually solitary but may be multiple. The most common site is the head and more specifically the pinna of the ear. The next most common site is the skin of the distal forelegs and forefeet. The remainder of the tumors are distributed over the neck, limbs, trunk, and tail.

**Gross Morphology.** This tumor seldom grows large and usually measures no more than 2 cm in diameter. The growths are usually domed or buttonlike in shape and tend to have an ulcerated surface. In cross section the deep margins of the tumor are well-defined but not encapsulated.

**Histiological Features.** The histiocytoma consists of uniform sheets of cells infiltrating the dermis and subcutis and displacing the collagen fibers and skin adnexa (figs. 2.9A and B). The cells are densely packed in the deeper layers of the dermis. Near the epidermis they are usually loosely ar-

ranged and often appear to be lined up in rows. The tumor cells are round to ovoid in shape and have large nuclei. The cytoplasm is pale staining and abundant.

A characteristic feature of this tumor is its high mitotic index; as many as 10 mitotic figures per high-power field have been observed.

In many of these lesions (presumably the older ones that are undergoing regression) there are focal areas of necrosis and lymphocytic infiltration. In those tumors in which the epidermis is ulcerated, the superficial tumor cells are mixed with an inflammatory exudate.

There may be difficulty in distinguishing canine cutaneous histiocytoma from small mastocytoma, and the use of Giemsa or toluidine blue stains may be necessary for differentiation.

**Etiology and Transmission.** Taylor *et al.* (1969) failed to isolate an etiological agent from canine cutaneous histiocytoma in tissue culture and could not transmit the growth with cell suspensions.

**Growth and Metastasis.** Canine cutaneous histiocytoma generally has a history of rapid growth, and most tumors develop in 1 to 4 weeks. Although this rapid growth and the high mitotic index suggest malignancy, histiocytoma is a benign tumor in all respects. It does not metastasize, and probably the great majority of tumors will spontaneously regress.

## Atypical Histiocytoma

**General Considerations.** Atypical histiocytoma is the name we have used to designate a neoplastic entity in the dog having light and electron microscopic similarities to the canine cutaneous histiocytoma. In the past this tumor has been given numerous other names such as cutaneous reticulum cell sarcoma, plasmacytoma, melanoma, and canine round cell tumor, as well as canine cutaneous histiocytoma. A neoplasm referred to as cutaneous myelocytoma in earlier editions of the book *Veterinary Pathology* by Smith and Jones (1966) may have been a description of atypical histiocytoma. The reference to cutaneous myelocytoma has been deleted from later editions.

At this time there is controversy concerning the cell of origin of atypical histiocytoma. To establish with certainty the histiocytic origin of this neoplasm will require further investigation. Regressing atypical histiocytosis (Flynn *et al.*, 1982), a cutaneous neoplastic process in humans, has many similarities to atypical histiocytoma in the dog. It has been shown to be composed of cells with histiocytic differentiation by the use of electron microscopy, immunologic cell markers, enzyme cytochemistry, and cytogenetics.

Nickoloff *et al.* (1985) in a report of 20 canine tumors initially classified as atypical histiocytomas concluded that they were neuroendocrine carcinomas resembling human Merkel cell tumors. This conclusion was based on finding cytoplasmic dense core granules in 3 of 4 tumors they studied using the electron microscope. This electron microscopic observation has not been confirmed by other investigators, leading to the suggestion that what we have called atypical histiocytoma may represent a group of similar appearing tumors having several different origins.

**Incidence, Age, Breed, and Sex.** Atypical histiocytoma occurs much less frequently than canine cutaneous histiocytoma and yet is more common than some of the skin appendage tumors. It occurs in middle to older aged dogs as opposed to the much younger age for canine cutaneous histiocytoma. The average age is approximately 8 years with a range of 4 to 16 years. Males appear to be more commonly affected; there is no recognized breed predilection.

**Sites.** Atypical histiocytoma can occur at any site in the skin, but the head, neck, and legs appear to be the more common locations. The oral cavity is also a frequent site; most develop on the gingiva or near the mucocutaneous junction of the lips. They have also been observed in the external ear canal and anus.

**Gross Morphology.** At the time of clinical detection or surgical removal, the tumors are usually 0.3 to 1.0 cm in diameter, although some as large as 2.5 cm in diameter have been observed. They are firm, usually ovoid or spherical, may be pedunculated or sessile, and are most often hairless when in the skin. The epithelial surface is occasionally ulcerated. They are usually described clinically as pink or red. On cross section the margins are well-demarcated from surrounding tissues, and they usually do not extend into the subcutis. Multiple atypical histiocytomas have been observed rarely in the skin.

**Histological Features.** The predominant cell type in atypical histiocytoma is medium sized and round, ovoid, or polygonal with fairly distinct cytoplasmic borders (figs. 2.10A–C). These tumor cells have a moderate amount of amphophilic, sometimes vacuolated or faintly granular cytoplasm. A perinuclear clear zone is occasionally present. The nuclei vary considerably in shape. They are usually round or ovoid, but many are bean shaped, folded, or lobulated. Some nuclei are eccentrically located in the cytoplasm. Nuclei have coarsely clumped chromatin, and most have large nucleoli. Mitotic figures vary from few to moderate in number.

Giant cells are the other characteristic cell type in atypical histiocytoma. They are similar to the smaller cells except for the presence of either a single round, lobulated, or folded giant nucleus or multiple nuclei. The number of giant cells can vary from few to numerous but they are never the predominant cell type.

observed principally in the periphery of lymphocytic follicles, especially in the spleen.

## Mast Cell Tumor of the Cat

**General Considerations and Classification.** Mast cell neoplasia in the cat usually occurs in two distinct forms. In one form, one or more tumors originate in the skin and may metastasize to regional nodes and other viscera. In the other form, the neoplasm arises in internal organs (spleen, liver, intestine, and mesenteric lymph nodes) without obvious cutaneous involvement.

**Incidence, Age, Breed, and Sex.** Mast cell tumors are less frequently encountered in the cat than in the dog. Various tumor surveys indicate that mast cell neoplasms account for less than 1 to 9% of all tumors in the cat (Head, 1958; Mulligan, 1951; Nielsen, 1964; Schmidt and Langham, 1967; Smith and Jones, 1957). Mast cell tumors account for approximately 2 to 3% of all forms of cutaneous tumors in the cat (Cotchin, 1961; Head, 1958).

Although most mast cell tumors occur in mature cats, they can develop at an early age. There appears to be no breed or sex predilection (Garner and Lingeman, 1970).

**Sites and Gross Morphology.** Cutaneous mast cell tumors in the cat most often involve the head, neck, and trunk regions. They are usually solitary, firm, discrete nodules 0.5 to 2.0 cm in diameter. Some are hairless and ulcerated. Occasionally, multiple mast cell tumors develop that can number in the hundreds and appear as small raised partially ulcerated tumors involving all regions of the skin.

**Histological Features.** Feline cutaneous mast cell tumors begin in the dermis and then extend into the superficial subcutis as they enlarge. In contrast to the dog, they tend to be well-circumscribed but never encapsulated. Most are composed of sheets of discrete round cells that can vary in their degree of differentiation like those in the dog.

Well-differentiated mast cell tumors are composed of uniform round cells with centrally or eccentrically placed nuclei and abundant eosinophilic, faintly granular to agranular cytoplasm. Cytoplasmic metachromatic granules are readily observed with toluidine blue stain. In less differentiated tu-

mors there tends to be considerable variation in cell and nuclear size. Some poorly differentiated tumors contain numerous giant cells which can be mono- or multinucleated. Metachromatic granules may be difficult or impossible to demonstrate in the less differentiated tumors.

Most feline cutaneous mast cell tumors contain a few lymphoid aggregates. Eosinophils are not present or are sparse. Collagen degeneration, vascular changes, and edema are not present.

**Growth and Metastasis.** Most solitary well-differentiated cutaneous tumors have low potential for recurrence and metastasis after complete surgical removal. Those less differentiated tumors having high mitotic rate, nuclear pleomorphism, anisocytosis, and tumor giant cells have high potential for metastasis to lymph nodes and internal organs.

When multiple tumors develop it is more difficult to predict their behavior. Two or three well-differentiated tumors developing at the same time suggests that more could develop in the future. When massive numbers of cutaneous tumors occur widespread metastasis should be expected.

## Mast Cell Tumor of the Horse

**Classification and Incidence.** Nodular mast cell lesions occasionally develop in the skin and subcutus of the horse (Altera and Clark, 1970; Cheville et al., 1972; Frese, 1969). The term *cutaneous mastocytosis* has been proposed for these growths to stress their apparent hyperplastic rather than neoplastic nature (Altera and Clark, 1970; Cheville et al., 1972). We feel that this lesion should be called mast cell tumor because of the varied usage of the term mastocytosis and because adequate criteria have not been developed to distinguish hyperplastic from neoplastic aggregates of mast cells in the horse's skin.

Two distinct forms of equine mast cell tumor have been observed. The most common form is a single cutaneous nodule. The much less common form consists of disseminated, multiple, focal mast cell lesions in the skin, which may be present at or shortly after birth (Cheville et al., 1972). This generalized form of mast cell disease in foals closely resembles urticaria pigmentosa of humans.

**Age, Breed, and Sex.** In the only large series of equine mast cell tumor, the mean age of affected animals was 7 years 4 months with a range of 1 year 6 months to 15 years (Altera and Clark, 1970). In one instance a foal was affected at birth (Cheville *et al.*, 1972). Male horses are affected much more frequently than females. No breed predilection has been observed.

**Sites and Gross Morphology.** Equine mast cell tumors can occur anywhere on the body, but they most frequently involve the head. The lesions appear as discrete nodular swellings varying from 2 to 20 cm in diameter. They usually are confined to the skin, but sometimes the underlying musculature is involved. The surface of the nodules can be normal in appearance, hairless, or ulcerated. The cut surface is usually white with multiple small, yellow to brown granular areas present.

**Histological Features.** The lesions consist of variable-sized aggregates of well-differentiated mast cells (fig. 2.12C). Mitotic figures are rare. The mast cell aggregates are often sharply delineated by fibrous connective tissue that sometimes produces a scirrhous appearance. The mast cells are almost invariably accompanied by mature eosinophils that may be scattered in diffuse and/or focal accumulations.

A characteristic feature of equine mast cell tumor is the presence of focal areas of necrosis. These foci contain intensely eosinophilic granular debris and sometimes intact but necrotic mast cells and eosinophils. Many necrotic foci are partially mineralized. Vascular lesions are common and consist of swollen endothelial cells, a primarily mononuclear cell infiltration affecting the walls and surrounding connective tissue of small blood vessels, and occasionally, fibrinoid degeneration of the media of small muscular arteries.

**Etiology and Transmission.** The etiology of equine mast cell tumor is unknown. Although *Onchocerca* sp. microfilariae can occasionally be observed in the surrounding connective tissue, they are not thought to be related to the tumor (Altera and Clark, 1970). Attempts to transmit equine mast cell tumor have been unsuccessful (Cheville *et al.*, 1972).

**Growth and Metastasis.** There is little information available on the behavior of equine mast cell tumor. Metastasis has not been reported. Spontaneous regression was observed in the case of gen-

eralized cutaneous mast cell tumors in a foal reported by Cheville *et al.* (1972).

## Mast Cell Tumor of Cattle, Pigs, and Sheep

There have been several reports of mast cell tumors in cattle (Dodd, 1964; Groth *et al.*, 1960; Head, 1958; McGavin and Leis, 1968; Migaki and Carey, 1972; Smith and Jones, 1957). Head (1958) estimated that mast cell tumors represent approximately 3% of the cutaneous and subcutaneous tumors of the bovine. The tumor occurs in calves as well as in mature animals (Dodd, 1964; Head, 1958). No sex or breed predilection has been noted. Mast cell tumors in cattle may originate in the skin or internal organs. The cutaneous mast cell tumors are usually multiple and appear as nodular masses generally from 1 to 10 cm in diameter. They are frequently located in the subcutaneous tissues. The majority of cutaneous mast cell tumors in the bovine are associated with aggregates of mast cells in the regional lymph nodes, liver, spleen, lungs, heart, and kidneys.

Bovine mast cell tumor also occurs in internal organs without cutaneous involvement. The condition has been observed in the tongue (Dodd, 1964), abomasum (Groth *et al.*, 1960), and omentum (Smith and Jones, 1957). Bovine mast cell tumors are similar microscopically to mast cell tumors in other species. Little information is available concerning growth and metastasis of this neoplasm.

There have been a few reports of mast cell tumors in pigs (Bundza and Dukes, 1982; Migaki, 1969; Migaki and Langheinrich, 1970). The reported cases have been in younger animals 6 to 18 months of age or referred to as slaughter animals. Porcine mast cell tumors in the skin may be single or multiple. The tumors appear as discrete nodules within the dermis, varying from 0.5 to 2.5 cm in diameter. Spleen, liver, and kidney involvement was observed by Bundza and Dukes (1982). Porcine mast cell tumor is similar microscopically to the same neoplasm in other species.

In the only reported case of ovine mast cell tumor, two sheep had mast cell tumors of the liver (Johnstone, 1972). It was not known if these neoplasms were primary or metastatic.

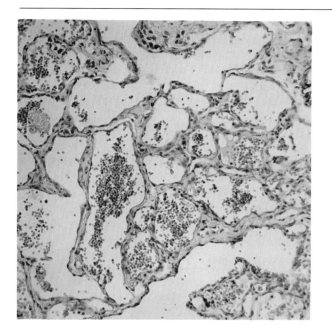

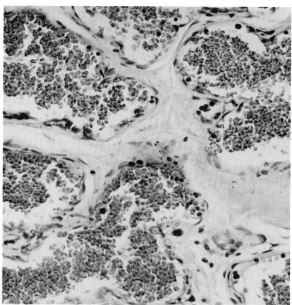

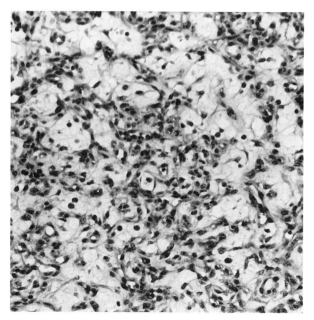

A|B  **FIGURE 2.13.** Hemangioma. A. Hemangioma of the
C|   skin in a cat showing multiple vascular spaces lined
by endothelium and containing blood cells. B. Hemangioma
of the skin of a dog showing large spaces filled with blood
and separated by collagenous stroma. C. Capillary hemangioma of the skin in a dog.

## Hemangioma

**General Considerations and Classification.**
Hemangioma is a benign tumor of endothelial
cells. They are usually classified as cavernous or capillary hemangiomas depending on the size of the
vascular spaces. Care must be taken in differentiating hemangioma from vascular malformations, excessively vascularized reparative and inflammatory
tissue, or from other highly vascularized neoplasms.

**Incidence, Age, Breed, and Sex.** Hemangiomas
are most common in the dog and are also found in
the cat, horse, cow, sheep, and pig. The average age
of affected dogs is 9 years, though the tumor may
develop in much younger dogs. Other affected animals are adult or aged. Congenital hemangiomas,
however, have been reported in the foal and calf
(Baker *et al.*, 1982; Sartin and Hodge, 1982).
There is no known breed or sex predisposition.

**Sites.** These tumors are usually solitary but may
be multiple. Since they arise from vascular endothelium, they can develop in any location in the
body. In the dog, however, they usually occur in
the dermis or subcutis of the leg, flank, neck, face,
and eyelid. In other species these tumors are also
found mainly in the skin and subcutis.

**Gross Morphology.** When hemangiomas are located in the subcutis, they are usually 0.5 to 3.0 cm in greatest dimension, ovoid or discoid in shape, moderately firm, and well-circumscribed. They are reddish black, and blood will ooze from the cut surface of the fresh specimen. The cut surface of the formalin-fixed tumor is black and dry. Hemangiomas in the dermis are usually smaller than those in the subcutis. They tend to be sessile or pedunculated and can be confused with melanomas.

**Microscopic Features, Growth, and Metastasis.** Hemangioma consists of blood-filled vascular spaces lined by single layers of well-differentiated flattened endothelial cells (figs. 2.13A–C). Thrombosis of vascular channels in hemangioma is frequent, particularly in the cavernous hemangioma. Broad, sometimes hyalinized, connective tissue septa may separate vascular spaces. The margins of the tumors are well-demarcated but not encapsulated. Hemangiomas do not recur after complete surgical removal.

## Hemangiomalike Lesions

**Skin of Cattle.** Bovine cutaneous angiomatosis (Cotchin and Swarbrick, 1963) is a hemangiomalike lesion occurring infrequently in the skin of dairy cattle in Great Britain. It has also been reported in France (Lombard and Levesque, 1964) and recognized in the United States in both dairy and beef cattle. A frequent site is the dorsum of the back, but the lesion can occur anywhere in the skin. One or several growths may be present on an individual animal. The growths are usually reddish gray to pink, soft, sessile or pedunculated masses, 0.5 to 2.5 cm in diameter. Most often the lesions are first detected because of recurring hemorrhage, which may in some cases be profuse. In Great Britain most of the cases occurred in cows averaging 5.5 years of age (Cotchin and Swarbrick, 1963).

Microscopically, the lesions arise in the dermis and consist of a nonencapsulated proliferation of vascular tissue. The vascular tissue appears as masses of thin-walled branching capillaries in some areas, while in other areas the tissue resembles arterioles or venules. There may also be areas of vasoformative tissue without conspicuous lumens. The stroma is composed of scattered fibroblasts and variable amounts of collagen in finely fibrillar or mucoid matrix. Inflammatory cells may be numerous with neutrophils predominating, particularly in areas adjacent to an ulcerated surface. Eosinophils and histiocytes are usually present in variable numbers.

Some of the lesions in the cow closely resemble the so-called pyogenic granuloma of human skin. In humans, pyogenic granuloma has been attributed to staphylococcal infection. Some of the causes suggested for bovine cutaneous angiomatosis are abnormal vascular repair following injury, highly vascular granulation tissue, a congenital vascular anomaly, and bacterial or viral infection.

**Scrotum in the Dog.** A lesion resembling hemangioma, sometimes referred to as "varicose tumor of the scrotum," was described by Weipers and Jarrett (1954) as a specific entity in the dog. They are solitary or multiple proliferations and strictly limited to the skin of the scrotum. They are most common in dogs past middle age and in breeds with pigmented skin, such as Scottish terriers, Airedales, Kerry blue terriers, and Labrador retrievers. These lesions may represent growth anomalies rather than true neoplasms, and they are not malignant.

The pathogenesis of this lesion is as follows. First it appears as a localized pigmented area that consists microscopically of collapsed capillaries and melanin pigmentation of the overlying skin. A plaque then forms as the capillaries become dilated with blood. Melanin pigmentation of the skin continues. The lesion then develops into a cavernous type of hemangioma with branching and communicating spaces lined by endothelium. Fibrous stroma is well developed, and the overlying epidermis is heavily pigmented with melanin. The proliferation may become traumatically ulcerated, and the dog licks it, causing periodic hemorrhage. Some growths recur after surgical removal, but this probably involves another vasoformative area of the scrotal skin rather than recurrence of the primary lesion. Cords of endothelial cells that become canalized at the periphery of these masses may give the impression of neoplastic invasion.

# Hemangiosarcoma

**Incidence.** Hemangiosarcoma (angiosarcoma or malignant hemangioendothelioma) is a malignant tumor of endothelial cells. It occurs most frequently in dogs. It is less common than hemangioma. Hemangiosarcoma occurs in other domestic species, particularly the cow (Sutton and McLennan, 1982; Zachary *et al.*, 1981), horse, and cat, but it is less common in these species than in the dog.

**Age, Breed, and Sex.** The average age for dogs with this neoplasm is 9 to 10 years. In other domestic animals it usually occurs in adulthood or old age. The German shepherd dog (Alsatian) is the breed most often affected, and the tumors occur more often in males than in females (Kleine *et al.*, 1970; Pearson and Head, 1976; Waller and Rubarth, 1967). There is no known breed or sex predisposition in other domestic animals.

**Clinical Characteristics.** Dogs with hemangiosarcoma exhibit a variety of clinical signs depending on the location of the primary and metastatic lesions, in addition to having nonspecific signs of malignant neoplastic disease. Heart failure, sometimes occurring suddenly, is caused by extensive neoplastic involvement of the heart or hemorrhage into the pericardial sac or both. Respiratory difficulties may be paramount because of extensive metastatic neoplasia in the lung or by hemothorax. Acute vascular collapse resulting from rupture of splenic hemangiosarcoma with massive hemorrhage into the peritoneal cavity can be the presenting clinical sign.

Dogs with hemangiosarcoma frequently exhibit borderline to severe anemia and have circulating nucleated red blood cells usually in numbers out of proportion to the degree of anemia. Reticulocytosis, basophilic stippling, leukocytosis with neutrophilia, and left shift are other common findings (Kleine *et al.*, 1970; Rebar *et al.*, 1980).

**Sites.** It is probable that hemangiosarcoma arises *de novo* rather than from preexisting hemangioma, since it occurs more commonly in internal sites than in the subcutis, the common site for hemangioma. In the dog the spleen and the right atrium and auricle of the heart are the most common sites. Since the tumor arises from vascular endothelium, it may occur at any site in the body, including such

areas as the bone, central nervous system, muscle, and gastrointestinal tract. When hemangiosarcoma arises in the skin of the dog, it has been reported that the lower abdomen, including the preputial skin and scrotum, are the most common sites (Culbertson, 1982).

**Gross Morphology.** The characteristic gross feature of hemangiosarcoma is its reddish black hemorrhagic appearance. In the subcutis the tumor is a soft or spongy, poorly circumscribed, infiltrating mass varying in size from less than 1 cm in diameter to as large as 10 cm in diameter. When the neoplasm is located in the heart, its endocardial surface may be covered by a thrombus, giving the tumor a reddish gray or yellow color. When located in the right atrium the tumor usually measures 2 to 5 cm in diameter, although in some cases the tumors are practically indistinguishable (Pearson and Head, 1976).

Hemangiosarcomas in the spleen can closely resemble nodular hyperplasia or hematoma of the spleen. The growths are usually spherical, reddish black, and can be 15 or 20 cm in diameter because of hemorrhage within the tumor. The cut surface of the tumor has reddish gray to reddish black spongy areas that represent neoplastic tissue. The areas of hemorrhage are usually clotted and may be dark red or yellow due to settling and lysis of red blood cells. Cysts containing red or clear yellow fluid may be present.

**Histological Features.** Hemangiosarcoma is composed of immature endothelial cells that generally form vascular spaces, often as small clefts but sometimes as cavernous channels, in the tumor tissue (figs. 2.14A and B). The vascular spaces contain variable amounts of blood and sometimes exhibit thrombi. In highly cellular tumors the vascular spaces must be identified to distinguish hemangiosarcoma from fibrosarcoma. The vessels formed by this neoplasm are fragile and frequently rupture, with hemorrhage resulting. Hemorrhage and necrosis are almost constant features of this growth.

The neoplastic cells vary in size and shape, but are usually elongated. The cells are larger and plumper than those of hemangioma. The nuclei are round or ovoid and very hyperchromatic. Mitotic figures are common. The connective tissue stroma

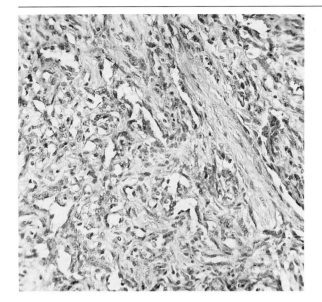

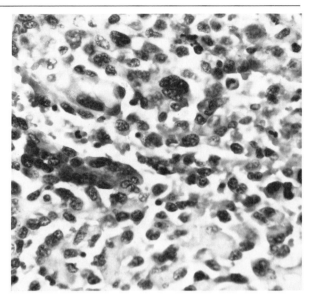

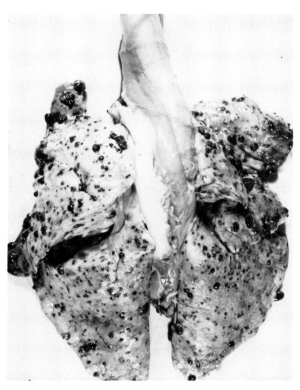

A|B
C|    **FIGURE 2.14.** Hemangiosarcoma. A. Immature endo-
thelial cells forming vascular spaces. B. Anaplastic
cells. C. Metastasis of hemangiosarcoma of the spleen to
the lungs in a dog.

in these growths is variable in amount and often difficult to distinguish from the tumor tissue. Macrophages filled with hemosiderin are common, as are infiltrations of polymorphonuclear leukocytes.

**Growth and Metastasis.** Hemangiosarcoma is a highly malignant neoplasm, readily metastasizing, and often recurring after surgery. Metastasis usually occurs early since the tumor cells have easy access to vascular channels. The lung is the most common site for metastasis, but metastasis can be found in almost any tissue (fig. 2.14C).

Hemangiosarcoma of the heart quickly showers the lungs with metastases, giving a characteristic radiographic appearance of many small, uniform, spherical nodules evenly scattered throughout the lung field. When hemangiosarcoma is found in multiple locations, such as spleen, liver, heart, skin, and bone, it may be difficult to determine the primary site of origin, and the possibility of multicentric origin is occasionally considered.

## Hemangiopericytoma

**General Considerations and Classification.** The canine hemangiopericytoma is a distinct neoplastic entity first described by Stout (1949) and later by Mulligan (1955) and Yost and Jones (1958).

Some controversy and reluctance to accept this tumor as a hemangiopericytoma has always existed since there has never been conclusive evidence that the tumor arises from pericytes. Although in humans it is classified as a vascular tumor, the canine tumor, as it is now known, bears little resemblance to that in humans. Blood vessels are not always a significant component, and the so-called occult or collapsed capillaries have been shown by electron microscopy to not exist in the centers of many of the whorls. Special stains to demonstrate these occult capillaries are of little value.

Many pathologists will classify the hemangiopericytoma as a Schwannoma or neurofibroma, and we must admit that in the absence of whorls there are few if any distinguishing differences. The differentiation between hemangiopericytoma, Schwannoma, and neurofibroma in practice is usually not a question of what is right or wrong, but rather is dependent on education, institutional philosophy, habit, inertia, or obstinacy. As with hemangiopericytoma, there have been no studies to prove that the so-called canine Schwannoma and neurofibroma arise from Schwann cells or perineural fibroblasts. In the World Health Organization classification by Weiss and Frese (1974), canine hemangiopericytoma is included as a subcategory of fibrosarcoma.

**Incidence, Age, Breed, and Sex.** The hemangiopericytoma occurs only in the dog. The report of its occurrence in other species (Brodey, 1970) is doubtful. It is one of the commonly occurring mesenchymal tumors, found less frequently than mast cell tumor, histiocytoma, and lipoma, but more commonly than fibroma, fibrosarcoma, and hemangioma.

Hemangiopericytoma usually appears in dogs older than 6 years, and most tumors occur in animals between 8 and 14 years of age. The female is more commonly affected than the male, and the boxer, German shepherd, and springer spaniel breeds are most commonly affected (Mills and Nielsen, 1967).

**Sites and Gross Morphology.** The most common site for the hemangiopericytoma is on the extremities, usually on the lateral surfaces. The neoplasms develop less frequently on the trunk and occur occasionally on the head, neck, and tail (Mills and Nielsen, 1967; Mulligan, 1955).

These neoplasms usually range from 2 to 10 cm

in greatest dimension, but occasionally attain a size of 25 cm in diameter. They tend to be firm and nodular. The skin rarely ulcerates and may be movable over the surface. The cut surface is gray to pink, often with large distinct lobules that easily separate from one another. Parts of the growth may be soft and moist and occasionally cystic.

**Histological Features.** The characteristic histological features of the hemangiopericytoma are the whorls around blood vessels and the "fingerprint" pattern formed by the tumor cells (figs. 2.15A–D). These features are very distinctive when present, but often there are few or no whorls to be found in an entire section. Instead, the tumor cells are arranged in short interlacing bundles and palisades. The lack of whorls is particularly evident in many recurrent tumors.

The tumor cells vary in their morphology. They are usually spindle shaped with short to long cytoplasmic processes, but may be round or ovoid with a moderate amount of pink-staining cytoplasm. Multinucleated cells are occasionally seen. Nuclei are usually ovoid with single, prominent, centrally located nucleoli and chromatin that is marginated along the nuclear membrane.

Blood vessels may be present in the centers of the whorls, but the numerous so-called occult or closed capillaries have not been demonstrated by electron microscopy. Blood vessels are present but usually not in numbers greater than expected to nourish and support the tumor cells. The amount of collagenous stroma varies greatly and is quite extensive in some tumors.

**Electron Microscopy.** Under electron microscope examination, the whorls in hemangiopericytoma are seen to consist of tumor cells and their cytoplasmic processes. These form concentric laminations not only around blood vessels but also around collagen bundles and fibroblasts. Nerves have not been seen in the centers of the whorls. The tumor cells lack a basal lamina and tight junctions that are usually seen in hemangiopericytoma of humans (Hahn *et al.*, 1973; Pantekoek and Schiefer, 1975) and in normal pericytes (Movat and Fernando, 1964). Cytoplasmic organelles consist of a well-developed Golgi apparatus, moderate to numerous mitochondria, and a moderate amount of granular endoplasmic reticulum. A distinctive feature is that most tumor cells contain bundles of

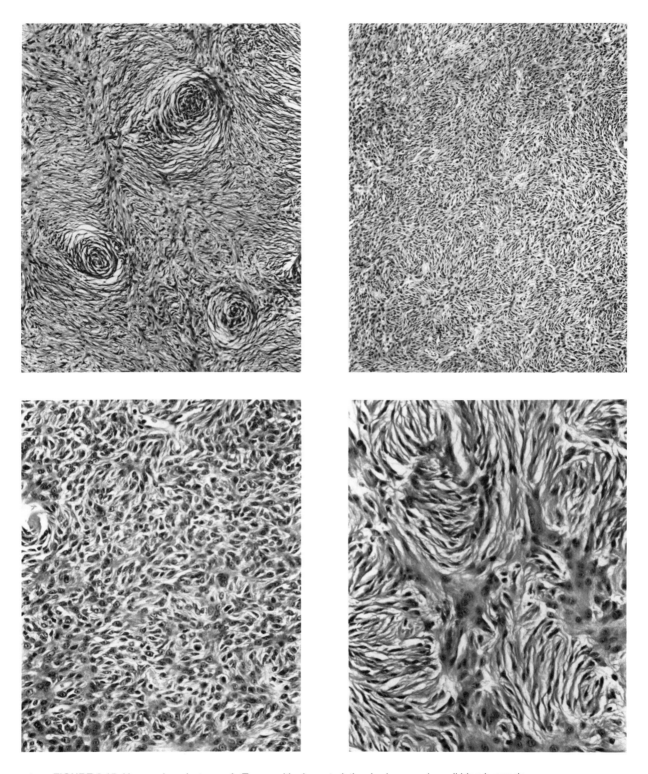

A|B
C|D  **FIGURE 2.15.** Hemangiopericytoma. A. Tumor with characteristic whorls around small blood vessels. B. Tumor cells arranged in short interlacing bundles. C. Poorly defined bundles without obvious vascular orientation. D. Elongated and ovoid-shaped cells in a storiform pattern.

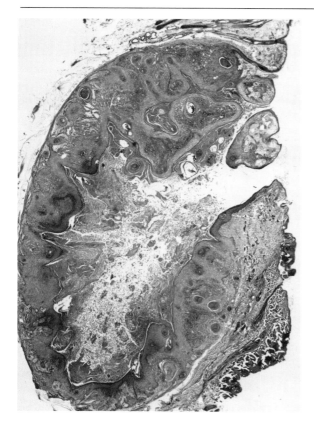

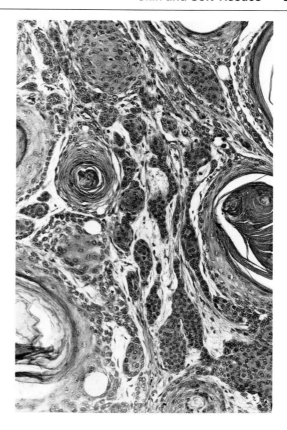

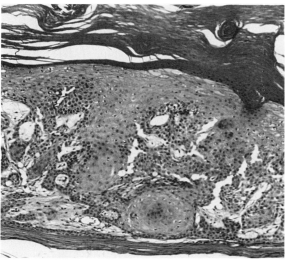

A|B
C|  **FIGURE 2.18.** Intracutaneous cornifying epithelioma in the dog. A. Cryptlike growth in the dermis and subcutis opens onto the skin surface. B. Anastomosing cords and nests of squamous epithelial cells. C. A portion of the wall of a cystic tumor.

timeters in diameter, opening onto the skin surface. The opening usually contains a hard keratinized plug. In some tumors the keratin plug is small and inconspicuous, whereas in others it is quite large and occasionally consists of a club-shaped mass of keratin with embedded hairs protruding above the skin surface. A few of the tumors are situated entirely within the dermis and subcutis with no communication to the surface of the skin.

**Histological Features.** Usually the tumors consist of a keratin-filled crypt in the dermis that opens onto the skin surface (figs. 2.18A–C). The wall of the crypt is composed of a thick folded layer of well-differentiated stratified squamous epithelium, with cells that maintain their usual polarity and orderly arrangement. Enclosed within the crypt are concentrically laminated masses of keratin. In most cases columns of squamous epithelial cells project peripherally from the basal surface of the wall, forming small epithelial nests, sometimes each with a central keratin mass and numerous anastomosing cords. The outer limits of the growth are well-demarcated and in most cases appear encapsulated because of compression of the surrounding dermal connective tissue by the expanding tumor mass.

In a few of the neoplasms there is no communication between the tumor and the skin surface. The tumors that lack this communication are composed of a large, central, keratin-filled cyst or are a solid epithelial growth with numerous small, concentrically laminated keratin masses, and many anastomosing cords of squamous epithelium. In the cystic form the neoplasm is lined in part by the thick complex wall observed in the more typical intracutaneous cornifying epithelioma, and the remainder of the cyst is lined by a thin layer of stratified squamous epithelium.

**Growth and Metastasis.** Intracutaneous cornifying epithelioma does not metastasize nor does it recur following surgical removal. In the generalized form a recurrent problem should be anticipated since the affected dogs will continue to develop new growths at other sites.

## Squamous Cell Carcinoma of the Skin

**Incidence, Age, Breed, and Sex.** Squamous cell carcinoma is a malignant tumor of squamous epithelial cells. It is a common neoplasm affecting all domestic animals, but most commonly the dog, cat, horse, and cow. Affected animals are mostly adults or aged. There is no known breed predilection, although it has been reported that squamous cell carcinomas arising on the digits of dogs occur more frequently in black Labrador retrievers and black standard poodles (Madewell *et al.*, 1982). There is no sex predisposition for squamous cell carcinoma of the skin.

**Sites.** Squamous cell carcinoma has been found in all areas of the skin of domestic animals, although most species have sites of predilection. The skin of the trunk, legs, scrotum, lips, and nail bed epithelium of the digits are particularly involved in the dog (Head, 1953). The mucocutaneous junctions are commonly involved in horses and cattle. Squamous cell carcinoma of the skin in cats is invariably found on the head, usually involving the pinna, the nasal planum, external nares, lips, or eyelids (Cotchin, 1961).

In all species there is a tendency for squamous cell carcinoma to develop in areas of unpigmented skin, especially squamous carcinomas of the pinna, eyelid, and nasal planum in cats; eyelids in cattle; and abdominal, inguinal, and scrotal areas in the dog.

**Gross Morphology.** The tumors may be productive or erosive. The productive types are papillary growths of varying size, many of which have a cauliflowerlike appearance. The surface tends to be ulcerated and bleeds easily. The more common erosive types initially appear as shallow, crusted ulcers which, if allowed to develop, can become deep and craterlike.

Squamous cell carcinomas involving the pinna(s) in white or white-eared cats have a characteristic appearance. The first sign is erythema involving the tips and margins of the pinna. Gradually there is a loss of hair, scaling, crust formation, and ulceration. The ulceration gradually increases in severity and eventually the entire pinna is destroyed.

**Histological Features.** The tumor is composed of irregular masses or cords of epidermal cells that proliferate downward and invade the dermis and subcutis (figs. 2.19 and 2.20A and B). The cell of origin is the keratinocyte, and thus a usual feature of these tumors is the formation of keratin. The amount of keratin produced depends on the degree of maturation of the neoplastic cells. In well-differentiated tumors, large numbers of "horn pearls" (cancer pearls) are present; these are composed of concentric layers of squamous cells showing gradually increasing keratinization toward the centers. In poorly differentiated tumors only an occasional individually keratinized cell can be seen. The individual cell undergoing keratinization is large and round and has a glassy, deeply eosinophilic cytoplasm and pyknotic nucleus.

The other characteristic feature of squamous cell carcinoma besides keratin formation is the presence of "intercellular bridges" that can readily be found in all but the most anaplastic tumors.

Mitotic figures are usually conspicuous in this neoplasm, and many mitotic figures are atypical in appearance.

**Growth and Metastasis.** In general, squamous cell carcinomas are locally invasive but slow to metastasize. In one report of 112 squamous cell carcinomas in the dog, metastasis occurred in 7 cases

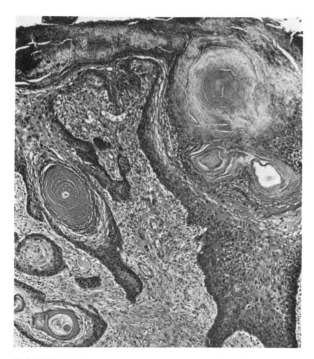

**FIGURE 2.19.** Squamous cell carcinoma of the skin. Irregular masses and cords of epidermal cells invading the dermis. "Horn pearl" formation is conspicuous.

and recurrence occurred in 8 cases (Strafuss *et al.,* 1976). When metastasis does occur, it is usually to the regional lymph nodes first and then to the lungs. Widespread metastasis is sometimes seen.

## Carcinoma in the Horn Core of Cattle

**General Considerations.** Carcinoma of the horn core in cattle is a neoplasm of stratified squamous epithelium first reported by Hewlett (1905). The exact site of origin has not been definitely determined. It probably arises from basal epithelium of the horn or possibly from the mucous membrane lining of the frontal sinus (Hewlett, 1905; Patra, 1959).

**Incidence.** This tumor occurs almost exclusively in India, where it affects approximately 1% of the cattle population (Naik *et al.,* 1969). A few cases have been reported from Sumatra (Burggraaf, 1935).

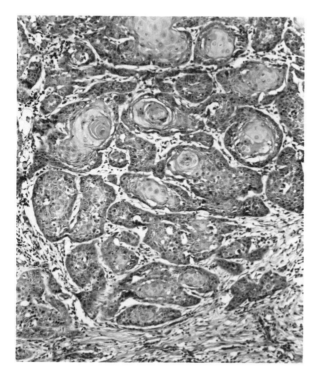
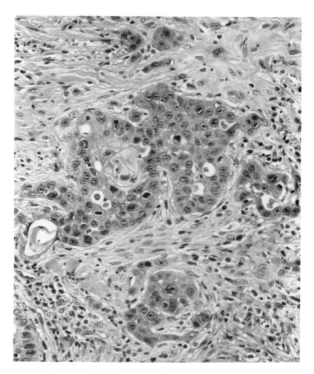

A|B   **FIGURE 2.20.** Squamous cell carcinoma. A. Variably sized masses of concentrically arranged squamous epithelial cells with "horn pearl" formation. B. Invasive tumor cells stimulating stromal fibrosis.

**Age, Breed, and Sex.** In a study of 6181 cases of horn core cancer in India, Lall (1953) found that 82% of the neoplasms were in animals 5 to 10 years old, 18% were in animals more than 10 years old, and the tumor was very rare in animals less than 5 years old. The tumors are most common in the breeds of cattle with large horns, such as the Kankrej breed. Purebred cattle are affected more often than are crossbreds (Naik *et al.*, 1969). Bullocks (castrated males) make up 95% and cows 5% of the affected animals (Kulkarni, 1953).

**Clinical Characteristics and Sites.** During the early stages of tumor growth, the animal exhibits pain by shaking its head, rubbing it against solid objects, and inclining it toward the affected horn. Eventually, the horn tilts to one side and hangs down by the side of the face. A cleft occurs between the horn and skin which often becomes infected. The horn finally becomes loose and can be removed by moderate traction, thereby exposing the cancerous horn core. The affected animals become emaciated and die in about 4 to 6 months. The occurrence of the neoplasms in the right and left horns is about equal. Rarely both horns are affected (Naik *et al.*, 1969).

**Gross Morphology and Histological Features.** After the horn is detached, the horn core reveals a fetid, grayish or yellowish cauliflowerlike growth. The tumor may invade the frontal sinuses and cranial bones. The tumor tissue is firm, but may be cut with a knife. The bony structure of the horn core is generally lost and no horn cavity remains. Sometimes the base of the growth is very vascular, and there may be secondary osteitis of the frontal bone.

Horn core carcinoma is a typical squamous cell carcinoma. In general, the histological appearance is one of low-grade malignancy.

**Etiology.** Trauma from paring of the outer horn layer of the horns of young animals to produce horns of uniform size and shape and trauma from constant striking of the horns against the yoke during plowing have been suggested as causes for the development of horn core cancer. Hormonal factors have also been suspect as a possible etiology on the basis of the high incidence of the neoplasm in castrated males, the low incidence in cows, and its absence in intact males (Lall, 1953). Also, on the basis of the successful treatment of five of nine

cattle with an autogenous vaccine, Pachauri and Pathak (1969) suggested that a virus may be involved.

**Growth and Metastasis.** The carcinoma almost invariably recurs after attempted surgical removal (Sahu, 1968). The tumor invades and destroys the tissues of the head but only rarely metastasizes (Naik *et al.*, 1969). In a few cases metastatic secondary tumors have been reported in the internal viscera (Kulkarni, 1953).

## Basal Cell and Appendage Tumors

**General Considerations.** The basal cell and appendage tumors are a very important group of skin tumors in the dog and cat, but are rare in other species of domestic animals. The basal cell tumor is a distinct undifferentiated epithelial tumor of the skin. The appendage tumor group includes tumors arising from or differentiating toward hair follicles and the various skin glands (sebaceous, sweat, ceruminous, and perianal).

During fetal development, the primary epithelial germ cells (hair germ or hair apparatus germ) give rise to the pilary complexes, each of which includes a hair follicle and a sebaceous and apocrine sweat gland. Basal cell tumors and the sebaceous and hair follicle tumors mimic the primary epithelial germ and its subsequent differentiation into a pilary complex.

The characteristic cell of basal cell tumor is the basal cell. This cell is not synonymous with the basal cells of the epidermis, which are a well-differentiated cell population and possess "intercellular bridges." In contrast, the basal cell of basal cell tumors and certain appendage tumors is a more primitive, pluripotential cell that lacks intercellular bridges. To stress the difference between these two basal cell populations, the terms *basaloma* and *basaloid cell* are sometimes used when discussing basal cell tumors in humans. The cells making up undifferentiated basal cell tumors can be considered somewhat analogous to the undifferentiated primary epithelial germ cells.

One group of appendage tumors mimics the primary epithelial germ and its differentiation into mature sebaceous glands. A continuous spectrum is often observed from tumors that are essentially

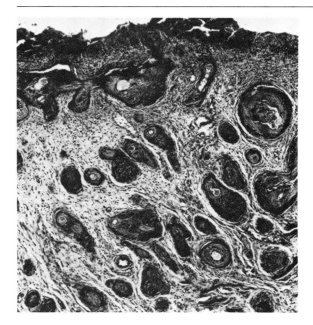

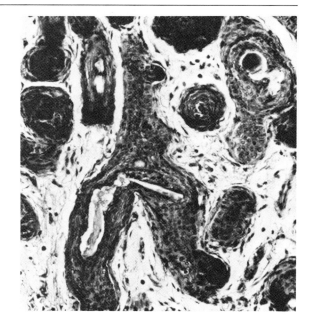

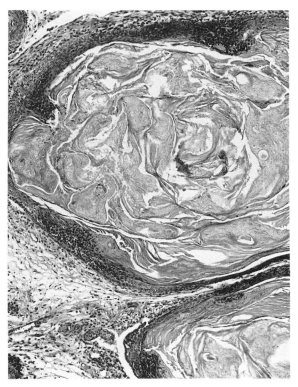

A|B **FIGURE 2.22.** Trichoepithelioma. A. Superficial tri-
C| choepithelioma (sometimes referred to as a baso-
squamous epithelioma). B. Rudimentary hair formation.
C. Horn cysts.

Sandersleben, 1964). Males and females appear to be equally affected.

**Sites.** Pilomatricoma involves the dermis and subcutis and almost always occurs as a solitary growth. In one series the growths were limited to the legs and shoulders of dogs (Nielsen and Cole, 1960), whereas in another survey it was observed that the legs and head of dogs were spared (von Sandersleben, 1964).

**Gross Morphology.** Pilomatricomas are very firm, well-circumscribed masses that are freely movable over the underlying structures. They vary from 2 to 10 cm in diameter. The overlying skin is usually thin, hairless, and frequently ulcerated. The cut surface is lobulated and contains white chalky areas of mineralization.

**Histological Features, Growth, and Metastasis.** Pilomatricomas consist of variably shaped masses of epithelial cells (figs. 2.23A and B). Two distinct cell types are present: "basophilic cells" and "shadow cells." The basophilic cells closely resemble the hair matrix cells found in the hair bulbs of actively growing hairs. They are small and deeply staining with only scant amounts of cytoplasm. The cellular borders are indistinct, and it appears as if the nuclei are embedded in a symplasmic mass.

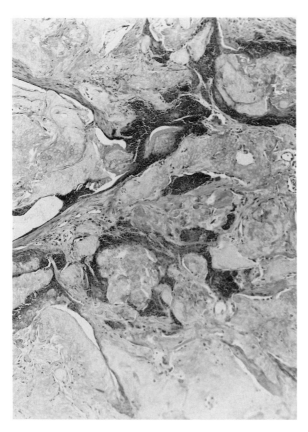

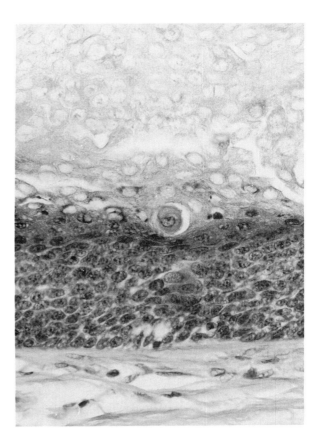

A|B  **FIGURE 2.23.** Pilomatricoma of the dog. A. Typical pilomatricoma consisting of variably shaped masses of epithelial cells. B. An area of transition from "basal cells" to "shadow cells" (top).

The fully keratinized shadow cells stain faintly eosinophilic with hematoxylin and eosin. They have a distinct border with a central unstained area at the site of the nucleus. In some areas the progression from basophilic to shadow cell can clearly be seen. An intermediate cell type is present that has undergone partial keratinization, but that still possesses a basophilic nucleus.

In tumors of recent origin the basophilic cells predominate, while in older lesions the shadow cells predominate and few basophilic cells can be found. A frequent but not constant feature of pilomatricomas is calcification within the areas of shadow cells; ossification occurs rarely. Usually, at least a portion of the tumor stroma shows a foreign-body giant cell reaction.

Pilomatricoma is a benign tumor in most respects. The tumors are slow growing, usually not invasive, and rarely metastasize (Goldschmidt *et al.*, 1981).

## Sebaceous Gland Tumor

**Classification and Incidence.** According to the level of maturation displayed by the cells, sebaceous gland growths can be divided into nodular hyperplasia, sebaceous adenoma, sebaceous epithelioma, and sebaceous adenocarcinoma. Although this is a more complex classification system than has normally been used in the past, it more accurately reflects the true spectrum of sebaceous gland growths that are encountered, and it standardizes the nomenclature used for sebaceous gland growths in humans and domestic animals.

Sebaceous gland growths are the most common epithelial skin tumors in the dog, accounting for approximately one-third of the total in one series (Nielsen and Cole, 1960). They occasionally occur in the cat and are rare in other species of domestic animals.

**Age, Breed, Sex, and Sites.** The mean age of

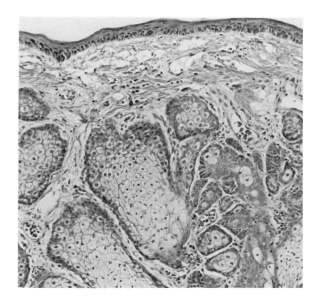

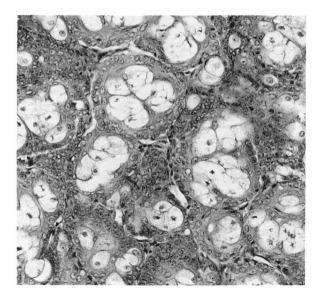

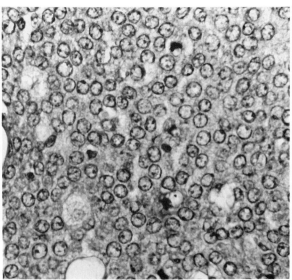

A|B
—|—
|C

**FIGURE 2.24.** Benign sebaceous gland tumors. A. Nodular sebaceous gland hyperplasia in the skin of a dog. B. Sebaceous adenoma showing undifferentiated, generative cells and mature sebaceous cells. C. Sebaceous epithelioma showing masses of "basal cells" with varying numbers of cells undergoing sebaceous differentiation.

dogs with sebaceous gland tumors is between 9 and 10 years (Nielsen and Cole, 1960; Strafuss, 1976b). The cocker spaniel is predisposed to develop these tumors (Nielson and Cole, 1960), but the tumors are also common in poodles (Strafuss, 1976b). Females appear to be more commonly affected (Strafuss, 1976b).

Sebaceous gland tumors may involve the skin anywhere on the body. The head, abdomen, and thorax are the most common sites (Mulligan, 1949; Nielsen and Cole, 1960; Strafuss, 1976b). One of the most frequent sites is the eyelid, where the growths arise from large modified sebaceous glands referred to as meibomian glands.

**Gross Morphology.** Sebaceous gland tumors may be single or multiple. The nodular sebaceous hyperplastic lesions are usually small, varying from 2 to 5 mm in diameter. They are discrete, lobulated, and normally yellow. Sebaceous gland adenomas tend to be larger and less lobulated than the hyperplastic lesions, ranging up to 2 cm in diameter. Sebaceous epitheliomas are similar to basal cell tumors and trichoepitheliomas in appearance, that is, they are firm, well-circumscribed masses that are easily movable over the underlying structures. The overlying skin is frequently hairless and often ulcerated.

There have not been enough sebaceous adenocarcinomas observed to provide an accurate picture of their gross appearance. Nevertheless, most of the features of a malignant neoplasm would be expected, such as rapid growth, ill-defined borders, and ulceration.

**Histological Features.** Nodular sebaceous hyperplasia consists of a greatly enlarged sebaceous gland composed of numerous lobules grouped around a centrally located, wide sebaceous duct (fig. 2.24A). Most lobules appear fully mature. In some lesions the duct that is composed of stratified squamous epithelium predominates, and the sebaceous gland lobules are inconspicuous.

Sebaceous adenomas are sharply demarcated from the surrounding tissue. They are composed of lobules that are irregular in size and shape. Two distinct types of cells are present in the lobules: undifferentiated generative cells and mature sebaceous cells (fig. 2.24B). Often there are some cells in a transitional stage of differentiation. The generative cells are identical to the cells present at the periphery of normal sebaceous glands. Some lobules contain mainly generative cells, while others contain mainly mature sebaceous cells. In many sebaceous adenomas there are foci with stratified squamous epithelium and keratinization, which represent areas of differentiation toward sebaceous gland duct structure.

Sebaceous epitheliomas are similar in most respects to basal cell tumors. The tumors are composed of irregularly shaped cell masses. The majority of cells are undifferentiated basal cells. In addition, there are varying numbers of transitional cells showing the start of fatty vacuolization of their cytoplasm (fig. 2.24C). Groups of mature sebaceous cells usually lie in the center of the cell masses. Cysts formed by the disintegration of cells and filled with amorphous material may also be present. As in the sebaceous adenomas, foci of stratified squamous epithelium and keratinization may be present. Many sebaceous epitheliomas are heavily pigmented, with large numbers of mature melanocytes interspersed among the basal cells. These pigmented sebaceous epitheliomas should not be confused with true melanocytic tumors. Finally, a dense infiltrate of lymphocytes and plasma cells may surround certain sebaceous epitheliomas.

Sebaceous adenocarcinoma must be differentiated from sebaceous epithelioma. There is a tendency to erroneously diagnose sebaceous epitheliomas as carcinomas, especially if they are poorly differentiated. Sebaceous adenocarcinoma consists of irregular lobular formations. Unlike the small, uniform basal cells in sebaceous epithelioma, the cells in sebaceous adenocarcinoma are large and exhibit considerable variation in size and shape of their nuclei (figs. 2.25A and B). The cytoplasm is eosinophilic and, in a few cells, is finely vacuolated. Focal areas of atypical keratinizing cells may also be present.

**Growth and Metastasis.** Nodular sebaceous hyperplasia and sebaceous adenoma are benign growths in all respects. Sebaceous epitheliomas are identical to basal cell tumors in their biological behavior: they are usually slow growing, tend to remain encapsulated, and rarely if ever metastasize, but will recur following incomplete surgical excision.

Sebaceous adenocarcinoma is a malignant tumor and like most carcinomas metastasizes to the regional lymph nodes and then to the lungs and other areas (Case *et al.,* 1969).

## Sweat Gland Tumor

**General Considerations.** In domestic animals apocrine glands make up the majority of the tubular skin glands. Merocrine (eccrine) sweat glands are confined mainly to the foot pads of dogs and cats.

The apocrine sweat glands are coiled tubular or saccular glands found mostly in association with hair follicles. The secretory parts are situated in the deeper parts of the dermis and in the subcutis. The excretory ducts pass up through the dermis and empty into the hair follicles above the ducts of the sebaceous glands. These glands are lined by a double layer of cells: an inner secretory and ductal epithelial cell layer and an outer myoepithelial cell layer interposed between the luminal epithelial cells and the basement membrane.

**Classification.** The classification scheme for sweat gland tumors in humans is very complex and many of the human tumor types (Lever and Schaumburg-Lever, 1975) have not been identified in animals. The classification used here for animals—cystic hyperplasia, adenoma, adenocarcinoma, and mixed tumor—is similar to that proposed by Nielsen and Cole (1960). In contrast to other classifications (Christie and Jabara, 1964; Weiss and Frese, 1974), skin tumors forming solid epithelial lobules or ribbons without lumens are classified as basal cell tumors since convincing evidence is lacking at this time as to their origin from apocrine sweat glands.

**Incidence, Age, Breed, and Sex.** Apocrine sweat gland tumors occur most frequently in the dog, but are among the least common of the epithelial skin tumors (Brodey, 1970), although Mul-

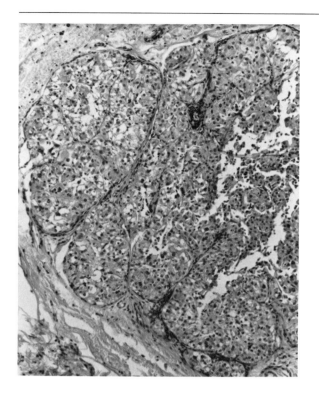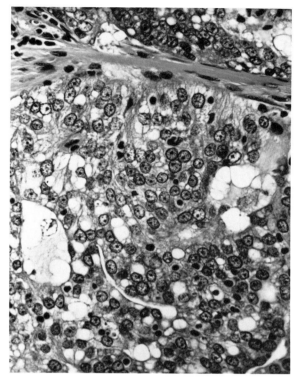

A|B **FIGURE 2.25.** Sebaceous gland adenocarcinoma. A. Irregular lobules of poorly differentiated sebaceous epithelial cells. B. Tumor cells with cytoplasmic lipid vacuoles forming glandular lumens.

ligan (1949) has suggested a higher relative incidence. His survey included tumors that we consider to be basal cell tumors. Sweat gland tumors are also uncommon in the cat (Cotchin, 1961; Schmidt and Langham, 1967) and are rare in other domestic animals. Merocrine sweat gland tumors are extremely rare in all species.

There is no apparent breed predisposition, and affected dogs and cats are usually 8 years of age or more. In dogs, males appear to be affected more frequently than females (Christie and Jabara, 1964).

**Sites and Gross Morphology.** Apocrine sweat gland neoplasms are usually solitary in the dog and cat and can occur at any site with no predilection for a specific area. Cystic hyperplasia in the dog, however, tends to occur more frequently on the head and neck.

The cystic lesions and benign tumors are well-circumscribed and usually 1 to 4 cm across, but are occasionally much larger. The tumors are generally firm but may have soft fluctuant areas. The cut surface is gray or light tan and solid or exhibits cysts of varying size and number. Cystic hyperplasia consists of single or multiple cysts filled with clear yellow or brown serous to gelatinous material that may coagulate when the specimen is fixed. The cysts often collapse completely when cut.

Carcinomas are often grossly indistinguishable from adenomas and mixed tumors. Some, however, are firm, poorly circumscribed masses diffusely infiltrating the skin, resulting in an ulcerated, moist, and sometimes hemorrhagic skin surface.

**Histological Features, Growth, and Metastasis.** The microscopic appearance of sweat gland tumors closely resembles that of mammary gland tumors (figs. 2.26A–D). This is understandable since the mammary gland is a modified apocrine sweat gland.

Sweat gland adenomas, which are sometimes further classified as cystadenomas or papillary cystadenomas, consist of multiple, often closely packed ducts or tubules with variably sized lumens. They are usually, but not always, lined by two layers of cells. The cells of the inner layer are cuboidal or columnar with basal nuclei and may exhibit apocrine secretory apices. The outer myoepithelial layer is either composed of inconspicuous flattened cells or small cuboidal cells having clear cytoplasm. There is often extensive intracystic papillary development. Mononuclear inflammatory cells and neutrophils may be numerous in the stroma, and neutrophils and macrophages are frequently found in the lumens of neoplastic ducts. Stromal invasion, mitoses, and anaplasia are not features of the adenoma.

In cystic hyperplasia the glands are numerous and cystic, yet the lining epithelial cells closely resemble those of the normal gland in various stages of secretory activity.

Mixed tumors occasionally occur and are characterized by myoepithelial cell proliferation in a mucinous stroma with chondroid metaplasia.

The ducts and intraluminal papillae of sweat gland adenocarcinoma are multilayered and usually of a single cell type. The cells are hyperchromatic and exhibit moderate to numerous mitotic figures. Invasion, which can be stromal, lymphatic, or both, is the single most important criterion for distinguishing sweat gland adenocarcinoma from adenoma. Stromal invasion is usually in the form of small cords and nests of cells that elicit a marked desmoplastic reaction. Extensive invasion in dermal lymphatics may result in edema, fibrosis, ulceration, and inflammation of the skin. The carcinomas have the capacity for rapid infiltrative growth and widespread metastasis.

## Ceruminous Gland Tumor

**General Considerations.** The ceruminous glands are a special variety of coiled tubular apocrine sweat gland occurring in the external auditory meatus. Each glandular tubule is surrounded by a thin network of myoepithelial cells. The ducts of ceruminous glands open either onto the free surface of the skin or with the sebaceous glands into the necks of hair follicles (Bloom and Fawcett, 1968). The combined secretion of ceruminous and sebaceous glands plus desquamated keratin make up the brown waxy material called cerumen in the ear canal.

**Incidence, Age, Breed, and Sex.** Ceruminous gland neoplasms, like the apocrine sweat gland tumors, are uncommon. They occur more frequently in the cat than in the dog. The average age in the cat is 13 years (Cotchin, 1961; Schmidt and Langham, 1967), much older than the usual tumor age. In a series of eight cases reported by Cotchin (1961), seven were in male cats. The tumor is extremely rare in other domestic species.

**Sites, Gross Morphology, and Histological Features.** Ceruminous gland tumors arise in the horizontal ear canal. They may be small nodular or pedunculated masses, although some attain a large size by invading through the cartilage of the horizontal ear canal and forming a mass at the base of the ear. The smaller masses must be differentiated from nodular hyperplasia of the ceruminous gland associated with chronic otitis externa. Otitis externa is frequently associated with ceruminous gland tumors, but it is not known if there is any direct relationship between the inflammation and development of the neoplasm. In the cat, pedunculated inflammatory polyps, which also must be differentiated from ceruminous gland tumors, are occasionally seen in the ear canal. These polyps originate from the middle ear as the result of chronic otitis media. Histologically, these polyps may contain ductlike structures lined by ciliated or mucus-producing epithelium.

Under microscopic examination ceruminous gland tumors are seen to closely resemble apocrine sweat gland tumors. The adenomas form acini or ducts (fig. 2.27). The ducts often become cystic, containing intraluminal papillary projections. A pinkish orange or copper colored secretion often containing inflammatory cells is usually present in the lumens. Mixed tumors containing foci of myoepithelial cell proliferation and cartilage formation also occur. Adenocarcinomas demonstrate cellular anaplasia and peripheral stromal and lymphatic invasion.

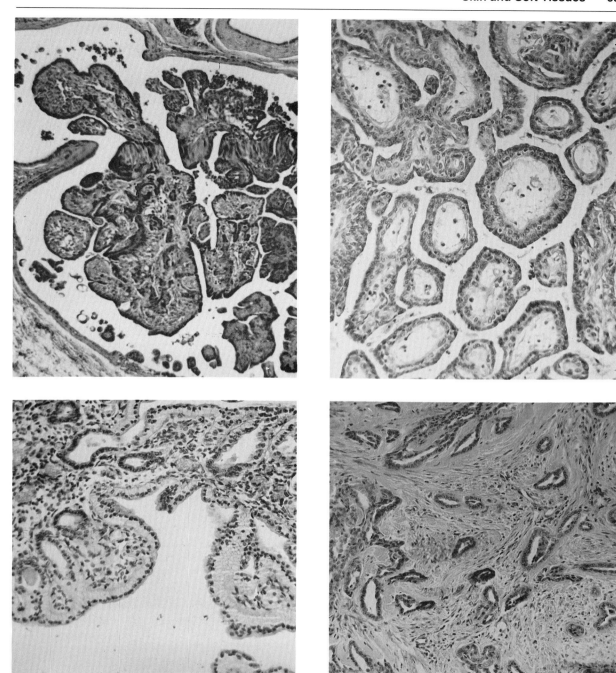

A|B  **FIGURE 2.26.** Sweat gland tumors. A. Adenoma
C|D  showing papillae growing into dilated tubule. B. Pa-
pillae in cross section. C. Irregular glands lined by cuboidal
cells. D. Adenocarcinoma showing invading tubular structures and fibrous stroma.

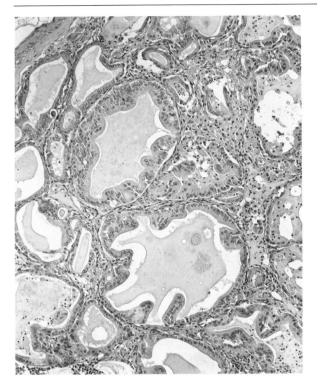

**FIGURE 2.27.** Ceruminous gland adenoma forming acini and ducts.

**Growth and Metastasis.** Nearly one-half of the ceruminous gland tumors in the cat are malignant. In the dog malignancy is much less frequent. Malignant ceruminous gland tumors invade into the parotid region and metastasize to regional lymph nodes and lungs. It may be difficult at times to differentiate between anaplastic ceruminous and parotid gland carcinomas.

## Perianal Gland Tumor

**General Considerations.** Three specialized glandular types occur around the anus in the dog. (1) The most important are the perianal (circumanal, hepatoid) glands, which are generally regarded as modified sebaceous glands (Trautmann and Fiebiger, 1957). They are located in the skin encircling the anus and are occasionally found in the skin of the sacral and lumbar regions, tail, thigh, and prepuce. The perianal glands are small at birth and continue to enlarge throughout life, probably under the influence of sex hormones (Baker, 1967; Nielsen and Aftosmis, 1964). It has been suggested by Baker (1967) that perianal glands are accessory sex glands in the dog and that they have an endocrine function. (2) Apocrine glands are found around the anus in two locations. They are in the skin of the anal canal where they open directly to the skin surface. In this location they are referred to as the anal glands. Apocrine glands also surround and empty into the anal sacs and are called anal sac glands. (3) The least abundant type of glands around the anus are sebaceous glands. These glands are found in association with the apocrine anal glands and superficial parts of the perianal glands. These specialized sebaceous glands empty directly onto the skin surface, into hair follicles, and into the neck of the anal sacs.

**Classification and Incidence.** Perianal gland growths are generally divided into three types: hyperplasia (which may be nodular or diffuse), adenoma, and carcinoma. Two mixed tumors, which may have actually been of apocrine gland origin, were found in a series of 300 perianal gland tumors studied by Nielsen and Aftosmis (1964).

Tumors arising from perianal glands are among the most common types of skin tumors in the dog (Brodey, 1970; Head, 1953). Nielsen and Aftosmis (1964) found that perianal gland tumors ranked third in frequency of all canine skin tumors, following mast cell tumors and mammary tumors.

Perianal gland tumors do not occur in other domestic species. One reported case in a cat (Weissman and Pulley, 1974) was probably a poorly differentiated sebaceous gland tumor arising from the sebaceous glands associated with the anus and anal sacs of the cat.

**Age, Breed, and Sex.** Perianal gland tumors are most common in male dogs 8 years of age and older, but a few have occurred in dogs as young as 2 years of age (Nielsen and Aftosmis, 1964). The average age in the series studied by Brodey (1970) was 11 years 4 months and the male:female ratio was 8.8:1. According to Hayes and Wilson (1977), males have 5.6 times the risk of females for developing perianal gland neoplasms, while intact males have 12 times the risk of intact females and spayed females have 3 times the risk of intact females.

In a study of 472 dogs with perianal gland neo-

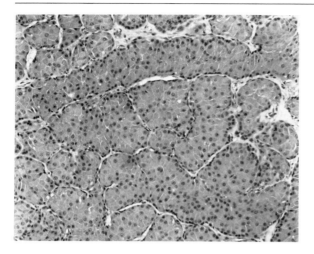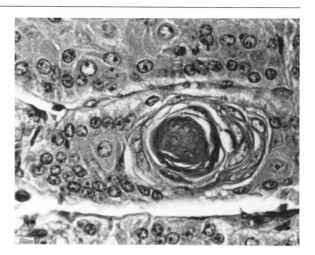

A|B    **FIGURE 2.28.** Perianal gland adenoma. A. Lobules and cords of large polyhedral cells surrounded
by small dark-staining reserve cells. B. Squamous metaplasia in the tumor; note small concentric
rings of keratin.

plasms, Hayes and Wilson (1977) observed the neoplasm in almost all breeds, and the cocker spaniel of both sexes, the English bulldog, the samoyed, and beagle males had the highest incidence.

**Sites and Gross Morphology.** Tumors of perianal glands are solitary or multiple. Most occur adjacent to the anus. They occasionally develop on the tail, perineum, prepuce, thigh, and dorsal sacral and lumbar areas. Older male dogs often develop diffuse hyperplasia, which forms a firm bulging ring around the anus. Nodular hyperplasia also occurs as multiple discrete nodules of varying sizes that are impossible to distinguish from adenomas.

Perianal gland tumors when small are ovoid or spherical. As they become larger (over 1 cm in diameter), they become multinodular and tend to ulcerate. They are usually well-circumscribed, but their margins may be difficult to distinguish when they are situated in firm, hyperplastic perianal gland tissue. Perianal gland tumors can attain a size as large as 10 cm in diameter. The cut surface is usually tan and lobulated, often with red mottling. Blood-filled cysts are occasionally observed.

**Histological Features.** It is difficult to distinguish nodular hyperplasia from adenoma, and this is why most nodular perianal gland masses are simply referred to as adenomas. Nodular hyperplasia closely resembles or is identical to a normal perianal gland except that it represents an expanding mass.

Adenomas appear as lobules or cords of large, discrete, round to polyhedral cells with abundant finely granular acidophilic cytoplasm (figs. 2.28A and B). Smaller, more basophilic, round or cuboidal cells are seen in varying numbers in the tumors. These small reserve or basal cells usually form a single row around the periphery of the lobules, as in the normal gland, and are often oriented around blood vessels. In some adenomas reserve cells make up the majority of the cells. The nuclei in both cell types are centrally located and mitotic figures are rare.

Small, round, laminated structures resembling cross sections of ducts are occasionally seen in tumor lobules. Squamous metaplasia can also occur. Delicate collagenous connective tissue stroma supports the lobules and many thin-walled vascular channels.

Inflammation (usually associated with an ulcerated surface), necrosis, hemorrhage, cholesterol clefts, and cyst formation are common. Considerable dense fibrous connective tissue may be present as the result of past inflammation and necrosis.

Malignant perianal gland tumors generally show disorderly growth and usually do not form discrete lobules (figs. 2.29A–B). Some carcinomas have no

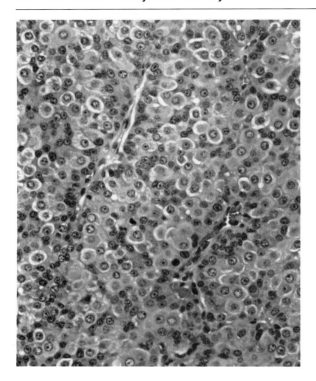
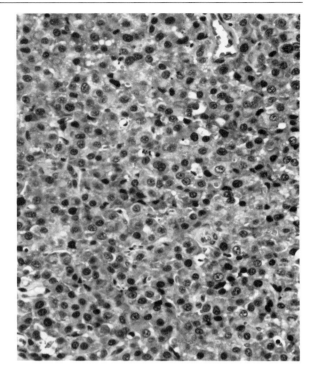

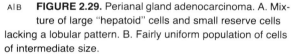 **FIGURE 2.29.** Perianal gland adenocarcinoma. A. Mixture of large "hepatoid" cells and small reserve cells lacking a lobular pattern. B. Fairly uniform population of cells of intermediate size.

distinct differentiation between the large polyhedral cells and the reserve cells, and there is just one pleomorphic cell type. In others, either the polyhedral cells or the reserve cells predominate. The reserve cells sometimes remain distinct and well oriented, even in metastatic sites. Mitotic figures may be uncommon or numerous.

The most important histological criterion of malignancy is the presence of tumor cell invasion. Clumps of tumor cells are common in lymphatics or in the supporting stromal connective tissue. Great care must be taken to distinguish lymphatic invasion from shrinkage artifact where there is a separation between the stroma and small isolated tumor lobules. Normally, perianal gland lobules are found between muscle bundles of the anal sphincter, and this also should not be interpreted as invasion.

**Growth and Metastasis.** Most perianal gland tumors are benign, and recurrence after complete removal is uncommon. Apparent recurrence is usually due to incomplete surgical excision or to development of a new separate tumor at or near the previous surgical site.

Of the 472 dogs with perianal gland neoplasms studied by Hayes and Wilson (1977), 59 were malignant and 7 of these metastasized. Out of 7 dogs with metastasis 6 were female. Also in this study, approximately one-half of the perianal gland tumors in females were malignant. Perianal gland carcinomas metastasize first to sacral and internal iliac lymph nodes; metastasis to lung, liver, kidney, and bone also occurs.

# Anal Sac Apocrine Gland Tumor

**General Considerations.** Tumors of anal sac apocrine gland origin have been recognized in the dog (Diamond and Garner, 1972; McGavin and Fishburn, 1975; Rijnberk *et al.*, 1978). They arise from the apocrine glands that surround and empty into the anal sacs of the dog and are often associated with the distinct clinicopathological syndrome of pseudohyperparathyroidism (Rijnberk *et al.*, 1978). These tumors are also discussed in chapter 13.

**Incidence, Age, Breed, and Sex.** Anal sac apocrine gland tumors have been reported only in the dog. They occur less frequently than other epithelial tumors of the skin and much less frequently than perianal gland tumors. In a series of 36 cases reported by Meuten *et al.* (1981) and another series of 14 cases reported by Goldschmidt and Zoltowski (1981), the average age of affected individuals was 10 years with a range of 7 to 16 years. A total of 44 cases occurred in females, 31 entire and 13 neutered, and 6 in males. There was no obvious breed predilection.

**Clinical Characteristics.** Most of the dogs with anal sac apocrine gland adenocarcinomas reported by Meuten *et al.* (1981) had pseudohyperparathyroidism. Serum calcium values were elevated (averaging 16.1 mg/dl), and serum phosphorus values were lowered (averaging 3.2 mg/dl). Parathyroid glands were inactive. Since tumor removal resulted in prompt return to normocalcemia while recurrence or growth of metastases were associated with an increase in serum calcium, it was concluded that the tumors produced a factor that induced hypercalcemia.

Clinical signs associated with this clinicopathological syndrome consist of weight loss, anorexia, lethargy, polyurea, and polydypsia (Goldschmidt and Zoltowski, 1981; Meuten *et al.*, 1981; Rijnberk *et al.*, 1978).

**Sites and Gross Morphology.** Most anal sac apocrine gland tumors are located in the subcutis lateral or ventral to the anus. The overlying epidermis is usually intact and freely movable. Ulceration is less common than with perianal gland neoplasms. The tumors are occasionally bilateral. Their growth is usually cranial into the pelvic canal as a single, large discrete mass. Separate tumor nodules may develop in the pelvic canal and abdominal cavity as the result of lymphatic extension or metastasis to sacral, iliac, and sublumbar lymph nodes. The size can vary greatly, but usually ranges from 1.0 to 8.0 cm at the time of clinical detection (Goldschmidt and Zoltowski, 1981; Meuten *et al.*, 1981). The cut surface of the tumor is tan, lobulated, and often has variably sized cysts containing yellow to blood-tinged serous fluid.

**Histological Features.** The anal sac apocrine gland tumors are usually composed of variably sized tubules and acini and of solid lobules separated by delicate fibrovascular septa. In some tumors the glandular pattern predominates, while others are primarily solid (Figs. 2.30A–D).

The glandular arrangement is characterized by well-defined acini and tubules lined by uniform columnar or cuboidal cells. These tumor cells usually have an abundant amount of eosinophilic cytoplasm, apical cytoplasmic blebs, and basally located round to oval nuclei. Mitotic figures are few to moderate in number.

In the solid pattern the tumor cells have ovoid vesicular nuclei and variable amounts of eosinophilic cytoplasm with indistinct borders. Pseudorosettes are conspicuous in some solid tumors and are characterized by columnar cells surrounding small blood vessels. On careful examination, some solid tumors also have a few very small acini or rosettes. With periodic acid–Schiff (PAS) stain most of the structures that appear to be rosettes can be shown to have lumens containing PAS positive secretory material.

Practically all anal sac apocrine gland tumors are carcinomas (Goldschmidt and Zoltowski, 1981; Meuten *et al.*, 1981; Rijnberk *et al.*, 1978). Although many appear well-circumscribed, careful inspection will usually reveal infiltrating individual and clumps of neoplastic cells in the surrounding stroma and within endothelial-lined spaces. In some tumors the infiltrating cells elicit a marked desmoplastic reaction.

**Electron Microscopy.** Meuten *et al.* (1982) demonstrated that the neoplastic apocrine gland cells had numerous profiles of rough endoplasmic reticulum, clusters of free ribosomes, and a well-developed Golgi apparatus. Electron dense granules having a limiting membrane and narrow submembranous space that resembled secretory gran-

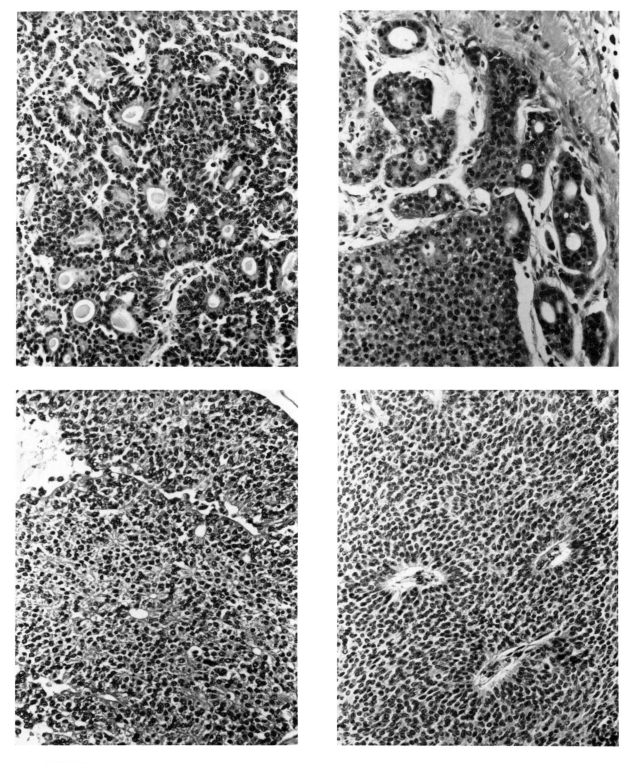

**FIGURE 2.30.** Anal sac apocrine gland carcinoma. A. Tumor cells arranged in acini with secretory material in the lumens. B. Tumor forming acini and solid lobules. C. Solid pattern with rosettes. D. Solid pattern with elongated cells arranged perpendicularly to blood vessels.

ules in polypeptide hormone-secreting endocrine cells were present. The tumor cells also contained microtubules, microfilaments, tonofilaments, and large lysosomelike dense bodies. Myoepithelial cells were absent in the tumors.

**Growth and Metastasis.** Practically all anal sac apocrine gland tumors show evidence of stromal and lymphatic invasion. Most will infiltrate along the side of the rectum into the pelvic canal. Metastasis to sacral, iliac, and sublumbar lymph nodes occurs in a high percentage of cases. Lung, liver, and spleen are other common sites for metastasis.

## Melanocytic Tumor

**General Considerations.** The melanocytic tumors of domestic animals include a group of neoplasms composed of melanin-producing cells. For purposes of discussion it is necessary to define several terms. A melanoblast is the cell that serves as the precursor of the melanocyte, the mature, melanin-synthesizing cell containing a specialized organelle, the melanosome. Normal melanocytes are dendritic cells. Within the epidermis they are located at the epidermal–dermal junction between the cells of the basal layer. Although their numbers are subject to variation in different species and regions, a ratio of one melanocyte per ten basal cells could be considered average.

The melanin pigment is formed in the cell body and is extruded outward along the dendritic processes where it is transferred to the surrounding basal cells. An analogous situation occurs in the hair bulbs. One of the main functions of melanin is the protection of the skin from the harmful effects of sunlight.

A nevus cell is an "altered" melanocyte. There is considerable confusion regarding the origin, structure, and function of the nevus cell. A melanophage is a phagocytic cell that has engulfed previously formed melanin; it is unable to synthesize melanin itself.

It is generally accepted that melanoblasts are of neuroectodermal origin. During fetal growth, the melanoblasts migrate to take up residence at the dermal–epidermal junction of the skin and in the hair bulbs (although a few of the melanoblasts fail to complete their migration and remain in the der-

mis). Having finished their migration, the cells are then referred to as melanocytes. Melanocytes are normally found in various ocular structures in addition to the skin, and they may also be present in the meninges, adrenal gland, and intima of the heart and blood vessels in some species.

Characteristically, melanocytes are endowed with a complex series of enzymes; one of them, tyrosinase, allows them to produce the brown pigment melanin from the amino acid tyrosine. A commonly used histochemical test to demonstrate the presence of tyrosinase is the DOPA reaction in which 3,4-dihydroxyphenylalanine is oxidized to black in the presence of the enzyme.

**Classification.** The simplistic nomenclature used in the past—benign or malignant melanoma—is clearly not adequate. Data are not available for animals, however, to justify the complex classification system of melanocytic tumors in humans. The classification of melanocytic tumors of domestic animals used in this discussion is presented in table 2.2. The terminology commonly used for the comparable growths in humans is also indicated. This classification may need to be expanded and refined in the future as more knowledge of melanomas in domestic animals is acquired.

The benign growths are subdivided on the basis of the presence or absence of junctional activity, which refers to "nests" of melanocytes situated primarily at the epidermal–dermal junction, but sometimes also involves the hair follicles. The benign melanocytic growths that exhibit junctional activity are referred to as junctional melanocy-

## TABLE 2.2. Melanocytic Tumors in Domestic Animals and Humans

| Domestic animals | Man |
| --- | --- |
| Junctional melanocytoma | Pigmented nevus |
| | Junctional |
| | Compound |
| | Dermal |
| Dermal melanocytoma | Blue nevus |
| Fibrous | Common |
| Cellular | Cellular |
| Malignant melanoma | Malignant melanoma |
| Epithelioid | Epithelioid |
| Spindle cell | Spindle cell |
| Mixed | Mixed |

tomas. This is the most common melanocytic tumor of humans and is referred to as a pigmented nevus or nevocellular nevus, since the cell involved is the so-called nevus cell or altered melanocyte. The terms *nevus* and *nevus cell* have been avoided in the present classification of melanocytic tumors of domestic animals. Their introduction would confuse rather than clarify an already poorly understood group of tumors.

It is customary to further divide the pigmented or nevocellular nevi in humans on the basis of the predominant location of the nests of nevus cells or melanocytes. In junctional nevi they are essentially limited to the epidermal–dermal junction. In compound nevi they are approximately equally divided between the epidermal–dermal junction and the dermis, and in dermal nevi the nests occur predominantly in the dermis. The location of the nests is related to the maturation of the tumor. Initially they are primarily epidermal–dermal in location and later predominantly dermal in location. A similar situation appears to exist with the junctional melanocytomas of the pig and possibly of the dog.

Dermal melanocytomas (blue nevi in humans) lack junctional activity. They are further subdivided as either fibrous or cellular. The classifications of malignant melanocytic tumors of domestic animals and humans are almost identical. In some classification systems several more subtypes of malignant melanoma are used than are shown in table 2.2.

**Incidence.** Melanocytic tumors are relatively common in the dog, horse, and certain breeds of swine. They are less frequently observed in cattle and goats and are quite rare in cats and sheep (Garna-Avina *et al.*, 1981).

Various tumor surveys indicate that melanocytic tumors in the dog represent from 4 to 7% of all tumors and from 9 to 20% of the skin tumors (Cotchin, 1954; Head, 1953; Jackson, 1936; Mulligan, 1949; Schwartzman and Orkin, 1962).

In the horse, melanocytic tumors represent 6% (Head, 1953) to 15% (Cotchin, 1960) of the skin tumors. There is a striking relationship between the incidence of melanocytic tumors and gray coats in the horse (Mangrulkar, 1944; Runnells and Benbrook, 1941), although they are occasionally found in horses with other hair color (M'Fadyean, 1933; Mostafa, 1953). There is a tendency for increasing development of melanocytic tumors as

the gray horses grow older, and approximately 80% of gray horses over 15 years of age have developed clinically recognizable melanocytic growths (M'Fadyean, 1933). It has been suggested that all gray horses eventually become affected with melanocytic tumors if they live long enough (M'Fadyean, 1933). Dermal melanocytoma is the most common melanocytic tumor of the horse.

Melanocytic lesions in the skin of swine are common. It has been estimated that 3 to 5% of slaughtered swine have pigmented skin lesions (Davis *et al.*, 1933), and in selected swine herds the incidence of melanocytic lesions has been over 20% (Nordby, 1933; Strafuss *et al.*, 1968). Junctional melanocytoma appears to be the most common melanocytic tumor of swine.

In cattle, melanocytic tumors represent less than 2% of all bovine tumors (Jackson, 1936), although they represent a significant proportion of all neoplasms of the skin and subcutis in this species. Cotchin (1960) reported that 17% and Head (1953) reported that 24% of these tumors were melanocytic.

Melanocytic tumors are quite rare in the cat. Tumor surveys indicate they constitute less than 1% of all feline tumors (Whitehead, 1967) and approximately 2% of all skin tumors in this species (Cotchin, 1961).

**Age, Breed, and Sex.** The incidence of melanocytic tumors is highest in dogs between 7 and 14 years of age. Scottish terriers, Boston terriers, Airedales, and cocker spaniels have a relatively higher incidence of melanocytic tumors than other breeds (Cotchin, 1955, 1956; Mulligan, 1961; Sastry, 1953). In general, incidence is higher in dogs with greater skin pigmentation (Conroy, 1967; Mulligan, 1949). Males appear to be affected more often than females (Conroy, 1967; Head, 1958; Mulligan, 1961).

Melanocytic tumors in horses less than 6 years of age are rare, but as mentioned earlier, there is a steadily increasing tendency for gray horses to develop these tumors after they become 6 years old. It has been stated that the Arabian breed has a high predisposition to develop melanocytic growths (Lerner and Cage, 1974). This may be a reflection of the high incidence of a gray coat color in this breed. No sex predilection has been observed in any horse breed.

Melanocytic growths in swine usually occur congenitally or in very young animals (Hjerpe and Theilen, 1964; Manning *et al.*, 1974; Strafuss *et al.*, 1968). Their occurrence is virtually limited to the Duroc–Jersey breed and the Hormel and Sinclair miniature swine (Flatt *et al.*, 1968, 1972; Hjerpe and Theilen, 1964; Manning *et al.*, 1974; Strafuss *et al.*, 1968). No sex predilection has been reported.

In cattle, melanocytic tumors usually occur in young animals (Cotchin, 1960; Head, 1953); they can also be congenital (Sividas *et al.*, 1971). These tumors are most commonly encountered in dark-haired cattle, especially the Aberdeen Angus breed. No sex predilection has been observed.

**Sites.** Melanocytic tumors can develop in the skin, the mucous membranes, and the eye. The melanocytic tumors arising from the iris, ciliary body, choroid, etc., are discussed separately in chapter 14, which covers tumors of the nervous system and eye.

Melanocytic tumors in the dog are usually solitary, and the skin is the most common site, followed by the oral cavity (Cotchin, 1955). The favored sites for cutaneous melanocytic tumors in the dog are the face (especially the eyelids), the trunk, and the extremities (Mulligan, 1961; Schwartzman and Orkin, 1962). The most common oral sites for melanocytic tumors in the dog are the gums, buccal mucosa, palate, and lips.

There is a striking difference in the behavior of canine melanocytic tumors depending on their location. At least 90% of oral melanocytic tumors are malignant (Gorlin *et al.*, 1959; Mulligan, 1961), whereas most cutaneous melanocytic tumors are benign with the notable exception of those on the digits (Conroy, 1967).

Melanocytic tumors in the horse are usually multiple and generally originate in the skin. The most common sites are the perineum and the underside of the root of the tail. Other areas are affected much less frequently.

These tumors in swine primarily originate in the skin but may also arise in internal organs (Flatt *et al.*, 1972; Manning *et al.*, 1974). In the Duroc–Jersey breed, the flank has been reported to be the most common site (Hjerpe and Theilen, 1964). In Hormel and Sinclair miniature pigs there is no site predilection.

The most common site for melanocytic tumors

in goats is the perineal region (Mustafa *et al.*, 1966). In cattle they are usually subcutaneous and no site predilection has been reported.

**Gross Morphology.** The melanocytic tumors range in gross appearance from inconspicuous black macules to large, rapidly growing masses that may be either amelanotic or dark brown to gray or black in color.

As indicated earlier, many junctional melanocytomas of domestic animals undergo a gradual evolution that parallels the life cycle of the pigmented or nevocellular nevi of humans. This has been best demonstrated in the pig and likely occurs also in the dog. Thus, the gross appearance of a junctional melanocytoma can vary depending on its stage of development. Initially they appear as flat, black macules. They slowly progress into elevated, firm, smooth or rough nodules that may be less than 0.5 cm to more than 1.0 cm in diameter. Although the degree of gross pigmentation can vary considerably, they are usually dark brown to black. Subsequently, the nodules flatten out and become less pigmented. In some cases the lesions nearly completely regress. It should be stressed that many junctional melanocytomas do not progress through all stages.

Dermal melanocytomas usually range from 0.5 to 2.0 cm in diameter, are darkly pigmented, dome shaped, and have a smooth, hairless surface. On the cut surface the tumors usually appear to be well-defined but are seldom encapsulated.

Malignant melanomas are normally larger than the melanocytomas, and the overlying skin or mucous membrane is frequently ulcerated and secondarily infected. Their color may vary from black to brown to light gray. Mulligan (1949, 1961) has stressed the importance of size in detecting gross evidence of benignancy or malignancy in melanocytic skin tumors of the dog. His data indicate that cutaneous melanocytic tumors less than 1.0 cm in diameter are usually benign, while those over 2.5 cm in diameter are usually malignant. According to studies by Bostock (1979) and Harvey *et al.* (1981), tumor volume has no significance in determining malignancy or survival rate.

**Histological Features.** The characteristic feature of junctional malanocytoma is junctional change in which melanocytes (or nevus cells), singly or in nests, can be seen dropping off the epidermis or

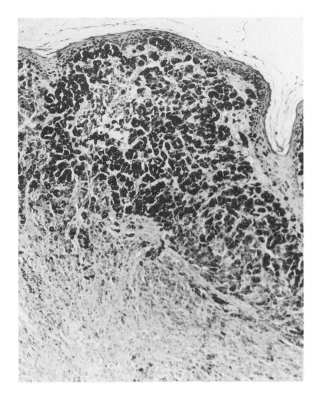

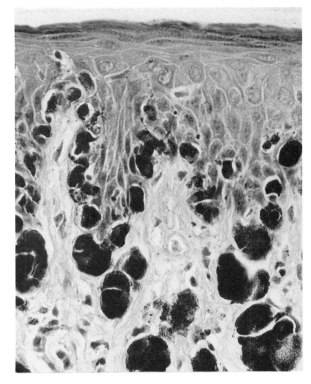

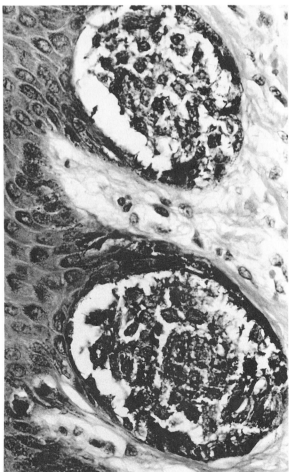

A | B
C
**FIGURE 2.31.** Junctional melanocytoma. A. Junctional melanocytoma of the skin in a dog showing nests of melanocytes at the epidermal–dermal junction and in the dermis. B and C. Nests of melanocytes at the epidermal–dermal junction.

hair follicles into the dermis (figs. 2.31A–C). The tumor cells that make up junctional melanocytomas show considerable variation in appearance and are often recognized by pigment content and arrangement in clusters or nests rather than by cellular characteristics. Within the epidermis the melanocytes may have a somewhat dense, dark-staining nucleus and a clear cytoplasm. In the upper dermis they usually are cuboidal or oval, resembling epithelioid cells. In the lower dermis the cells are usually elongated and possess spindle-shaped nuclei resembling fibroblasts. In general, the pigment content tends to diminish from the surface downward. Probably all junctional melanocytomas have an epidermal and a dermal component, although the proportions of these two components vary greatly. In some junctional melanocytomas nearly all of the tumor cells are situated at the epidermal–dermal junction, while in others the junctional activity is very slight and nearly all the tumor cells are located in the dermis.

Dermal melanocytomas, in contrast to junctional melanocytomas, lack junctional change and appear to arise in the dermis (figs. 2.32A–C). They may spare the upper dermis or lie directly against the epidermis. Most dermal melanocytomas can be classified as either fibrous or cellular, although some exhibit features of both types. In the fibrous dermal melanocytoma, the dendritic or flattened melanocytes lie grouped in irregular bundles admixed with fibroblasts, often in an interlacing pattern. The cells usually lie parallel to the epidermis. Melanophages are usually present in varying numbers and tend to be larger and contain coarser melanin granules than the actual tumor cells. The distribution of melanin may be uniform or patchy, but is usually prominent near the surface and around blood vessels.

In cellular dermal melanocytoma there are islands of densely packed, rounded, or spindle-shaped cells. The larger islands are often subdivided into alveolar cell groups. Conroy (1967) pointed out that certain melanocytic tumors in the dog appear to be cellular dermal melanocytomas and have melanocytes migrating from the hair follicles. The significance of this is unknown.

Malignant melanomas may originate from normal melanocytes in the epidermis and oral epithelium and from the junctional or dermal elements of benign melanomas. In malignant melanomas originating at the epidermal–dermal junction, there is considerable junctional activity with downward streaming of anaplastic melanocytes from the epidermis into the dermis. There are numerous anaplastic melanocytes in the lower epidermis lying singly or in irregularly shaped nests (figs. 2.33A–D). The tumor cells often invade the upper epidermis to such an extent that the epidermis disintegrates, resulting in ulceration. Once within the dermis, the tumor cells may exhibit considerable pleomorphism and range in shape from cuboidal to fusiform. The cells tend to lie in alveolar formations or irregular branching strands. Malignant melanomas (especially the amelanotic ones) are formed predominantly of fusiform cells and resemble fibrosarcomas. Malignant melanomas in which epitheliallike cells predominate resemble undifferentiated carcinomas. Mitotic figures are usually present in

small numbers, although they can be extremely numerous in some tumors. Bizarre giant cells may be present.

The melanin content in malignant melanomas varies greatly. In most tumors considerable amounts of melanin are found. Occasionally, a malignant melanoma will show no evidence of melanin in hematoxylin- and eosin-stained tissues. In those cases, staining with ammoniated silver nitrate may be of help. If fresh tissue is available the DOPA reaction can be carried out. This should show a positive reaction in at least part of the tumor. It should be stressed that the amount of melanin present is not necessarily a reliable indicator of malignancy. The belief that the more melanin present, the less malignant the tumor, is probably unfounded.

The two major diagnostic problems involving malignant melanomas are (1) differentiating an early malignant melanoma arising at the epidermal–dermal junction from a junctional melanocytoma, and (2) recognizing early malignant transformation of a junctional melanocytoma. For humans, the following findings favor a diagnosis of malignant melanoma: diffuse scattering of the tumor cells in the lower epidermis rather than in nests, pleomorphism of the tumor cells, the presence of tumor cells in the upper epidermis, and the presence of an inflammatory infiltrate not adequately explained by either trauma or infection (Lever and Schaumburg-Lever, 1975). These criteria appear to be applicable to domestic animals as well.

A remaining diagnostic problem is the recognition of malignant transformation of a dermal melanocytoma. In addition to the standard features of malignancy, such as invasion and nuclear pleomorphism, the two most reliable indicators of malignant transformation are the presence of mitotic figures and areas of necrosis. In humans, it appears that the fibrous dermal melanocytoma (common blue nevus) is without malignant potential. Among domestic animals this appears to hold true for at least the dog (Conroy, 1967).

**Etiology and Transmission.** For the most part, the etiology of melanocytic tumors, like most tumors in domestic animals, is unknown. Passey (1938) induced the formation of a malignant melanoma in the skin of a dog by applying a tar extract at weekly intervals for 6 to 7 years. McCullough *et al.* (1972) were able to induce both malig-

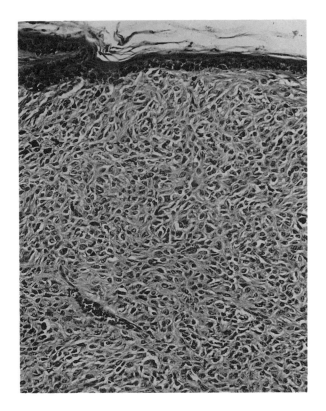

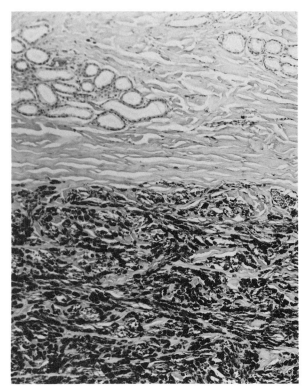

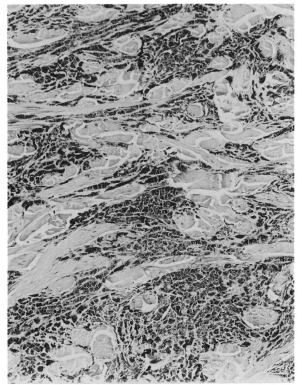

**FIGURE 2.32.** Dermal melanocytoma. A. Cellular type dermal melanocytoma in a dog. Tumor cells lie directly against the epidermis. B. Cellular type dermal melanocytoma in a horse. The tumor spares the upper dermis. C. Fibrous type dermal melanocytoma in a horse.

nant melanomas and fibrosarcomas with the Gardner strain of feline fibrosarcoma virus. The exact role of this virus in production of melanocytic tumors is uncertain because other investigators have not been able to confirm this finding.

Genetic factors appear to be important in melanocytic tumors of swine since the occurrence of these neoplasms can be dramatically increased by selective breeding (Millikan *et al.*, 1973; Nordby, 1933).

**Growth and Metastasis.** Most melanocytomas have a completely benign course. As mentioned earlier, junctional melanocytoma and cellular dermal melanocytoma may occasionally undergo malignant transformation. Fibrous dermal melanocytoma apparently lacks a malignant potential.

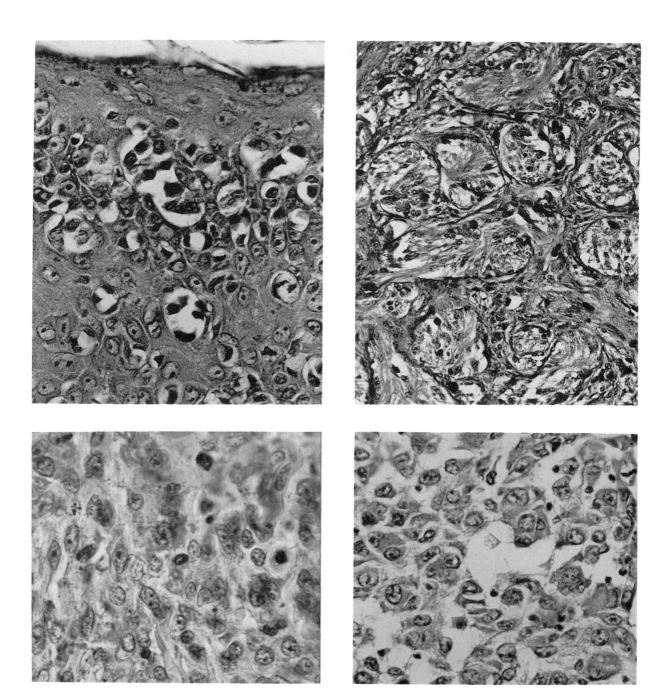

**FIGURE 2.33.** Malignant melanoma. A. Anaplastic
melanocytes, singly and in nests, at the epider-
mal−dermal junction and invading the upper epidermis.
B. Tumor cells arranged in alveolar formations. C. Malignant
melanoma comprised of fusiform cells resembling fibrosarcoma. D. Epitheliallike tumor cells.

Malignant melanomas can metastasize via lymph channels and blood, probably regardless of their origin. Regional lymph nodes are commonly the first sites affected. The lung is the most common site of visceral involvement. Widespread metastasis occurs in many cases.

Again it should be emphasized that malignant potential for melanocytic tumors in the dog is greatly influenced by their location. Those from the oral cavity, lip, and digits have a much higher potential for malignancy than those from other sites. In the horse, once melanocytic tumors start to develop they tend to be multiple, and eventually (usually years later) metastasis will occur in the majority of cases.

## REFERENCES

Alexander, J. W., Riis, R. C., and Dueland, R. (1975) Extraskeletal Giant Cell Tumor in a Cat. *Vet. Med. Small Anim. Clin.* 70, 1161–1166.

Altera, K., and Clark, L. (1970) Equine Cutaneous Mastocytosis. *Path. Vet.* 7, 43–55.

Bagdonas, V., and Olson, C. (1953) Observations on the Epizootiology of Cutaneous Papillomatosis (Warts) of Cattle. *J. Amer. Vet. Med. Assoc.* 122, 393–397.

Baker, J. C., Hultgren, B. D., and Larson, V. L. (1982) Disseminated Cavernous Hemangioma in a Calf. *J. Amer. Vet. Med. Assoc.* 181, 172–173.

Baker, K. P. (1967) The Histology and Histochemistry of the Circumanal Hepatoid Glands of the Dog. *J. Small Anim. Pract.* 8, 639–647.

Belhorn, R. W., and Henkind, P. (1967) Ocular Nodular Fasciitis in a Dog. *J. Amer. Vet. Med. Assoc.* 150, 212–213.

Black, P. H., Hartley, J. W., Rowe, W. P., and Huebner, R. J. (1963) Transformation of Bovine Tissue Culture Cells by Bovine Papilloma Virus. *Nature* 199, 1016–1018.

Blackwell, J. G. (1972) Unusual Adipose Tissue Growth in a Colt. *J. Amer. Vet. Med. Assoc.* 161, 1141–1142.

Bloom, W., and Fawcett, D. W. (1968) *A Textbook of Histology.* 9th ed. W. B. Saunders (Philadelphia).

Bostock, D. E. (1973) The Prognosis Following Surgical Removal of Mastocytomas in Dogs. *J. Small Anim. Pract.* 14, 27–40.

———. (1979) Prognosis after Surgical Excision of Canine Melanomas. *Vet. Path.* 16, 32–40.

Bostock, D. E., and Dye, M. T. (1980) Prognosis after Surgical Excision of Canine Fibrous Connective

Tissue Sarcomas. *Vet. Path.* 17, 581–588.

Bowles, C. A., Kerber, W. T., Rangan, S. R. S., Kwapien, R., Woods, W., and Jensen, E. M. (1972) Characterization of a Transplantable, Canine, Immature Mast Cell Tumor. *Cancer Res.* 32, 1434–1441.

Brobst, D., and Hinsman, E. J. (1966) Electron Microscopy of the Bovine Cutaneous Papilloma. *Path. Vet.* 3, 196–207.

Brodey, R. S. (1970) Canine and Feline Neoplasia. *Adv. Vet. Sci.* 14, 309–354.

Brown, N. O., Patnaik, A. K., Mooney, S., Hayes, A., Harvey, H. J., and MacEwen, E. G. (1978) Soft Tissue Sarcomas in the Cat. *J. Amer. Vet. Med. Assoc.* 173, 744–749.

Bundza, A., and Dukes, T. W. (1982) Cutaneous and Systemic Porcine Mastocytosis. *Vet. Path.* 19, 453–455.

Burggraaf, H. (1935) Kanker aan de basis van de hoorns bij zebus. *T. Diergeneesk.* 62, 1121–1136.

Cadéac, C. (1901) Sur la transmission expérimentale des papillomes des diverses espèces. *Bull. Soc. Sci. Vet.* (Lyon) 4, 333–341.

Case, M. T., Bartz, A. R., Bernstein, M., and Rosen, R. A. (1969) Metastasis of a Sebaceous Gland Carcinoma in the Dog. *J. Amer. Vet. Med. Assoc.* 154, 661–664.

Cheevers, W. P., Roberson, S. M., Brassfield, A. L., Davis, W. C., and Crawford, T. B. (1982) Isolation of a Retrovirus from Cultured Equine Sarcoid Tumor Cells. *Amer. J. Vet. Res.* 43, 804–806.

Cheville, N. F. (1966) Studies on Connective Tissue Tumors in the Hamster Produced by Bovine Papilloma Virus. *Cancer Res.* 26, 2334–2339.

Cheville, N. F., and Olson, C. (1964) Epithelial and Fibroblastic Proliferation in Bovine Cutaneous Papillomatosis, *Path. Vet.* 1, 248–257.

Cheville, N. F., Prasse, K., van der Maaten, M., and Boothe, A. D. (1972) Generalized Cutaneous Mastocytosis. *Vet. Path.* 9, 394–407.

Christie, G. S., and Jabara, A. G. (1964) Canine Sweat Gland Growths. *Res. Vet. Sci.* 5, 237–244.

Confer, A. W., Enright, F. M., and Beard, G. B. (1981) Ultrastructure of a Feline Extraskeletal Giant Cell Tumor (Malignant Fibrous Histiocytoma). *Vet. Path.* 18, 738–744.

Conroy, J. D. (1967) Melanocytic Tumors of Domestic Animals with Special Reference to Dogs. *Arch. Derm.* 96, 372–380.

Cook, R. H., and Olson, C. (1951) Experimental Transmission of Cutaneous Papilloma of the Horse. *Amer. J. Path.* 27, 1087–1097.

Cotchin, E. (1954) Further Observations on Neoplasms in Dogs, with Particular Reference to Site of Origin and Malignancy. *Brit. Vet. J.* 110, 218–230.

———. (1955) Melanotic Tumours of Dogs. *J. Comp. Path.* 65, 115–129.

———. (1956) Further Examples of Spontaneous Neoplasms in the Domestic Cat. *Brit. Vet. J.* 112, 263–272.

———. (1960) Tumours of Farm Animals: A Survey of Tumours Examined at the Royal Veterinary College,

London, During 1950–60. *Vet. Rec.* 72, 816–823.

———. (1961) Skin Tumours of Cats. *Res. Vet. Sci.* 2, 353–361.

Cotchin, E., and Swarbrick, O. (1963) Bovine Cutaneous Angiomatosis: A Lesion Resembling Human Pyogenic Granuloma (Granuloma telangiectaticum). *Vet. Rec.* 75, 437–444.

Creech, G. T. (1929) Experimental Studies of the Etiology of Common Warts of Cattle. *J. Ag. Res.* 39, 723–737.

Culbertson, M. R. (1982) Hemangiosarcoma in Canine Skin and Tongue. *Vet. Path.* 19, 556–558.

Davis. C. L., and Kemper, H. E. (1936) Common Warts (Papillomata) in Goats. *J. Amer. Vet. Med. Assoc.* 88, 175–179.

Davis, C. L., Leeper, R., and Shelton, J. E. (1933) Neoplasms Encountered in Federally Inspected Establishments in Denver, Colorado. *J. Amer. Vet. Med. Assoc.* 83, 229–237.

Diamond, S. S., and Garner, F. M. (1972) Multiple Perianal Neoplasms in a Dog. *Modern Vet. Pract.* 53, 44–45.

Dionne, P. G., and Seemayer, T. A. (1974) Infiltrating Lipomas and Angiolipomas Revisited. *Cancer* 33, 732–738.

Diters, R. W., and Goldschmidt, M. H. (1983) Hair Follicle Tumors Resembling Tricholemmomas in Six Dogs. *Vet. Path.* 20, 123–125.

Diters, R. W., and Walsh, K. M. (1984) Feline Basal Cell Tumors: A Review of 124 Cases. *Vet. Path.* 21, 51–56.

Dodd, D. C. (1964) Mastocytoma of the Tongue of a Calf. *Path. Vet.* 1, 69–72.

England, J. J., Watson, R. E., Jr., and Larson, K. A. (1973) Virus-like Particles in an Equine Sarcoid Cell Line. *Amer. J. Vet. Res.* 34, 1601–1603.

Flatt, R. E., Middleton, C. C., Tumbleson, M. E., and Perez-Mesa, C. (1968) Pathogenesis of Benign Cutaneous Melanomas in Miniature Swine. *J. Amer. Vet. Med. Assoc.* 153, 936–941.

Flatt, R. E., Nelson, L. R., and Middleton, C. C. (1972) Melanotic Lesions in the Internal Organs of the Miniature Swine. *Arch. Path.* 93, 71–75.

Flynn, K. J., Dehner, L. P., Gajl-Peczalska, J., Dahl, M. V., Ramsy, N., and Wang, N. (1982) Regressing Atypical Histiocytosis. *Cancer* 49, 959–970.

Ford, H. G., Empson, R. N., Plopper, C. G., and Brown, P. H. (1975) Giant Cell Tumor of Soft Parts: A Report of an Equine and a Feline Case. *Vet. Path.* 12, 428–433.

Fowler, E. H., Wilson, G. P., Roenigk, W. J., and Koestner, A. (1966) Mast Cell Leukemia. *J. Amer. Vet. Med. Assoc.* 149, 281–285.

Frenz (1941) Ausgedehnte Papillomatose in einem Jungrinderbestand. *Dtsch. Tierärztl. Wschr.* 49, 158–160.

Frese, K. von (1969) Mastzellentumoren beim Pferd. *Berl. Münch. Tierärztl. Wschr.* 18, 342–344.

Fu, Y. S., Gabbiani, G., Kay, G. I., and Lattes, R. (1975) Malignant Soft Tissue Tumors of Probable Histiocytic Origin (Malignant Fibrous Histiocytomas): General Considerations and Electron Microscopy and Tissue Culture Studies. *Cancer* 35, 176–198.

Fujimoto, Y., and Olson, C. (1966) The Fine Structure of the Bovine Wart, *Path. Vet.* 3, 659–684.

Garna-Avina, A., Valli, V. E., and Lumsden, J. H. (1981) Cutaneous Melanomas in Domestic Animals. *J. Cutaneous Pathol.* 8, 3–24.

Garner, F. M., and Lingeman, C. H. (1970) Mast Cell Neoplasms of the Domestic Cat. *Path. Vet.* 7, 517–530.

Gleiser, C. A., Jardine, J. H., Raulston, G. L., and Gray, K. N. (1979a) Infiltrating Lipomas in the Dog. *Vet. Path.* 16, 623–624.

Gleiser, C. A., Raulston, G. L., Jardine, J. H., and Gray, K. N. (1979b) Malignant Fibrous Histiocytoma in Dogs and Cats. *Vet. Path.* 16, 199–208.

Goldschmidt, M. H., and Zoltowski, C. (1981) Anal Sac Gland Adenocarcinoma in the Dog: 14 Cases. *J. Small Anim. Pract.* 22, 119–128.

Goldschmidt, M. H., Thrall, D. E., Jeglum, K. A., Everett, J. I., and Wood, M. G. (1981) Malignant Pilomatricoma in a Dog. *J. Cutaneous Pathol.* 8, 375–381.

Gordon, D. F., and Olson, C. (1968) Meningiomas and Fibroblastic Neoplasia in Calves Induced with the Bovine Papilloma Virus. *Cancer Res.* 28, 2423–2431.

Gorlin, R. J., Barron, C. N., Chaudhry, A. P., and Clark, J. J. (1959) The Oral and Pharyngeal Pathology of Domestic Animals: A Study of 487 Cases. *Amer. J. Vet. Res.* 20, 1032–1061.

Gourley, I. M., Popp, J. A., and Park, R. D. (1971) Myelolipomas of the Liver in a Domestic Cat. *J. Amer. Vet. Med. Assoc.* 158, 2053–2057.

Groth, A. H., Bailey, W. S., and Walker, D. F. (1960) Bovine Mastocytoma: A Case Report. *J. Amer. Vet. Med. Assoc.* 137, 241–244.

Gründer, H. D. (1959) Sammelreferat: Die Tierpapillomatosen. *Dtsch. Tierärztl. Wschr.* 66, 159–162.

Hahn, M. J., Dawson, R., Easterly, J. A., and Joseph, D. J. (1973) Hemangiopericytoma: An Ultrastructural Study. *Cancer* 31, 255–261.

Harvey, H. J., MacEwen, E. G., Braun, D., Patnaik, A. K., Withrow, S. J., and Jongeward, S. (1981) Prognostic Criteria for Dogs with Oral Melanoma. *J. Amer. Vet. Med. Assoc.* 178, 580–582.

Hayes, H. M., and Wilson, G. P. (1977) Hormone Dependent Neoplasms of the Canine Perianal Gland. *Cancer Res.* 37, 2068–2071.

Head, K. W. (1953) Skin Diseases: Neoplastic Diseases. *Vet. Rec.* 65, 926–929.

———. (1958) Cutaneous Mast Cell Tumours in the Dog, Cat, and Ox. *Brit. J. Derm.* 70, 389–408.

———. (1965) Some Problems Involved in the Investigation of Mast Cells in Pathological Processes. In: *Comparative Physiology and Pathology of the Skin.* F. A. Davis (Philadelphia).

Hewlett, K. (1905) Cancer of the Horn-Core of Cattle. *J. Comp. Path.* 18, 161–163.

Hjerpe, C. A., and Theilen, G. H. (1964) Malignant

Melanomas in Porcine Littermates. *J. Amer. Vet. Med. Assoc.* 144, 1129–1131.

Hottendorf, G. H., and Nielsen, S. W. (1966) Collagen Necrosis in Canine Mastocytomas. *Amer. J. Path.* 49, 501–513.

———. (1967) Pathologic Survey of 300 Extirpated Canine Mastocytomas. *Zbl. Vet. Med.* (A) 14, 272–281.

———. (1968) Pathologic Report of 29 Necropsies on Dogs with Mastocytoma. *Path. Vet.* 5, 102–121.

Hottendorf, G. H., Nielsen, S. W., and Kenyon, A. J. (1965) Canine Mastocytoma. I. Blood Coagulation Time in Dogs with Mastocytoma. *Path. Vet.* 2, 129–141.

Howard, E. B. (1967) Immunologic Defeat in Mastocytoma-Bearing Dogs. *J. Amer. Vet. Med. Assoc.* 151, 1308–1310.

Howard, E. B., and Nielsen, S. W. (1969) Cutaneous Histiocytomas of Dogs. *Nat. Cancer Inst. Monogr.* 32, 321–327.

Howard, E. B., Sawa, T. R., Nielsen, S. W., and Kenyon, A. J. (1969) Mastocytoma and Gastroduodenal Ulceration. *Path. Vet.* 6, 146–158.

Ikede, B. O., and Downey, R. S. (1972) Multiple Hepatic Myelolipomas in a Cat. *Can. Vet. J.* 13, 160–163.

Jackson, C. (1936) The Incidence and Pathology of Tumours of Domesticated Animals in South Africa: A Study of the Onderstepoort Collection of Neoplasms with Special Reference to Their Histopathology. *Onderstepoort J. Vet. Sci. and Anim. Indust.* 6, 1–460.

James, V. S. (1968) A Family Tendency to Equine Sarcoids. *S. West. Vet.* 21, 235–236.

Johnstone, A. C. (1972) Two Cases of Hepatic Mastocytomas in Sheep. *Vet. Path.* 9, 159–163.

Kleine, L. J., Zook, B. C., and Munson, T. O. (1970) Primary Cardiac Hemangiosarcomas in Dogs. *J. Amer. Vet. Med. Assoc.* 157, 326–337.

Konwaler, B. E., Keasbey, L., and Kaplan, L. (1955) Subcutaneous Pseudosarcomatous Fibromatosis (Fasciitis): A Report of 8 Cases. *Amer. J. Clin. Path.* 25, 241–252.

Kulkarni, H. V. (1953) Carcinoma of the Horn in Bovines of the Old Baroda State. *Indian Vet. J.* 29, 415–421.

Lall, H. K. (1953) Incidence of Horn Cancer in Meerut Circle, Uttar Pradesh. *Indian Vet. J.* 30, 205–209.

Lanfranchi, A., and Seren, E. (1938) Ricerche su la trasmissione sperimentale e su la immunizzazione nella papillomatosi cutanea dei bovini. *Nuova Vet.* 16, 32–43.

Lattes, R. (1982) Malignant Fibrous Histiocytoma. *Amer. J. Surg. Pathol.* 6, 761–771.

Lavignette, A. M., and Carlton, W. M. (1974) A Case of Nodular Fasciitis in a Dog. *J. Amer. Anim. Hosp. Assoc.* 10, 503–506.

Lee Chin Hua (1957) Haemangioendotheliomata in a Herd of Pure-Bred Middle White Swine. *J. Malay. Vet. Med. Assoc.* 1, 164–167.

Lee, K. P., and Olson, C. (1968) Response of Calves to Intravenous and Repeated Intradermal Inoculation of Bovine Papilloma Virus. *Amer. J. Vet. Res.* 29, 2103–2112.

———. (1969) Precipitin Response of Cattle to Bovine Papilloma Virus. *Cancer Res.* 29, 1393–1397.

Lerner, A. B., and Cage, G. W. (1974) Melanomas in Horses. *Yale J. Biol. Med.* 46, 646–649.

Lever, W. F., and Schaumburg-Lever, G. (1975) *Histopathology of the Skin.* J. B. Lippincott (Philadelphia).

Liess, J. (1934) Zur Genese und Behandlung der Papillomatose des Rindes. *Dtsch. Tierärztl. Wschr.* 42, 521–526.

Lombard, C., and Levesque, L. (1964) A New Disease in France; Hemangiomatosis of the Skin and Nasal Mucosa in Normandy Cows. *C. R. Acad. Sci.* (Paris) 258, 3137–3138.

Lombard, L. S., Moloney, J. B., and Rickard, C. G. (1963) Transmissible Canine Mastocytoma. *Ann. N.Y. Acad. Sci.* 108, 1086–1105.

Madewell, B. R., Pool, R. R., Theilen, G. H., and Brewer, W. G. (1982) Multiple Subungual Squamous Cell Carcinomas in Five Dogs. *J. Amer. Vet. Med. Assoc.* 180, 731–734.

Makino, S. (1963) Some Epidemiologic Aspects of Venereal Tumors of Dogs as Revealed by Chromosome and DNA Studies. *Ann. N.Y. Acad. Sci.* 108, 1106–1122.

Mangrulkar, M. Y. (1944) Melanomata in Domesticated Animals. *Indian J. Vet. Sci.* 14, 178–185.

Manning, P. J., Millikan, L. E., Cox, V. S., Carey, K. D., and Hook, R. R. (1974) Congenital Cutaneous and Visceral Melanomas of Sinclair Miniature Swine: Three Case Reports. *J. Nat. Cancer Inst.* 52, 1559–1566.

McChesney, A. E., Stephens, L. C., Lebel, S., Snyder, S., and Ferguson, H. R. (1980) Infiltrative Lipoma in Dogs. *Vet. Path.* 17, 316–322.

McCullough, B., Schaller, J., Shadduck, J. A., and Yohn, D. S. (1972) Induction of Malignant Melanomas Associated with Fibrosarcomas in Gnotobiotic Cats Inoculated with Gardner-Feline Fibrosarcoma Virus. *J. Nat. Cancer Inst.* 48, 1893–1896.

McEntee, K. (1952) *Transmissible Fibropapillomas of the External Genitals of Cattle.* Report of New York Veterinary College, 1950–1951. Cornell University (Ithaca, New York), 28.

McGavin, M. D., and Fishburn, F. (1975) Perianal Adenoma of Apocrine Origin in a Dog. *J. Amer. Vet. Med. Assoc.* 166, 388–389.

McGavin, M. D., and Leis, T. J. (1968) Multiple Cutaneous Mastocytomas in a Bull. *Aust. Vet. J.* 44, 20–22.

Meuten, D. J., Capen, C. C., Kociba, G. J., Chew, D. J., and Cooper, B. J. (1982) Ultrastructural Evaluation of Adenocarcinomas Derived from Apocrine Gland of the Anal Sac Associated with Hypercalcemia in Dogs. *Amer. J. Path.* 107, 167–175.

Meuten, D. J., Cooper, B. J., Capen, C. C., Chew, D. J., and Kociba, G. J. (1981) Hypercalcemia Associated with an Adenocarcinoma Derived from the Apocrine Glands of the Anal Sac. *Vet. Path.* 18, 454–471.

M'Fadyean. J. (1933) Equine Melanomatosis. *J. Comp. Path.* 46, 186–204.

Migaki, G. (1969) Hematopoietic Neoplasms of Slaughter Animals. In: Lingeman, C. H., and Garner, F. M., eds., *Comparative Morphology of Hematopoietic Neoplasms.* National Cancer Institute Monograph 32. Government Printing Office (Washington, D.C.), 121–151.

Migaki, G., and Carey, A. M. (1972) Malignant Mastocytoma in a Cow. *Amer. J. Vet. Res.* 33, 253–256.

Migaki, G., and Langheinrich, K. A. (1970) Mastocytoma in a Pig. *Path. Vet.* 7, 353–355.

Millikan, L. E., Hook, R. R., and Manning, P. J. (1973) Gross and Ultrastructural Studies in a New Melanoma Model: The Sinclair Swine. *Yale J. Biol. Med.* 46, 631–645.

Mills, J. H. L., and Nielsen, S. W. (1967) Canine Hemangiopericytoma: A Survey of 200 Tumors. *J. Small Anim. Pract.* 8, 599–604.

Montpellier, J. R., Dieuzeide, R., and Badens, P. (1939) Greffe d'une Tumeur Schwannienne chez le Mulet. *Bull. Acad. Vet. Fr.* 12, 91.

Mostafa, M. S. F., (1953) A Case of Malignant Melanoma in a Bay Horse. *Brit. Vet. J.* 109, 201–205.

Moulton, J. E. (1954) Cutaneous Papillomas on the Udders of Milk Goats. *N. Amer. Vet.* 35, 29–33.

Moulton, J. E., Garg, S. P., and Frazier, L. M. (1966) Morphological Changes in Cells Transformed *In Vitro* by Bovine Papilloma Virus. *Cornell Vet.* 56, 427–433.

Movat, H. Z., and Fernando, N. V. P. (1964) The Fine Structure of the Terminal Vascular Bed. IV. The Venules and Their Perivascular Cells (Pericytes, Adventitial Cells). *Exp. Molec. Pathol.* 3, 98–114.

Mulligan, R. M. (1948) Neoplastic Diseases of Dogs. II. Mast Cell Sarcoma, Lymphosarcoma, Histiocytoma. *Arch. Path.* 46, 477–492.

———. (1949) Neoplastic Diseases of Dogs. I. Neoplasms of Melanin-Forming Cells. *Amer. J. Path.* 25, 339–355.

———. (1951) Spontaneous Cat Tumors. *Cancer Res.* 11, 271.

———. (1955) Hemangiopericytoma in the Dog. *Amer. J. Path.* 31, 773–789.

———. (1961) Melanoblastic Tumors in the Dog. *Amer. J. Vet. Res.* 22, 345–351.

Mustafa, I. E., Cerna, J., and Cerny, L. (1966) Melanoma in Goats. *Sud. Med. J.* 4, 113–118.

Naik, S. N., Balakrishnan, C. R., and Randelia, H. P. (1969) Epidemiology of Horn Cancer in Indian Zebu Cattle: Breed Incidence. *Brit. Vet. J.* 125, 222–230.

Nickoloff, B. J., Hill, J., and Weiss, L. M. (1985) Canine Neuroendocrine Carcinoma: A Tumor Resembling Histiocytoma. *Am. J. Dermatopath.* 7, 579–586.

Nielsen, S. W. (1952a) Extraskeletal Giant Cell Tumor in a Cat. *Cornell Vet.* 42, 304–311.

———. (1952b) Clinical Aspects of Mastocytoma in Dogs. *Proc. Amer. Vet. Med. Assoc. 89th Meeting,* 212–218.

———. (1964) Neoplastic Diseases. In: Catcott, E. J., ed., *Feline Medicine and Surgery.* American Veterinary Publications (Wheaton, Ill. and Santa Barbara, Calif.).

Nielsen, S. W., and Aftosmis, J. (1964) Canine Perianal Gland Tumors. *J. Amer. Vet. Med. Assoc.* 144, 127–135.

Nielsen, S. W., and Cole, C. R. (1958) Canine Mastocytoma. A. Report of One Hundred Cases. *Amer. J. Vet. Res.* 19, 417–432.

———. (1960) Cutaneous Epithelial Neoplasms of the Dog—A Report of 153 Cases. *Amer. J. Vet. Res.* 21, 931–948.

Nordby, J. E. (1933) Congenital Melanotic Skin Tumours in Swine. *J. Hered.* 24, 361–364.

Ochoa, R. (1972) Hibernoma in a Dog. *Cornell Vet.* 62, 138–144.

Olson, C., Jr., (1948) Equine Sarcoid, a Cutaneous Neoplasm, *Amer. J. Vet. Res.* 9, 333–341.

Olson, C., Jr., and Cook, R. H. (1951) Cutaneous Sarcoma-like Lesions of the Horse Caused by the Agent of Bovine Papilloma. *Proc. Soc. Exp. Biol. Med.* 77, 281–284.

Olson, C., Jr., Segre, D., and Skidmore, L. V. (1959) Immunity to Bovine Cutaneous Papillomatosis Produced by Vaccine Homologous to the Challenge Agent. *J. Amer. Vet. Med. Assoc.* 135, 499–502.

———. (1960) Further Observations on Immunity to Bovine Cutaneous Papillomatosis. *Amer. J. Vet. Res.* 21, 233–242.

Orkin, M., and Schwartzman, R. M. (1959) A Comparative Study of Canine and Human Dermatology. II. Cutaneous Tumors: The Mast Cell and Canine Mastocytoma. *J. Invest. Derm.* 32, 451–466.

Pachauri, S. P., and Pathak, R. C. (1969) Bovine Horn Cancer: Therapeutic Experiments with Autogenous Vaccine. *Amer. J. Vet. Res.* 30, 475–477.

Pantekoek, J. F. C. A., and Schiefer, B. (1975) Metastasising Canine Fibrosarcoma Originally Diagnosed as Hemangiopericytoma. *J. Small. Anim. Pract.* 16, 259–265.

Papp, E., and Williams, D. J. (1970) Bovine Lipomatosis. *Zbl. Vet. Med.* (A) 17, 735–742.

Passey, R. D. (1938) Experimental Tar Tumours in Dogs. *J. Path. Bact.* 47, 349–351.

Patnaik, A. K., Ehler, W. J., and MacEwen, E. G. (1984) Canine Cutaneous Mast Cell Tumor: Morphologic Grading and Survival Time in 83 Dogs. *Vet. Path.* 21, 469–474.

Patnaik, A. K., MacEwen, E. G., Black, A. P., and Luckow, S. (1982) Extracutaneous Mast Cell Tumor in the Dog. *Vet. Path.* 19, 608–615.

Patra, B. N. (1959) Observations on Horn Cancer in Cattle. *Vet. Rec.* 71, 844–846.

Pearson, G. R., and Head, K. W. (1976) Malignant Hemangioendothelioma in the Dog. *J. Small. Anim. Pract.* 17, 737–745.

Peiffer, R. L., Gelatt, K. N., and Gwin, R. M. (1976) Proliferative Episcleritis in the Dog. *Vet. Med. Small Anim. Clin.* 71, 1273–1278.

Peters, J. A. (1969) Canine Mastocytoma: Excess Risk as

Related to Ancestry. *J. Natl. Cancer Inst.* 42, 435–443.

Post, J. E., Noronha, F., and Rickard, C. G. (1969) *Canine Mast Cell Leukemia.* In: Dutcher, R. M., ed., Proceedings of the Fourth International Symposium on Comparative Leukemia Research, 1969. *Bibl. Haemat.* 36. S. Karger (Basel and New York), 425–429.

Price, E. B., Silliphant, W. M., and Shuman, R. (1961) Nodular Fasciitis: A Clinicopathologic Analysis of 65 Cases. *Amer. J. Clin. Path.* 35, 122–136.

Pulley, L. T., Shively, J. N., and Pawlicki, J. J. (1974) An Outbreak of Bovine Cutaneous Fibropapillomas Following Dehorning. *Cornell Vet.* 64, 427–434.

Ragland, W. L., and Spencer, G. R. (1968) Attempts to Relate Bovine Papilloma Virus to the Cause of Equine Sarcoid: Immunity to Bovine Papilloma Virus. *Amer. J. Vet. Res.* 29, 1363–1366.

———. (1969) Attempts to Relate Bovine Papilloma Virus to the Cause of Equine Sarcoid: Equidae Inoculated Intradermally with Bovine Papilloma Virus. *Amer. J. Vet. Res.* 30, 743–752.

Ragland, W. L., Keown, G. H., and Gorham, J. R. (1966) An Epizootic of Equine Sarcoid. *Nature* 210, 1399.

Ragland, W. L., Keown, G. H., and Spencer, G. R. (1970a) Equine Sarcoid. *Eq. Vet. J.* 2, 2–11.

Ragland, W. L., McLaughlin, C. A., and Spencer, G. R. (1970b) Attempts to Relate Bovine Papilloma Virus to the Cause of Equine Sarcoid: Horses, Donkeys and Calves Inoculated with Equine Sarcoid Extracts, *Eq. Vet. J.* 2, 168–172.

Rebar, A. H., Hahn, F. F., Halliwell, W. H., Denicola, D. B., and Benjamin, S. A. (1980) Microangiopathic Hemolytic Anemia Associated with Radiation-Induced Hemangiosarcomas. *Vet. Path.* 17, 443–454.

Richardson, R. C., Render, J. A., Rudd, R. G., Shupe, R. E., and Carlton, W. W. (1983) Metastatic Canine Hemangiopericytoma. *J. Amer. Vet. Med. Assoc.* 182, 705–706.

Rijnberk, A., Elsinghorst, A. M., Koeman, J. P., Hackeng, W. H. L., and Leguin, R. M. (1978) Pseudohyperparathyroidism Associated with Perirectal Adenocarcinomas in Elderly Female Dogs. *T. Diergeneesk.* 103, 1069–1075.

Robl, M. G., and Olson, C. (1968) Oncogenic Action of Bovine Papilloma Virus in Hamsters. *Cancer Res.* 28, 1596–1601.

Rosenberger, G. (1941) Ursache und Behandlung der Papillomatose des Rindes. *Dtsch. Tierärztl. Wschr.* 49, 177–181.

Rosenberger, G., and Gründer, H. D. (1959) Untersuchungen über die Immunitätsbildung und Immuntherapie bei der Papillomatose des Rindes. *Dtsch. Tierärztl. Wschr.* 66, 661–666.

Rudolph, R., Gray, A. P., and Leipold, H. W. (1977) Intracutaneous Cornifying Epithelioma ("Keratoacanthoma") of Dogs and Keratoacanthoma of Man. *Cornell Vet.* 67, 254–264.

Runnels, R. A., and Benbrook, E. A. (1941) Connective Tissue Tumors of Horses and Mules. *Amer. J. Vet. Res.* 2, 427–430.

Sahu, S. (1968) The Effectiveness of the Advocated Methods of Treatment of Horn Cancer in Bovine—A Report of 27 Cases. *Indian Vet. J.* 45, 965–970.

Sanford, J. (1965) The Pharmacology of the Mast Cell. In: *Comparative Physiology and Pathology of the Skin.* F. A. Davis (Philadelphia).

Sartin, E. A., and Hodge, T. G. (1982) Congenital Dermal Hemangioendothelioma in Two Foals. *Vet. Path.* 19, 569–571.

Sastry, G. A. (1953) Melanomata in Dogs. *Indian Vet. J.* 29, 482–491.

Schmidt, R. E., and Langham, R. F. (1967) A Survey of Feline Neoplasms. *J. Amer. Vet. Med. Assoc.* 151, 1325–1328.

Schwartzman, R. M., and Orkin, M. (1962) *A Comparative Study of Skin Diseases of Dog and Man.* Charles C. Thomas (Springfield, Ill.).

Segre, D., Olson, C., and Hoerlein, A. B. (1955) Neutralization of Bovine Papilloma Virus with Serums from Cattle and Horses with Experimental Papillomas. *Amer. J. Vet. Res.* 16, 517–520.

Seiler, R. J., and Wilkinson, G. T. (1980) Malignant Fibrous Histiocytoma Involving the Ilium in a Cat. *Vet. Path.* 17, 513–517.

Sividas, C. G., Nair, M. K., Rajan, A., and Ramachandran, K. M. (1971) Congenital Melanoma in a Calf: A Review and Case Report. *Brit. Vet. J.* 127, 289–293.

Smith, H. A., and Jones, T. C. (1957) *Veterinary Pathology.* Lea and Febiger (Philadelphia).

———. (1961) *Veterinary Pathology.* 2nd ed. Lea and Febiger (Philadelphia).

———. (1966) *Veterinary Pathology.* 3rd ed. Lea and Febiger (Philadelphia).

Stannard, A. A., and Pulley, L. T. (1975) Intracutaneous Cornifying Epithelioma (Keratoacanthoma) in the Dog: A Retrospective Study of 25 Cases. *J. Amer. Vet. Med. Assoc.* 167, 385–388.

Stout, A. P. (1949) Hemangiopericytoma: A Study of Twenty-Five New Cases, *Cancer* 2, 1027–1054.

Strafuss, A. C. (1976a) Basal Cell Tumors in Dogs. *J. Amer. Vet. Med. Assoc.* 169, 322–324.

———. (1976b) Sebaceous Gland Adenomas in Dogs. *J. Amer. Vet. Med. Assoc.* 169, 640–642.

Strafuss, A. C., Cook, J. E., and Smith, J. E. (1976) Squamous Cell Carcinoma in Dogs. *J. Amer. Vet. Med. Assoc.* 168, 425–427.

Strafuss, A. C., Dommert, A. R., Tumbleson, M. E., and Middleton, C. C. (1968) Cutaneous Melanoma in Miniature Swine. *Lab. Anim. Care* 18, 165–169.

Sutton, R. H., and McLennan, M. W. (1982) Hemangiosarcoma in a Cow. *Vet. Path.* 19, 456–458.

Tams, T. R., and Macy, D. W. (1981) Canine Mast Cell Tumors. *Compend. Contin. Educ.* 3, 869–878.

Taylor, D. O. N., Dorn, C. R., and Luis, O. H. (1969) Morphologic and Biologic Characteristics of the

Canine Cutaneous Histiocytoma. *Cancer Res.* 29, 83–92.

Trautmann, A., and Fiebiger, J. (1957) *Fundamentals of the Histology of Domestic Animals.* Comstock Publishing Associates (Ithaca, N.Y.).

von Sandersleben, J. (1958) Über epitheliale Neubildungen in der Haut des Hundes. *Berl. Münch. Tierärztl. Wschr.* 71, 287–290.

———. (1964) Gutartige epitheliale Neubildungen in der Haut des Hundes. *Zbl. Vet. Med.* 11, 702–728.

Voss, J. L. (1969) Transmission of Equine Sarcoid. *Amer. J. Vet. Res.* 30, 183–191.

Waller, T., and Rubarth, S. (1967) Hemangioendothelioma in Domestic Animals. *Acta Vet. Scand.* 8, 234–261.

Watrach, A. M. (1969) The Ultrastructure of Canine Cutaneous Papilloma. *Cancer Res.* 29, 2079–2084.

Watson, R. E., Jr., and Larson, F. A. (1974) Detection of Tumor-Specific Antigens in an Equine Sarcoid Cell Line. *Inf. and Immunol.* 9, 714–718.

Weber, W. T., Nowell, P. C., and Hare, W. C. D. (1965) Chromosome Studies of a Transplanted and a Primary Canine Venereal Sarcoma. *J. Nat. Cancer Inst.* 35, 537–547.

Weipers, W. L., and Jarrett, W. F. H. (1954) Haemangioma of the Scrotum of Dogs. *Vet. Rec.* 66, 106–107.

Weiss, E. (1965a) The Pathology of the Tissue Mast Cell in Domestic Animals. In: *Comparative Physiology and Pathology of the Skin.* Blackwell Scientific Publications (Philadelphia).

———. (1965b) Intranuclear and Intracytoplasmic Inclusions of Glycogen in Canine Mast Cell Tumours. *Path. Vet.* 2, 514–519.

Weiss, E., and Frese, K., (1974) VII. Tumors of the Skin. *Bull. Wld. Hlth. Org.* 50, 79–100.

Weiss, S. W., and Enzinger, F. M. (1978) Malignant Fibrous Histiocytoma: An Analysis of 200 Cases. *Cancer* 41, 2250–2266.

Wiessman, S., and Pulley, L. T. (1974) Perianal Gland Adenocarcinoma. *Fel. Pract.* 4, 25.

Whitehead, J. E. (1967) Neoplasia in the Cat. *Vet. Med. Small Anim. Clin.* 62, 357–358.

Yost, D. H., and Jones, T. C. (1958) Hemangiopericytoma in the Dog. *Amer. J. Vet. Res.* 19, 159–163.

Zachary, J. F., Mesfin, M. G., and Wolff, W. A. (1981) Multicentric Osseous Hemangiosarcoma in a Chianina–Angus Steer. *Vet. Path.* 18, 266–70.

# 3

*Thomas J. Hulland*
## Tumors of the Muscle

---

Although a very large part of the animal body consists of smooth or striated muscle fibers, tumors and their precursors are relatively rare in these fibers. Tumors in the smooth and striated muscle of mature animals may seem to have too little in common to be combined in the same chapter. They are similar in anatomic ubiquity, however, and have a common embryonic origin. Consequently, tumors of either smooth or striated muscle arise occasionally from the same unusual sites. Additionally, striated muscle tumors, whether occurring naturally or induced experimentally, often appear to pass through a developmental stage that is morphologically indistinguishable from sarcoma of smooth muscle.

Despite their rarity in animals, tumors of both smooth and striated muscle have now been described often enough for patterns to emerge. This chapter summarizes some of those patterns.

## TUMORS OF SMOOTH MUSCLE

The wide distribution of smooth muscle fibers in blood vessels throughout the mammalian body might lead to the supposition that smooth muscle tumors could arise almost anywhere. However, apart from the rare glomangioma (perhaps a modified smooth muscle tumor), the cardiovascular system of domestic animals seems to be exceptionally free of tumors derived from vascular smooth

muscle. More correctly, when they occur, their origins may not be recognized as vascular. In any case, some tissues that are mainly smooth muscle obviously do give rise to smooth muscle tumors. Examples include the intestinal tract and reproductive tract, but even there the incidence of tumors is uneven (Cordes and Shortridge, 1971; Schmidt and Langham, 1967). Some regions, such as the lower gut, are apparently affected very rarely, while other parts, such as the body of the uterus, have a relatively high incidence of tumors. Furthermore, some tissues with very little smooth muscle fiber (e.g., lungs and kidneys) develop smooth muscle tumors with some regularity (Shortridge and Cordes, 1971).

## Classification

Smooth muscle tumors can be categorized as benign or malignant, but it is becoming apparent in extensive studies in humans that such a classification cannot adequately take into account newer information on the wide range of different cell origins of these tumors (Eimoto *et al.*, 1979; Wick *et al.*, 1982). It also does not allow recognition of the sometimes capricious malignant habits of benign-looking tumors or the benign habits of some that appear malignant on morphological grounds (Chiotasso and Fazio, 1982). Adequately described examples of leiomyoblastoma in animals have not yet been published nor have the techniques for immunohistochemical differentiation been adapted for animal tissues. These steps might allow a more sophisticated subdivision of smooth muscle tumors. For this reason we recognize only the fibroleiomyoma as a subdivision or variant of the smooth muscle group of tumors in animals, in addition to the benign and malignant identification.

In contrast to the situation in humans, smooth muscle neoplasms in animals tend to have a predominantly benign growth pattern and metastasize or invade slowly. This is generally true even if one excludes the large proportion of smooth muscle tumors that are of benign mixed fibrous and smooth muscle type and that arise in the vagina and vulva of the bitch and queen (female cat). These fibroleiomyomas may represent a reversible reaction of tissue rather than a true neoplastic transformation. This difference in the proportion of malignant tumors between animals and humans is consistent with the fact that many of the more malignant smooth muscle tumors arise in humans of old age.

## Leiomyoma

**Incidence, Age, Breed and Sex.** Benign smooth muscle tumors are uncommon in domestic species. Leiomyomas constitute 1 to 2% of all neoplasms found in cattle, sheep, and pigs, although surveys of tumor incidence in abattoir and diagnostic laboratories have obvious built-in errors of sampling, not the least of which is the relative youth of the animals sampled (Anderson and Sandison, 1969b). In the urogenital tract, leiomyomas constitute about one-tenth to one-half of all reported tumors in the female reproductive tract of the large domestic animals and about one-fifth of the bladder tumors of the dog.

In contrast to that of human males, the reproductive tract of male animals seems rarely to be the site of smooth muscle tumors. In cattle, sheep, and pigs this incidence may merely reflect the fact that many more breeding females than males reach old age; however, leiomyomas occur in the genital tract of the bitch and the queen but seem to be absent from the dog and tom (Brodey, 1966; Brodey, 1970). For purposes of description, fibroleiomyomas of the dog and cat are considered separately from leiomyomas in this chapter. If we define fibro-

leiomyomas as mixed fibrous and smooth muscle tumors of the lower reproductive tract of intact females, there remains a small group of true leiomyomas of the uterus and uterine horns, urinary bladder, upper intestinal tract, and esophagus. Only those in the uterus reflect a significant influence from sex, breed, or geography. Most of these tumors have been discovered in mature animals.

The pathogenesis of leiomyoma is not well understood, except that the tumors arise from the muscularis mucosae of the intestinal tract or from the outer smooth muscle coats of the esophagus, gut, gall bladder, urinary bladder, or uterus, and only rarely from scattered smooth muscle fibers in organ capsules or trabeculae. Exceptional smooth muscle tumors in humans arise from vascular pericytes, now recognized as pluripotent mesenchymal cells (Eimoto et al., 1979; Wick et al., 1982), myoepithelial cells of glandular structures (Cameron et al., 1973), or myofibroblasts (Scully, 1981). No common preparatory event seems to be required, and although some breeds of cattle are supposed to be more susceptible than others, incidence studies have not confirmed this.

**Clinical Characteristics and Sites.** Clinical manifestations of leiomyoma are related almost completely to the physcial obstruction of normal function. Reports exist of a leiomyoma obstructing the pregnant uterus of a mare (Grant, 1964) and the urinary bladder of dogs and cats (Osborne et al., 1968; Strafuss and Dean, 1975). A pedunculated smooth muscle tumor led to torsion of a cow's uterus (Arbeiter and Geigenmüller, 1966), and one in the lower esophagus of a dog led to persistent vomiting (Campbell and Pirie, 1965). Reproductive failure may be associated with a leiomyoma, although rarely a tumor and a fetus have been found coexisting in a cow's uterus, and a cervical leiomyoma in a doe was no impediment to a normal twin kid parturition (Ramadan and El Hassan, 1975).

Too few leiomyomas have been described adequately to establish firm patterns of site incidence. The only permissible generalizations are that in large animals leiomyomas are almost certain to be uterine or vaginal, whereas in the dog or cat they are seen in many more sites. Leiomyomas of the digestive tract are more likely to be located in the upper rather than the lower tract (Kohler, 1971).

**Gross Morphology.** The gross appearance of

leiomyomas in domestic animals depends on site and vascularity. The tumors may protrude in or out of the hollow viscus in which they have developed or may remain enclosed within the wall. Muscosal and serosal surfaces are intact, and the most obvious feature of the mass is its bulk. Leiomyomas may be pedunculated, particularly on the uterus of the cow, and most are solitary. The cut surface of the tumor is usually firmer than the surrounding tissue, and lighter in color (off-white to pink). Some lobulation may be apparent. Leiomyomas generally have an indistinct line of separation from the surrounding tissues, but may have a compression line. True encapsulation does not occur.

**Histological Features.** Under microscopic examination, leiomyomas are shown to be composed of interlacing bundles of straplike smooth muscle fibers that tend to intersect at right angles rather than blend in curving bundles. Stroma is minimal but variable from region to region, and degenerative changes are infrequent. Mitotic figures are exceptional. In cross section of fibers, the presence of a central nucleus confirms the identity. In the longitudinal plane the nuclei are ordinarily cigar shaped and have rounded blunt ends rather than angulated ones. Smooth muscle tumors can be usefully demonstrated with a connective tissue stain, such as van Gieson's stain or Masson's trichrome stain for identifying muscle cells and Masson's trichrome or phosphotungstic acid hematoxylin stain for identifying myofibrils after rapid fixation.

## Fibroleiomyoma

These tumors of the reproductive tract are described here only for dogs and cats. Fibroleiomyoma is a special type of leiomyoma that has a significant fibrous component, occurs only in mature intact females, and is usually multicentric. It is probably incorrect to use the term *fibroid* in referring to this tumor.

**Incidence, Age, Breed, and Sex.** Fibroleiomyoma is by far the most frequent tubular genital tract tumor in the dog and cat. In one large study (Brodey and Roszel, 1967) it constituted about 80% of tumors of the uterus, vagina, and vulva of the bitch.

Studies in the queen, although not nearly as extensive, clearly indicate that the incidence is much lower than in the bitch.

The age range of susceptibility in the bitch is from 2 years to senility, although in one series the average age was over 10 years. Only boxers seem to be disproportionately represented. Also, aside from the obvious sex relationship, the tumors were almost twice as common in bitches that had had one or more litters as in bitches that had not borne a litter.

**Clinical Characteristics.** Clinical signs of fibroleiomyoma are usually few unless the tumor protrudes visibly from the vulva. There is ordinarily no significant deviation in estrus periods, nor is there likely to be an increase in pseudopregnancies. It is frequently suggested that these tumors represent a tissue reaction in response to hormonal malfunction that induces hormonal imbalance such as hyperestrinism. Proliferating pluripotent myofibroblasts have been discovered in a wide variety of lesions of the female reproductive tract, particularly those that enlarge during hyperestrinism or pregnancy (Scully, 1981). The presence of these myofibroblasts may explain many of the changes seen in fibroleiomyomas. Both fibrous tissue and smooth muscle tissue can be derived from myofibroblasts. All three cell types are present both in Müllerian duct remnants and in the sexually mature uterus, vagina, vulva, and ovary, and in the peritonium in varying proportions. Their presence makes it easy to understand why the cellularly labile female reproductive tract is frequently a site of aberrant cellular proliferations. Bitches with fibroleiomyomas are unlikely to conceive, but this may reflect the underlying hormonal problem rather than the physical presence of the tumors.

**Gross Morphology.** As with leiomyomas, fibroleiomyomas may protrude inward or outward or result in lenticular swellings of the uterine or vaginal wall. These tumors are usually multiple in the bitch and solitary in the queen. They are often found in the uterus, cervix, vagina, or vulva.

Examination of the intact surface and fusiform enlargement shows no distinct demarcation, other than color and perhaps texture, between tumorous and normal tissue. The neoplasm is likely to be lighter in color than normal tissue, but resembles the uterine or vaginal wall in texture even when large.

**Histological Features, Growth, and Metastasis.** On a microscopic level the admixture of smooth muscle, collagen, and fibroblastic cells varies from tumor to tumor and from one area to another within a single tumor. Cellular components are essentially normal in appearance, although they are disoriented. Mitotic figures can be found, but they are normal and not numerous.

Fibroleiomyomas may recur if removed surgically, although removal of large tumors plus ovariectomy will lead to cure. Small tumors strink almost completely after spaying.

## Leiomyosarcoma

**Incidence, Age, Breed, and Sex.** Malignant smooth muscle tumors constitute only about one-tenth of the total smooth muscle tumors reported, and even some of these tumors may really have been leiomyomas. These smooth muscle sarcomas often arise in the same sites as their benign counterparts (e.g., in the uterus), suggesting that a leiomyoma has undergone malignant transformation. Leiomyosarcomas also occur where leiomyomas have not been found (e.g., in the kidney, ovary, and skeletal muscle).

There seems to be no sex or breed predisposition, except that some tumors arise in the uterine or vaginal wall. Young adult animals are involved most often. Cats have been reported as having a disproportionate number of leiomyosarcomas, although this may simply reflect the marked tendency of the cat to have malignant rather than benign tumors of most types. No geographic patterns seem to exist.

**Clinical Characteristics.** Descriptions of this tumor are too few to allow analysis of clinical manifestations. Surgical biopsy and histological examination can establish the identity of the tumor, but cannot accurately predict the probability of invasion or metastasis. The tumors that have been examined demonstrate local invasion with destruction of adjacent tissue and a tendency toward late metastasis to the lungs and other distant organs. The primary tumor, however, can sometimes be successfully removed surgically, followed by clinical recovery if metastasis has not occurred. In one case, surgical removal of a kidney extensively affected by leiomyosarcoma was followed by recovery. Nonobstructive perforation of the gut has been reported (Eckerlin, 1974). Irradiation and other types of therapy are unlikely to be successful modes of treatment (Chiotasso and Fazio, 1982).

**Gross Morphology.** The gross appearance of a leiomyosarcoma will depend on the extent of degenerative processes in the tumor. Some of these tumors are extensively necrotic and cavitated, whereas others do not differ greatly from the typical leiomyoma. Those arising in the urinary bladder may infiltrate the wall and obstruct urine flow. Leiomyosarcomas in the uterus and urinary bladder are usually multiple, whereas ones in the kidney may be solitary masses (fig. 3.1A).

**Histological Features.** On a microscopic level, cells vary from the normal straplike smooth muscle fibers to anaplastic rounded cells that can be classified only as sarcoma (figs. 3.1B and C). Its clinical behavior does not have much bearing on its degree of anaplasia; one that metastasized to the lungs of a cow showed well-differentiated smooth muscle cells (Maeda *et al.*, 1971).

Distinguishing among fibrosarcoma, rhabdomyosarcoma, and leiomyosarcoma may be difficult. Leiomyosarcoma can be identified by cigar-shaped central nuclei. The presence of myofibrils is also helpful in diagnosis, but the absence of striated fibrils is not conclusive. It is not necessary to demonstrate metastasis or local invasion to support a diagnosis of leiomyosarcoma. Diagnosis should be based on all available evidence: site, growth characteristics, cell morphology, etc. The electron microscopic demonstration of attachment plaques, pinocytotic vesicles, and dense bodies with or without filaments provides strong support for a diagnosis of leiomyosarcoma (Bundtzen and Norback, 1982), but these findings cannot be considered conclusive. For the future, immunocytochemical techniques promise greater precision and confidence in diagnosis (Bures *et al.*, 1981).

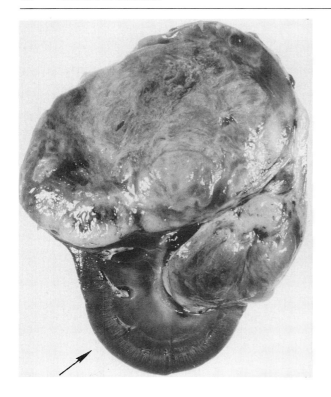

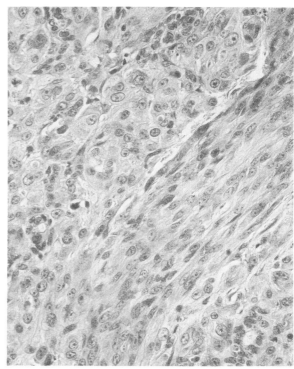

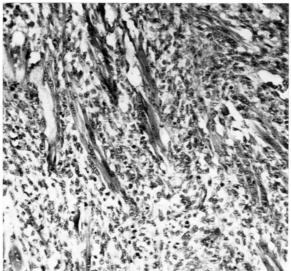

**FIGURE 3.1.** Leiomyosarcoma of the dog. A. Neoplasm retained within the kidney; the normal pole of the kidney (arrow) can be seen. B. Neoplasm in the spleen showing bundles of elongated cells; the nuclei are often blunted on the ends. There is greater cellularity in this tumor than in the benign form. C. Tumor in the stomach. Observe elongated muscle fibers intermixed with smaller tumor cells.

## TUMORS OF STRIATED MUSCLE

### General Considerations

Striated muscle tumors are rare in any animal population. In sharp contrast to this low natural incidence is the ease with which striated muscle tumors can be induced in experimental animals in the laboratory.

Muscle tumors, like many other neoplasms, are unlikely to arise from a fully developed and specialized parent cell. We look then for an immature cell of origin with potential for developing into either normal or neoplastic tissue. It has long been suggested that some forms of striated muscle tumor arise from embryonic remnants of myotomes left behind in the development of muscle masses, or from pluripotent cells of embryological structures such as the Müllerian or Wolffian ducts (Stamps and Harris, 1968). That suggestion is supported by the clearly congenital nature of many striated muscle tumors and also by instances of striated muscle tumors arising from organs that normally contain no striated muscle fibers. For example, striated muscle tumors arise from the urinary bladder, kidney, uterus, and lungs, but these organs do not contain skeletal muscle (Donnelly and Hamilton, 1972). In a similar category are teratomatous neoplasms of the testicle and ovary, in which striated fibers apparently arise from pluripotent cells capable of fetal developmental differentiation.

Not all animal muscle tumors, however, seem to fit this pattern of origin from a fetal cell, so perhaps neoplastic transformation of a myoblast can occur where degeneration and repair changes are taking place. The few instances of muscle tumor origin coinciding with chronic traumatic damage to muscle suggest a possible cause and effect relationship in some cases.

Striated muscle tumors cover a full range of growth characteristics. Congenital rhabdomyomas of the heart seem to be benign, with no potential for malignant transformation. Malignant rhabdomyosarcomas, in contrast, are among the most aggressive and destructive tumors in animals, readily able to metastasize by either lymphatic or venous routes. Muscle tumors metastasize to skeletal muscle, so multiple nodules in muscles support diagnosis.

## Rhabdomyoma

**Classification.** Benign striated muscle tumors are reported to be about half as common as malignant ones. The great majority of these benign tumors have been found in the heart of animals and are probably of the congenital type. Although no convincing reports are yet found, it is likely that examples of extracardiac rhabdomyomas will be found in domestic animal populations. The one reported case (Day, 1922) should perhaps be rejudged as a rhabdomyosarcoma. It is possible, however, that some of these tumors reported as malignant, but without metastasis or invasiveness, should have been originally classified as benign. The paucity of examples of extracardiac rhabdomyoma in animals is probably only a reflection of low numbers of muscle tumor cases studied. In the future we might anticipate finding rhabdomyomas in other sites, such as the head, urogenital tract, or limb extremities of young or young adult animals.

### Cardiac Rhabdomyoma

**Incidence.** About one-third of all striated muscle tumors reported in domestic animals have been found in the heart myocardium. The various species affected include the pig, cow, sheep, and dog. Although some tumors were not discovered until the animal had reached maturity, several were reported in neonates and it is likely that these were congenital in origin. The pathogenesis of these tumors in humans has been the subject of numerous studies (see Silverman et al., 1976). It has been suggested that they are neoplasms, hamartomas, developmental anomalies, expressions of a storage disease, or examples of cellular gigantism. Cells contained in the lesions have been identified as fibroblasts, Purkinje cells, myofibers, myofibroblasts, satellite cells, or mixtures of these components (Silverman et al., 1976; Trillo et al., 1978). Evidence presently seems to favor the inclusion of cardiac rhabdomyomas as hamartomatous growths having a mixed benign cellular population; this view reflects the feeling that a pluripotent embryonic cell is the most likely cell of origin. It has been argued that the absence of mitotic figures indicates that the mass is not neoplastic and that any increase in size occurs by hypertrophy, not hyperplasia, of individual cells (Bradley *et al.*, 1980). This conclusion seems to be at odds with the finding that large rhabdomyomas can occupy half of the volume of an adult steer's heart. Skarpa (1966) reported amitotic division of some cells in a pig's heart, but it is clear that some form of cellular hyperplasia takes place as the animal grows. No sex, breed, or regional variations of cardiac rhabdomyoma incidence seem apparent, although Kast and Hanichen (1968) suggested that there may be a familial predisposition in pigs. Since clinical manifestations of the heart tumor are minimal, most findings have been incidental to slaughter.

**Gross Morphology.** Cardiac rhabdomyomas usually do not exceed one-sixth of the heart volume, but rarely can occupy half of the heart mass; they may be multiple or solitary in pigs but are usually solitary in other species. The tumors may be pedunculated or completely embedded in the heart muscle (fig. 3.2A). The cardiac ventricles are often affected, with the interventricular septum being the most common site. The tumor is grossly visible because of its mass, which irregularly increases the size of the myocardium, and by its difference in color from the surrounding or adjacent myocardium. The usual color of the neoplasm is yellow to brown. The tumor usually has no sharp demarcation from normal myocardium, but it may be encapsulated.

**Histological Features.** The microscopic features of congenital rhabdomyoma are variable, but a consistent finding is a population of large mononuclear or binuclear cells with abundant granular vacuolated cytoplasm (so-called spider cells). Nuclei are round to oval, contain prominent nucleoli, and are centrally situated. The cells are pleomorphic and vary from fibroblastlike cells to multinucleate cells having clear fibrillar cross striations (fig. 3.2B). The usual signs of rapid cell turnover are absent except for the variation in cell size. Mitotic figures are sparse. The most characteristic neoplastic cell is large and vacuolated and has a high glycogen content comparable to levels in similar tumors in children. Bradley *et al.* (1980) demonstrated diastase—labile, periodic acid—Schiff positive granules in cardiac rhabdomyomas in sheep and pigs. The high glycogen content (as high as 30%) may help to identify the tumor.

Electron microscopic studies have not been done on cardiac rhabdomyomas of domestic animals, but have been done in humans. The neoplasm in children shows abnormal cells with abundant myofilaments and visible sarcomeres. Also, intercalated disc junctions may be seen and glycogen granules are numerous.

## Rhabdomyosarcoma

Malignant tumors of striated muscle constitute a majority of voluntary muscle tumors in domestic animals, but still represent less than 1% of all spontaneous tumors in each domestic species. No sex, breed, or regional predisposition seems to exist. The age range is broad, although the mean age of 2 to 3 years is considerably lower than for most tumors.

**Classification.** Malignant striated muscle tumors can be grouped in several different ways, but historically, a commonly used classification was based on tissue of origin. Tumors arising from striated muscle were designated as rhabdomyosarcomas and tumors arising in tissues that ordinarily contain no striated muscle were called metaplastic rhabdomyosarcomas. It is now evident that morphologically similar tumors can be found in both groups, that epidemiological and biological behavior patterns do not conform to this grouping, and that some tumors arising in skeletal muscle are apparently derived from a progenitor cell other than a muscle fiber or myoblast. As an alternative, an anatomical classification is sometimes used because, at least in humans, most rhabdomyosarcomas are found in the head and neck region, the urogenital tract, or the limb muscles. This categorization has little to recommend it since morphologically similar tumors are derived from all three sites. The most frequently used classification that seems to be practical for tumors of both humans and animals is based on cell morphology. In this scheme, three major types are recognized: alveolar, embryonal, and pleomorphic. No clearly identifiable examples of the alveolar type have been reported as a naturally occurring tumor of domestic animals. The histological and electron microscopic features of the three types are considered in greater detail below.

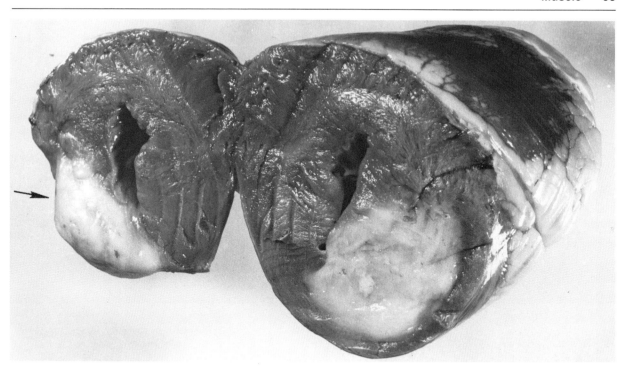

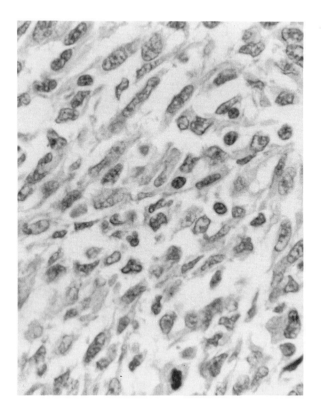

FIGURE 3.2. Rhabdomyoma. A. Rhabdomyoma in the heart of a sheep. The abnormal tissue (**arrow**) has no sharp line of demarcation from the normal myocardium. B. Rhabdomyoma in the heart of a steer. Cells vary in shape, size, and orientation. (A, courtesy of Dr. D. Cordes and the *N. Z. Vet. J.*)

The rhabdomyosarcomas of the urinary bladder of the dog are of special interest because they are more common than other forms of this neoplasm. These tumors are considered separately below, although their histomorphology corresponds to that in similar tumors found elsewhere.

**Incidence.** Rhabdomyosarcomas arising in skeletal muscles are uncommon in domestic animals, and no clear pattern of site incidence has appeared. Several have been found in the limbs, a few on the tongue and cheeks, and single tumors in the pharynx, esophagus, thorax, brisket, uterus, and ovary (Ladds and Webster, 1971; Torbeck *et al.,* 1980; White, 1966). At least 15 rhabdomyosarcomas have been found in the urinary bladder of the dog. Tumors in this site have also been reported in the cow, sheep, horse, dog, and cat, but not the pig (Anderson and Sandison, 1969a; Whitehead, 1967).

**Clinical Characteristics.** Clinical manifestations of rhabdomyosarcoma include lameness and irregular swelling of the leg when the tumor arises from or metastasizes to skeletal muscles of the leg. Any tumors that encroach physically on the oral cavity or elsewhere in the digestive tract lead to anorexia. These tumors may also lead to uterine or urinary bladder obstruction.

Clinical examination is likely to reveal palpable masses in the skeletal muscles. Rhabdomyosarcomas generally metastasize early and widely, and the tumor is usually inoperable, although early amputation of the limb has been effective in selected cases. (Clinical manifestations of urinary bladder rhabdomyosarcomas are considered below.)

**Gross Morphology.** Spherical nodules of pinkish gray tumor are visible on gross inspection of body tissues, and as the nodules grow over 1 cm in diameter there is likely to be progressive evidence of necrosis and hemorrhage.

The term *botryoid* has been frequently used to identify the appearance of rhabdomyosarcomas that protrude from mucous membranes. Rhabdomyosarcomas with a botryoid form arise in the urinary bladder and uterus particularly where a thin tissue cover allows the rapid, nodular tumor growth to take its natural form.

The site of origin of a metastatic rhabdomyosarcoma may not be apparent. Metastasis spreads to lymph nodes, lungs, heart, spleen, adrenal glands, kidneys, and skeletal muscles. In neither primary tumors nor metastases is there likely to be any evidence of encapsulation or supporting connective tissue stroma.

The tumor is highly invasive, and compression lines are overrun by tumor cells that borrow the stroma of adjacent parenchymal tissues and frequently engulf a few normal cells.

**Histological Features.** The microscopic appearance of rhabdomyosarcoma is variable. The cells show marked differences in a single tumor or in different tumors (figs. 3.3A–D and 3.4A–D). These differences probably result from the marked variation in ploidy among cells (Yamashiro *et al.*, 1980), but may also occur because of the (presumed) derivation of these cells from pluripotent cells, best exemplified by the embryonal cell type of rhabdomyosarcoma. This cellular difference is expressed in nucleolar size, contour, and number; in cytoplasmic granularity and vacuolation; and in the presence of recognizably cross-striated fibrils.

Alveolar types of rhabdomyosarcomas are composed of dark-staining, round or oval cells arranged in an acinar pattern. A small number of these neoplasms have cells that contain cross-striated fibrils in their cytoplasm. The cells tend to be smaller and more regular than those in other types of rhabdomyosarcomas.

The embryonal type of rhabdomyosarcoma shows little or no organization, but consists of irregularly lobulated sheets of cells showing marked pleomorphism. Cells may be small and round, oval, or racket-shaped, or may be large and mono- or multinucleated, containing cytoplasmic vacuoles or striated myofibrils. Intermediate cell forms, including "strap" cells or ribbon-shaped myoblasts without fibrils, may be present. Sometimes the cells are separated from one another by a myxoid stroma. At least half of the rhabdomyosarcomas of this type reveal cross striations of fibrils, as seen by light microscopy.

In the pleomorphic type of rhabdomyosarcoma highly irregular cell types grow in irregular sheets. Small round cells may be present, but the predominant cell is a large angular cell with variation in the size of the nucleus. In some areas of the neoplasm, these cells may become elongated (so-called ribbon cells with centrally located nuclei appearing in rows). Multiple nuclei are common and giant cells may contain as many as a dozen nuclei. Some large vacuolated cells ("spider" cells) may also be present. Large cells with abundant cytoplasm should be examined for cross-striations through use of some special stains, although only a minority of cells will show striations.

The most useful diagnostic characteristic of tumor cells in the embryonal and pleomorphic types of rhabdomyosarcoma is the irregular angularity of the cells, including an extreme range in the size of the nuclei. Mitotic figures are often numerous and may be irregular in shape. Both the primary and metastatic tumors contain cells with an increased or decreased number or a highly irregular number of chromosomes.

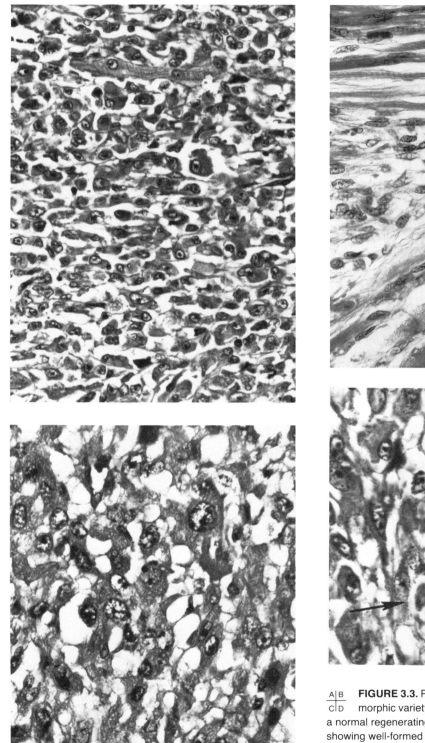
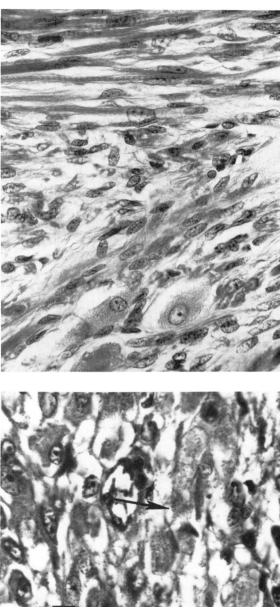

A | B
C | D

**FIGURE 3.3.** Rhabdomyosarcoma in the dog. A. Pleo-morphic variety. This metastatic tumor has surrounded a normal regenerating muscle fiber. B. Embryonal tumor showing well-formed striated myofibrils and "spider cells." C. Embryonal tumors showing racket-shaped cells, nuclear pleomorphism, polyploidy, and vacuolation. D. Several tumor cells (**arrows**) show intact myofibrillar sarcomeres.

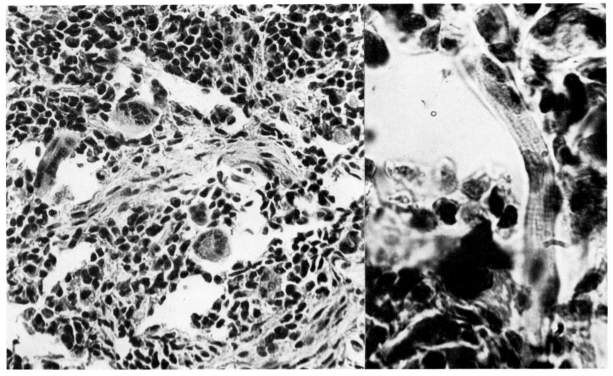

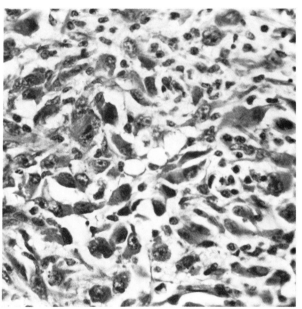

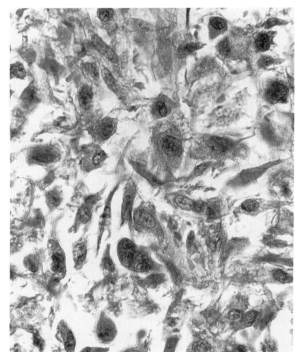

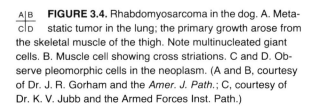 **FIGURE 3.4.** Rhabdomyosarcoma in the dog. A. Metastatic tumor in the lung; the primary growth arose from the skeletal muscle of the thigh. Note multinucleated giant cells. B. Muscle cell showing cross striations. C and D. Observe pleomorphic cells in the neoplasm. (A and B, courtesy of Dr. J. R. Gorham and the *Amer. J. Path.*; C, courtesy of Dr. K. V. Jubb and the Armed Forces Inst. Path.)

The presence of fibrillar cross-striations is the most important criterion for demonstrating the muscle origin of a pleomorphic rhabdomyosarcoma. Some rhabdomyosarcomas fail to show convincing striations, even on exhaustive search by light microscopy (Bundtzen and Norback, 1982; Peter and Kluge, 1970), so diagnosis may be a problem. The display of cross and longitudinal striations can be improved by using special stains such as Heidenhain's iron hematoxylin, phosphotungstic acid hematoxylin, or silver. The use of semi-thin plastic embedded sections may improve resolution (Meyvisch *et al.,* 1977; Pletcher and Dalton, 1981). Two other techniques that can improve diagnostic performance are electron microscopy and immunocytochemistry for demonstrating the presence of cellular myoglobin (Brooks, 1982). The latter technique has not yet been applied to animal tissues.

The most important criterion for accepting a tumor as a rhabdomyosarcoma by electron microscopy is the demonstration of subcellular structures that are present only in muscle cells. It has been proposed that the confirmation of diagnosis must rest on the demonstration of more than one sarcomere component in the tumor cell since single sarcomere components can be found in cells of other tumors, notably in fibrous histiocytoma and smooth muscle tumors. Sarcomere filaments are confirmatory if they are arranged in alternate linear sequence or if thin filaments are arranged hexagonally around thick filaments. Rhabdomyosarcomas can be identified by thick and thin filaments along with a Z-line, by thin filaments with a Z-line and I-band, or by thin filaments inserted into a Z-line. The presence of only disorganized thick and thin filaments indicates a myogenous cell but does not distinguish between smooth and striated muscle tumor cells. Other subcellular components such as abundant glycogen, free ribosomes associated with dilated endoplasmic reticulum profiles, and numerous indentations of the nuclear membrane are characteristic of skeletal muscle tumor cells.

It must be remembered that the electron microscope is only an aid to diagnosis and that all factors must be considered before a neoplasm can be called a rhabdomyosarcoma. The microscopist must also remember that invasive tumors may incorporate normal muscle fibers that are difficult to distinguish from neoplastic muscle fibers.

Rhabdomyosarcoma cells apparently undergo changes in antigenicity. Corbeil (1968) reported on the different muscle-specific antigens found in these cells. There is little evidence, however, to suggest that these tumor antigens initiate immunological containment or regression of the tumor.

## Rhabdomyosarcoma in the Urinary Bladder of the Dog

This tumor deserves separate consideration because it constitutes nearly two-thirds of reported rhabdomyosarcomas in the dog. These tumors are likely to constitute less than 1% of all bladder tumors in the dog, however, so they are important only as an occasional diagnostic problem.

The origin of these tumors is thought to be from pluripotent or myoblastic cells of mesenchymal origin that ensheath the developing Müllerian or Wolffian ducts. Reviews of several cases have been reported (Kelly, 1973; Meyvisch *et al.,* 1977; Pletcher and Dalton, 1981).

**Age, Breed, and Sex.** Seven of ten reported cases of these tumors involved female dogs and only one of the dogs was older than 2 years of age. Large breeds, particularly the Saint Bernard, were overrepresented among cases.

**Clinical Characteristics.** Affected dogs usually have hematuria and dysuria for 4 weeks to 6 months. Cystitis is a frequent complication, and weight loss and secondary anemia occur when the disease course is long. The tumors are demonstrable radiographically as large intravesicular masses. Careful examination of urine sediment may reveal neoplastic cells among predominantly inflammatory debris. Hypertrophic osteoarthropathy in the absence of pulmonary metastasis has been observed in dogs with rhabdomyosarcoma of the urinary bladder (Halliwell and Ackerman, 1974).

**Gross Morphology.** These tumors are usually located in the neck of the bladder. They are large, generally polypoid, nodular or grapelike and are firm or soft and friable, and white, grayish tan or pink in color. The mucosal surface overlying the tumor is usually ulcerated.

**Histological Features, Growth, and Metastasis.** These tumors consist microscopically of fusiform and polygonal cells with scanty cytoplasm. Multinucleated cells with prominent granules or fibrillar eosinophilic cytoplasm are common.

Microscopic features of these tumors are similar to those of rhabdomyosarcoma located in other sites. Many of these tumors are of pleomorphic type. Clearly recognizable cross-striations in the tumor cells have been reported in less than half of the neoplasms.

Surgical removal of the tumor has been unrewarding since the tumors tend to recur or metastasize. It would appear that surgery should be attempted only in dogs with early or slow-growing tumors in accessible sites since postsurgical death often occurs from complications associated with radical surgery.

## Granular Cell Myoblastoma

**Incidence.** The name *granular cell myoblastoma* implies a myoblast origin, although this is now in some doubt (see also chap. 7, Tumors of the Respiratory System). Sobel *et al.* (1973) claimed to demonstrate a similarity of the tumor cells in myoblastoma to Schwann cells and suggested a common cell of origin. The only cases reported in animals have been in the tongue of the dog (Giles *et al.*, 1974; Wyand and Wolke, 1968) and in the laryngeal muscles and lungs of the horse (Parodi *et al.*, 1974). The tumor apparently occurs in mature or old animals.

**Gross Morphology.** Myoblastoma seems to be less malignant than most other tumors of muscle; it may be locally invasive, but apparently does not metastasize. This tumor is pink to yellow and well-demarcated from surrounding normal tissue but not encapsulated.

**Histological Features.** Microscopically, the tumor cells are uniformly elongated with granular cytoplasm. Nuclei are regular in size and shape and resemble the nuclei of mesenchymal cells rather than those of muscle tumors. Cross-striations are not present and longitudinal fibrils are rare. Collagen is relatively abundant, and the tumor tissue may be freely admixed with normal tissue components such as muscle fibers and blood vessels.

Clinically, granular cell myoblastoma often ap-

pears as a bulging mass on the surface of the tongue and may cause masticatory problems. The clinical course is usually protracted.

## REFERENCES

Anderson, L. J., and Sandison, A. T. (1969a) Tumors of the Female Genitalia in Cattle, Sheep and Pigs Found in a British Abattoir Survey. *J. Comp. Path.* 79, 53–63.

———. (1969b) Tumors of Connective Tissue in Cattle, Sheep and Pigs. *J. Path.* 98, 253–263.

Arbeiter, K., and Geigenmüller, H. (1966) Gebärmuttertumor beim Rind als Ursache einer Torsio uteri. *Dtsch. Tierärztl. Wschr.* 73, 588–590.

Bradley, R., Wells, G. A. H., and Arbuckle, J. B. R. (1980) Ovine and Porcine So-called Cardiac Rhabdomyoma (Hamartoma). *J. Comp. Path.* 90, 551–558.

Brodey, R. S. (1966) Alimentary Tract Neoplasms in the Cat: A Clinicopathologic Survey of 46 Cases. *Amer. J. Vet. Res.* 27, 74–80.

———. (1970) Canine and Feline Neoplasia. *Adv. Vet. Sci.* 14, 309–354.

Brodey, R. S., and Roszel, J. R. (1967) Neoplasms of the Canine Uterus, Vagina and Vulva: A Clinicopathologic Survey of 90 Cases. *J. Amer. Vet. Med. Assoc.* 151, 1294–1307.

Brooks, J. J. (1982) Immunohistochemistry of Soft Tissue Tumors, Myoglobin as a Tumor Marker for Rhabdomyosarcoma. *Cancer* 50, 1757–1763.

Bundtzen, J. L., and Norback, D. H. (1982) The Ultrastructure of Poorly Differentiated Rhabdomyosarcomas. *Human Path.* 13, 301–313.

Bures, J. C., Barnes, L., and Mercer, D. (1981) A Comparative Study of Smooth Muscle Tumors Utilizing Light and Electron Microscopy, Immunocytochemical Staining and Enzymatic Assay. *Cancer* 48, 2420–2426.

Cameron, H. M., Hamperl, H., and Warambo, W. (1974) Leiomyosarcoma of the Breast Originating from Myothelium (Myoepithelium). *J. Path.* 114, 89–92.

Campbell, J. R., and Pirie, H. M. (1965) Leiomyoma of the Oesophagus in a Dog. *Vet. Res.* 77, 624–626.

Chiotasso, J. P., and Fazio, W. (1982) Prognostic Factors of 28 Leiomyosarcomas of the Small Intestine. *Surg. Gynecol. Obstet.* 155: 197–202.

Corbeil, L. B. (1968) Antigenicity of Rhabdomyosarcomas Induced by Nickel Sulfide (Ni$_3$S$_2$). *Cancer* 21, 184–189.

Cordes, D. O., and Shortridge, E. H. (1971) Neoplasms of Sheep: A Survey of 256 Cases Recorded at Ruakura Animal Health Laboratory. *N. Z. Vet. J.* 19, 55–64.

Day, L. E. (1922) Rhabdomyoma of the Lungs of a Sheep. *J. Amer. Vet. Med. Assoc.* 61, 436.

Donnelly, W. J. C., and Hamilton, A. F. (1972) Fatal Pulmonary Rhabdomyosarcoma in a Lamb. *Vet. Rec.* 91, 280–285.

Eckerlin, R. H. (1974) Perforated Duodenum Associated with Nonobstructive Leiomyosarcoma in a Dog. *J. Amer. Vet. Med. Assoc.* 165, 449–450.

Eimoto, T., Miyake, M., and Sasaki, T. (1979) Vascular Leiomyoblastoma of the Stomach. *Acta. Path. Jpn.* 29(2), 277–288.

Giles, R. C., Montgomery, C. A., and Izen, L. (1974) Canine Lingual Granular Cell Myoblastoma: A Case Report. *Amer. J. Vet. Res.* 35, 1357–1359.

Grant, D. L. (1964) Uterine Tumor in a Mare—Leiomyoma. *Vet. Rec.* 76, 474–475.

Halliwell, W. H., and Ackerman, N. (1974) Botryoid Rhabdomyosarcoma of the Urinary Bladder and Hypertrophic Osteoarthropathy in a Young Dog. *J. Amer. Vet. Med. Assoc.* 165, 911–913.

Kast, A., and Hanichen, T. (1968) Rhabdomyome in Schweineherzen. *Zbl. Vet. Med.* B 15, 140–150.

Kelly, D. F. (1973) Rhabdomyosarcoma of the Urinary Bladder in Dogs. *Vet. Path.* 10, 375–384.

Kohler, H. (1971) Leiomyom in Jejunum eines Hundes. *Dtsch. Tierärztl. Wschr.* 78, 548.

Ladds, P. W., and Webster, D. R. (1971) Pharyngeal Rhabdomyosarcoma in a Dog. *Vet. Path.* 8, 256–259.

Maeda, T., Hayashi, T., Sasaki, T., and Tsumura, I. (1971) Tumors of the Genital Organs in Domestic Animals. I. Uterine and Vaginal Tumors in Cows and a Sow. *J. Jap. Vet. Med. Assoc.* 24, 226–231.

Meyrisch, C., Thoonen, H., and Hoorens, J. (1977) The Ultrastructure of Rhabdomyosarcoma in a Dog. *Zbl. Vet. Med.* 24A, 542–551.

Osborne, C. A., Low, D. G., Perman, V., and Barnes, D. M. (1968) Neoplasms of the Canine and Feline Urinary Bladder: Incidence, Etiologic Factors, Occurrence and Pathologic Features. *Amer. J. Vet. Res.* 29, 2041–2055.

Parodi, A. L., Tassin, P., and Rigoulet, J. (1974) Myoblastome à cellules granuleuses. Trois nouvelles observations à localisation pulmonaire chez le cheval. *Rec. Méd. Vét.* 150, 489–494.

Peter, C. P., and Kluge, J. P. (1970) An Ultrastructural Study of a Canine Rhabdomyosarcoma. *Cancer* 26, 1280–1288.

Pletcher, J. M., and Dalton, L. (1981) Botryoid Rhabdomyosarcoma in the Urinary Bladder of a Dog. *Vet. Path.* 18, 695–697.

Ramadan, R. O., and El Hassan, L. M. (1975) Leiomyoma in the Cervix and Hyperplastic Ectopic Mammary Tissue in a Goat. *Aust. Vet. J.* 51, 362.

Schmidt, R. E., and Langham, R. F. (1967) Survey of Feline Neoplasms. *J. Amer. Vet. Med. Assoc.* 151, 1325–1328.

Scully, R. E. (1981) Smooth Muscle Differentiation in Genital Tract Disorders. *Arch. Path. Lab. Med.* 105, 505–507.

Shortridge, E. H., and Cordes, D. O. (1971) Neoplasms in Cattle: A Survey of 372 Neoplasms Examined at the Ruakura Veterinary Diagnostic Station. *N. Z. Vet. J.* 19, 5–11.

Silverman, J. F., Kay, S., McCue, C. M., Lower, R. R., Brough, A. J., and Change, C. H. (1976) Rhabdomyoma of the Heart. Ultrastructural Study of Three Cases. *Lab. Invest.* 35, 596–605.

Škarpa, M. (1966) Rabdomiom Srca Svinje. *Vet. Arch.* 36, 137–141.

Sobel, H. J., Schwart, R., and Maraquet, E. (1973) Light- and Electron-Microscopic Study of the Origin of Granular-Cell Myoblastoma. *J. Path.* 109, 101–111.

Strafuss, C., and Dean, M. J. (1975) Neoplasms of the Canine Urinary Bladder. *J. Amer. Vet. Med. Assoc.* 166, 1161–1163.

Stamps, P., and Harris, D. L. (1968) Botryoid Rhabdomyosarcoma of the Urinary Bladder of a Dog. *J. Amer. Vet. Med. Assoc.* 153, 1064–1068.

Torbeck, R. L., Kittleson, S. L., and Leathers, C. W. (1980) Botryoid Rhabdomyosarcoma in the Uterus of a Filly. *J. Amer. Vet. Med. Assoc.* 176, 914–916.

Trillo, A. A., Hollman, I. L., and White, J. T. (1978) Presence of Satellite Cells in a Cardiac Rhabdomyoma. *Histopath.* 2, 215–225.

White, A. E. (1966) Skeletal Muscle Tumor (Rhabdomyosarcoma) in a Puppy. *Mod. Vet. Pract.* 47, 74.

Whitehead, J. E. (1967) Neoplasia in the Cat. *Vet. Med. Small Anim. Clin.* 62, 357–358.

Wick, M. R., Scheithauer, B. W., Piehler, J. M., and Pairolero, P. C. (1982) Primary Pulmonary Leiomyosarcomas. *Arch. Path. Lab. Med.* 106, 510–514.

Wyand, D. S., and Wolke, R. E. (1968) Granular Cell Myoblastoma of the Canine Tongue: Case Reports. *Amer. J. Vet. Res.* 29, 1309–1313.

Yamashiro, S., Gilman, J. P. W., Hulland, T. J., and Abandowitz, H. M. (1980) Nickel Sulphide-Induced Rhabdomyosarcomata in Rats. *Acta Path. Jpn.* 30, 9–22.

**4**

*Roy R. Pool*

# Tumors and Tumorlike Lesions of Joints and Adjacent Soft Tissues

Tumors as well as nonneoplastic growths of undetermined etiology may be centered in joints, tendon sheaths, bursae, and fasciae. Although many of these lesions originate in synovioblastic mesenchyme, they can also arise from any of several supporting tissues of the synovium or fascia, including fibrous, adipose, vascular, or nervous tissue. Fascia is included in this group of lesions because synovial neoplasms may arise in intermuscular fascia at a considerable distance from joints and tendon sheaths (Hale and Calder, 1970; Roth *et al.*, 1975). Other lesions centered in fascia that are included here are fibrotic myopathy and musculo-aponeurotic fibromatosis of horses and malignant giant cell tumor of soft parts and malignant mesenchymoma of dogs.

Synovial sarcoma is the most common and best understood of this rare group of tumors and tumorlike lesions occurring in or around the joints of animals. In dogs and cats malignant synovial tumors of joints outnumber benign joint lesions, but more tendon sheath tumors are benign than malignant in these species. Most synovial growths in horses have a benign behavior. These tumors are rarely reported in other domestic species.

No treatise on neoplasms of joints and related structures in domestic animals currently exists. There are only two published reviews of joint tumors in animals (Lipowitz *et al.*, 1979; Madewell and Pool, 1978), and both reports deal primarily with synovial sarcomas of canine joints. The World Health Organization classification of the tumors of bones and joints of animals provides a brief description of the main features of only three putative types of synovial tumors: synovial sarcoma, fibroxanthoma (fibrous histiocytoma), and the malignant giant cell tumor of soft tissue (Misdorp and Van der Heul, 1976). An attempt will be made here to describe this uncommon group of lesions by relying on personal experience with original case material and on published case reports.

## GENERAL CONSIDERATIONS

### Diagnostic Considerations

To reach a correct diagnosis the pathologist must review and correlate the clinical, radiographic, and pathological findings in the case. Many synovial tumors go unrecognized as such for two reasons. First, the exact anatomical location of the lesion is not determined by careful dissection at time of biopsy or surgical extirpation, and second, most pathologists are unfamiliar with the variety of histological patterns produced by these tumors.

### Clinical Characteristics

Synovial tumors typically present as solitary lesions in older animals. They may be confused on clinical examination with a resolving infection, an organizing hematoma, synovial osteochondromatosis, tumoral calcinosis, or one of the idiopathic proliferative lesions of the synovium affecting a tendon sheath or a joint. Anatomical location of the lesion and the species of the animal affected are important diagnostic considerations. For example, villonodular synovitis affects only the metacarpophalangeal joint of racing thoroughbreds or quarter horses. Benign synovial tumors of tendons and tendon sheaths primarily involve the extensor and flexor tendons of the distal part of the limbs of dogs and cats, whereas malignant synovial tumors of joints occur mainly in the large weight-bearing joints of canine limbs.

### Radiographic Evaluation

Radiographic examination using at least two views is helpful in accessing the approximate size and location of the lesion. The examination usually distinguishes between a tumor centered in a joint and one in a tendon sheath. It will indicate the extent and character of the disturbance in adjacent bony tissue. Sequential radiographs are helpful in estimating the rate of growth of the synovial tumor. Benign synovial lesions involving bone organs evoke "nonaggressive" radiographic signs (Morgan, 1979). For example, villonodular synovitis of horses produces a characteristic abruptly bordered depression in the dorsal cortex of the distal end of the cannon bone at the insertion line of the joint capsule of the fetlock joint. Malignant tumors of joints usually produce "aggressive" radiographic signs of bone destruction (Morgan, 1979) and are first detected as indistinct areas of osteolysis along the joint capsule insertion lines in the ends of bones on both sides of a diarthrodial joint. Radiographs may not distinguish, however, between primary and metastatic tumors of joints or tendon sheaths.

### Pathological Considerations

Knowledge of the exact anatomical location of a synovial tumor may be critical for making a definitive diagnosis because microscopic patterns of synovial tumors may mimic those of other soft tissue neoplasms. Pathologists must rely on the observations of the surgeon who resected the mass or must carefully dissect out the lesion themselves. It should also be remembered that certain members of this group of tumors may arise in unexpected sites. For example, synovial tumors may arise in intermuscular fasciae unassociated with joints and tendon sheaths (Hale and Calder, 1970; Roth *et al.,* 1975). In support of this finding, Ackerman and Rosai (1974) stated that most synovial sarcomas of humans do not arise from synovial cells but rather from mesenchymal cells with the capacity to differentiate into synovioblasts.

To fully appreciate the assortment of histological patterns one encounters in the examination of tumors and tumorlike lesions of joints and related structures, the pathologist should be familiar with the microscopic appearance of joints, tendons and tendon sheaths, bursae, ligaments, fasciae, and adjacent soft tissues in animals of all age groups. Synoviocytes not only line the surface of synovial membranes, but they are also the most common cell type found in the subsynovial tissue (fig. 4.1). Cells with light and electron microscopic features of synoviocytes are also found in intermuscular fascia and in the interfascicular framework of muscles, tendons, and ligaments where they produce proteoglycan which provides the suppleness of these soft tissues. In response to trauma, chronic irritation, and other nonspecific influences, this cell population may undergo metaplasia to form fibrous tissue and cartilage. Fibrocytes of tendons and ligaments commonly undergo metaplasia to produce chondroid tissue within tendons, ligaments, and the fibrous layer of joint capsules that have been subjected to chronic trauma or degenerative joint diseases. Synovial chondromas arise from metaplasia of synoviocytes in the synovial lining of joints with chronic degenerative joint disease. Some chondrosarcomas arising in soft tissues possibly originate in nests of metaplastic chondrocytes.

## BENIGN TUMORS AND TUMORLIKE LESIONS IN AND AROUND JOINTS

These lesions are uncommon and their clinicopathological features are incompletely characterized in domestic animals. The animal lesions are generally named after human disorders perceived to be their analogs. This classification procedure has two

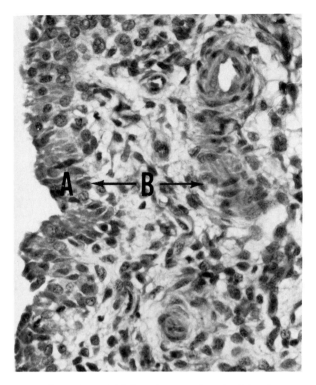

**FIGURE 4.1.** Synovial lining of a normal equine joint. Synoviocytes not only line the intimal layer (A) of the synovial membrane, but they are also the most common cell type in the subintimal layer (B).

### TABLE 4.1. Benign Tumors and Tumorlike Lesions In and Around Joints of Domestic Animals

Benign synovioma
Idiopathic proliferative lesions of the synovium
    Pigmented villonodular synovitis of joints
    Localized nodular synovitis of joints
    Villonodular synovitis of the equine metacarpo-
        phalangeal joint
    Localized nodular tenosynovitis
    Benign giant cell tumor of tendons and tendon sheaths
    Fibroma of tendons and tendon sheaths
    Metabolic disorders of the synovium
    "Myxoma" of the synovium
Synovial hemangioma of horses
Synovial chondroma and osteochondroma
Tumoral calcinosis
Ganglia, synovial cysts, and adventitious bursitis
Heterotopic, metaplastic, and reactive bone formation in soft
    tissues
Fibrotic myopathy and ossifying myopathy of horses
Localized myositis ossificans of the dog and cat
Generalized myositis ossificans of the pig and cat

defects. First, the nomenclature for this group of human lesions has not been standardized (Ackerman and Rosai, 1974; Fechner, 1976; Lattes, 1982), and second, appropriate detailed comparative studies of the morphology and biological behavior of these lesions have not been done. In this section the author has attempted, where applicable, to follow the morphological criteria used for the diagnosis of comparable disease processes in humans (Ackerman and Rosai, 1974; Fechner, 1976; Lattes, 1982; Spjut *et al.*, 1971). The benign tumors and reactive lesions covered in this chapter are given in table 4.1.

## Benign Synovioma

Tumorlike nodules occasionally found in the joint capsule of the human knee joint are regarded as foci of reactive synovial hyperplasia. Microscopically, these lesions are composed of complex, slitlike cavities lined by hyperplastic, but otherwise normal, synovial cells. Lining cells are supported by well-differentiated fibrous tissue usually infiltrated with chronic inflammatory cells. The use of the term *benign synovioma* for these lesions is discouraged in human medicine (Lattes, 1982).

Benign synoviomas also probably do not exist in domestic animals (Misdorp and Van der Heul, 1976). We have seen a number of focal soft tissue masses occurring in the synovium of joints and tendon sheaths of horses, dogs, and goats that resemble the tumorlike synovial nodules of humans. The infrapatellar pouch of the stifle joint is a common location for such lesions in dogs (fig. 4.2). On histological examination, these "tumors" include foci of chronic synovitis, foci of villous hyperplasia without a major inflammatory cell response, and hematomas in varying stages of organization. Additional benign lesions to be considered in a differential diagnosis are listed in table 4.1.

## Idiopathic Proliferative Lesions of the Synovium

The synovium is a complex tissue composed of synoviocytes arising from synovioblastic mesenchyme and of supporting subsynovial soft tissues such as blood vessels, nerves, fat cells, and fibroblasts. Well-differentiated benign tumors (e.g., hemangiomas, Schwannomas, lipomas, and fibromas) may arise from the supporting cell population. Tumors of supporting tissue have the same morphological appearance and clinical behavior as tumors arising in other soft tissue sites. Although benign tumors of subsynovial soft tissues are apparently rare in animals, their origin in subsynovial tissue most likely goes unrecognized unless the lesion is carefully dissected. By contrast, idiopathic proliferative responses and tumors and the synovium arise only from cells of synovioblastic mesenchyme, and the synovial origin of these lesions is more apparent because of their unique morphology.

## Villonodular Synovitis of Joints and Tendon Sheaths

**General Considerations.** This disorder produces a diffuse pigmented villonodular lesion or a localized nodular lesion in the joint capsule of a

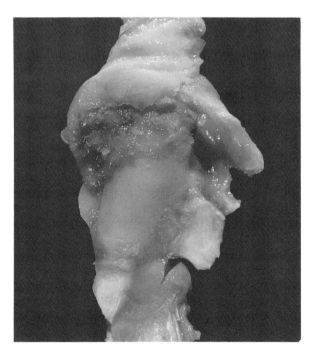

**FIGURE 4.2.** Tumorlike lesion of chronic synovial hyperplasia in the infrapatellar pouch of a canine stifle joint. The term *benign synovioma* should not be used for these reactive lesions.

knee, ankle, hip, or shoulder joint, or a localized nodular lesion in a tendon sheath (i.e., nodular tenosynovitis) in the hands or feet of young adults or middle-aged persons (Ackerman and Rosai, 1974). A lesion of nodular tenosynovitis (also called localized villonodular tenosynovitis, giant cell tumor of the tendon sheath, benign giant cell tumor of soft tissue, or xanthofibroma) may be attached to a tendon, to a tendon sheath, or to muscle fascia. It may also arise in deep fibrous tissue (Lattes, 1982).

Grossly, the diffuse lesion is a brown, papillary spongy mass with nodular areas, and it derives its color from hemosiderin pigment. The solitary lesions are nodular and lobulated and may also have brown pigmentation.

Histologically, the diffuse and solitary lesions are similar except for the prominence of villous structures in the diffuse lesion of joints. Papillary projections and fibrous tissue are intermixed with a pleomorphic population of synoviocytes, foamy cells, and hemosiderin-laden macrophages. Mitotic figures are easily found in the proliferating synoviocytes, and multinucleated giant cells are invariably present (Fechner, 1976).

Clinically, there is swelling, pain, and limitation of motion of the affected part. Erosion of adjacent bony structures may occur. Treatment involves surgical excision, but local recurrence is a frequent problem (Spjut *et al.*, 1971). Progression to malignancy does not occur (Ackerman and Rosai, 1974).

The etiology of this disorder is unknown (Spjut *et al.*, 1971). Lack of understanding of the nature of this disorder causes a dilemma in classifying the lesion in humans. Certain pathologists believe that these synovial lesions in and around joints and tendon sheaths of humans are reactions to repeated synovial trauma and bleeding (Jaffee *et al.*, 1941; Spjut *et al.*, 1971). This opinion is supported in part by the production of similar lesions in the stifle joints of dogs and rabbits following repeated injections of fresh blood or saline (Roy and Ghadially, 1969; Young and Hadacek, 1954). Unlike the natural disease, however, experimental lesions regress following cessation of injections (Collins, 1951). Other pathologists have begun to consider these lesions to be a variant of benign fibrous histiocytoma (Ackerman and Rosai, 1974; Lattes, 1982). Ackerman and Rosai (1974) reviewed the hypotheses regarding tumors of probable histiocytic origin and devised a classification scheme in which these synovial lesions are included. Lattes (1982) referred to the localized nodular lesions of villonodular synovitis occurring in and around joints and tendon sheaths as "benign giant cell tumors of soft tissue." He indicated that the diffuse villonodular lesion of joints known as pigmented villonodular synovitis is a variant of benign fibrous histiocytoma involving a larger surface area of the synovium and having features of granulomatous inflammation.

### Pigmented Villonodular Synovitis of Joints

**Classification.** It is undetermined whether this lesion in animals is a reaction to chronic injury and hemarthrosis or whether it is a benign tumor, that is, a variant of benign fibrous histiocytoma. On the basis of the few cases examined by the author, the lesion in animals appears to be a unique synovial response and possibly a variant of fibrous histiocytoma.

**Incidence, Age, Breed, and Sex.** The author could find no published reports describing the spontaneous disease in animals. We have seen what we consider to be animal analogs of this disease in older dogs of both sexes from large and medium breeds. One putative lesion arose in the hock joint of an old male goat.

**Clinical Characteristics.** The lesion is first recognized because of joint distention or gradual onset of lameness. The affected joint is not initially warm or painful. Later, if there has been bony erosion along joint margins, pain due to joint instability may be recognized. The cases we have examined were initially thought to be examples of very low grade synovial sarcomas. In one older dog long-term "cure" followed limb amputation. The goat with this lesion was destroyed because of marked lameness brought about by chronic degenerative joint disease affecting several joints, including the joint with the synovial lesion.

**Sites.** Pigmented villonodular synovitis may potentially occur in any major weight-bearing joint. In dogs three lesions were in hip joints, two in stifle joints, and one in the antebrachiocarpal joint. The caprine lesion was located in a hock joint.

**Gross Morphology.** Most of the synovium of the joint was replaced by a thick, tan to dark brown, shaggy mat of villi. Amber-colored joint fluid was excessive in amount but retained its normal viscosity. In two dogs the abnormal synovial tissue produced superficial erosions in the femoral neck along the joint capsule insertion line. Bone erosion was not apparent in the other canine lesions. While all of the affected canine joints had mild gross changes of degenerative joint disease, similar degenerative changes were also present in the same joint of the opposite leg. In the goat, however, pigmented villonodular synovitis occurred in a hock joint affected with severe chronic degenerative joint disease. Marked fibrosis of the joint capsule and chronic adhesive tenosynovitis of the flexor tendons caudal to the hock joint suggested that joint infection probably preceded the development of the degenerative joint disease. The role, if any, that severe degenerative joint disease played in the development of pigmented villonodular synovitis in this joint was undetermined.

**Radiographic Appearance.** Several small and smoothly contoured erosions were present in the cortical surface of the femoral neck along the joint capsule insertion line of the hip joints in two canine cases. Periarticular bone destruction was a more prominent feature in the tarsus of the goat. All affected joints that were radiographed showed distention of the joint capsule.

**Histological Features.** The affected synovium is several times greater than the normal thickness (fig. 4.3A). Most surfaces are covered by complex villous formation, while in other areas fused villi form a nodular surface. Deep areas have either a solid pattern or a pattern with numerous irregular slits lined by synovial cells. The subsynovial cells are isochromic and without anaplastic features (fig. 4.3B). Mitotic figures are occasionally found by searching for them. Many synovial cells are ovoid, whether located on a surface or within the stroma, and some histiocytelike synoviocytes contain fine granules of hemosiderin in their cytoplasm (fig. 4.3C). Other synovial cells located within the stroma have a fusiform shape and cannot always be distinguished from fibroblasts. Binucleate synoviocytes are not uncommon. A few multinucleated giant cells appearing to arise from the fusion of synovial cells are present within the depths of the lesion. Macrophages, some of which are filled with hemosiderin, and small lymphocytes are scattered diffusely in small numbers throughout the lesion. Occasionally,

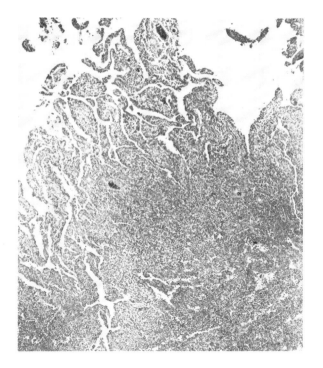

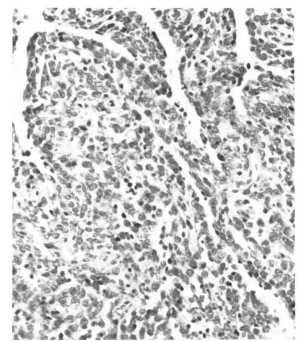

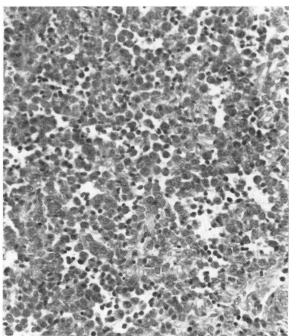

A|B
C| **FIGURE 4.3.** Pigmented villonodular synovitis in the antebrachiocarpal joint of a dog. A. Hyperplastic synovium having a villous surface and both solid and slitlike patterns in deep tissues. B. Villi and clefts lined by synoviocytes. Subintimal synoviocytes and stromal cells are without anaplastic features. C. Solid area of subintima is populated by numerous large synoviocytes resembling histiocytes and by small lymphocytes.

both types of inflammatory cells will form in dense clusters, especially at the border of the lesion. Proliferative synoviocytes spread into the fibrous layer of the joint capsule. They do not, however, extend beyond the joint capsule and do not invade the adjacent soft tissues in the specimens that we have examined. In some cases the synovial response enters vascular channels in the periarticular bone along joint capsule insertion lines and mediates bone resorption by osteoclasts.

Differential diagnosis would include chronic infectious synovitis, synovitis in response to hemarthrosis, reactive synovitis in response to osteoarthrosis, and low-grade synovial sarcoma.

**Growth and Metastasis.** These are proliferative lesions that demonstrate slow but progressive enlargement. In humans these lesions do not undergo malignant progression and do not metastasize (Ackerman and Rosai, 1974). In none of the animal lesions was there evidence of local vessel invasion or metastasis to local lymph nodes or to internal body organs. Long-term follow-up was available in only one case, a dog with pigmented villonodular synovitis of the hip joint. This dog was without local or systemic recurrence 6 years following amputation at the hip joint.

## Localized Nodular Synovitis of Joints

Animal analogs of this human disorder have not been reported. The only purported example of this human disease is villonodular synovitis of the equine metacarpophalangeal joint (discussed in the following section). The author believes that this unique equine lesion is a synovial reaction to chronic trauma and is not a variant of fibrous histiocytoma, as has been proposed for humans (Ackerman and Rosai, 1974; Lattes, 1982).

## Villonodular Synovitis of the Equine Metacarpophalangeal Joint

**Classification.** This condition is thought to be a chronic, reactive, inflammatory response of the synovium resulting from trauma (Nickels *et al.,* 1976). It more closely resembles "green osselets" (Adams, 1974; Rooney, 1974) of horses than localized nodular synovitis of human joints, considered by some to be a variant of benign fibrous histiocytoma (Ackerman and Rosai, 1974; Lattes, 1982).

**Incidence, Age, Breed, and Sex.** This condition was first reported in the literature in 1976 (Nickels *et al.,* 1976), and since then, several cases per year are seen in any busy equine clinic treating race horses. Lesions are more commonly seen in racing thoroughbreds than in racing quarter horses. Nickels *et al.* (1976) reported that both sexes are affected equally and that the horses range in age from 2 to 13 years.

**Clinical Characteristics.** Horses are presented because of a soft tissue swelling over the dorsal surface of the distal end of the third metacarpal bone. The fetlock joint is distended and stiff. The degree of pain and lameness is accentuated when the joint is flexed and the horse is made to jog. In many cases prior to diagnosis, the joint has been treated unsuccessfully by firing, blistering, intraarticular injections of corticosteroids, and rest.

**Gross Morphology.** Lesions vary greatly in size and appearance, but all are centered on a synovial pad of fibrous and adipose tissue located between the dorsal articular margin of the distal end of the third metacarpal bone and the proximal insertion line of the fetlock joint capsule on the distal end of that bone. The lesion appears to be caused by trauma when the pad is struck by the dorsal articular margin of the first phalanx during excessive dorsiflexion of the fetlock joint. We have seen large lesions of a relatively short duration having the gross appearance of an organizing hematoma of the synovial pad. Most lesions are pale, rubbery, lobulated, and pedunculated (fig. 4.4A). They may involve the envire synovial pad or be located only on one side of the midline. In our experience many lesions are located on the medial side of the sagittal ridge of the cannon bone. The traumatized synovial pad with its pedunculated mass will often extend over the articular margin. When the lesion is removed, the underlying articular cartilage is pitted and the surface of the dorsal cortex of the cannon bone is eroded.

**Radiographic Appearance.** The characteristic finding is a smoothly contoured erosion in the dorsal cortex of the distal end of the third metacarpal bone located just proximal to the articular margin. An intraarticular soft tissue mass centered in the proximal recess of the dorsal part of the fetlock joint can be demonstrated by positive contrast arthrography.

**Histological Features.** Microscopic appearance varies with the duration of the lesion. Acute lesions may have the features of an organizing hematoma. In these cases immature granulation arising from the traumatized synovial pad invades the borders of the hematoma. Hemosiderin-laden macrophages are prominent. Subacute lesions (fig. 4.4B) still have areas of necrosis and organizing hematoma, but the granulation tissue is orderly and mature. Chronic lesions are composed primarily of poorly vascularized, dense, irregular fibrous tissue covered on the joint surface by a thin layer of synoviocytes. Inflammatory cells are invariably present, but their numbers and types are reflections of the size and duration of the lesion on the traumatized synovial pad. Large numbers of histiocytes are not present and multinucleated giant cells have not been observed.

**Growth and Metastasis.** Most of these lesions enlarge over a period of a few weeks. Lesions with a history of rapid growth over a few days usually result from a hematoma. These lesions appear to have a traumatic basis. There is no morphological evidence of neoplasia. Excision of the mass appears to

ance presented by the giant cell population. Until proper studies are done, however, the well-recognized caution in attempts to grade giant cell tumors of bone (Spjut *et al.,* 1971) should also pertain to giant cell tumors of tendons and tendon sheaths.

**Growth and Metastasis.** Individual tumors will vary in their rate of growth after first recognition. These tumors are not believed to have metastatic potential nor are they considered to undergo continuous malignant progression. Too few cases, however, have been followed closely to make that assumption with confidence. The major clinical problem is local recurrence following attempts at surgical removal.

## Fibroma of Tendons and Tendon Sheaths

**Classification.** Solitary or multiple, discretely bordered nodular masses of dense fibrous tissue resembling fibromas of the dermis and subcutis of animals (Stannard and Pulley, 1978) may arise from mesenchyme in the paratendon or tendon sheath. These tumors have been described in humans (Flynn, 1975) and in the horse (Adams *et al.,* 1982). Whether these are unique tumors or sclerotized variants of localized nodular tenosynovitis has not been determined.

**Incidence, Age, Breed, and Sex.** These uncommon lesions have been described in two immature quarter horse fillies (Adams *et al.,* 1982). Our series also includes three fibromas of tendons occurring in a 4-year-old male Welsh Corgi dog.

**Clinical Characteristics.** Fibromas of tendons or tendon sheaths demonstrate slow but progressive enlargement over a period of several months. They may cease growth and remain asymptomatic. An animal may have more than one fibroma affecting the same tendon, or solitary fibromas may affect tendons of different legs in the same animal. These nodules are typically first discovered during grooming of the animal. Skin over the lesion is normal and freely movable. Fibromas are firm but are not warm or painful to palpation. They do not cause lameness. Their major importance is that of a blemish.

None of the three fibromas in the dog recurred following surgical removal.

Incomplete removal of tendon fibromas on the dorsomedial surface of the hock of one horse was followed by regrowth of the lesion to its original size during the course of a year. However, no further enlargement of the recurrent tumor mass or lameness subsequently occurred. The second horse returned to racing 7 months after surgical removal of a solitary tendon fibroma on a foreleg. The tumor did not recur.

**Sites.** Extensor tendons at the level of the carpus and tarsus were affected in two horses. The Welsh Corgi had three separate fibromas, two involving the digital branches of the extensor tendon lying over the metacarpus of a forefoot and one involving the Achilles tendon of a hindleg.

**Gross Morphology.** Fibromas have distinct borders and may appear to have a fibrous capsule. They are not firmly attached to adjacent soft tissue structures. Tumors are ovoid to fusiform in shape. In one horse with multiple tendon fibromas the nodules varied from 2 to 4 cm in diameter. The solitary nodule in the second horse measured 3.5 × 5.5 cm. The largest of the three nodules in the dog was 1.5 cm in diameter. On cut surface the tumor tissue is white, firm, and solid.

In horses the fibromas were so firmly attached to the tendon that the tumor could not be removed without causing tendon damage. All three tendon fibromas in the dog were freed from their tendon attachment by blunt dissection. While none of the fibromas had cavitations, canine tendon fibromas appeared to have remnants of synovial lining between tendon attachment sites.

**Radiographic Appearance.** Tendon fibromas produce nodular soft tissue masses. In one horse (Adams *et al.,* 1982) a tendon fibroma caused a depression in the cortex of the underlying radius.

**Histological Features.** These discretely bordered nodular tumors consist of solid masses of dense fibrous tissue having a low capillary density. In some lesions a histological pattern of coarse interwoven bundles of dense collagenous tissue predominates. Entrapped cells are mostly mature spindle-shaped fibroblasts. In other lesions (figs. 4.8A and B) polygonal and fusiform cells are set in unpatterned fields of dense fibrous tissue. While cleft formation was not observed within the tendon fibromas of the horse and dog, remnants of a synovial surface, probably the lining of a synovial sheath, were pres-

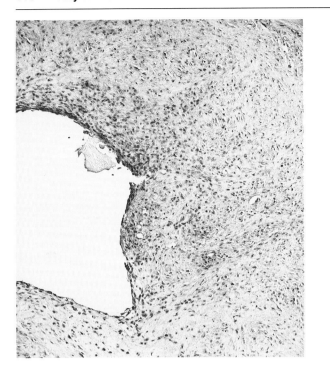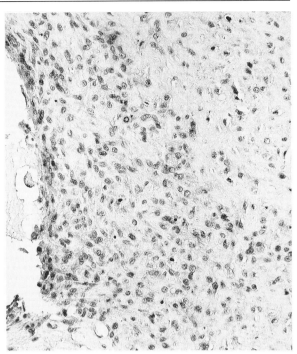

A | B    **FIGURE 4.8.** Fibroma of a tendon sheath of a dog. A. Solid mass of unpatterned dense fibrous tissue lined by synovium. B. Polygonal and fusiform tumor cells are without anaplastic features and some resemble synovial lining cells.

ent in cross sections through the canine fibromas. No synoviocytes, hemosiderin-laden macrophages, xanthoid cells, multinucleated giant cells, or adipose cells were recognized within the tumor masses. Inflammatory cells were also absent in these lesions.

A differential diagnosis would include a fibrosed lipoma, a sclerotic variant of localized nodular tenosynovitis, a sclerotic Schwannoma, or a healed focal area of chronic tendon injury or infection.

**Growth and Metastasis.** Fibromas of tendons and tendon sheaths typically show slow progressive growth over a period of months and then maintain their size and shape indefinitely. Since these nodular tumors do not produce lameness, their importance is as a blemish. Total surgical excision of a fibroma may not be possible without producing a substantial disruption of the tendon, as was the case in one horse (Adams *et al.*, 1982). Incomplete re-

moval of the tendon fibroma was followed by local regrowth of the nodule to its original size over a period of a few months. In the Welsh Corgi described here and in one horse (Adams *et al.*, 1982) surgical removal was curative. No malignant change was encountered in any of the fibromas.

## Metabolic Disorders of the Synovium

Biopsy tissues have been examined from several dogs with slowly progressive lameness centered in either a solitary joint or a pair of major limb joints. The dogs were of different breeds, including a standard poodle, a Doberman pinscher, an Irish setter, and a Labrador retriever. Both sexes were represented. The joints were not warm or very painful on palpation, but were distended with joint fluid of

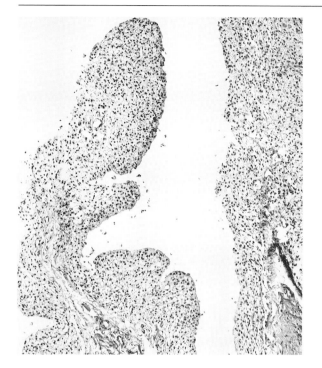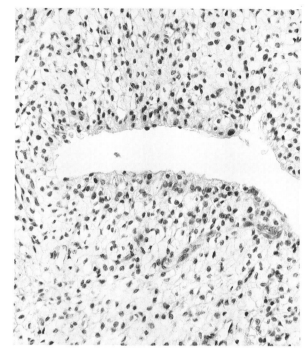

A|B   **FIGURE 4.9.** Metabolic disorder of the synovium in the elbow joint of a dog. A. Hypertrophic villus of joint is heavily infiltrated with foamy cells. B. Foamy cells fill the subintima of the synovium.

normal color and consistency. During arthrotomy to obtain an excisional biopsy, the clinicians observed marked villous hyperplasia of synovium in affected joints. Bilateral elbow joint disease in the poodle was progressive over a 2-year period, and the dog was euthanized without a necropsy or gross examination of the elbow joints. The Doberman pinscher and the Irish setter were lost to follow-up. The Labrador retriever was the only immature dog in this group, and he was necropsied because marked epiphyseal dysplasia affected all major epiphyses of the long bones.

The histological appearance of the synovium varied among the several cases, but all affected joints had a thickened synovium with villous hypertrophy. The synovium was distended by a localized proliferation of pale, foamy cells, presumably synoviocytes (figs. 4.9A and B). Inflammatory cells and multinucleated giant cells were absent. The cases differed primarily in the morphological appearance of the foamy synoviocytes. These differences included the location of the nucleus in the cell, the number and size of the cytoplasmic vacuoles, and whether there was granular material present within the cytoplasm. In the puppy with epiphyseal dysplasia the pale granular material occurring in the foamy cytoplasm of synoviocytes was also present in chrondrocytes of the deformed epiphyses. No similar foamy cells were present in lymph nodes draining the appendicular skeleton or in the bone marrow of this dog.

While we do not know the cause of these synovial lesions and can only assume that they have a metabolic basis, our intention in presenting them here is for a differential diagnosis for synovial tumors.

## Myxoma of the Synovium

**Classification.** We have observed a morphologically unique lesion centered in the synovial linings of joints from three dogs. This lesion does not seem to belong to any of the existing categories of tumors or tumorlike conditions of animal joints. We have used the term *myxoma of the synovium* to identify this disorder until more is learned about the nature of this condition. The term *myxoma* reflects both the gross and microscopic appearance of the lesion and its biological behavior.

**Incidence, Age, Breed, and Sex.** A recent review of the tumors of soft tissues in humans (Lattes, 1982) did not include a comparable entity. We can find no previous reports of this condition in animals.

Myxoma of the synovium was found in synovial joints of three dogs. The affected dogs included a mature male Doberman pinscher, a 16-year-old spayed female Doberman pinscher, and a 9-year-old spayed female English spaniel.

**Clinical Characteristics.** In two cases the tumors produced cool, initially painless swellings that apparently caused mechanical lameness. In both of these Doberman pinscher dogs, the synovial tumors involved a single stifle joint. In the mature male dog, synovectomy of the affected femoropatellar joint sac was apparently curative. Within a few months after surgery, the dog resumed its daily jogging routine with its owner. No local or systemic disease has been observed in 2 years since surgery. The stifle lesion in the older female Doberman was locally infiltrative and resulted in limb amputation. No local recurrence at the amputation stump or metastatic disease was found at necropsy a short time later.

The tumor in the English spaniel arose in ipsolateral apophyseal (synovial) joints of the second and third cervical vertebrae. Lesions in this case did not produce signs and were discovered during a general necropsy for an unrelated condition. Tumor tissue had infiltrated beyond the joint capsule and had extended into adjacent muscle fascia making surgical extirpation impossible.

**Sites.** Tumors affected a stifle joint from each of two dogs and involved two adjacent ipsolateral apophyseal joints of C-2 and C-3 in the cervical spine of a third dog.

**Gross Morphology.** Myxomas of the synovium were composed of multiple nodules of pale gelatinous tissue that replaced the synovial lining of the affected joints (fig. 4.10A). There was no destruction of articular cartilage or of the joint margins. Joint fluid was excessive in amount but normal in color and consistency. In two cases the myxoid tumor tissue was observed to extend beyond the fibrous layer of the joint capsule and to infiltrate along fascial planes of adjacent musculature.

**Radiographic Appearance.** There was no radiographic evidence of destruction of joint margins or periarticular new bone formation.

**Histological Features.** Most of the normal synovial architecture is replaced by pale, poorly vascularized myxoid nodules (fig. 4.10B). These nodules are formed by stellate mesenchymal cells set in a loose matrix of delicate collagen fibrils and a large volume of proteoglycan. Large nodules arise by coalescence of smaller nodules. Cellularity and density of collagen fibrils increase at the borders of intrasynovial nodules. Once the tumor penetrates beyond the fibrous layer of the joint capsule, however, the border of the neoplasm is indistinct and tumor tissue extends along fascial planes. In parts of the synovium not replaced by myxoid nodules, the synovium is infiltrated with clusters of macrophages and other mononuclear inflammatory cells (fig. 4.10C). This inflammatory response was a striking feature in the synovium of the male Doberman pinscher whose joint was successfully treated by synovectomy.

Lattes (1982) indicated that true myxomas must be differentiated from areas of myxomatous change in Schwannomas, liposarcomas, rhabdomyosarcomas, mesenchymomas, and fibrous tumors. He pointed out that a true myxoma has a striking paucity of vessels. He also indicated that in the areas of secondary fibrosis that may occur in a true myxoma most of the tumor cells will retain their stellate shape. Both of these requirements for a diagnosis of myxoma were met in these canine neoplasms.

**Growth and Metastasis.** Growth is slow but progressive. Once tumor tissue has extended beyond the fibrous layer of the joint capsule, it infiltrates along muscle fascial planes. In one case synovectomy appeared to be curative possibly because tumor tissue was still confined to the synovial lining and was removed along with the synovial membrane. Local recurrence should be anticipated and

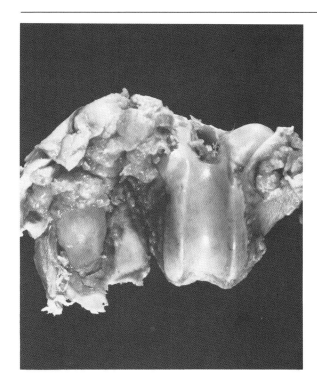

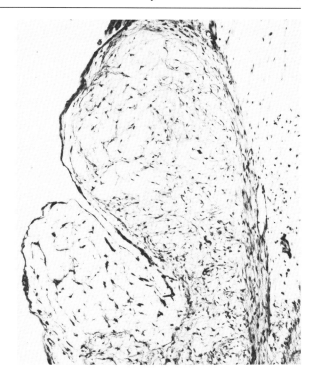

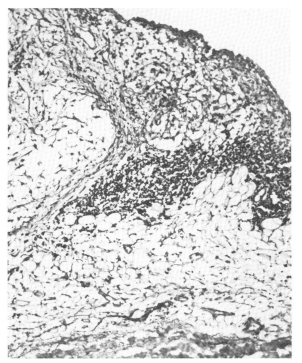

A|B
C|

**FIGURE 4.10.** "Myxoma" of the synovium of a canine stifle joint. A. Multinodular, pale gelatinous tissue replaces the normal synovial membrane. Note lack of articular cartilage destruction. B. Normal synovial subintima is replaced by nodular aggregations of poorly vascularized mucoid connective tissue. C. Area of chronic lymphocytic inflammation in a synovial myxoma.

amputation should be considered in advanced cases. Metastases in true myxomas are exceedingly rare in humans (Lattes, 1982). We anticipate that the metastatic potential for these canine lesions is also low.

## Synovial Hemangioma in the Tendon Sheath of the Horse

These are solitary vascular lesions centered in the recesses of tendon sheaths of horses. It has not been determined whether these lesions are true hemangiomas or are developmental defects of the blood vascular system, that is, vascular hamartomas. Heman-

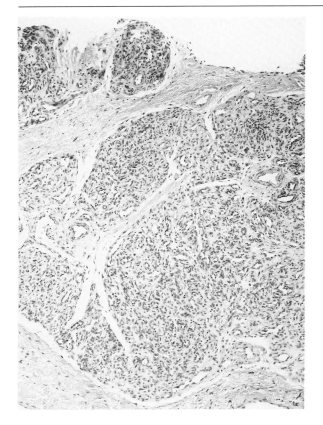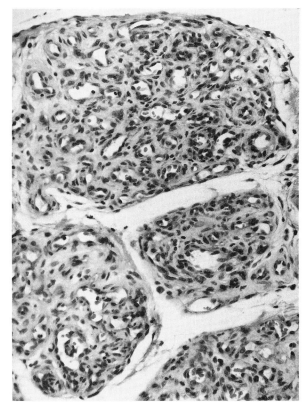

A|B    **FIGURE 4.11.** Synovial hemangioma of a tendon sheath. A. Sessile tumor is covered by flattened synovial lining cells (top). Nodular clusters of vessels are separated by thin septa of mature fibrous tissue. B. Endothelial cells are without anaplastic features, and there is no fibroplasia in the supporting stroma.

giomas have been reported to occur in the tendon sheaths of humans (Rodnan, 1966).

We have observed this condition in the carpal and digital sheaths of forelegs of immature horses. Multiple lesions of tendon sheaths were not present in these animals. Affected breeds included an American quarter horse, an American saddle horse, and an Arabian horse.

The condition was recognized because of filling of the affected sheaths with a blood-stained fluid. No pain or lameness was evident. Surgical removal was attempted but severe bleeding was a major problem.

On surgical exploration of the tendon sheath, the tumor appeared as a solitary, deep red, multi-

nodular structure that arose in the synovial lining of a recess in the tendon sheath. Clotted blood sometimes adhered to the surface of the tumor. Bleeding into the sheath was apparently due to the trauma of locomotion.

Microscopic examination shows that well-differentiated small caliber vessels tend to grow in nodular aggregations mimicking glomerular tufts (figs. 4.11A and B). Vascular nodules are randomly separated by septae of mature fibrous tissue. Endothelial cells lining the vessel walls do not have anaplastic features. Mitotic figures are uncommon.

These vascular lesions appear to be benign. They exhibit little or no enlargement after being recognized and do not appear to locally infiltrate the tendon sheath. Their major importance is their tendency to bleed into the tendon sheath and keep it distended. Surgical removal is difficult because of the tumor location and the problem in controlling hemorrhage.

## Synovial Chondroma and Synovial Osteochondroma

**Classification.** Synovial chondromas are metaplastic nodules of hyaline cartilage that develop in the synovial linings of bursae, tendon sheaths, and synovial joints. The stimulus for the metaplastic transformation of synovial cells into chondrocytes is unknown (Jeffreys, 1967). Synovial osteochondromas are synovial chondromas that have undergone endochondral ossification.

Synovial chondromatosis is a condition in which the synovial lining of a bursa, tendon sheath, or joint has numerous synovial chondromas. If the majority of these metaplastic cartilage nodules have undergone bony replacement, the term *synovial osteochondromatosis* should be used to describe the lesion.

In humans it is unclear whether synovial chondromatosis is a true neoplastic disease (Smith, 1977) or whether synovial chondromas develop secondary to trauma, chronic irritation, inflammation, or other disturbances of the synovium (Jeffreys, 1967; Spjut *et al.,* 1971). Primary (i.e., idiopathic) and secondary forms of the disorder occur in animals, with the secondary form being the more common condition.

**Incidence, Age, Breed, and Sex.** Primary synovial chondromatosis and osteochondromatosis are rarely encounted in animals. One case involved the femorotibial bursa of a 16-year-old quarter horse mare (Kirk, 1982). We have seen a 5-month-old Arabian colt with synovial osteochondromatosis of both stifle joints. In humans the condition is twice as common in males as in females.

Lesions of secondary synovial chondromatosis and synovial osteochondromatosis are commonly encountered as incidental findings at necropsy in major limb joints of older horses and dogs affected with chronic secondary osteoarthritis. Sex and breed do not appear to be important factors in the secondary form of the disorder.

**Clinical Characteristics.** Neither horse with primary synovial osteochondromatosis exhibited lameness or pain on palpation of the affected structures. Lesions were recognized by local enlargement of the synovial structure that resulted primarily from increased amounts of synovial fluid and palpation of firm, nodular masses. Potential for creating painful or mechanical lameness exists. Treatment in the horse with involvement of the femorotibial bursa (Kirk, 1982) was complete surgical excision. The lesion did not recur. No treatment was attempted in the young Arabian colt because there was extensive involvement of both stifle joints and because the femoropatellar pouches of the horse are not accessible to the surgeon for the extensive exposure that was required for this case.

In contrast to animals, affected humans experience pain and limitation of motion. Synovial resection is the treatment of choice for humans (Smith, 1977) and is probably the appropriate therapy for symptomatic lesions in animals. Local recurrence is a problem in human cases (Smith, 1977) and should be anticipated in animals since new nodules may continue to develop in the synovium.

Animals with the more common secondary form of the disorder often have pain, lameness, and limitation of motion probably resulting from chronic degenerative joint disease. The nodular lesions (i.e., synovial chondromas or synovial osteochondromas) may be trapped between articular surfaces or break free to become joint bodies and produce painful or mechanical lameness. Surgeons may not recognize the origin of these lesions and may consider them to be loose fragments of articular cartilage. Surgical removal of the attached nodules or free joint bodies may give temporary relief, but will not alter the predisposing condition.

**Sites.** Rare lesions of the primary form of synovial osteochondromatosis involved the femorotibial bursa of the left stifle region of an older horse (Kirk, 1982) and the femoropatellar synovial sacs of both stifle joints of a colt from our collection.

In the secondary form of this disorder, solitary or multiple synovial chondromas and/or synovial osteochondromas may arise in any structure lined by a chronically irritated synovium. In dogs these synovial lesions are typically found in the linings of joints with advanced secondary osteoarthritis. These would include shoulder joints having untreated lesions of osteochondrosis of the proximal humerus and elbow joints having a long-standing ununited anconeal or fragmented coronoid process. Synovial nodules and free bodies in horses are found in shoulder and stifle joints affected by chronic secondary osteoarthritis often due to osteochondrosis. Solitary osteochondromas arising in traumatized synovium along the dorsal articular margin of the metacarpophalangeal joints of the forelegs of horses are often mistaken for displaced chip fractures of the proximal end of the first phalanx. Metaplastic cartilage nodules are also found in unstable stifle joints of dogs and horses with long-standing cruciate ligament disease. They are also found in the synovial lining of any chronically irritated bursa (e.g., cases of bicipital bursitis) or in the linings of adventitious bursae.

**Gross Morphology and Radiographic Appearance.** Synovial chondromas and osteochondromas are pale hard nodules with smooth borders that are set in a thickened synovial membrane. They are small in dogs, ranging from microscopic dimensions to about 1 to 3 mm in diameter. In horses they will sometimes reach 2 cm in diameter and may appear in grapelike clusters. Large solitary nodules may be pedunculated and are attached to the synovium by a thin fibrous thread. Sometimes numerous nodules with the appearance of rice grains will be set randomly within the synovium. Both large and small nodules can become free bodies within the affected joint, sheath, or bursa. Many cases of the secondary form of this disease are missed at necropsy unless the synovial membrane is removed and examined carefully.

On radiographic examination of the affected part, the primary form of the disorder is suspected when radiodense nodules are recognized in the lining of a synovial structure in which there is no evidence of a chronic primary disease process. In the secondary form of the disorder, the radiodense nodules cannot usually be distinguished radiographically from avulsion fractures of articular cartilage in a chronic osteoarthritic joint. Tumoral calcinosis involving the femorotibial joint capsule of horses probably cannot be distinguished from synovial osteochondromatosis without a biopsy.

**Histological Features.** The diagnosis of this condition depends on the demonstration of cartilaginous metaplasia within the synovial membrane (Smith, 1977). Foci of metaplastic cartilage may

range in size from a cluster of a few chondrocytes set within a thickened synovial membrane to large pedunculated nodules covered by flattened synovial lining cells. In any given case, none, some, or most of the synovial chondromas will have undergone endochondral ossification to form synovial osteochondromas (fig. 4.12A). Actively growing chondromas are cellular. Chondrocytes grow in clusters or chondrones. Some chondrocytes will be enlarged and binucleate cells are not uncommon. These cytological features in synovial chondromas are considered to reflect active cartilage growth and are not indicative of malignancy as would be the case if these features were found in a central cartilage tumor of bone (Spjut *et al.*, 1971) (fig. 4.12B).

In synovial osteochondromas much of the original cartilage nodule may be replaced by cancellous bone. The intervening marrow spaces may contain hematopoietic cells. Like the synovial chondroma, the attached synovial osteochondroma is covered by flattened synovial lining cells.

It is usually possible to distinguish detached synovial chondromas or osteochondromas from free fragments of articular cartilage that have become separated from deteriorated joint margins of osteoarthritic joints. Metaplastic cartilage of the synovial nodules does not have the precise histological arrangement found in articular cartilage. The unique structure of articular cartilage usually remains recognizable in detached fragments of articular surfaces. Bony spicules in synovial osteochondromas do not show the arrangement and maturity of bone tissue found in subchondral bone of marginal articular fractures. In both cases the bone tissue and marrow spaces become ischemic after separation from their blood supply.

The cartilage tissue of free joint bodies originating from a detached fragment of a chronically damaged articular surface may continue to grow because cartilage derives its nutrition from joint fluid. New cartilage tissue is deposited in concentric lamellae on the original cartilage tissue by proliferation of cells lying adjacent to the surface. The deeper tissue becomes necrotic and mineralizes when nutrients cannot reach the chondrocytes by simple diffusion. Small detached articular cartilage fragments may also be entrapped by the synovium and undergo resorption by granulation tissue. It is generally recognized that synovial cartilage meta-

thors (Spjut *et al.*, 1971) believe that the lesion in humans is initiated by trauma to paraskeletal tissues including muscle. The traumatized area contains a hematoma, disrupted fascia, and damaged muscle tissue. This area undergoes a unique pattern of organization and repair having a zonal arrangement in which metaplastic bone tissue forms at the periphery of the lesion. The name of this disorder was poorly chosen since muscle tissue is not always involved, no inflammation may be present, and bone formation is a late event in the development of the lesion (Ackerman and Rosai, 1974; Spjut *et al.*, 1971). The pathologist should be aware of this disorder since a biopsy specimen containing tissue from the center of a forming lesion may be confused with osteosarcoma.

**Incidence, Age, Breed, and Sex.** This condition is thought to be uncommon based on the paucity of reports in the veterinary medical literature; however, since it is not a life-threatening disease and resolves eventually into a firm mass, few animals would be euthanized and submitted for postmortem examination because of the lesion. Liu and Dorfman (1976) reported two cases in 7- and 8-year-old male German shepherd dogs. Liu *et al.* (1974) recognized the condition in a 2-year-old female Siamese cat.

**Clinical Characteristics.** The affected animals had progressive weakness, muscle atrophy, pain, and loss of range of movement in the joints of the affected limbs. One of the dogs had a history of trauma to the affected leg about 2 months prior to presentation for this disorder. Surgical excision was not attempted in either dog (Liu and Dorfman, 1976).

The cat had similar bilateral lesions. Firm nodular swellings were palpated in the common tendon of the triceps brachii muscle just proximal to its insertion onto the olecranon process of the ulna. Neither lesion recurred following surgical removal (Liu *et al.*, 1974).

**Sites.** Both dogs had unilateral lesions involving the gluteal musculature just caudal to the femoral neck of the right hind leg (Liu and Dorfman, 1976). The cat developed bilateral nodular swellings involving the soft tissues surrounding the common tendon of the triceps brachii muscle proximal to its insertion onto the olecranon process of the ulna (Liu *et al.*, 1974).

**Gross Morphology.** The partially ossified masses removed from the gluteal musculature of the right hindlegs of both dogs measured 4.5 × 3.2 × 2.9 cm. and 24 × 6.9 × 10.8 cm, respectively (Liu and Dorfman, 1976). The larger mass had a huge central hematoma. Adjacent muscle tissue was pale and fibrotic.

In the cat the ossified masses in both forelegs measured about 1.4 × 2.5 cm, and they were centered on the soft tissues investing the common tendon of the triceps brachii muscle proximal to its insertion line on the olecranon of the ulna (Liu *et al.*, 1974).

**Radiographic Features.** A paraarticular soft tissue radiodensity was located just caudal to the femoral neck of the right femur of each dog (Liu and Dorfman, 1976). Radiographs of a necropsy specimen showed zonation in the mass with maximum radiodensity occurring at the periphery.

Radiographic studies of the cat showed radiodense masses located in the soft tissues proximal to the olecranon processes of both ulnas. Also present was a mild periosteal bony response on the left proximal ulna and a marked periosteal bony reaction on the distal humerus and proximal ulna of the right leg (Liu *et al.*, 1974).

No cortical destruction of adjacent bones was observed in any of the affected animals.

**Histological Features.** A zonal pattern was evident histologically in the lesions of the dogs (Liu and Dorfman, 1976) and the cat (Liu *et al.*, 1974). An organizing hematoma is commonly found in the center of a lesion of localized myositis ossificans. The hematoma is bordered by a highly cellular and rapidly proliferating population of mesenchymal cells. Some cells have bizarre nuclei, and they may be found in areas where osteoid and cartilage matrix are being produced. Biopsy specimens taken from this area share many histological features with osteosarcoma. The proliferative zone is covered by a more mature fibrovascular response within which the osteoid is more abundant and orderly. In the maturing lesion the mass is covered by a thin bony shell formed by anastomotic trabeculae of woven bone. Peripheral to the shell of metaplastic bone the soft tissues are fibrotic and may contain atrophic muscle fibers.

**Growth and Metastasis.** This is a rare and unique reactive lesion occurring in traumatized paraskeletal tissues. The lesion is self-limiting in humans (Spjut *et al.*, 1971) and probably also in animals. Pathologists should be aware of this lesion and distinguish it from parosteal osteosarcoma and extraosseous osteosarcoma.

## Generalized Myositis Ossificans of the Pig and Cat

**Classification.** This is a nonneoplastic disease of the supporting connective tissues of muscle organs, attachments, fasciae, and aponeuroses. It is characterized by an abnormal proliferation of primitive connective tissue elements that undergo metaplastic bone formation and produce secondary degenerative changes in muscle tissue (Adams, 1975; McKusick, 1966). Examples of this rare disorder of children have been reported in a group of related pigs (Siebold and Davis, 1967) and a domestic cat (Norris *et al.*, 1980).

The etiology of this disorder is unknown. In children there is evidence that the disease may be hereditary (Eaton *et al.*, 1957; Mair, 1932), as is the case reported in swine (Siebold and Davis, 1967). When the disease in children is recognized in the early fibroproliferative stage before ossification has begun, it is sometimes called progressive myositis fibrosa or hereditary polyfibromatosis (Lattes, 1982).

**Incidence, Age, Breed, and Sex.** The disease is rare in children and animals. Age of onset varies in children from infancy to adolescence (Adams, 1975). The boar was 9 months of age, and its 34 affected offspring ranged from 2 to 6 months of age at the time of initial onset of signs (Siebold and Davis, 1967). The breed of swine was not reported. The diseases affected both male and female pigs sired by this boar.

The female domestic long-haired cat was 10 months old at the time the disease was discovered (Norris *et al.*, 1980).

**Clinical Characteristics.** The pigs developed rapidly progressive hindleg paresis and loss of condition. Stiffness and reluctance to move accompanied the appearance and rapid growth of firm swellings in the soft tissues and musculature along the spine, hindlegs, neck, shoulders, and tarsal regions (Siebold and Davis, 1967).

The cat had a history of stiffness, pain, and progressive posterior paresis. A firm lump removed at 4 months of age from the musculature over the

thoracic vertebrae recurred 3 months later. At this time numerous masses were also recognized in the musculature of all legs and later in the musculature of the ventral abdomen and back. Popliteal lymph nodes were greatly enlarged, and there was a neutrophilia with a left shift (Norris *et al.*, 1980).

In humans only striated skeletal muscle is involved; striated muscle of the diaphragm and heart are not affected (McKusick, 1966). This also appears to be the case in the swine and the cat.

**Sites.** Location of bony masses varied in different pigs, but major sites affected in decreasing order of frequency were the musculature overlying the caudal thoracic and lumbar vertebrae, neck, shoulder, and tarsal regions (Siebold and Davis, 1967).

In the cat, musculature of the back, ventral abdomen, shoulders, forelegs, and caudal thighs contained numerous nodular masses of heterotopic bone (Norris *et al.*, 1980).

**Gross Morphology.** Lesions described in the pigs and cat are basically similar (Norris *et al.*, 1980; Siebold and Davis, 1967). There is widespread replacement of muscle tissue by masses of cancellous bone and fibrous connective tissue. It is not always possible to distinguish between an extraosseous bony mass and the adjacent bone organ since they appear to fuse at some sites.

**Histological Features.** In sites of soft tissue involvement, muscle tissue is replaced by fibrous tissue and bone. Fatty tissue and some fibrous tissue fill the marrow spaces. In sites of bone organ involvement, the masses of heterotopic bone are continuous with the bony elements of the skeleton without obvious intervening remnants of the original cortex of periosteum. The boundary can usually be recognized by the abrupt transition from hematopoietic marrow filling the marrow spaces of the bone organ to fatty marrow filling the cancellous bone spaces of the heterotopic bone (Siebold and Davis, 1967). Union of the heterotopic bone formed in the soft tissues to the adjacent bone organ apparently is the result of remodeling activities. Along the borders of the developing bony masses there are cells in the fibrous tissue response resembling fibroblasts that undergo metaplasia to osteoblasts. Soft tissues adjacent to the bony masses are fibrotic and often contain degenerating (Norris *et al.*, 1980) and atrophic (Siebold and Davis, 1967) muscle fibers.

**Growth and Metastasis.** This is a progressive, nonneoplastic, and fatal disorder of the interstitial tissue of muscle organs. McKusick (1966) reports that late in the course of the human disorder the person becomes a virtual "stone man" due to union of bony masses in different muscle groups and formation of periarticular bony bridges that prevent joint motion. Eventually death results from progressive involvement of the musculature of the thoracic cage leading to respiratory failure or fatal pneumonia. None of the animals in the two reports were permitted to live to the end stage described for humans.

## MALIGNANT TUMORS AND TUMORLIKE LESIONS IN AND AROUND JOINTS, TENDONS, AND DEEP FASCIAE

These disorders are uncommon and their clinicopathological features are incompletely characterized in animals. The animal lesions are generally named after human disorders perceived to be their analogs. This section attempts to follow the morphological criteria used for the diagnosis of comparable disease processes in humans (Ackerman and Rosai, 1974; Fechner, 1976; Lattes, 1982). The malignant tumors and tumorlike lesions covered in this chapter are given in table 4.2.

This author believes that most of the tumors and tumorlike lesions discussed in this section arise from undifferentiated mesenchyme found in the superficial and deep fasciae, synovium of joints, bursae and tendon sheaths, paratenon, and other deep connective tissues. These primitive cells are the surviving remnants of that portion of the fetal mesenchyme that underwent partial necrobiosis during the formation of cavities in joints and tendon sheaths and of fascial planes separating muscle groups. In a normal animal these cells are recognized as a nondescript population of primitive cells varying in shape from ovoid to fusiform. The cells form the major cellular component of the subsynovial tissue, paratenon, and loose connective tissue of fascia. Normally some of these cells produce proteoglycan to maintain suppleness and permit gliding movement within soft tissues. Some of the cells resemble fibroblasts and have a sustentacular role. They assume the role of synoviocytes when located in the subsynovial tissues. If the environment of this cell population becomes edematous following trauma or inflammation, many cells transform into facultative fibroblasts and produce a fibrillar matrix.

As a pathologist who looks daily at soft tissue changes caused by a variety of conditions occurring in and around the joints and attachments of lame animals, this author cannot help but reflect on the range of morphological alterations shown by perturbed cells in the subsynovial tissues of joints and tendon sheaths. We have injected a sterile irritant and carbon particles into the joints of horses and observed the ultrastructural changes in cells of the synovial lining at intervals up to 4 days. The A-synoviocytes located on the surface as well as in the subintima and bearing an ultrastructural resemblance to tissue macrophages were observed to take up carbon particles. The B-synoviocytes recognized by their ovoid shape and abundant profiles of rough endoplasmic reticulum often appeared to transform into fusiform cells with ultrastructural features resembling fibroblasts. It seems most reasonable to consider that the dual cell populations characterizing many of the malignant tumors and tumorlike conditions discussed in this section arise from a single population of local primitive mesenchymal cells rather than from local mesenchymal cells and histiocytes, as has been proposed for malignant fibrous histiocytoma and malignant giant cell tumor of soft parts (Guccion and Enzinger, 1972; O'Brien and Stout, 1964). In humans these tumors continue to be regarded as tumors of probable histiocytic origin in which some histiocytes become facultative fibroblasts. Ackerman and Rosai (1974) reviewed the evidence supporting the histiocytic origin of these tumors and classified the soft tissues of probable histiocytic origin in humans.

## TABLE 4.2. Malignant Tumors and Tumorlike Lesions In and Around Joints, Tendons, and Deep Fasciae of Domestic Animals

Synovial sarcoma of joints
Synovial sarcoma of tendons and tendon sheaths
Malignant fibrous histiocytoma
Malignant giant cell tumor of soft parts or
    malignant giant cell tumor of the tendon sheath
Hemangiosarcoma of the tendon sheath
Musculo-aponeurotic fibromatosis of the pectoral region of
    horses
Malignant mesenchymoma of the dog

The following generalities may be helpful to pathology and oncology residents attempting to learn about this group of lesions for the first time. Synovial sarcomas of joints, tendon sheaths, and bursae of humans and animals are composed of two variously intermingled cellular elements: a synovioblastic or epithelioid element and a fibroblastic element. These tumor cells are not phagocytic. Tumor giant cells, while absent from human tumors, are frequently present in animal tumors. Fibroblastic and histiocytic cellular elements arranged in a storiform ("whirligig") pattern characterize the malignant fibrous histiocytoma of soft tissues. Giant cells and a mixed inflammatory cell component may also be present in these tumors. Malignant giant cell tumor of soft parts is believed to be a variant of malignant fibrous histiocytoma in which the tumor giant cells are the predominant feature. In humans the malignant giant cell tumor of tendon sheath is no longer recognized as a distinct entity, and those malignant giant cell tumors involving tendons in humans are currently regarded as deeply seated forms of malignant giant cell tumors of soft parts. Since these tumors occur in both deep connective tissue sites and in tendon sheaths of animals, this author has elected to discuss the two lesions as separate entities, but under a combined heading (see Malignant Giant Cell Tumors of Soft Parts and Malignant Giant Cell Tumors of Tendon Sheath).

## Synovial Sarcoma

**General Considerations.** Synovial sarcoma is a relatively uncommon tumor of animals (Lipowitz *et al.*, 1979; Madewell and Pool, 1978) and humans (Cadman *et al.*, 1965; Fechner, 1976; Lattes, 1982). This malignant disease has been thoroughly described for humans using a large number of cases from major medical centers (Cadman *et al.*, 1965; Haagensen and Stout, 1944; Tillotson *et al.*, 1951). There are no comparable studies of synovial sarcoma in various animal species available that would permit a similar in-depth characterization of this neoplasm in animals. Frequently in veterinary medicine those of us who are involved in comparative oncological pathology too often anticipate that an animal neoplasm will have the same clinical, pathological, and behavioral characteristics as the coun-

terpart human tumor. When the animal tumor deviates from the expected behavior or shows unique features, we often tend to question the observation or doubt the validity of recognizing the tumor as an animal analog of the human neoplasm. Since veterinary pathologists and oncologists are conditioned to compare animal with human tumors, it seems appropriate to briefly summarize the synovial sarcoma of humans because of the number of misconceptions about major features of synovial sarcoma that exist in the veterinary medical literature. For a more detailed description of synovial sarcoma in humans, the reader is referred to the following papers: Cadman *et al.* (1965), Fechner (1976), Haagensen and Stout (1944), Lattes (1982), and Tillotson *et al.* (1951).

**Synovial Sarcoma in Humans.** This is a very malignant tumor in humans and it has a highly variable duration from onset of symptoms to death (5 months to 16 years) resulting from metastasis in the majority of patients. Unfortunately, in one of the early descriptions of this neoplasm Smith (1927) applied the term *synovioma*, which has a benign connotation for this malignant neoplasm. Since there is no benign counterpart to the synovial sarcoma, the term *synovioma* has no significance and its use is discouraged in human medicine (Lattes, 1982) and veterinary medicine (Misdorp and Van der Heul, 1976).

While the term *synovial sarcoma* implies that the tumor originates from the synovium of joints, tendons, bursae, or adventitious bursae, this has never been substantiated (Cadman *et al.*, 1965). These tumors often arise in close proximity to the aforementioned synovial structures in humans, but they rarely involve the synovial membrane except by extension (Ackerman and Rosai, 1974; Lattes, 1982). Synovial sarcomas infrequently arise in soft tissue sites unassociated with synovial-lined structures in the musculature of the neck, nasopharynx, and abdominal wall (Lattes, 1982). Synovial sarcomas appear to arise *de novo* from undifferentiated mesenchyme, which in the clinical neoplasm is capable of producing at best a crude caricature of synovial tissue (Cadman *et al.*, 1965).

Clinical features of the human tumor include involvement of males slightly more than females; the age of onset in most cases is young adulthood (mean age is 32 years). Presenting symptoms and signs are a palpable mass or swelling (in 97% of cases) accompanied by pain or tenderness in slightly more than half of the cases (Cadman *et al.*, 1965; Lattes, 1982). Cadman *et al.* (1965) found that 95% of the lesions occurred in the extremities and about 70% were in the lower extremities. Regions involved in decreasing order of frequency are the thigh, knee, foot, hand, and leg. Ackerman and Rosai (1974) also include soft tissue sites of the shoulder, elbow, and hip. Less common sites of involvement are the musculature of the neck, nasopharynx, and torso (Lattes, 1982).

Synovial sarcomas of humans are solid tumors often having sharply circumscribed borders (Lattes, 1982). Extension along fascial planes is common, but infiltration of adjacent muscle tissue or fascia is unusual (Cadman *et al.*, 1965). Tumors may have gritty areas resulting from calcification of tumor tissue. The joint space is rarely invaded (Fechner, 1976), and if an intraarticular mass is encountered, then the tumor is probably not a synovial sarcoma (Murray, 1977).

On radiographic examination there was no reaction in adjacent bone organs. Tumors were recognized as partially lobulated masses having discrete margins and radiodensity of muscle tissue (Murray, 1977). Calcification of tumor tissue was recognized in about 30% of the radiographic studies in one report (Cadman *et al.*, 1965). In about 20% of the cases, one of two patterns of bone destruction was evoked by synovial sarcomas (Craig *et al.*, 1955). In one pattern the areas of bone loss had sharp sclerotic margins that were attributed to pressure from the expanding tumor mass. Cortical destruction secondary to bone invasion characterized the second pattern.

Human synovial sarcomas are composed of two differing but inextricably intermingled cellular components (Lattes, 1982). The synovioblastic or epithelioid element is formed by moderately large polygonal and cylindrical cells that may grow in cords or short tubes and may line slitlike spaces, thus giving the tumor a glandular appearance. The spindle cell component usually predominates and may produce a stromal pattern indistinguishable from fibrosarcoma (Fechner, 1976). Tissue culture and ultrastructural studies have confirmed that the two components are morphological variations of the malignant synovioblast (Lattes, 1982). Al-

though tumor cells have ultrastructural features not found in normal synoviocytes, these features may be found in synoviocytes of nonneoplastic inflammatory and degenerative responses of the synovium (Fechner, 1976). The epithelioid cells may secrete a mucicarminophilic acid mucopolysaccharide that stains positive with periodic acid—Schiff stain. Cadman *et al.* (1965) emphasized that histological diagnosis depends on recognizing the nature of the tumor cells and does not depend on finding synovial slits and villous projections. Tumor cells are not phagocytic, and tumor giant cells are not found in human synovial sarcomas. Cadman's report also concludes that there is no relationship between the histological appearance of the tumor and its clinical behavior.

Growth rates of synovial sarcomas and their clinical course are highly variable, with the mean duration of the disease from onset of symptoms to death being about 6.5 years (Cadman *et al.*, 1965). Metastasis can occur to the lungs (81%), regional lymph nodes (23%), and bones (20%).

**Classification of Malignant Synovial Tumors of Animals.** No apparent distinction is made in humans among synovial sarcomas arising in the vicinity of joints, tendon sheaths, bursae, and extrasynovial sites (Ackerman and Rosai, 1974; Cadman *et al.*, 1965; Fechner, 1976; Lattes, 1982). This author, however, has chosen to present synovial sarcomas of joints and tendon sheaths as separate entities, if for no other reason than to emphasize the much greater frequency with which the malignant tendon sheath tumors are seen in animals as compared to humans. Many of the synovial sarcomas of joints and tendon sheaths of animals do not appear to have the same degree of malignant behavior as is reported for humans. This could be because many of the animals are euthanized after diagnosis and are not permitted to die from the direct effects of the tumor. While tumor giant cells are not a feature of human synovial sarcomas, many of the synovial sarcomas of joints and tendon sheaths of animals have a variable component of giant cells. When the tumor giant cells are the predominant component of a malignant tendon sheath tumor of an animal, the author regards this tumor as a malignant giant cell tumor of the tendon sheath. The author is unaware of the existence of a malignant giant cell tumor centered entirely on the joint capsule of an animal. Malignant giant cell tumors of the tendon sheath in humans are currently regarded as examples of malignant giant cell tumor of soft parts which involve tendon sheaths and thus would be morphological variants of malignant fibrous histiocytoma.

### Synovial Sarcoma of Joints

**Classification.** Synovial sarcomas of joints are malignant tumors arising in synovioblastic mesenchyme found in deep connective tissue adjacent to the joint capsule of synovial joints. Use of the terms *synovioma* or *malignant synovioma* for these lesions is discouraged in both human medicine (Lattes, 1982) and veterinary medicine (Misdorp and Van der Heul, 1976). For more detailed information about the neoplasm in dogs, refer to papers by Lieberman (1956), Lipowitz *et al.* (1979), Madewell and Pool (1978), Mitchell and Hurov (1979), and Reed *et al.* (1978).

**Incidence, Age, Breed, and Sex.** These are infrequently diagnosed tumors occurring primarily in dogs (Madewell and Pool, 1978) and rarely in cattle (Dungworth *et al.*, 1964; Gupta and Singh, 1978). The mean age of dogs at time of diagnosis is about 8 years (range 12 months to 12 years), and more males are affected than females (Lipowitz *et al.*, 1979; Madewell and Pool, 1978). No breed predilection is apparent. Large but not giant breeds of dogs are primarily affected. The two cattle with tumors were a 3-year-old Jersey cow and a 10-year-old bullock.

**Clinical Characteristics.** Most dogs are presented because of lameness associated with a non-painful palpable mass located in the vicinity of a major weight-bearing joint in one of the legs. The tumor mass is firm, but may have soft fluctuant areas. A few tumors will pursue an indolent course and slowly destroy the joint over a period of several months to more than 1 to 2 years. Conversely, a few tumors will suddenly appear and pursue a fulminating course ending in euthanasia or death within a few weeks to a month. Most tumors, however, will be slow-growing masses for several weeks to months and suddenly increase in size over a period of 2 to 3 weeks. The degree of lameness can usually be correlated with the degree of bone involvement seen radiographically (Lipowitz *et al.*,

1979). Seven of 18 dogs in the report by Madewell and Pool (1978) had extensive joint destruction. Local recurrence following surgery and metastatic disease are common developments, but some dogs will remain free of tumor following amputation.

**Sites.** In dogs the tumors are located at or near major weight-bearing joints of the legs. The stifle joint is the most frequent site, followed in decreasing frequency by the elbow, shoulder, antebrachiocarpal, talocrural, and hip joint. It is unusual for tumors to develop at joints distal to the carpus and tarsus, but tumors may occasionally occur in interphalangeal joints of dogs. We have recently found a synovial sarcoma involving an apophyseal synovial joint of a cervical vertebra in a dog.

Two synovial sarcomas reported in cattle involved the right hock joint of a cow and the soft tissues on the medial side of the leg of a bullock.

**Gross Morphology.** Synovial sarcomas of joints appear to be composed of confluent lobules of firm tan-colored tissue. The borders are distinct and seem to be encapsulated (fig. 4.18A). The cut surface exposes smooth textured tissue often containing dark staining areas of hemorrhage and pale areas of necrosis. Cystic spaces filled with mucinous fluid are prominent features of a few lesions. Tumor tissue infiltrates along fascial planes leading away from the affected joint. Most of the synovial membrane of the joint is infiltrated and effaced by tumor tissue. Unlike human tumors the synovial sarcomas of dogs commonly encroach on the joint cavity in most of the cases that we have examined. The tumor does not appear to produce any direct damage to the articular cartilage. With aggressive tumors, however, the neoplastic tissue destroys the joint by eroding the articular margins and by invading the subchondral bone. Tumor tissue reaches the subchondral bone by infiltrating the joint capsule insertion line. Tumor tissue frequently gains access to the epiphyseal cancellous bone by entering the bony vascular channels of the epiphyseal vessels. This process may lead to vessel occlusion and infarction of segments of the subchondral bone and the epiphyseal spongiosa. We have rarely encountered calcified tumor tissue in the canine synovial sarcomas that we have dissected, unlike the finding in some human joint tumors.

**Radiographic Appearance.** Most synovial sarcomas of canine joints appear as large nodular masses with discrete borders, often eccentrically oriented on a major joint of a limb. The tumor mass usually has a radiodensity similar to that of muscle tissue. In a few cases, and early in the course of many tumors, there are no radiographic signs of bone involvement. With aggressive tumors there are multiple foci of osteolysis involving the ends of all bones forming the joint (fig. 4.18B). The two major radiographic patterns of permeative and punctate bone loss seen in affected joints of humans may occur as separate or combined patterns in canine joint tumors. It is our experience that when one examines the radiographs of a major limb joint of an older large breed dog and finds destructive lesions in the ends of the bones forming the joint, one should think first of synovial sarcoma. We have seen a few examples where metastatic tumors to the synovium of a joint have mimicked the pattern of a primary malignant joint tumor. Cases of osteomyelitis or inflammatory joint disease do not normally produce radiographic signs resembling malignant joint disease.

We occasionally encounter atypical cases of synovial sarcoma in which clinical progression is very slow and the radiographic changes reflect this indolent behavior. Radiographs of these lesions show numerous discrete areas of bone resorption with sclerotic borders involving several bones of the affected joint (fig. 4.18C). The ovoid radiolucencies appear to be the enlarged bony foramens of vessels entering the bone organs along joint capsule insertion lines. Tumor tissue apparently mediates the bone resorption and in doing so creates a pathway for entering the ends of the bones.

**Histological Features.** Synovial sarcomas of joints are characterized histologically by the presence in varying proportions of two intermingled cellular elements: the synovioblastic or epithelioid component and the fibroblastic component. The proportion of these two components is highly variable from tumor to tumor or even within the same tumor (fig. 4.19A–D). Cells of the synovioblastic component have hyperchromatic cytoplasm, an eccentric nucleus, and ovoid, angular, or fusiform profiles. Synovioblastic cells may be the predominant cell in sheetlike areas of the tumor (fig. 4.19D). They may grow in packets and short cords (fig. 4.20A) or be interspersed with the fibroblastic component. Cavitary areas lined by epithelioid tu-

mor cells may develop within some of the packets of synovioblastic cells (fig. 4.19A). Areas with clefts and tubular spaces lined by epithelioid cells are uncommon in most canine synovial sarcomas. It is also difficult to find mucicarminophilic or periodic acid–Schiff positive staining of amorphous material in the cystic spaces, clefts, and pseudoglandular structures of animal tumors. When the fibroblastic component predominates and forms interwoven bundles of spindled cells, such areas may be indistinguishable from fibrosarcoma (fig. 4.20B). The degree of anaplasia and the mitotic index are highly variable features in the canine tumors. Numbers of tumor giant cells vary greatly between tumors and even in different microscopic fields of the same tumor. Tumor giant cells, however, were not the predominant cell type in any of the canine joint tumors that we examined. Tumor giant cells are often associated with major fibroblastic areas of the tumor, especially those areas with a high mitotic index. Areas of necrosis are usually found in large aggressive tumors.

In certain cases of synovial sarcoma of the canine joint demonstrating a longer than usual clinical course, tumor tissue may be composed of primitive mesenchymal cells without pronounced anaplastic features or a high mitotic index (fig. 4.20C). These tumors are not very cellular, and the microscopic appearance resembles the subintimal tissue of the synovial membrane. Tumor cells may be widely separated by poorly staining amorphous matrix and they rest in a delicate fibrillar stroma. Some fields resemble mucoid connective tissue. In aggressive areas of the tumor the pattern may resemble myxosarcoma (fig. 4.20D). This innocuous tumor tissue may infiltrate fascial planes, penetrate the fibrous layer of the joint capsule, and extend along vascular channels into bone organs. We have not seen metastatic disease develop from synovial sarcomas having this pattern.

We agree with Cadman *et al.* (1965) who found no relationship between the histological appearance of a synovial sarcoma and its biological behavior.

**Growth and Metastasis.** There is considerable variation in the rate of growth of the tumors following the onset of lameness. The clinical course of the disease may vary from less than 1 month to 1 or more years. Apparently the metastatic potential of the canine synovial sarcoma (about 25%) is less than

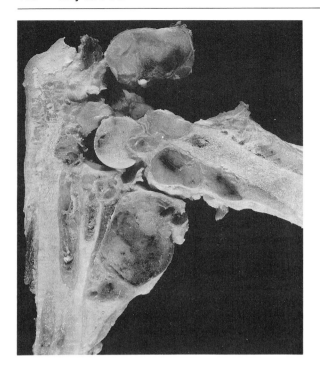

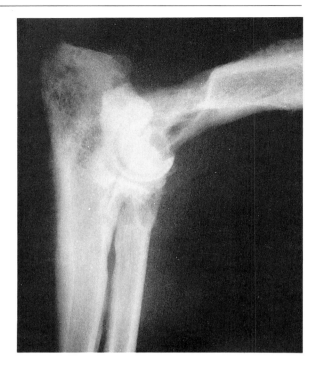

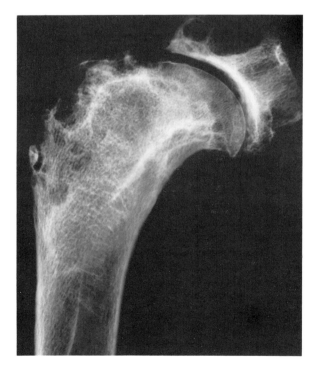

FIGURE 4.18. Synovial sarcoma of joints. A. Synovial sarcoma in a dog involving the elbow joint. B. Radiograph showing destructive lesions in ends of all bones forming the elbow joint. C. Radiograph from the shoulder joint of a dog showing clinical signs for over 14 months and slow clinical progression of the tumor. The sclerotic borders of the multiple areas of bone resorption reflect the indolent behavior of this canine synovial sarcoma.

that in humans, as judged by reports of Lipowitz *et al.* (1979) and Madewell and Pool (1978). These authors indicated that local recurrence following excision or amputation is common. However, not all operated dogs subsequently developed metastatic disease even after multiple surgeries. Perhaps if more affected dogs were permitted to live longer with their clinical disease or live longer after local recurrence following surgery, the metastatic rate would be higher. Regional lymph nodes, lungs, and other locations including the skeleton may be sites of metastatic disease (Lieberman, 1956; Lipowitz *et al.*, 1979; Madewell and Pool, 1978).

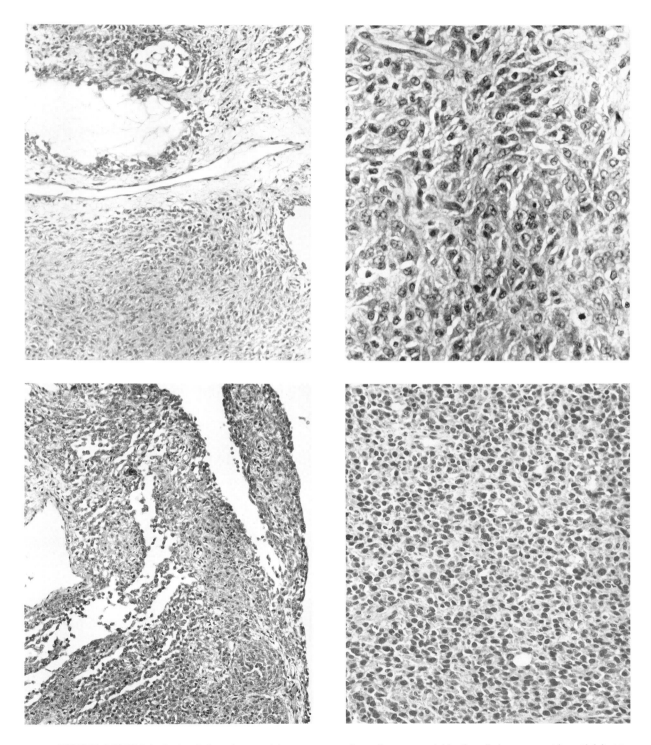

A | B
─────
C | D

**FIGURE 4.19** Histological variations in synovial sarcoma of joints. A. Tumor with a predominance of the synovioblastic or epithelioid component in which spaces lined by tumor cells are formed. B. Higher magnification shows these synovioblastic cells have eccentric nuclei, hyperchromatic cytoplasm, and angular profiles. C. Synovioblastic cells form both slitlike and solid patterns. D. Epithelioid cells in this tumor form a sheetlike mass of cells.

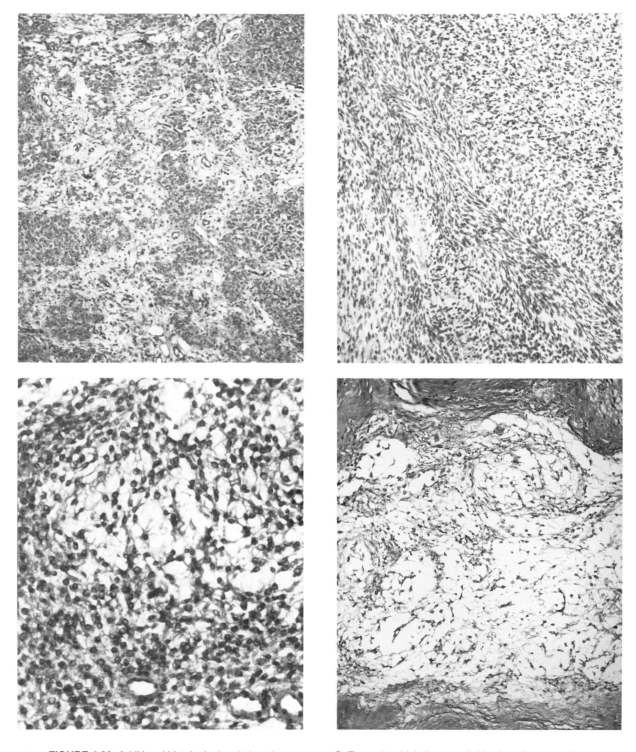

$\frac{A|B}{C|D}$ **FIGURE 4.20.** Additional histological variations in synovial sarcoma of joints. A. Tumor in which synovioblastic cells form packets and short irregular cords. B. Area of joint tumor in which the fibroblastic component predominates and mimics the interwoven pattern of fibrosarcoma.

C. Tumor in which the synovioblastic cells were without anaplastic features, but which slowly destroyed the joint by local bone invasion. D. Joint tumor forming histological patterns mimicking myxosarcoma.

## Synovial Sarcoma of Tendons and Tendon Sheaths

**Classification.** Synovial sarcomas of tendons and tendon sheaths are malignant tumors arising in synovioblastic mesenchyme in and around tendon sheaths and paratenon sites where sheaths are absent. Reports indicate that this a rare neoplasm in animals (Madewell and Pool, 1978; Schiefer *et al.*, 1973). In humans these tumors are included under the general topic of synovial sarcomas (Lattes, 1982). Although we assume that in animals these tumors arise from essentially the same primitive mesenchyme as joint tumors, we wish to present synovial sarcomas of tendons and tendon sheaths as a separate entity to distinguish them from the more common benign giant cell tumors of tendons and tendon sheaths and from the equally rare malignant giant cell tumors of tendon sheaths.

**Incidence, Age, Breed, and Sex.** These are rare animal neoplasms. Schiefer *et al.* (1973) reported one case in a 6-year-old male bulldog. I have five examples in my collection. These tumors occurred in both sexes of dogs of different medium and large breeds; ages ranged from 5 to 15 years. The real incidence may be higher since synovial sarcomas of flexor tendons that extend into the carpal or tarsal canals would probably be regarded clinically as joint tumors unless an anatomical dissection was done to determine the precise location of the tumor mass.

**Clinical Characteristics.** These neoplastic tumors of tendons and their sheaths develop insidiously with the first clinical signs being a slowly progressive lameness. At some point in the clinical course a slowly growing mass becomes apparent. The tumor is painless on palpation and feels firm except for soft fluctuant areas that are present in the larger masses. The tumors form a nodular fusiform lesion in the soft tissues typically overlying the ends of one of the long bones of a limb or occasionally overlying the metacarpus or metatarsus of a foot. Early in the course of the disease the skin over the mass is movable, but the tumor remains fixed to the deep structures of the leg. Eventually, as the mass enlarges, there is swelling and pitting edema of the leg, and the skin becomes fixed to the tumor. By this time the dog uses the leg very little, if at all. In two of the cases observed, radiographic evidence of bone destruction and secondary extension into a nearby joint occurred as a late event. One dog treated by local resection of the tumor mass experienced local regrowth of the tumor mass about 3 weeks later (Schiefer *et al.*, 1973). This dog was alive but with local tumor recurrence at the time the report was made. Combined chemotherapy by limb perfusion and radiation therapy was ineffective in controlling continued local tumor growth in a second dog. Limb amputation was not done in any of the dogs, and the owners had the dogs euthanized in five cases because of the local disease. Clinically undetected metastasis to a regional lymph node was found at necropsy in one case, but complete necropsies were permitted only in two dogs.

**Sites.** Four of six tumors involved locations proximal to the carpus and tarsus. One tumor arose in tendon sheaths in the region of the right elbow joint (Schiefer *et al.*, 1973). Three tumors involved a tendon and/or tendon sheath located on the lateral or caudal surface of the distal tibia, which include tendons and tendon sheaths of the superficial digital flexor muscle, the deep digital flexor muscle, and the gastrocnemius muscle.

Two tumors were located on the surface of the metatarsus. One tumor entrapped the main body and the origin of all digital branches of the common digital extensor tendon in a hindfoot. A second tumor involved both flexor tendons of the fourth digit in the hindfoot of another dog.

**Gross Morphology.** Four of the tumors located proximal to the carpus or tarsus were fusiform masses composed of confluent nodules of soft tissue. Each one was centered on the tendon and tendon sheath apparatus of a large caliber tendon. While the major tumor mass appeared to have a distinct border, tumor tissue extended along fascial planes and dissected between the underlying bone surfaces and the adjacent musculature. On cut surface (fig. 4.21A) tumor tissue was smooth and tan-colored except for dark areas of hemorrhage and necrosis. Small cystic spaces often contained viscous fluid. One mass on the foot formed a padlike structure that entrapped all of the digital branches of the common digital extensor tendon. Sheetlike extensions from the main tumor attached to the indurated edematous tissue in the subcutis beneath the lesion. The other metatarsal lesion was a lobulated, fusiform mass enclosing both digital branches of the flexor tendons of the fourth digit. On cut

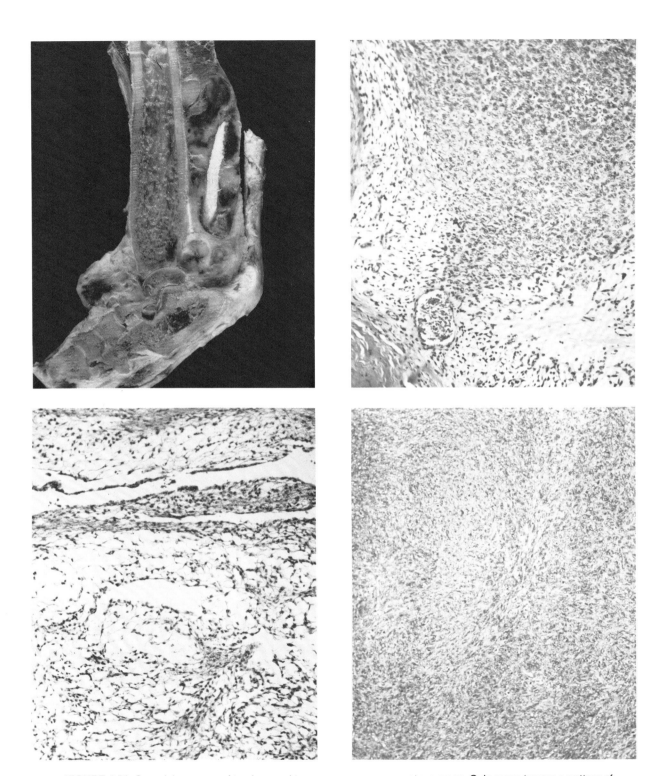

**FIGURE 4.21.** Synovial sarcoma of tendons and tendon sheaths. A. Tumor centered on the deep digital flexor tendon of a dog. B. In this tumor solid areas of synovioblastic and fibroblastic cellular components predominated over myxomatous areas. C. In some tumors a pattern of loose myxomatous tissue with slitlike spaces predominates. D. Anaplastic spindle cell pattern predominated in this locally aggressive tumor.

section the center of this tumor was filled with soft, pale, gelatinous tissue and viscous fluid. Small, irregular nodules of pale mucoid tumor tissue infiltrated beyond the borders of the tumor, especially along the course of the tendon proximal to the main tumor mass. Complete necropsies were done without finding metastases in two dogs. The entire tumor-bearing limbs and regional lymph nodes were available for dissection from two additional dogs. Metastasis to a regional lymph node was found in only the dog with the tendon sheath tumor in the fourth digit.

**Histological Features.** The histological appearance of these tumors was variable among the different tumors and within the same tumor, as was the case with the joint tumors. Both the synovioblastic and fibroblastic elements were present, but were not always as obvious as in the joint tumors (fig. 4.21B). The bulk of the tumor tissue in several lesions was composed of irregularly sized nodules of loose myxomatous tissue having numerous slitlike spaces (fig. 4.21C). This loose tissue contained pale-staining primitive mesenchymal cells without apparent anaplastic features and having a low mitotic index. Cells from this innocuous myxomatous element, however, metastasized to the regional lymph node in a dog with a tendon sheath tumor of the fourth digit. The largest and most locally aggressive tumor, which was centered on the tendon apparatus of the gastrocnemius muscle, had large, irregular, confluent nodular masses composed mostly of a dense population of highly anaplastic synovioblasts with a variable component of anaplastic spindle cells (fig. 4.21D). Infiltration, high mitotic index, necrosis, bone lysis, and secondary joint invasion were major features of this lesion, but metastatic disease was not found at necropsy.

Tumor giant cells are less common in the synovial sarcomas of tendon sheaths than in the synovial sarcomas of canine joints. Giant cells were small multinucleated cells with only two to four nuclei. None of the tumors described here had areas with a storiform pattern, xanthoma cells, or histiocytes, which are features seen in malignant fibrous histiocytoma of soft tissues. Only the tumor involving the tendon of the gastrocnemius muscle had an inflammatory cell component. The exudate in this tumor was usually located in the vicinity of necrotic tumor tissue. This tendon sheath tumor was also the only tumor with areas that could be mistaken for a poorly differentiated fibrosarcoma.

**Growth and Metastasis.** In all of these cases the synovial sarcomas of tendons and tendon sheaths grew slowly over a period of 3 to 6 months into large masses. A short period of rapid growth was only observed in two tumors. Malignancy of these tumors was determined by their biological behavior. All of the tumors extensively infiltrated adjacent soft tissues. Bone destruction and joint involvement were late events in two cases. Metastasis to a regional lymph node occurred in one dog. No systemic metastases were found in the only two dogs submitted for necropsy examination. We agree with the comment made by Cadman *et al.* (1965) that there is little or no relationship between the histological appearance of synovial sarcomas and their biological behavior.

## Malignant Fibrous Histiocytoma of Soft Tissue

**General Considerations and Classification.** The malignant fibrous histiocytoma is a pleomorphic sarcoma centered more often in deep than in superficial connective tissues of adult humans. In its classic form the tumor is characterized by the presence of spindled (fibroblastlike) cells arranged in a storiform (cartwheel or whirligig) pattern and rounded (histiocytelike) cells that are accompanied by pleomorphic multinucleated giant cells and occasionally by inflammatory cells (Lattes, 1982; Weiss and Enzinger, 1978). Some mononuclear cells and giant cells may have foamy cytoplasm and, along with a few spindle cells, may show phagocytosis of hemosiderin, lipid droplets, and erythrocytes. Animal tumors diagnosed as being examples of malignant fibrous histiocytoma are reported in increasing numbers in the veterinary literature (Confer *et al.*, 1981; Gleiser *et al.*, 1979; Renlund and Pritzker, 1984). Unfortunately, no attempt has been made in these reports to distinguish the less common animal tumors having the so-called classic pattern of malignant fibrous histiocytoma from the more common variants of this tumor called malignant giant cell tumor of soft parts, in which category the malignant giant cell tumors of tendon sheaths are included.

It is suggested that, as additional cases of malignant fibrous histiocytoma are recognized in animals, the pathologist in reporting the case should attempt to distinguish between the different histological variants of this neoplasm as has been done with human tumors (Lattes, 1982). In the initial characterization of malignant fibrous histiocytoma in animals, pathologists should be looking for differences among tumor variants, such as species predilection, anatomical location, age, breed, sex, biological behavior, and response to different therapeutic modalities. Perhaps after a sufficient number of cases are evaluated, veterinary oncological pathologists will come to the same conclusion reached by Lattes (1982): that the varieties of the human tumor frequently overlap and that there is no difference in prognosis.

With this in mind, when evaluating the published descriptions of malignant fibrous histiocytoma of animals, this author placed the five feline tumors described by Confer *et al.* (1981), Gleiser *et al.* (1979), and Renlund and Pritzker (1984) in the section "Malignant Giant Cell Tumors of Soft Parts and Malignant Giant Cell Tumors of Tendon Sheaths" later in this chapter. As far as I am aware, this leaves the two canine tumors reported by Gleiser *et al.* (1979) as the only published examples of the classic form of malignant fibrous histiocytoma of soft tissues in animals.

Since these animal tumors are considered to be analogs of the human neoplasm on the basis of their purported similarity in microscopic appearance, it seems appropriate to briefly summarize the other important features of this tumor in humans. Weiss and Enzinger (1978) reported the clinicopathological findings in 200 cases in humans. The tumor mass was located in an upper extremity (in 19% of cases), in a lower extremity (49%), or in the abdominal cavity or retroperitoneum (16%) of adult humans (peak incidence at 61 to 70 years of age). Tumors involved primarily the subcutis (7%), deep fascia (19%), or skeletal muscles (59%). No tendon sheath tumors having the histological features of the classic pattern of malignant fibrous histiocytoma were found in the large survey. However, 32 cases of deeply seated tumors having tumor giant cells as the predominant feature were recognized as a giant cell variant of malignant fibrous histiocytoma named "malignant giant cell tumor of

soft parts." Because of its unique histological appearance, this tumor was reported as a separate entity (Guccion and Enzinger, 1972). Rates of local recurrence (44%) and metastasis (42%) were similar. The most common sites for metastasis were the lungs (82%) and lymph nodes (32%). Several factors influencing metastatic potential were depth of lesion, size, and the presence of an inflammatory cell component. Small tumors located superficially and having a prominent inflammatory cell component metastasized less frequently than large, deeply seated tumors, especially those involving muscles and having a meager inflammatory cell response.

The histogenesis of this tumor is uncertain. The original concept that this was a purely histiocytic neoplasm with some histiocytes modulating into facultative fibroblasts (O'Brien and Stout, 1964; Ozzello *et al.*, 1963) continues to have advocates (Ackerman and Rosai, 1974; Lattes, 1982). Weiss and Enzinger (1978) believe that malignant fibrous histiocytoma is a tumor of primitive mesenchyme giving rise mainly to tumor cells with the structural and functional properties of histiocytes and fibroblasts. Ackerman and Rosai (1974) reviewed the hypothesis proposed to explain the dual composition of these tumors.

**Malignant Fibrous Histiocytoma in Dogs.** Gleiser *et al.* (1979) diagnosed this tumor in two dogs. The first was a 7-year-old male mixed breed dog with a large (7 × 12 × 9 cm), unencapsulated, fleshy mass infiltrating the musculature and invading the cervical vertebrae on the left side of the neck. The dog was killed because of rapid loss in condition. No metastases were found at necropsy. The second case was a 9-year-old female German shepherd cross with a discrete but unencapsulated firm mass on the lateral aspect of the elbow of the right foreleg. The mass that was partially fused to the epimysium of a muscle organ was removed by surgical dissection and had not recurred at the time of the report.

On microscopic examination, both tumors were characterized by fibroblastic cells arranged in a storiform pattern, mononuclear cells, and nonsuppurative inflammatory cells. Tumor cells from the aggressive lesions in the male dog were more anaplastic and had a higher mitotic index than cells in the tumor of the female dog. The female dog was diagnosed as having a malignant fibrous histiocytoma of low-grade malignancy. A neoplastic cell line derived by culturing the tumor of the male dog was composed primarily of multinucleated giant cells. Tumor cells from this canine neoplasm did not contain stellate cells having phagocytic properties capable of migration and transformation, which characterize the human tumor (Ozzello *et al.*, 1963). This finding caused Gleiser *et al.* (1979) to speculate that the canine tumor may be derived from a different cell of origin than the human neoplasm.

**Malignant Fibrous Histiocytoma in Cats.** The feline tumors reported in the literature that have this diagnosis by Confer *et al.* (1981), Gleiser *et al.* (1979), and Renlund and Pritzker (1984) are considered here to be morphological variants of malignant fibrous histiocytoma called "malignant giant cell tumors of soft parts" and are discussed in the following section.

## Malignant Giant Cell Tumors of Soft Parts and Malignant Giant Cell Tumors of Tendon Sheaths

**Classification.** Malignant giant cell tumor of soft parts is a malignant tumor of superficial and deep connective tissue that has some of the microscopic features of malignant giant cell tumor of bone. Guccion and Enzinger (1972) first used the term to describe 32 cases of this unique extraskeletal neoplasm in humans. This tumor has also been reported in domestic animals (Alexander *et al.*, 1975; Confer *et al.*, 1981; Danks and Olafson, 1939; Ford *et al.*, 1975; Gleiser *et al.*, 1979; Neilsen, 1952; Render *et al.*, 1982).

The exact tissue of origin has not been determined. Earlier descriptions of this neoplasm in humans (Ackerman, 1953) and in cats (Nielsen, 1952) indicated that some of the deeply seated tumors in the group may have originated in tendons or their sheaths, and at that time the term *malignant giant cell tumor of the tendon sheath* was applied to those lesions (Guccion and Enzinger, 1972). Evidence accumulated since that time, however, has led Fechner (1976) to conclude that malignant giant cell tumors of the tendon sheath have not been convincingly documented as a specific category of tumors, at least not in humans. In support of the argument, Guccion and Enzinger (1972)

found that although some deeply seated tumors involved the tendon apparatus, no tumor was completely localized to a tendon or tendon sheath. In fact the majority of the human tumors involved only deep fascia and skeletal muscles. These authors also observed that the malignant giant cell tumor of soft parts should not be regarded as the malignant counterpart of the benign giant cell tumor of tendons and tendon sheaths, and they pointed out that the two tumors occur in different anatomical sites.

Guccion and Enzinger (1972) were unable to draw firm conclusions on the histogenesis of malignant giant cell tumors of soft parts in humans. However, they found a close resemblance between the neoplastic mononuclear cells and the normal histiocytes, and they observed phagocytic activity in both the mononuclear and multinucleated giant cells of the tumor. They believe that these microscopic findings strongly indicate that the tumor originates from histiocytes or their precursors. Ackerman and Rosai (1974) and Lattes (1982) believe that the malignant giant cell tumor of soft parts is a variant of malignant histiocytoma.

Ultrastructural findings in animal analogs of this tumor occurring in two horses and two cats suggest that these tumors probably arise from pluripotential mesenchyme in the connective tissue (Confer *et al.*, 1981; Ford *et al.*, 1975; Render *et al.*, 1982). Ford *et al.* (1975) found little similarity between giant cells of the tumor and giant cells arising from histiocytes. Small mononuclear cells in the feline tumor had ultrastructural features more closely resembling osteoblasts and chondroblasts than histiocytes.

In writing this chapter this author was faced with a dilemma as to how to deal with this tumor category. I have recognized an example of malignant giant cell tumor of soft parts occurring in skeletal muscle of a dog unassociated with a tendon apparatus; however, other examples of malignant giant cell sarcoma have centered in tendon sheaths. A similar case was reported in a cat by Nielsen (1952). Therefore, a dilemma exists. The existence of malignant giant cell sarcoma of tendon sheaths as a separate and distinct tumor category could be perpetuated. The tendon sheath tumor could be regarded as a giant cell variant of synovial sarcoma of tendons and tendon sheaths. Finally the malignant giant cell tumor of tendon sheaths could be considered as an example of a malignant giant cell tumor of soft parts, in other words, a variant of malignant fibrous histiocytoma, which occasionally arises within the mesenchyme of tendons and tendon sheaths of animals. Until more is known about these tumors in animals, the last of the three alternatives seems best for describing this tumor category.

**Incidence, Age, Breed, and Sex.** Seven cases of malignant giant cell tumors of soft parts have been reported in mature equidae (one in a mule, three in quarter horse geldings, two in standardbred mares, and one in a standardbred stallion), and three cases were reported in 7-, 9-, and 10-year-old male and female domestic cats (Alexander *et al.*, 1975; Confer *et al.*, 1981; Danks and Olafson, 1939; Ford *et al.*, 1975; Render *et al.*, 1982). We have seen one example of this tumor in an 8-year-old female Doberman pinscher. It was difficult to determine from the report of Gleiser *et al.* (1979) whether all three of their feline cases had malignant giant cell tumors of soft parts or if only their second cat case was an example of this neoplasm.

Nielsen (1952) reported a case of a malignant giant cell tumor thought to be of tendon sheath origin in an 8-year-old male domestic cat. It is possible that the first and third cats in the report of Gleiser *et al.* (1979) were also afflicted with malignant giant cell tumors of the tendon sheath. We would also place the tumor involving the digit of a 2-year-old male cat described by Renlund and Pritzker (1984) in this category. The two examples of this tumor in our collection occurred in mature male dogs.

**Clinical Characteristics.** Malignant giant cell tumors of soft parts appear in horses as firm, raised, solitary masses firmly attached to superficial subcutaneous tissue (Ford *et al.*, 1975; Render *et al.*, 1982). Although none of these tumors metastasized, excision was followed by local recurrence in three of seven cases. In two of three cats (Alexander *et al.*, 1975; Ford *et al.*, 1975) and in the dog of our collection the tumors were located in deep fascia. In one cat (Confer *et al.*, 1981) the tumor formed a movable subcutaneous mass. The tumor recurred six times in this cat following surgery. Metastatic disease was not reported in the cats, and at the time of this writing the dog is asymptomatic following removal of the tumor mass. In humans (Guccion and Enzinger, 1972) the superficial tu-

mors are small, occur in the subcutis and superficial fascia, recur frequently after excision, and metastasize infrequently. The deep tumors are large and involve skeletal muscle, deep fascia, and tendons. About 70% of human patients with deeply seated tumors develop metastatic disease.

Malignant giant cell tumors of the tendon sheath form a painless cylindrical swelling of soft tissues following the course of a muscle–tendon apparatus. Usually, there is a history of rapid swelling and a rapidly progressive mechanical lameness. On initial examination the lesion is often thought to be an infection. Metastatic disease developed in one dog from our collection. Early diagnosis and amputation may control the tumor.

**Sites and Gross Morphology.** The superficial lesions of malignant giant cell tumors of soft parts reported in horses were located in the superficial fascia and subcutis of the jugular groove of the neck (two), thigh (two), stifle region (two), and shoulder (one) (Ford *et al.*, 1975; Render *et al.*, 1982). The tumors were solitary, firm, raised, incompletely lobulated, ovoid masses, 1 to 4 cm in diameter, and had a capsule. On cut surface they were pale and firm and had multiple small areas of hemorrhage and necrosis. The superficial lesion in one cat (Confer *et al.*, 1981) was a mass 2 cm in diameter located in the subcutaneous tissue of the back between the shoulder blades.

The deep lesions of malignant giant cell tumors of soft parts formed a large (3 × 4 × 12 cm), glistening, lobulated mass obliterating the femoral canal on the medial side of the right hindlimb of one cat (Ford *et al.*, 1975) and a large mass involving the soft tissues of the right shoulder and axilla of a second cat (Alexander *et al.*, 1975). A firm, nodular, ovoid mass (2.5 cm in diameter) was located in the body of the triceps muscle of the left foreleg of a dog in our collection. Small hemorrhages were present in the cut section of both tumors. Mineralized tissue was present within and at the borders of the canine tumor.

The malignant giant cell tumor of tendon sheaths in the cat (Nielsen, 1952) produced a cylindrical soft tissue swelling that extended from the elbow region to the carpus on the caudal side of the right foreleg. In our collection the tumor produced a flattened, saclike, doughy mass containing the digital flexor tendons on the plantar surface of the left metatarsal region of one dog and a fusiform swelling involving the tendon of the biceps brachii muscle and the biceps bursa in the second dog (fig. 4.22A). All three tumors were incompletely lobulated. Multiple hemorrhages were present in the sectioned tumors. The feline tumor was very firm. Both canine lesions were formed of soft, fleshy, tan to grayish white tissue. No mineralized tissue was apparent in any of the three tendon sheath tumors.

**Histological Features.** The characteristic cytological features occurring in both the malignant giant cell tumors of soft parts and malignant giant cell tumors of tendon sheaths include large multinucleated tumor giant cells, large pleomorphic mononuclear cells, histiocytes, neoplastic spindle cells, and fibroblasts (figs. 4.22B, C, and D). The multinucleated giant cells had as many as 60 nuclei per cell and appeared to arise from large mononuclear tumor cells or their precursors. Anaplastic features could be found in the multinucleated giant cells, the large mononuclear cells, and the spindle cell component. The later cells often formed areas of fibrosarcomatous stroma at the periphery of the mass or in septa that partially divided the tumor into incomplete lobules.

Malignant giant cell tumors of soft parts in humans (Guccion and Enzinger, 1972), which are located in superficial connective tissue, are relatively small. Mononuclear tumor cells have slight to minimal anaplastic features and a relatively low mitotic index. These features correlate with a low degree of malignancy of the superficial tumors in humans. Malignant bone tissue was formed in 4 of the 12 superficial human tumors. The pattern of the tumors described in horses (Render *et al.*, 1982) bore a striking similarity to the superficial human tumors, but no osteogenic tissue was found in the equine tumors.

The deep types of malignant giant cell tumors of soft parts in humans (Guccion and Enzinger, 1972) are large. The mononuclear tumor cells in these tumors exhibit moderate to marked anaplastic features and have a higher mitotic index than the superficial tumors. The amount of the fibrosarcomatous component is also increased. Areas of differentiation to malignant cartilage and bone were seen in 11 of the 20 deep tumors. It is likely that the deep types of tumors in the cat (Alexander *et al.*, 1975; Confer *et al.*, 1981; Ford *et al.*, 1975)

and the dog of our collection are counterparts to the deeply seated tumors of humans. The dog had areas of metaplastic bone formed both within and at the borders of the tumor (fig. 4.22B). We could find no evidence of malignant bone or cartilage tissue in the tumor.

The malignant giant cell tumors of two cats (Nielsen, 1952; Renlund and Pritzker, 1984) and of two dogs in our collection had histological features similar to that described for the deep types of malignant giant cell tumors of soft parts, with the exception that bone and cartilage tissues were absent. Although multinucleated giant cells and large mononuclear tumor cells were prominent features of these tumors, there were also large areas of spindle cell sarcoma that had the interwoven pattern of fibrosarcoma, especially along the borders and the poles of the fusiform tumor mass.

**Growth and Metastasis.** The superficial types of malignant giant cell tumors of soft parts as reported in horses (Ford *et al.*, 1975; Render *et al.*, 1982) and humans (Guccion and Enzinger, 1972) tend to be smaller, grow slower, and are less infiltrative than the more deeply seated types found in two cats (Alexander *et al.*, 1975; Ford *et al.*, 1975), the dog of our collection, and humans (Guccion and Enzinger, 1972). A superficial tumor in one cat (Confer *et al.*, 1981), however, recurred six times after local resection. Both the superficial and deep tumors tend to recur following surgery, but the deep form, at least in humans (Guccion and Enzinger, 1972), has a much higher metastatic potential.

The malignant giant cell tumors of tendon sheaths of two cats (Nielsen, 1952; Renlund and Pritzker, 1984) and the two dogs of our collection grew rapidly in a few weeks' time. All four tumors appeared grossly to have a defined border, but infiltration of adjacent soft tissues was present microscopically in both canine cases. Metastasis to abdominal lymph nodes occurred in one of the dogs.

## Hemangiosarcoma of Tendon Sheaths

**Classification.** Hemangiosarcoma (also called angiosarcoma or malignant hemangioendothelioma) is a malignant tumor of the endothelial cells of blood vessels. These tumors are commonly found in the internal organs and skin of older animals, es-

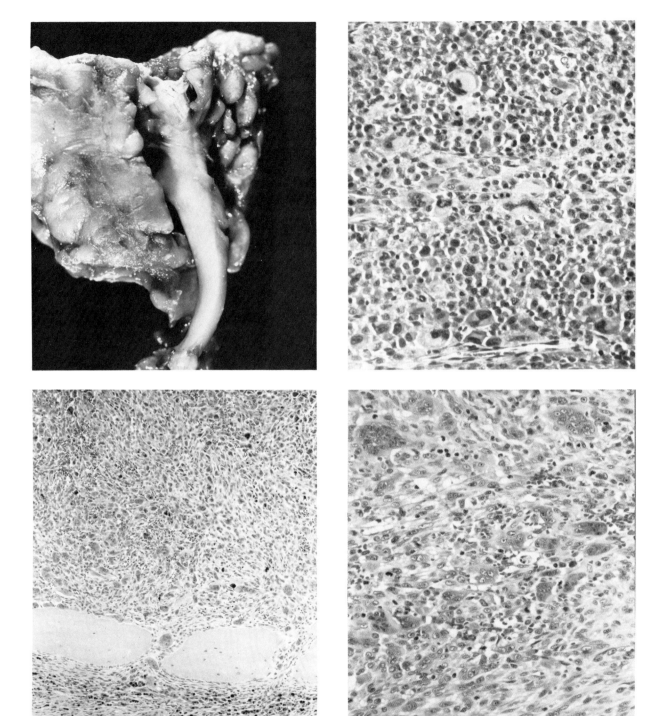

A|B
C|D

**FIGURE 4.22.** Malignant giant cell tumors of soft parts and of tendon sheaths. A. Malignant giant cell tumor of the biceps bursa in a dog. Synovial lining of the bursa has nodular infiltrates of tumor cells. B. Numerous bizarre multinucleated tumor giant cells are among the infiltrate of large and small mononuclear cells. C. Low magnification of a ma-

lignant giant cell tumor of soft parts located in the triceps muscle of a dog. Plates of metaplastic bone are located at the border of the tumor. D. Pleomorphic mononuclear cells, multinucleated giant cells, and spindled cells are major features of this sarcoma.

Flynn, J. E. (1975) *Hand Surgery.* 2d ed., Williams and Wilkins Co. (Baltimore).

Ford, G. H., Empson, R. N., Plopper, C. G., and Brown, P. H. (1975) Giant Cell Tumor of Soft Parts: A Report of an Equine and a Feline Case. *Vet. Path.* 12, 428–433.

Gleiser, C. A., Raulston, G. L., Jardine, J. H., and Gray, K. N. (1979) Malignant Fibrous Histiocytoma in Dogs and Cats. *Vet. Path.* 16, 199–208.

Goulden, B. E., and O'Callaghan, M. W. (1980) Tumoral Calcinosis in the Horse. *N. Z. Vet. J.* 28, 217–219.

Guccion, J. G., and Enzinger, F. M. (1972) Malignant Giant Cell Tumor of Soft Parts: An Analysis of 32 Cases. *Cancer* 29, 1518–1529.

Gupta, P. P., and Singh, B. (1978) Synovial Sarcoma in a Bullock. *Indian Vet. J.* 55, 831–832.

Haagensen, C. D., and Stout, A. P. (1944) Synovial Sarcoma. *Ann. Surg.* 120, 825–842.

Hale, J. E., and Calder, J. M. (1970) Synovial Sarcoma of the Abdominal Wall. *Br. J. Cancer* 24, 471–474.

Hulse, E. V. (1966) A Benign Giant Cell Synovioma in a Cat. *J. Path. Bact.* 91, 269–271.

Ihrke, P. J., Cain, G. R., and Stannard, A. A. (1983) Fibromatosis in a Horse. *J. Amer. Vet. Med. Assoc.* 10, 1100–1102.

Jaffee, H. L. (1968) *Tumors and Tumorous Conditions of Bones and Joints.* Lea and Febiger (Philadelphia).

Jaffee, H. O., Lichtenstein, L., and Sutro, C. J. (1941) Pigmented Villonodular Synovitis, Bursitis and Tenosynovitis. *Arch. Path.* 31, 731–765.

Jeffreys, T. E. (1967) Synovial Chondromatosis. *J. Bone Joint Surg.* 49B, 530–534.

Johnson, A. D., and Parisien, M. V. (1979) Soft Tissue Tumors about the Knee. *Orthop. Clin. N. Amer.* 10, 253–279.

Kirk, M. D. (1982) Radiographic and Histologic Appearance of Synovial Osteochondromatosis of the Femorotibial Bursae in a Horse: A Case History Report. *Vet. Radiol.* 23, 168–170.

Lattes, R. (1982) Tumors of Soft Tissue. In: *Atlas of Tumor Pathology.* 2d Series, Fascicle 1, revised. Armed Forces Institute of Pathology (Washington, D.C.).

Lieberman, L. L. (1956) Synovioma in a Dog. *J. Amer. Vet. Med. Assoc.* 128, 263–264.

Lipowitz, A. J., Fetter, Q. W., and Walker, M. A. (1979) Synovial Sarcoma of the Dog. *J. Amer. Vet. Med. Assoc.* 174, 75–81.

Liu, S. K. (1981) Tumors of Bone and Cartilage. In: Bojrab, M. J., ed., *Pathophysiology in Small Animal Surgery.* Lea and Febiger (Philadelphia).

Liu, S. K., and Dorfman, H. F. (1976) A Condition Resembling Localized Myositis Ossificans in Two Dogs. *J. Small Anim. Pract.* 17, 371–377.

Liu, S. K., Dorfman, H. D., and Patnaik, A. K. (1974) Primary and Secondary Bone Tumors in the Cat. *J. Small Anim. Pract.* 15, 141–156.

Madewell, B. R., and Pool, R. R. (1978) Neoplasms of Joints and Related Structures. *Vet. Clin. N. Amer.* 8, 511–521.

Mair, W. F. (1932) Myositis Ossificans Progressiva. *Edinburgh Med. J.* 39, 13–36; 69–92.

Mason, J. B. (1930) Desmoid Tumors. *Ann. Surg.* 92, 444–453.

McKusick, V. (1966) *Heritable Disorders of Connective Tissue.* C. V. Mosby Co. (St. Louis).

Misdorp, W., and Van der Heul, R. O. (1976). Tumors of Bones and Joints. *Bull. Wld. Hlth. Org.* 53, 265–282.

Mitchell, M., and Hurov, L. I. (1979) Synovial Sarcoma in a Dog. *J. Amer. Vet. Med. Assoc.* 175, 53–55.

Moore, R. W., Snyder, S. P., Houchens, J. W., and Folk, J. J. (1983) Malignant Mesenchymoma in a Dog. *J. Amer. Vet. Med. Assoc.* 19, 187–190.

Morgan, J. P. (1979) Systemic Radiographic Interpretation of Skeletal Diseases in Small Animals. *Vet. Clin. N. Amer.* 4, 611–626.

Murray, J. A. (1977) Synovial Sarcoma. *Orthop. Clin. N. Amer.* 8, 963–972.

Nickels, F. A., Grant, B. D., and Lincoln, S. D. (1976) Villonodular Synovitis of the Equine Metacarpophalangeal Joint. *J. Amer. Vet. Med. Assoc.* 168, 1043–1046.

Nielsen, S. W. (1952) Extraskeletal Giant Cell Tumor in a Cat. *Cornell Vet.* 42, 304–311.

Norris, A. M., Pallet, L., and Wilcock, B. (1980) Generalized Myositis Ossificans in a Cat. *J. Amer. Anim. Hosp. Assoc.* 16, 659–663.

O'Brien, J. E., and Stout, A. P. (1964) Malignant Fibrous Xanthomas. *Cancer* 17, 1445–1455.

Ozzello, L., Stout, A. P., and Murray, M. P. (1963) Cultural Characteristics of Malignant Histiocytomas and Fibrous Xanthomas. *Cancer* 16, 331–344.

Pedersen, N. C., Pool, R. R., and Morgan, J. P. (1983) Joint Diseases of Dogs and Cats. In: Ettinger, S. J., ed., *Textbook of Veterinary Internal Medicine, Diseases of the Dog and Cat.* 2d ed. W. B. Saunders Co. (Philadelphia).

Reed, J. R., Weller, R. E., and Hornoff, W. J. (1978) Synovial Sarcoma in a Dog. *Mod. Vet. Pract.* 59, 605–608.

Render, J. A., Harrington, D. D., Wells, R. E., Dunstan, R. W., Turek, J. J., and Boosinger, T. R. (1982) Giant Cell Tumor of Soft Parts in Six Horses. *J. Amer. Vet. Med. Assoc.* 183, 790–793.

Renlund, R. C., and Pritzker, K. P. H. (1984) Malignant Fibrous Histiocytoma Involving the Digit in a Cat. *Vet. Path.* 21, 442–444.

Rodnan, G. P. (1966) Tumors of Synovial Joints, Bursae and Tendon Sheaths. In: Hollander, J. L., ed., *Arthritis and Allied Conditions,* 7th ed. Lea and Febiger (Philadelphia), 1135–1147.

Rooney, J. R. (1974) *The Lame Horse, Causes, Symptoms and Treatment.* A. S. Barnes and Co., Inc. (South Brunswick, New Jersey).

Roth, J. A., Enzinger, F. M., and Tannenbaum, M. (1975) Synovial Sarcoma of the Neck: A Follow-up Study of 24 Cases. *Cancer* 35, 1243–1253.

Roy, S., and Ghadially, F. N. (1969) Synovial Membrane in Experimentally Produced Chronic Haemarthrosis. *Ann. Rheum. Dis.* 28, 402–411.

Schiefer, B., Neitzke, J. P., and Gray, M. D. (1973) Synovioma in a Dog. *Can. Vet. J.* 14, 225–227.

Siebold, H. R., and Davis, C. L. (1967) Generalized Myositis Ossificans (Familial) in Pigs. *Path. Vet.* 4, 79–88.

Smith, C. F. (1977) Synovial chondromatosis. *Orthop. Clin. N. Amer.* 10, 861–868.

Smith, L. W. (1927) Synovialmata. *Am. J. Path.* 3, 355–363.

Spjut, H. J., Dorfman, H. D., Fechner, R. E., and Ackerman, L. V. (1971) Tumors of Bone and Cartilage. In: *Atlas of Tumor Pathology.* 2d Series, Fascicle 5. Armed Forces Institute of Pathology (Washington, D.C.).

Stannard, A. A., and Pulley, L. T. (1978) Tumors of the Skin and Soft Tissues. In: Moulton, J. E., ed., *Tumors of Domestic Animals.* 2d ed. University of California Press (Berkeley), 16–74.

Stout, A. P. (1948) Mesenchymoma: The Mixed Tumor of Mesenchymal Derivatives. *Ann. Surg.* 127, 278–290.

———. (1954) Juvenile Fibromatosis. *Cancer* 7, 953–978.

Thoday, K. L. (1972) Benign Tendon Sheath Tumor in a Cat [Letter to the Editor]. *J. Small Anim. Pract.* 13, 399–402.

Tillotson, J. F., McDonald, J. R., and Janes, J. M. (1951) Synovial Sarcomata. *J. Bone Joint Surg.* 33A, 459–473.

Turner, A. S., and Trotter, G. W. (1984) Fibrotic Myopathy in the Horse. *J. Amer. Vet. Med. Assoc.* 184, 335–338.

Van Pelt, R. W., Langhan, R. F., and Gill, H. E. (1972) Multiple Hemangiosarcomas in the Tarsal Synovial Sheath of a Horse. *J. Amer. Vet. Med. Assoc.* 161, 49–52.

Weiss, S. W., and Enzinger, F. M. (1978) Malignant Fibrous Histiocytoma: An Analysis of 200 Cases. *Cancer* 41, 2250–2266.

Young, J. M., and Hudacek, A. G. (1954) Experimental Production of Pigmented Villonodular Synovitis in Dogs. *Amer. J. Path.* 30, 799–812.

# 5

*Roy R. Pool*
# Tumors of Bone and Cartilage

Any tissue present within a bone organ may undergo neoplastic transformation. The most common tumors arise in mesenchymal precursors of osseous and cartilaginous tissues. Tumors of fibrous connective tissue and vascular tissue occur much less frequently. Tumors arising from hematopoietic and fatty marrow elements are exceedingly rare. In the dog benign neoplasms of bone are much less common than primary sarcomas. In cats about equal numbers of benign and malignant bone tumors are found, whereas benign tumors of bone exceed sarcomas in horses and cattle (Priester and Mantel, 1971).

When compared with the incidence of neoplasia in other organ systems of domestic animals, primary bone cancer is uncommon (Dorn *et al.,* 1968). In veterinary medicine bone cancer is a malignant disease primarily of domestic dogs. Other than cartilaginous tumors of sheep (Sullivan, 1960), bone sarcomas of livestock are so exceptional that they are regarded as novelties.

A number of references were selected to provide the reader with a greater understanding of bone tumors in animals than space in this chapter permits. Tumors and tumorlike conditions of the mammalian skeleton are the subject of two monographs (Jacobson, 1971; Owen, 1969) that provide an extensive review of the world literature on this subject. The typical clinical, radiographic, and pathological findings in primary bone sarcomas of dogs are well documented (Brodey and Riser, 1969; Brodey *et al.,* 1959; Morgan, 1972; Nielsen *et al.,*

1954; Owen, 1962). Early diagnosis with interpretation of biopsy specimens is emphasized in two studies (Ling *et al.,* 1974; Wykes *et al.,* 1985). Few reports on bone neoplasia in cats are available (Liu *et al.,* 1974; Turrel and Pool, 1982); however, impressions of feline bone cancer can be gained from surveys of feline neoplasia (Cotchin, 1957; Engle and Brodey, 1969; Nielsen, 1964). Additional references may be indicated with each topic.

## General Considerations

**Diagnostic Considerations.** The pathologist greatly enhances his opportunity to make a correct diagnosis of a bone lesion by reviewing the clinical and radiographic findings before he begins a microscopic examination of tissue specimens. Correlation of these three parameters is important not only for correct diagnosis but, in the case of bone sarcomas, for assessment of the degree of malignancy.

**Clinical Characteristics.** Important clinical data include species, breed, age, skeletal site and number of bones involved, duration of bone disease, clinical evaluation of lesion, and general condition of the animal. It is important to know if the animal recently had a systemic disease or had surgery or therapy for soft tissue tumors during the previous year.

**Radiographic Appearance.** The pathologist is trained to evaluate gross specimens and to interpret tissue sections. Radiographs provide important additional information about the entire lesion as it presents within the intact bone specimen. Patterns of architectural alterations within the diseased area, along the borders of the lesion where it adjoins normal bone, and in soft tissue surrounding the lesion can be recognized, interpreted, and correlated with histological findings.

Radiographs that show at least two views of the lesion and that permit evaluation of both soft and hard tissue changes are invaluable aids to the pathologist in characterizing the lesion. The precise location of the disease process in the bone (epiphysis, metaphysis, or diaphysis; periosteum, cortex, or medulla), the number of skeletal sites involved (monostotic or polyostotic disease), and whether or not there is joint or soft tissue involvement should be determined. These features may be obscured by normal structures or by reactive tissue and may be missed or not fully appreciated during gross inspection.

The character of the periosteal response and structural alterations at the margins of the lesion are important measures of the degree of "aggressive" behavior (Morgan, 1974) exhibited by the disease process, and of the ability of adjacent bone tissue to contain and react to the disease process. Within the area of perturbed morphology, the changes can usually be described as destructive (lytic), mixed, or productive (sclerotic).

Benign bone tumors and other "nonaggressive" bone lesions (Morgan, 1974) from which they must be differentiated show a slow rate of development. Adjacent bony structures have time to remodel and respond to the destructive process. This is reflected by a sclerotic intraosseous margin delimiting the lesion and an intact, evenly contoured periosteal border. The "zone of transition" (Morgan, 1974) between affected and normal bone is abrupt, and limits of the lesion are obvious on the radiograph.

Primary bone sarcomas, secondary bone tumors such as locally invasive soft tissue tumors and metastatic tumors, and certain cases of bone infection may all exhibit aggressive radiographic changes as evidenced by the presence of poorly defined borders and rapid alteration of the lesion in sequential examinations. The cortical shadow may be partially lost. Periosteal new bone is irregular and may be incomplete over the surface of the lesion. The disease process may extend into adjacent soft tissue. The long zone of transition between altered and normal bone indicates that the rate of bone destruction exceeds repair. The permeative radiographic pattern and indistinct borders of aggressive lesions reflect both the enlargement of normal vascular channels in bone to accommodate increased blood flow to the affected area and osteoclastic bone resorption within and at the margins of the lesions. Tongues of tumor tissue in bone sarcomas, granulation tissue accompanying infiltrating carcinoma, or exudate from an inflammatory process extend through pathways of least resistance within bone organs, that is, along vascular channels and marrow spaces.

While radiographic diagnosis may not provide the definitive diagnosis, since few radiographic changes are of themselves pathognomonic of a specific disease entity, radiographic findings usually indicate the category of bone disease present: (1) congenital, (2) developmental, (3) metabolic and nutritional, (4) traumatic, (5) infectious, or (6) neoplastic. As a practical matter it is sometimes impossible on radiographic appearance alone to distinguish among primary tumors, secondary tumors, and inflammation of bone, particularly in certain destructive monostotic lesions when they happen to occur in a skeletal site without a high predilection for primary bone tumor. In cases of low-grade fibrosarcoma and chondrosarcoma of bone, however, radiographs are often better indicators of benign or malignant behavior than are microscopic sections. Radiographs may also indicate early malignant change in benign bone tumors, such as osteochondromas.

Collaboration with a radiologist in characterizing a bone lesion is a highly recommended and mutually beneficial experience. For the pathologist operating without a consulting radiologist, two helpful published sources on radiographic interpretation of skeletal diseases of domestic animals are recommended (Morgan, 1972, 1974).

**Pathologic Examination.** A primary requirement for making a correct microscopic diagnosis of a bone lesion is familiarity with the basic microscopic responses of bone and cartilage within the various categories of skeletal disease. Equally important are properly fixed and decalcified tissue sections that can be oriented to the lesion *in situ*. Where the possibility exists, the pathologist should participate in selection of the biopsy site and take responsibility for processing the specimen so that optimal preservation of structure and orientation of the specimen is maintained. The reader is referred elsewhere (Ling *et al.*, 1974; Wykes *et al.*, 1985) for a discussion of biopsy procedures, site selection, causes of unsatisfactory results, and problems of differential diagnosis. A good gross description of the lesion, including the appearance of the tumor tissue and the adjacent normal tissue observed at surgery or necropsy, contributes to making a definitive diagnosis.

Without an adequate clinical and radiographic evaluation of the lesion and in the absence of tissue sections that can be structurally oriented to the bone abnormality, the pathologist may overinterpret or underdiagnose the bits and pieces of tissue presented for microscopic examination. Sections made tangential to an active front of granulation tissue or through exuberant callus of an unstable fracture may be highly suggestive of primary bone sarcoma. Oblique tissue sections through an active, benign, periosteal response (e.g., a bony callus, a cuff of reactive bone, an actively forming osteophyte, an organizing subperiosteal hematoma, or the healing tract of a biopsy punch) may mimic the cellular features and stromal patterns of osteosarcoma. This may also be true of fragmented tissue sections from a benign endosteal response obtained with a trephine, for example, the active stage of canine panosteitis or the forming wall of a bone abscess in the spongiosa. Hemangiosarcoma of bone may go undetected in pieces of tissue from the site of a pathologic fracture, and conversely, small pieces of tissue taken from a large organizing hematoma in a spontaneous fracture may resemble hemangiosarcoma. The low cellularity, abundant fibrillar matrix component, and normochromic and isochromic properties of the spindle cells in a low-grade fibrosarcoma of bone may belie its malignant behavior. Osteochondromas require proper orientation to determine their biphasic morphology and to distinguish them from exostoses. A most important consideration that the pathologist should keep in mind when the final diagnosis is made is whether the morphological diagnosis is consistent with the clinical and radiographic findings in the case.

## TABLE 5.1. Benign Tumors and Tumorlike Lesions of Bone in Domestic Animals

Osteoma
Ossifying fibroma
Fibrous dysplasia
Myxoma/myxosarcoma of the jaw
Osteochondroma, solitary and multiple (osteochondromatosis) of the developing skeleton
Feline osteochondromatosis
Enchondroma, solitary and multiple (enchondromatosis)
Primary chondroma of bone
Primary hemangioma of bone

## BENIGN TUMORS AND TUMORLIKE LESIONS OF BONE

Benign bony, fibroosseous, and cartilaginous lesions of animal bone are relatively uncommon and usually of no great clinical concern or economic significance. As a result these lesions have been neglected by veterinary pathologists and consequently are inadequately documented, and their biological behavior is uncertain. Yet pathologists encounter tissue sections of these lesions with disconcerting regularity. Probably no single veterinary teaching institution has a sufficiently large collection of these conditions to permit any individual to make an authoritative characterization of these entities as they occur in the various domestic species. The descriptions and opinions offered in this section result from an examination of only a few specimens from the following categories of lesions and may not accurately reflect the range of morphological variations or biological behavior that occur in any large population of animals. Fibroosseous lesions are included here with benign tumors of bone because of problems in differential diagnosis. In this section the author has followed the morphological criteria used for diagnosis of comparable disease entities in humans (Spjut *et al.*, 1971). Benign bone lesions covered in this chapter are indicated in table 5.1.

### Osteoma, Ossifying Fibroma, and Fibrous Dysplasia

**General Considerations.** Osteoma, ossifying fibroma, and fibrous dysplasia form a miscellaneous group of poorly understood benign lesions found primarily in intramembranous bone where abnormal tissue of varying degrees of differentiation and compactness arises from osteogenic connective tissue to alter the shape and function of affected bones. A certain degree of morphological similarity is shared by the three entities. All three diseases may occur in the jaw, but only ossifying fibroma seems to be restricted to that location. Osteomas are lesions composed of dense accumulations of well-differentiated cancellous or compact bone with delicate intervening fibrous and vascular tissue (fig. 5.1A and B). In contrast, fibrous dysplasia has a major component of fibrovascular stroma separating equidistant, tenuous, curved trabeculae of poorly differentiated bone (fig. 5.1C). These trabeculae arise by metaplasia of fibrous connective tissue and are not typically lined by osteoblasts. The ossifying fibroma shows an intermediate architecture (fig. 5.1D). Some osteomas have features common to all three entities, which suggests the possibility that osteoma may be an end stage of more than one process. In fact, some physician pathologists consider that certain osteomas of the human skull are mature lesions of fibrous dysplasia and that ossifying fibroma is a form that fibrous dysplasia assumes in the mandible. This confounding problem in humans is not readily resolvable at present in animals. However, it is important that veterinary pathologists be aware of the morphology of these benign, proliferative, fibroosseous processes if for no other reason than to not overdiagnose these lesions as a sarcoma of bone.

## Osteoma

**Classification.** Smoothly contoured, solitary, benign bony growths of substantial size protruding from the surfaces of bones, typically formed by intramembranous ossification, are called osteomas. There is doubt whether these are true tumors, and they are regarded by some pathologists as hamartomas (Aegerter and Kirkpatrick, 1968). They may resemble exostoses in structure, and at times, the two entities probably cannot be differentiated by microscopic examination.

**Incidence, Age, Breed, and Sex.** These uncommon tumors appear in all domestic species, but are more often recognized in horses and cattle. Most so-called osteomas of the canine head are really examples of multilobular tumors (discussed later in this chapter with primary sarcomas of bone). Ossified canine epulides or tumors of tooth germ origin are excluded from this category as well as craniomandibular osteopathy of intramembranous bones of terrier puppies. Too few cases of osteoma are documented to permit proper evaluation of the influence of age, breed, or sex.

**Clinical Characteristics.** Osteomas demonstrate slow but progressive growth over a period of months and then may cease growth and remain quiescent for years. They cause disfigurement, obstruct natural passages in the head, place pressure on adjacent structures, disturb normal breathing, and interfere with prehension, mastication, and deglutition of food. They may recur locally following incomplete surgical removal.

**Sites.** Mandible, maxilla, nasal sinuses, and bones of the face and cranium are the most common sites of involvement in domestic animals. Massive benign bony growths resulting from unexplained chronic periosteal hyperplasia are occasionally found on the limbs, sternum, ribs, and skull of cats. These feline osteomas (see Parosteal Osteosarcoma) can be distinguished from osteochondromas and osteophytosis of vitamin A intoxication of cats on the basis of morphology, distribution, and history.

**Gross Morphology and Radiographic Appearance.** Osteomas typically have evenly contoured borders covered by a moderately vascularized layer of connective tissue, which tends to be mucoid or edematous in osteomas of the nasal cavity. In horses and cattle osteomas may attain remarkable size. One nasal osteoma in a bull (fig. 5.2) was more than 14 cm in diameter (Rumbaugh *et al.*, 1978). Osteomas are so dense that they must be sectioned with a saw. On cut surface, mature osteomas are found to be composed of densely packed cancellous bone with fibrous and adipose connective tissue filling the marrow spaces.

Osteomas are typically monostotic, sclerotic lesions. They blend into contiguous normal bone structure and protrude from the bone surface while maintaining a distinct and regularly contoured border.

**Histological Features.** Osteomas are bony growths initially formed of cancellous bone that

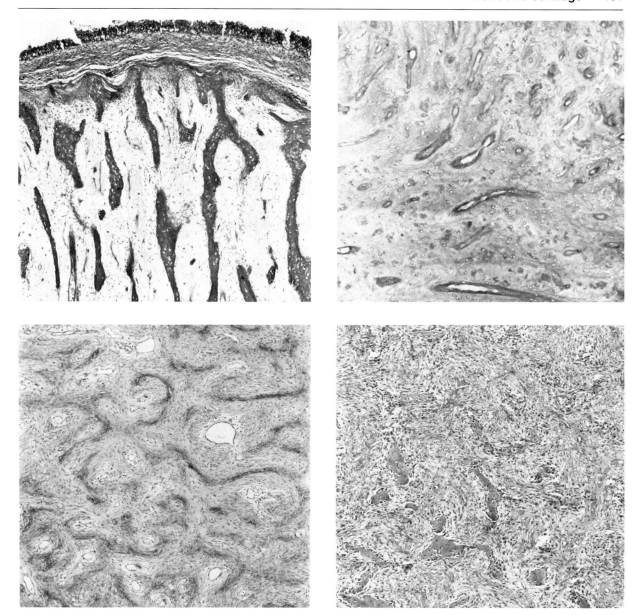

A|B  **FIGURE 5.1.** Fibroosseous tumorlike lesions of bone.
C|D  A. Developing nasal osteoma. B. Eburnated osteoma
of maxilla. C. Fibrous dysplasia of femur. D. Ossifying fibroma of mandible.

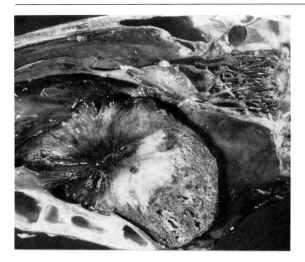

**FIGURE 5.2.** Sagittal section of the skull of a bull with the nasal septum removed showing an osteoma of the nasal cavity. Smoothly contoured tumor has compressed the turbinates.

may become increasingly compact with time (figs. 5.1A and B; 5.3A and B). Soft tissue spaces intervening between bony trabeculae contain one or more centrally located small caliber blood vessels, a sparse population of spindle cells, and a moderately fibrillar connective tissue matrix. The matrix of nasal osteomas frequently has a mucoid appearance. Actively growing osteomas are bordered by a layer of connective tissue resembling the periosteum. Newly formed bony trabeculae are slender and oriented perpendicular to the surface of the osteoma. Less superficial older trabeculae are thicker and may show no surface orientation. Sclerotic or eburnated osteomas are produced by growth in diameter of individual bony trabeculae at the expense of tissue spaces (fig. 5.1B). In mature osteomas bony fusion of peripheral trabeculae produces a cortical margin of compact bone. Osteomas as a group show a variety of deviations from this pattern.

Many osteomas have an orderly zonal architecture. In actively growing osteomas the periosteum is well-differentiated and is composed of both fibrous and osteogenic layers. Peripheral trabeculae are formed of woven bone deposited by a border of typical osteoblasts. Deeper trabeculae are broader structures formed of finely fibered lamellar bone

that partially or completely replaces woven bone following normal remodeling activity.

The pathologist will also encounter a number of less well structured osteomas (figs. 5.3C and D). In some of these osteomas the periosteal covering is poorly differentiated and resembles only the fibrous layer of the periosteum. Recognizable osteoblasts are not present in the periosteum or on trabecular surfaces. The thin fibrous layer gives rise to peripheral trabeculae of immature woven bone by osseous metaplasia of fibrous connective tissue. Trabeculae are irregular in shape and size and show little or no orientation to the surface of the lesion. Even the older and deeper trabeculae are composed almost entirely of woven bone (fig. 5.3B). Remodeling and replacement by lamellar bone is infrequent. Spindle cells in the mucoid matrix filling the tissue spaces account for appositional growth of the cancellous bone.

**Growth and Metastasis.** Osteomas typically show slow progressive growth over a period of months and then may maintain this size and shape indefinitely. Some nasal osteomas appear to arise by bony metaplasia of the fibrous stroma in nasal polyps. Such lesions not arising from skeletal tissues should probably not be designated as osteomas, but rather as metaplastic lesions. Site, size, and weight of the osteomas cause clinical problems. Neoplastic transformation is unreported and not anticipated.

## Ossifying Fibroma

**Classification.** This is a fibroosseous lesion producing a tumorlike disease in the jaws of animals. The nomenclature of this entity is complex because of disagreement among pathologists as to the nature of the lesion. In humans this disease has also been called fibrous osteoma, osteofibroma, osteogenic fibroma, and osteoid fibroma. Some physician pathologists have considered similar jaw lesions in humans as variants of fibrous dysplasia or variants of osteoblastoma. Other pathologists have expressed concern that the lesion is no more than a postextraction granuloma. Only one veterinary pathologist (Owen, 1969) has recognized the occurrence of a case of osteoblastoma in animals and it was found in the scapula of an older cat. In humans

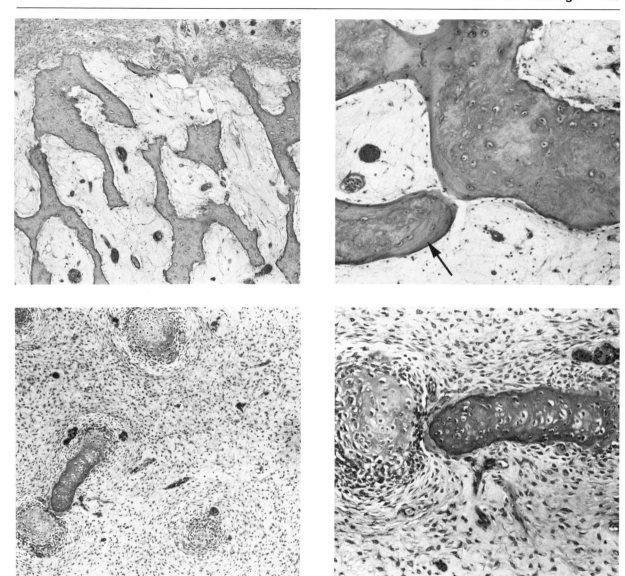

A|B  **FIGURE 5.3.** Osteoma of the head. A. Nasal osteoma
C|D  with poorly differentiated periosteal membrane. A few
flattened cells line bone surfaces. B. Minimal remodeling of
woven bone with replacement by lamellar bone (**arrow**).
C. Mandibular osteoma possibly arising from ossifying fibroma. D. Higher magnification of C showing condensation
of cells along margins of crude bone spicules.

ossifying fibroma can be distinguished from fibrous dysplasia on a clinical and morphological basis (Spjut *et al.*, 1971). It seems reasonable for veterinary pathologists to attempt to differentiate between these two entities in animals because the indications for therapy are different in humans.

**Incidence, Age, Breed, and Sex.** Ossifying fibroma is a rare tumorlike lesion occurring primarily in the jaws of horses, ruminants, cats, and possibly other species (Boever *et al.*, 1977; Turrel and Pool, 1982). Because of certain morphologic similarities between the two lesions, it is possible that some ossifying fibromas may mature into osteomas. Until this area of confusion is resolved the incidence of this disease remains unclear.

**Clinical Characteristics and Sites.** These large, solitary lesions in the jaw may replace alveolar and cortical bone. The disease causes loosening and loss of teeth, interference with mastication of food, and predisposition of the jaw to pathological fracture. Either the maxilla or mandible may be involved. Lesions may be bilateral.

**Gross Morphology and Radiographic Appearance.** Ossifying fibroma, unlike an osteoma that arises from a sessile base on the surface of a bone, produces an expansile lesion of the jaw bone and replaces normal bone tissue with fibroosseous stroma. The abnormal tissue is dense and may be too well mineralized to be cut with a knife.

Ossifying fibroma presents as a sharply demarcated, solitary, mixed to moderately radiolucent lesion that expands the normal contours of the affected bone at the area of involvement (fig. 5.4A). If the fibroosseous process extends into adjacent soft tissue, the border of the lesion may be irregular, but without fingerlike projections or a brush border. Possibly some of the more exuberant, large, productive bony lesions occasionally encountered at the mandibular symphysis of horses are examples of ossifying fibroma rather than osteoma or osteosarcoma.

**Histological Features, Growth, and Metastasis.** Irregularly shaped spicules of osteoid and bone rimmed with osteoblasts are randomly formed in a moderately vascularized, fibroosseous stroma (fig. 5.4B). The proliferative element is composed of isochromic spindle cells resembling fibroblasts that undergo transformation to osteoblasts along the margins of developing bone spicules (fig. 5.4C).

Cartilage is not formed in the lesion. As the name of the disease implies, the morphology of the process is that of a fibroma in which bone forms by osseous metaplasia of the fibrous connective tissue component. Therefore, tissue spaces between bony trabeculae have a greater density of cells and fibers in ossifying fibroma than do the marrow spaces of an osteoma.

Zonation in the lesion if present is not obvious and no recognizable periosteal membrane borders the lesion. Ossification occurs randomly through the lesion. Bone spicules are composed almost entirely of woven bone. In a few scattered areas a few large, well-developed, irregularly shaped bony trabeculae may be found. These may show evidence of osteoclastic resorption and have some patchy deposits of lamellar bone. Soft tissue between bone spicules shows a loss of cell and fiber density, so that in these small areas of the lesion there are foci resembling the major structure of the osteoma.

Proliferative tissue extends into adjacent soft tissue along a contoured front restrained in part by layers of compressed connective tissue. Within the jaw preexisting bone is removed by osteoclastic activity.

Cellular and stromal microscopic features distinguish ossifying fibroma from osteosarcoma. In osteosarcoma the malignant cells have a high mitotic index and are more pleomorphic and hyperchromatic than cells in ossifying fibroma. Well-structured trabecular bone is seldom produced in osteosarcoma.

Ossifying fibromas destroy preexisting bone structure and produce expansile lesions of affected bones. They are not considered to be premalignant lesions.

## Fibrous Dysplasia

**Classification.** Smoothly contoured expansile deformities of bone are caused by an unexplained failure in maintenance of cancellous bone structure and its replacement by a fibroosseous matrix of characteristic morphology. Extraskeletal manifestations, including endocrine disturbances and patchy pigmentation of the skin seen in humans, have not been reported to occur in animals with fibrous dysplasia. Like ossifying fibroma this disease is also

thologist, however, may see surgical specimens of solitary osteochondromas more often in horses because of their greater economic value.

Typically, osteochondromatosis is first recognized in immature dogs and horses during the period of active bone growth when exostoses are most likely to cause clinical abnormalities. Osteochondromas in most dogs and horses respond to the same trophic influences as do growth plates and gradually cease growth at skeletal maturity. No breed or sex predilection has been indicated for any domestic species.

**Clinical Characteristics.** Clinical disease includes disfigurement, lameness, pain, paresis, and paralysis. Clinical signs result from distortion and compression of normal structures. Lesions on limbs may interfere with the function of tendons, muscles, vessels, and nerves in the area, resulting in lameness and pain. Vertebral involvement, especially in dogs, causes spinal cord compression and attendant neurologic deficits. Many animals have clinically silent osteochondromatosis in which case the lesions may go undiscovered or be found during routine care of the animal. Malignant transformation sometimes occurs in osteochondromas of dogs and may arise from either clinically silent or symptomatic long-standing lesions (Banks and Bridges, 1956; Owen and Bostock, 1971).

**Sites.** Osteochondromas may form in any bone of endochondral origin and should never arise from the flat bones of the skull of intramembranous origin. Scapulae, ribs, vertebrae, and the pelvis are the most commonly affected sites. Bilateral lesions of the limbs occur regularly in dogs and horses.

Self-limiting metaplastic proliferations of cartilage occurring in soft tissues may undergo endochondral ossification and acquire the biphasic morphology of an osteochondroma. Such lesions are commonly found in the synovium of joints with chronic degenerative joint disease and in the trachea of dogs (Gourley *et al.*, 1970). Although the term *osteochondroma* is applied to these lesions, they should be distinguished from the developmental skeletal lesions and identified as osteochondromas of the synovium, trachea, and other areas.

**Gross Morphology.** An osteochondroma is an evenly contoured outgrowth from the surface of a bone with a bony base and a cap of hyaline cartilage (fig. 5.7A). Lesions on limbs tend to be pedunculated. They are located on the cortical surface in the metaphyseal region or toward the end of the diaphysis of a long bone, but they always spare the epiphysis. Osteochondromas on flat bones typically are bulky ovoid structures with a sessile base. They often form eccentric cuffs around the shafts of ribs and tend to be found adjacent to the costochondral junction. The outer surface of an osteochondroma is white to bluish white, reflecting the presence of the cartilaginous component. The thin cortex of the bony base of the exostosis blends imperceptibly with the cortex of the affected bone. Spongy bone and marrow spaces of the osteochondroma are continuous with those of the host bone.

**Radiographic Appearance.** Osteochondromas are exostoses with regular contours that merge into the substance of the bone from which they arise (fig. 5.7B). Radiodensity of the tumor reflects the component of cancellous bone, while radiolucent areas represent areas of hyaline cartilage yet to undergo endochondral ossification. Loss of smooth contour with bone destruction or production along the margin or base of an osteochondroma may indicate malignant transformation in the lesion. Large osteochondromas during the active growth phase may occasionally have an ominous mottled radiographic pattern and be initially suggestive of malignant bone tumor. Sequential radiographic studies or a bone biopsy will clarify the nature of the lesion.

**Histological Features.** Osteochondromas are orderly biphasic growths with an apical margin of hyaline cartilage and a bony base of cancellous bone and intervening marrow spaces (fig. 5.7C). In young developing lesions the cartilage cap is a distinctive structure, but in maturing lesions the cap is discontinuous. In actively growing lesions the cartilage cap mimics a growth plate and produces bone by orderly endochondral ossification. Islands of cartilage, however, may be retained in cancellous bone within the base of the exostosis. Multiple islands of calcified cartilage scattered through large, rapidly growing osteochondromas produce a mottled radiographic pattern that may give concern for the presence of malignant bone tumor. A membrane continuous with the periosteum of the host bone covers the surface of the osteochondroma. Chondrogenic activity of the membrane followed by endochondral ossification accounts for most of the growth of the osteochondroma. Some enlargement

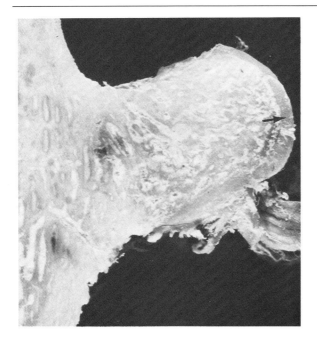

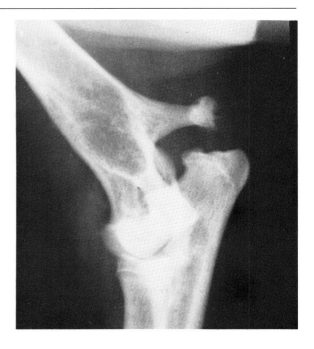

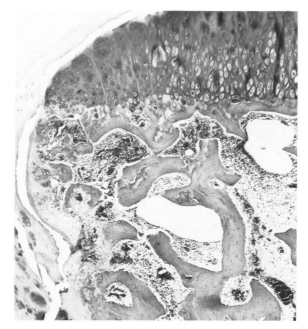

FIGURE 5.7. Osteochondroma. A. Cartilage cap (**ar-row**) covers bony stalk. Note how marrow spaces of stalk blend with those of the bone organ. B. Evenly contoured stalk of osteochondroma blends smoothly into cortical surface of distal humerus. C. Cartilage cap gives rise to cancellous bone of stalk by endochondral ossification.

of the bony base is due to appositional growth by the periosteum.

Biopsies of osteochondromas must be properly oriented to reveal the architecture of the lesion. Sections taken tangentially through the cartilage gap of an actively growing lesion can be misleading and suggestive of chondrosarcoma. The pathologist should also realize that in mature osteochondromas, endochondral ossification may be completed with little or no cartilage remaining at the apical surface. In some cases the cartilage that remains is hyalinized and the chondrocytes are poorly stained, necrotic, ghostlike remnants that can easily be overlooked.

**Growth and Metastasis.** Growth of an osteochondroma typically is in synchronization with skeletal maturation, so that most osteochondromas do not become obvious or present clinical problems until the last half of the period of active skeletal growth. Growth of an osteochondroma should cease at about the time of skeletal maturity. Malignant transformation to chondrosarcoma and osteosarcoma can occur in dogs.

# Feline Osteochondromatosis

**Classification.** Osteochondromatosis of cats is presented separately from the disorder in dogs and horses bearing the same name because the disease in cats has a different clinical setting, a different skeletal distribution, and apparently a different cause. Unlike the cartilage-capped exostoses of dogs and horses, which are developmental disturbances that cease growth at skeletal maturity, the osteochondromas of cats show progressive enlargement, which is a feature of true tumors.

Viral particles resembling the agent causing feline leukemia and transmissible feline sarcoma have been found consistently in the cartilage caps of cats with multiple cartilaginous exostoses (Pool, 1981; Pool and Carrig, 1972; Pool and Harris, 1975). Although the significance of the virus in the pathogenesis of the lesions is undetermined, a viral etiology with hematogenous localization in the periosteum at random sites could explain the different pattern of distribution and clinical setting of the disease in cats compared to dogs and horses.

**Incidence, Age, Breed, and Sex.** The incidence of osteochondromatosis in cats is unknown. Fewer cases of this disease have been reported in cats (Brown *et al.,* 1972; Pool, 1981; Pool and Carrig, 1972; Pool and Harris, 1975; Riddle and Leighton, 1970) than in dogs. Affected cats ranged in age from 16 months to 8 years, but most cats were young adults 2 to 4 years old at the time the exostoses were first discovered. There is no evidence of a breed or sex predilection. No hereditary pattern has been reported in cats.

**Clinical Characteristics.** Initially the lesions are asymptomatic. In most instances owners discovered the nodules while petting or grooming the cat and only became concerned when one or more of the slowly growing lesions suddenly enlarged. Continued growth of the nodules caused disfigurement, pain, encroachment on joints and tendons, and muscle atrophy. All cats were afebrile and most had normal hemograms. All cats tested for feline leukemia virus infection were positive. All of these cases appeared in animals with mature skeletons, and once the exostoses appeared, they demonstrated progressive enlargement, a feature that is characteristic of a true tumor.

**Sites.** Unlike osteochondromatosis in dogs, skeletal lesions in cats had a random distribution, including the development of exostoses in bones of the skull formed by intramembranous ossification. Sites of skeletal involvement in decreasing order of frequency are the rib cage, scapulae, vertebral column, skull, pelvis, and bones of the limbs. When exostoses occur on long bones, the lesions are random in distribution with no affinity for the metaphysis.

**Gross Morphology.** Most feline osteochondromas are bulky masses, sometimes appearing to be formed by a coalescence of smaller nodules, that are attached to the bone by a sessile base (fig. 5.8A). Most of the mass is formed of cancellous bone, but a pale surface layer of cartilage can usually be recognized on cut surface.

**Radiographic Appearance.** Usually osteochondromas of cats arise from bone surfaces as sessile excrescences with well-defined, bosselated borders. Often the outer third of a rapidly growing exostosis has an amorphous, mottled appearance. An aggressive radiographic pattern was present in an osteochondroma of a cervical vertebra. Malignant transformation to osteosarcoma was demonstrated by histopathology.

**Histological Features.** Feline osteochondromas usually have a biphasic pattern with a cover of cartilage giving rise to a bony base by endochondral ossification. However, it is not uncommon for the hyperplastic layer of periosteum to directly form bone instead of cartilage, a feature not seen in canine osteochondromas. Even when cartilage is formed by the periosteum, the cartilage tissue differs from that of the cartilage cap of the dog in being more cellular, forming fewer chondrones, and producing less ground substance. Endochondral ossification is less orderly than in the dog, and the cancellous bone is composed mostly of woven bone tissue (fig. 5.8B). In time the bony structures of many feline osteochondromas undergo remodeling and the architecture becomes increasingly disorganized with some stromal cells acquiring atypical features (fig. 5.8C).

**Growth and Metastasis.** Growth of feline osteochondromas is continuous. In a cat with numerous nodules of varying size and duration, lesions can be identified that undergo progressive transformation from periosteal hyperplasia to parosteal sar-

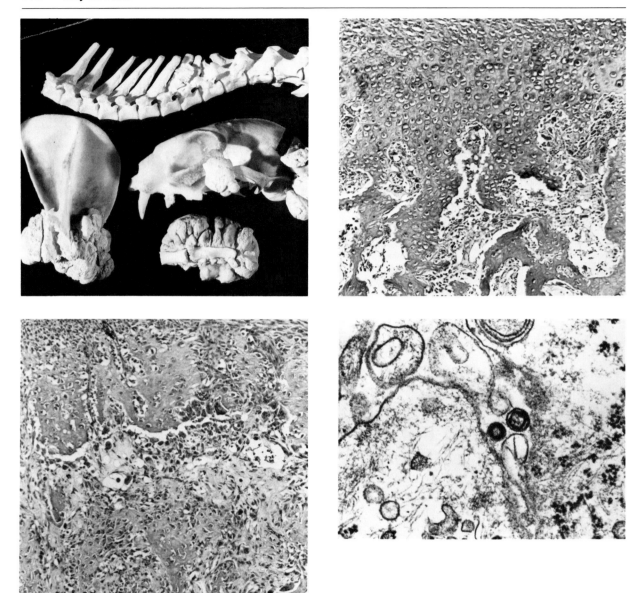

A|B
C|D  **FIGURE 5.8.** Feline osteochondromatosis. A. Multiple, sessile, cartilage-capped, bony growths are randomly distributed on several bones including the skull of a cat. B. Orderly endochondral ossification along base of cap. C. Disorganized architecture of osteochondroma with pleomorphism of stromal cells. D. Virus particles bud from plasmalemma of a chondrocyte in the cartilage cap.

coma. The proliferative response is thought to be caused by virus acting on cells of the periosteum (fig. 5.8D). A grave prognosis should be given for any cat with this neoplasm since new lesions continue to appear in the skeleton throughout the course of the disease. Owners usually have the cat euthanized because of disfigurement and lameness caused by the enlarging lesions. Malignant transformation occurred in an osteochondroma of a cervical vertebra in one cat.

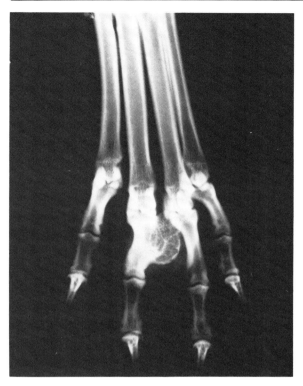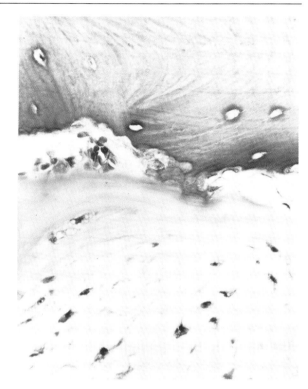

A | B    **FIGURE 5.9.** Enchondroma of the dog. A. Expansile growth of a radiolucent, benign cartilage tumor in a metatarsal bone in the foot of a dog. B. Slow encroachment of chondroma on compact bone of the inner cortical surface of a metatarsal bone.

## Enchondroma

An enchondroma is a benign cartilaginous tumor originating within the medullary cavity of a bone. In animals enchondromas may produce monostotic (Brodey *et al.*, 1959; Folger, 1917; Morgan, 1974) or polyostotic (McGrath, 1960; Nieberle and Cohrs, 1967) patterns of skeletal involvement. An animal with a single lesion has a solitary enchondroma of bone, while one with multiple tumors has enchondromatosis. These benign central cartilage tumors should not be confused with osteochondromas, which arise from the surface of the bone and are a developmental disorder. Enchondromas are much less commonly reported in animals than osteochondromas, and the two entities probably do not coexist in the same individual.

An enchondroma is an autonomous growth of hyaline cartilage arising within a bone. It is unclear whether enchondromas have their origin in cartilage remnants that escaped endochondral ossification, in areas of cartilaginous metaplasia of bone marrow stroma, or as hamartomas. Expansile growth of the tumor attenuates the cortex and expands the surface of the affected bone (fig. 5.9A) (Morgan, 1972). The lesion is radiolucent with well-demarcated borders. The cortical surface over the lesion is smooth. Lameness caused by pain and pathological fracture may be the presenting sign. Tumor tissue resembles hyaline cartilage. Chondrocytes are smaller, less numerous, and more isomorphic than those of chondrosarcoma (fig. 5.9B). There are no good histological criteria to distinguish enchondroma from a chondroma of bone, but it is important to recognize that the lesion is benign. The diagnosis of enchondromatosis, however, can be made with confidence since the finding of an animal with multiple primary chondromas is unlikely. Malignant transformation of an enchondroma sometimes occurs in humans (Spjut *et al.*, 1971) and probably occurs in animals. One can only speculate on the role of solitary enchondromas in the histogenesis of central chondrosarcomas in animals.

Too few cases of enchondroma have been reported in animals to permit an adequate description of this neoplasm. The intent here is to present a few features of this entity so that the pathologist will consider this tumor in his differential diagnosis when a nonaggressive, radiolucent, expansile lesion of a bone containing benign cartilage is presented.

## Primary Chondroma of Bone

**Classification.** A chondroma is a benign neoplasm of cartilage. In veterinary medicine the term *chondroma* often has been used to include all benign proliferations of cartilage including a number of clinical entities such as extraskeletal chondromas, especially those originating in canine mammary mixed tumors, synovial and bursal chondroma and osteochondroma, multilobular tumors of the canine skull, osteochondroma, enchondroma, and a large group of unclassified chondromas of bone. Periosteal chondroma (juxtacortical chondroma) has not been reported in animals. To be a meaningful term, primary chondroma of bone must refer to a distinctive clinicopathological entity that can be differentiated from other specific types of chondromas. Unfortunately, the term *chondroma* often has been used for benign growths of cartilage in cases in which there were inadequate clinical, radiographic, and gross descriptions of the lesion and limited tissue sections for proper evaluation. Many lesions diagnosed as chondromas may have been enchondromas, low-grade chondrosarcomas, and self-limiting metaplastic proliferations of cartilage associated with cartilaginous structures of the larynx, trachea, and bronchi or the synovial lining of tendon sheaths. Veterinary pathologists will continue to use the term *primary chondroma of bone* as the diagnosis for those rather rare benign cartilaginous tumors of the turbinates, flat bones, sternal–costal cartilage complex, and limbs of animals until the nature of these lesions is clarified. There is a distinct possibility that once the nature of these various benign cartilaginous proliferations in animals is

understood, chondroma as an entity will no longer exist (Aegerter and Kirkpatrick, 1968).

**Incidence, Age, Breed, and Sex.** Primary chondroma of bone is a rare lesion that has been reported in all domestic animals (Sullivan, 1960). These benign neoplasms are less common than their malignant counterparts. Most tumors have been reported in mature to aged dogs and sheep. There is no known breed or sex prevalence.

**Clinical Characteristics, Sites, and Gross Morphology.** Chondromas demonstrate slow growth and deform affected bones. Clinical signs are related to size and location of the tumor. Flat bones are more commonly involved than long bones.

Tumors vary in size. They are firm and generally have evenly contoured borders covered by a fibrous capsule. On cut surface chondromas are bluish white to milk white and have a multilobular structure.

**Radiographic Appearance.** Chondromas produce expansile bone lesions that attenuate the cortex while maintaining a smooth but discrete border (Morgan, 1972). Evidence of osteolysis, production of reactive bone, soft tissue response, and change in radiographic appearance in a 2-week interval may indicate either malignant transformation or traumatic injury of the tumor.

**Histological Features.** Benign tumors are formed of irregular lobules of hyaline cartilage. Neoplastic cartilage is composed of innocuous chondrocytes tending to be rather uniform in size and shape set in a matrix that on occasion has more fibrous stroma than is found in normal hyaline cartilage (fig. 5.10). Histological distinctions between chondroma and low-grade chondrosarcoma are often equivocal in specific cases. Once the pathologist appreciates the limitations of microscopic interpretation in these instances, he will rely heavily on clinical and radiographic findings in making the final diagnosis. Commonly the biological behavior of a cartilaginous bone tumor is evaluated better by sequential radiographic studies than by biopsy.

**Growth and Metastasis.** Primary chondromas of bone grow by expansion. Since the relationship between enchondroma and primary chondroma of bone in animals is uncertain and since so few cases of either are well-documented, one can only speculate on the percentage of cases of either tumor that give rise to chondrosarcoma. It is currently believed that most chondrosarcomas of dogs arise *de novo*

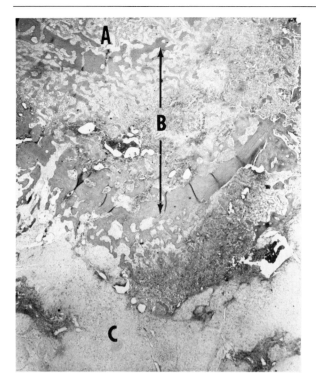

FIGURE 5.12. Osteosarcoma of a dog's tibia. Transverse section through the cranial cortex at the tibial crest shows an osteosarcoma arising in the medullary cavity (A), invading the cortex (B), and producing malignant cartilage on the surface (C) of the bone.

graphic studies; and the category of bone sarcoma, which, as previously mentioned, indicates the rapidity of the clinical course and the anticipated fate of the patient. There is disagreement regarding the validity of histological grading of osteosarcoma as a useful indicator of anticipated survival rate in humans (Spjut et al., 1971), although grading does appear correlated with survival rates in human fibrosarcoma and chondrosarcoma. Human patients with well-differentiated chondrosarcomas and fibrosarcomas of bone have a better prognosis than those with poorly differentiated tumors. By contrast, most reports indicate that the level of differentiation in human osteosarcoma has no prognostic value (Spjut et al., 1971). In studies by Dahlin (1967) working with human osteosarcoma patients

in the United States and in other studies on patients in the Netherlands (Netherlands Committee on Bone Tumors, 1966) it was found that the fibroblastic subtype of osteosarcoma is associated with a more favorable prognosis than are the other subtypes. Spjut et al. (1981) have recognized another subtype of human osteosarcoma called an intraosseous well-differentiated osteosarcoma that when treated by wide resection or amputation offers a good prognosis. Misdorp and Hart (1979) report that the fibroblastic form of osteosarcoma in dogs also has a more favorable prognosis in that species of animal.

Details of malignant bone disease in most domestic animals are cursory, but initial epidemiological studies have improved the estimates of the frequency with which the various types of bone sarcomas are distributed among the major animal species of veterinary concern (Dorn et al., 1968; Misdorp and Hart, 1979; Priester and Mantel, 1971). Bone cancer is not a common disease in the animal population. One animal neoplasm survey found an incidence rate for bone cancer of 7.9 for dogs and 4.9 for cats per 100,000 individuals (Dorn et al., 1968). The disease is too rare in the other domestic species to determine an incidence rate. Of the major classes of animal bone sarcoma (table 5.2), osteosarcoma is by far the most common type occurring in dogs (Brodey and Riser, 1969; Brodey et al., 1963; Jacobson, 1971; Owen, 1962) and in cats (Engle and Brodey, 1969; Liu et al., 1974; Turrel and Pool, 1982).

In the dog, osteosarcoma (80%) and chondrosarcoma (10%) are the most common histological types. Fibrosarcoma and hemangiosarcoma together account for approximately 7% of the tumors. Lymphoid and myeloid tumors of the marrow (Osborne et al., 1968) are seen infrequently. Parosteal osteosarcoma (Banks, 1971; Jacobson, 1971; Liu et al., 1974; Turrel and Pool, 1982) and liposarcoma of bone marrow (Brodey and Riser, 1966) are very rare tumors of the dog and cat skeleton.

As the importance of breed variations in the development of primary bone neoplasia becomes better understood, clinicopathological studies will appear in the literature that will characterize the skeletal distribution of different breeds. It has long been recognized that certain breeds of dogs are predisposed to bone neoplasia, and one study (Brodey *et al.*, 1963) has indicated that the pattern of skeletal involvement varies among several breeds of dogs. Certainly, the size of the dog is a major predisposing factor in the development of bone cancer (Tjalma, 1966). Most skeletal maps depicting sites of predilection of canine bone sarcoma apply to large and giant breeds of dogs. Similar maps need to be made for the smaller canine breeds.

Influence of tumor site within the skeleton on biological behavior has not been fully evaluated. Osteosarcomas in humans located below the knee and elbow joints and occurring in the jaws are usually less aggressive and have less metastatic potential than osteosarcomas of other sites (Dahlin and Unni, 1977). Misdorp and Hart (1979) in their study on dogs from the Netherlands found that osteosarcomas of the hindlegs have a poorer prognosis than those arising in other skeletal sites. It is not known whether bone sarcomas of comparable histological appearance have the same growth rate and metastatic potential when located in the manus or pes as when situated in a more proximal site in the appendicular skeleton. With the recent interest in cancer therapy for animal bone tumors, new demands are being placed on the pathologist to characterize these tumors precisely and to provide morphological support in determining the efficacy of treatment of the several categories of mesenchymal neoplasms encountered in animal bone.

## SARCOMA OF CENTRAL OR MEDULLARY ORIGIN

### Osteosarcoma

Sarcomas arising within the bone organs are more common and exhibit a consistently greater malignant behavior than sarcomas of periosteal origin. Osteosarcoma of central or medullary origin as it occurs in the dog is the most common primary bone tumor seen by the veterinary pathologist, and consequently, it is the only sarcoma of bone for which large numbers of cases have been available for gross and microscopic study. The description of osteosarcoma in this chapter pertains mainly to the disease as it appears in dogs.

**Classification.** The classification scheme used here (table 5.2) for central bone tumors is a modified version of the one developed by Dahlin and Unni (1977) for categorizing primary bone tumors of humans. Osteosarcomas are primary malignant bone tumors in which the neoplastic cells produce tumor osteoid and tumor bone, that is, calcified tumor osteoid. Osteosarcomas are not a homogeneous group of tumors. They vary greatly in the amount and quality of matrix and in histological patterns, and they produce a wide range of radiographic changes. Often the radiographic and histological patterns will mimic those of the other major classes of primary bone tumor. Although there are no large studies in animals that conclusively prove differences in clinical behavior among the several subclasses of osteosarcoma, this classification scheme is useful for acquainting the veterinary pathology resident with the range of histological patterns produced in these tumors. Misdorp and Hart (1979) have found in their study of 144 dogs with naturally occurring osteosarcomas of the skeleton that dogs with the fibroblastic type of osteosarcoma have a better prognosis than dogs having one of the other subclasses of osteosarcoma.

**Incidence, Age, Breed, and Sex.** The incidence of bone neoplasia is higher in the dog (6.5 per 100,000 cases) than in the cat (3.1 per 100,000 cases) (Schneider, 1978). Comparable data are not available for the other domestic animals since primary bone neoplasia is so uncommon in those species (Jacobson, 1971). Osteosarcoma accounts for about 80% of the malignant bone tumors in dogs (Brodey and Riser, 1969) and about 70% in cats (Turrel and Pool, 1982).

In dogs the average age at time of first clinical recognition of the tumor is about 7 years 6 months with a range of from a few months to 18 years. Affected giant breeds of dogs are generally younger than dogs of smaller breeds (Misdorp and Hart, 1979). Tumors of ribs also tend to occur more often in slightly younger adult dogs (Owen, 1962), whereas osteosarcomas of the skull tend to appear at a later age than those in the appendicular skeleton (Hardy *et al.*, 1967). The average age of dogs developing primary osteosarcomas of the vertebral column is 7 years (Morgan *et al.*, 1980). Five breeds of dogs (boxers, Great Danes, Saint Bernards, German shepherds, and Irish setters) accounted for two-thirds of the cases in a study of dogs from Pennsylvania (Brodey and Riser, 1969),

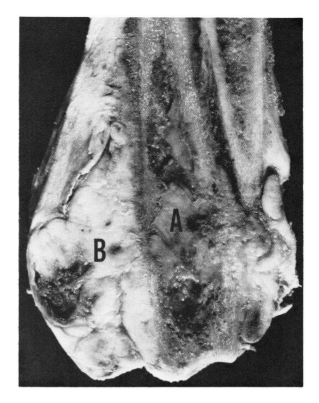

**FIGURE 5.14.** Moderately productive osteoblastic osteosarcoma of the distal radius replaces the normal metaphyseal spongiosa (A), penetrates the cortex, and forms a large soft tissue mass (B) on the surface of the cranial cortex.

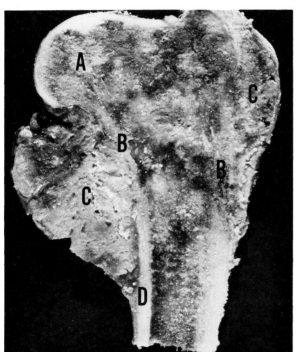

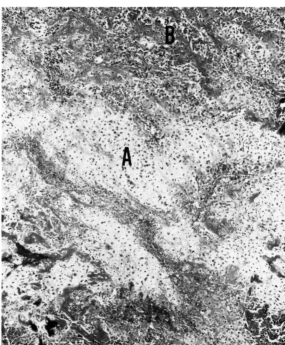

A|B  **FIGURE 5.15.** Chondroblastic osteosarcoma of the proximal humerus. A. Sectioned proximal humerus showing nodular areas (A) of neoplastic bone and cartilage, cortical bone destruction (B), extraosseous tumor (C), and periosteal elevation (Codman's triangle) (D). B. Tumor cells produce an admixture of malignant cartilage (A) and bone (B) tissue.

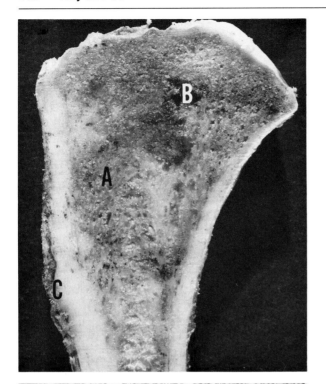

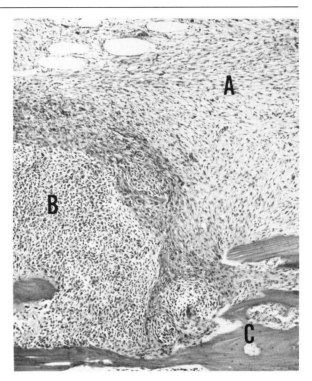

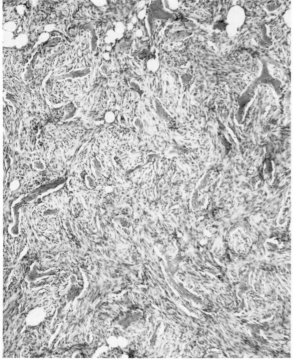

A | B
C |     **FIGURE 5.16.** Fibroblastic osteosarcoma of the proximal tibia. A. In this early lesion, tumor tissue primarily infiltrates marrow spaces of the metaphyseal spongiosa (A) without producing much bone lysis (B), and without provoking a prominent periosteal bony response (C). B. In relatively early cases the neoplasm is primarily a spindle cell sarcoma (A), and areas of osteosarcomatous differentiation (B) with tumor bone matrix formation may be uncommon. Note residual lamellar bone of cortex (C). C. In more advanced cases, tumor osteoid and bone production may be a prominent feature in older areas of the neoplasm.

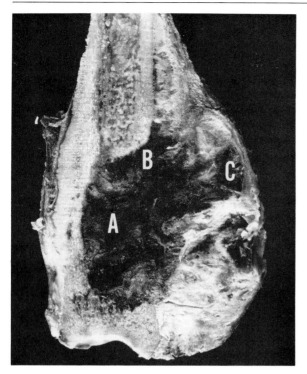

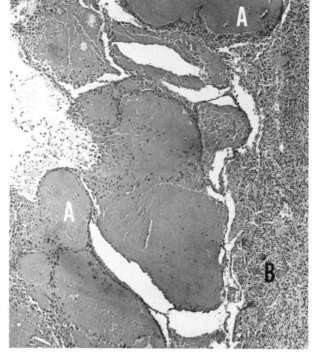

AIB   **FIGURE 5.17.** Telangiectatic osteosarcoma of the distal radius. A. Soft bloody tumor tissue replaces the metaphyseal spongiosa (A), and the medial cortex (B). Tumor almost penetrates the periosteal cuff of reactive bone (C) covering the medial surface of the bone. B. Numerous large blood-filled spaces (A) lined by tumor cells, and small spicules of tumor bone matrix (B) produced by tumor cells, are characteristic findings in this osteosarcoma subtype.

comas (fig. 5.15A), about half of the fibroblastic osteosarcomas, and most of the combined types of osteosarcoma. On gross inspection of sectioned fresh bone specimens, the prosector cannot often distinguish between moderately productive osteoblastic osteosarcoma and fibroblastic osteosarcoma or between chondroblastic osteosarcoma (fig. 5.15A) and the combined type of osteosarcoma. However, one can often recognize a tumor from the latter pair if they contain enough glistening cartilage matrix.

Only a few osteosarcomas form primarily productive lesions (fig. 5.13C). Macerated specimens of these tumors show a dense, bony tumor centered in a bone organ often having a flat surface, such as the scapula, ilium, ischium, or mandible. While the tumor destroys and penetrates the cortex, it spares enough compact bone that the cortex can be recognized on cut surface. Amorphous bone tumor matrix fills the medullary cavity. Tumor bone on the periosteal surface, however, is orderly arranged perpendicular to the cortical surface in a pattern that mimics a massive overgrowth of periosteal new bone seen following trauma and infection. This pattern presents a major diagnostic problem for the radiologist when a productive osteoblastic osteosarcoma arises in the diaphysis of a long bone (fig. 5.19D). During the development of this tumor, the blood supply to the medullary cavity and cortex is lost and tumor tissue within the diaphysis as well as the diaphysis itself is infarcted. Viable tumor and reactive periosteal new bone form a cuff of bone around the surface of the diaphysis. This confusing pattern may be misinterpreted as osteomyelitis, including fungal infection of the bone. The only subtype of osteosarcoma capable of forming this pattern is a productive osteoblastic osteosarcoma.

Representatives from any of the subtypes of osteosarcoma may occur at any skeletal site. In long bones of the limbs the tumors are typically centered

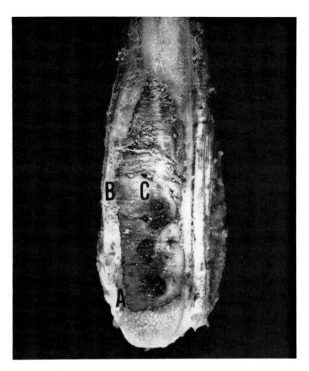
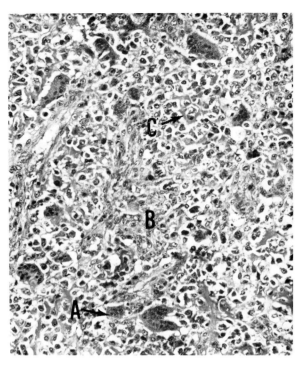

FIGURE 5.18. Giant cell type of osteosarcoma of the distal radius. A. This expansile bone tumor has destroyed the cranial cortex (A), but the tumor is covered by a smooth shell of periosteal new bone (B). The soft pale tumor tissue (C) has necrotic areas containing blood. B. Tumor is characterized by numerous multinucleated tumor giant cells (A), stroma of undifferentiated sarcoma (B), and fields of malignant osteoblasts producing tumor bone matrix (C).

⟶

FIGURE 5.19. Radiographic patterns of canine osteosarcoma. A. Osteolytic lesion in distal radius with minimal periosteal new bone or tumor bone production. B. Mixed lesion in proximal humerus with destruction of cranial and caudal cortices as well as the metaphyseal spongiosa. There is also pathological fracture and extension of bone matrix-producing tumor tissue into adjacent soft tissues. C. Productive lesion of ischium in which radiodense tumor tissue of ischium in which radiodense tumor tissue forms a contoured mass centered on the bone organ, but does not substantially destroy the cortical outline. D. Productive lesion of the proximal humerus characterized by no significant loss of bone architecture and by production of a radiodense bony collar on the cortical surface that histologically is an admixture of tumor bone and periosteal reactive bone.

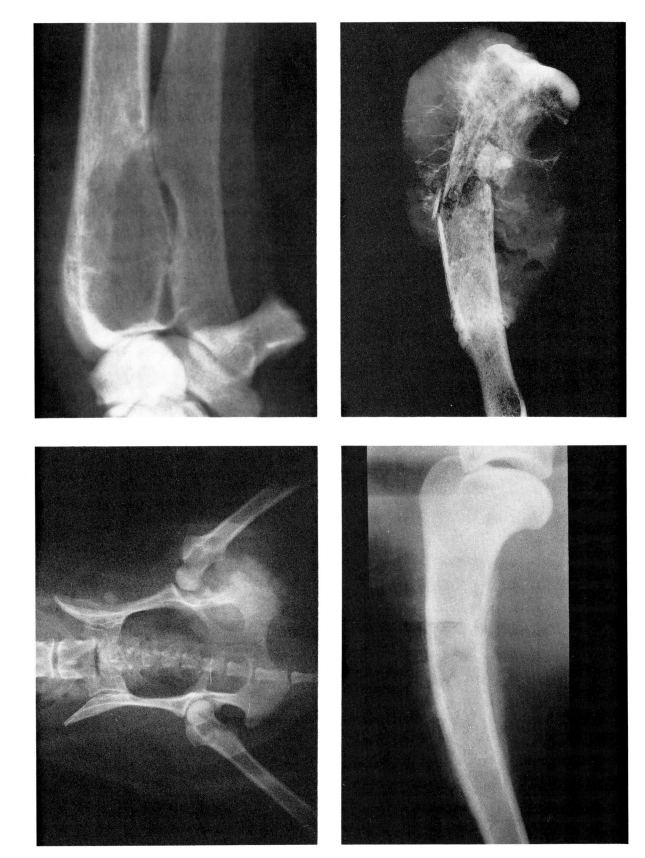

in the metaphysis. Most tumor subtypes that produce osteolytic lesions destroy the bone organ very rapidly. The bone lesion is often quite advanced by the time the animal shows signs, and pathological fracture may develop early in the disease. In the author's experience the tumor subtypes associated with this aggressive course are poorly differentiated osteosarcoma, the nonproductive type of osteoblastic osteosarcoma, and telangiectatic osteosarcoma. In these lesions the tumor rapidly penetrates the cortex before significant periosteal and endosteal responses are made. The clinical course in untreated dogs with lytic osteosarcoma is usually shortened by the locally aggressive behavior of the tumor in the limb rather than by early development of metastatic disease. There is no evidence to indicate that dogs with lytic tumors develop metastatic disease earlier or more frequently than dogs with mixed or productive lesions caused by osteosarcoma. In contrast, the giant cell type of osteosarcoma that also produces a lytic pattern usually forms a much less aggressive, expansile bone lesion (fig. 5.18A and B). Apparently, this tumor grows slowly, destroying the inner cortical surface at a rate that can be matched by periosteal new bone production. The periosteum lays down a thin shell of bone over the slowly expanding cortical surface of the affected bone. After a few weeks to months the tumor penetrates the neocortex and pathological fracture can result.

Most tumor subtypes forming the mixed patterns of production and destruction have a relatively slower initial growth rate than the more aggressive tumors forming the lytic bone lesions. The slow initial growth rate permits the bone organ to mount a periosteal containment similar to a periosteal callus to keep pace, at least temporarily, with cortical destruction. The bony endosteal abutment that develops across the medullary cavity, like the periosteal response, eventually becomes incapable of blocking the extension of tumor tissue. Often a continuous core or tongue of tumor tissue extends from the tumor mass along the medullary cavity of the bone for a few centimeters beyond the limits of the tumor as seen in radiographs. "Skip" metastases, which are tumors that spread within the medullary cavity of the bone organ, occur infrequently in human patients (Enneking and Kagan, 1975) and in dogs.

**Radiographic Appearance.** Moderately advanced cases of primary bone sarcoma of dogs can usually be recognized quite accurately as malignant by clinical and radiological examination, but the final diagnosis rests on histological findings since osteosarcoma, chondrosarcoma, and fibrosarcoma of bone do not produce pathognomonic radiographic patterns. In the initial stages of clinical bone disease, all three of these tumors produce similar radiographic changes: cortical destruction and periosteal response (Ling *et al.*, 1974).

As discussed in the previous section, the various subtypes of osteosarcoma can produce lytic, mixed (destructive and productive), or productive bone lesions, which are best distinguished by radiographic examination of the tumors. Unfortunately for the diagnostician, some of these patterns may also be formed by other primary bone tumors as well as by metastatic tumors of bone. For example, malignant primary bone tumors that may produce indistinguishable osteolytic radiographic patterns (fig. 5.19A) include fibrosarcoma, hemangiosarcoma, giant cell sarcoma of bone, poorly differentiated osteosarcoma, a few of the chondroblastic osteosarcomas, about half of the fibroblastic osteosarcomas, most telangiectatic and giant cell type osteosarcomas, and some of the combined type osteosarcomas. Malignant bone tumors that may produce indistinguishable mixed radiographic patterns (fig. 5.19B) include some higher-grade chondrosarcomas, most moderately productive osteoblastic osteosarcomas, most chondroblastic osteosarcomas, about half of the fibroblastic osteosarcomas, and most of the combined type osteosarcomas. A primarily productive radiographic pattern (fig. 5.19C) is produced almost exclusively by the productive type of osteoblastic osteosarcoma, although this pattern can rarely be formed by a chondrosarcoma. In these tumors the matrix is so dense that it causes ischemic necrosis of the tumor as well as of the normal medullary and cortical structures. Viable tumor tissue along with the periosteal new bone forms a bony response of the cortical surface that has an almost orderly appearance mimicking ones seen following trauma or infection. The cortical shadow persists (fig. 5.19D) because of bone ischemia. There is an insufficient blood supply to provide the osteoclasts necessary to destroy the compact bone of the cortex.

Most osteosarcomas are monostotic metaphyseal

lesions in one of the sites of high predilection in the limbs of a large or giant breed dog. These tumors commonly show several of the following radiographic signs of an aggressive bone lesion (Morgan, 1974): the lesion is poorly delimited since there is a long zone of transition between abnormal and normal bone and there is no sclerotic border at the margin of the lesion; normal metaphyseal architecture is lost; the cortical shadow is partially or completely effaced; the regular periosteal elevation (Codman's triangle) on either side of the lesion is irregular and discontinuous over the lesion, and spicular or amorphous patterns of mineralized matrix may fill the breach in the periosteal response; and the adjacent soft tissue swelling may show invasion of the neoplastic process. The periosteal response on the cortical surface of a canine osteosarcoma more often has an amorphous radiographic pattern than a sunburst or brush pattern (Ling *et al.*, 1974).

Osteosarcomas are dynamic structures that may show a dramatic alteration in radiographic appearance in as little as 7 to 10 days. Because these tumors present constantly evolving patterns, one report has indicated that there is little correlation between the type of radiographic pattern (i.e, osteolytic, mixed, or productive) and either the biological age or degree of malignancy of the tumor (Ling *et al.*, 1974). The same report also provides a detailed discussion of variations in the radiographic appearance of osteosarcoma in different regions of the canine skeleton.

Most osteosarcomas of the axial skeleton have radiographic features similar to those already described for the appendicular skeleton, with the exception of tumors located in the canine skull. The following observations were made in a study of bone tumors of the dog (Ling *et al.*, 1974). Osteosarcomas of vertebrae tend to be osteolytic and are often overlooked because of problems of positioning, exposure, and soft tissue shadows. Tumors of the ribs are located near the costochondral junction and are often osteoblastic. In the head, tumors of the maxilla and zygomatic arch are usually osteolytic while those in the mandible tend to be osteoblastic. Osteosarcomas of the paranasal sinuses and calvarium are exclusively osteoblastic tumors. These dense bony masses have less aggressive features than osteosarcomas of the limbs. Borders of

the tumor are often smooth, but brush patterns when present are pronounced. These unique semi-aggressive osteoblastic osteosarcomas of the canine calvarium were described in another report (Hardy *et al.*, 1967) as containing evenly distributed granular calcific densities and as having a regular, well-defined border. A review by the author of the tissue sections from the skull tumors of one report (Ling *et al.*, 1974) indicates that a few of the osteosarcomas of the canine calvarium and paranasal sinuses have areas containing the histological pattern characteristic of multilobular sarcoma of the canine skull.

**Histological Features.** Osteosarcoma is a primary sarcoma of bone in which malignant tumor cells produce fibrillar stroma, tumor osteoid, and tumor bone. Sometimes neoplastic cartilage is also formed, but the tumor is still designated osteosarcoma since the osteogenic mesenchyme has the greatest malignant potential. Any one of these malignant matrices may predominate in a particular tumor; thus, an osteosarcoma could mimic other primary bone tumors such as fibrosarcoma or chondrosarcoma.

Malignant osteoid and bone may take a variety of microscopic forms. Osteoid may be irregularly deposited as spicules between small spindled cells resembling neoplastic reticular cells of bone marrow stroma (fig. 5.20A) or between larger pleomorphic cells more closely resembling osteoblasts (fig. 5.20B). Tumor osteoid may be formed in sheets and entrap fields of malignant osteoblasts (fig. 5.20C). At times tumor osteoid and bone can closely resemble reactive bone so that it may be difficult or nearly impossible to distinguish between the two on a biopsy specimen. Periosteal collars of new bone often do not contain tumor tissue, which may be confined to the medullary cavity and cortex (Ling *et al.*, 1974). Nonneoplastic woven bone produced in response to destruction of metaphyseal spongiosa by a tumor is poorly appreciated in osteosarcoma because of the difficulty in distinguishing it from tumor bone. It is instructive, however, for the pathologist to examine tissue sections from a bone lesion of comparable radiographic appearance caused by a metastatic carcinoma where the component of reactive bone can be appreciated.

The neoplastic tissue of osteosarcoma, in addition to resembling fibrosarcoma and chondrosar-

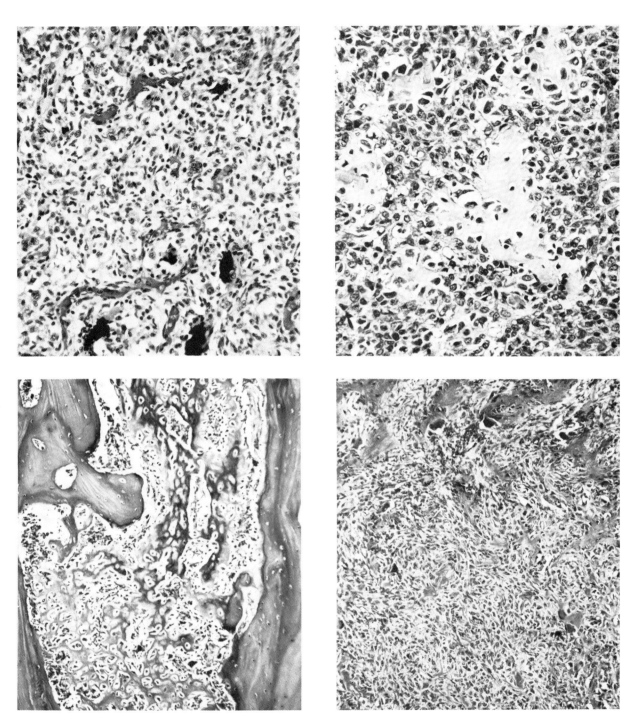

A|B<br><abbr>C|D</abbr> **FIGURE 5.20.** Some histological patterns of canine osteosarcoma. A. Poorly differentiated osteosarcoma in which small spindle cells resembling reticular cells of bone marrow stroma produce thin spicules of tumor osteoid and bone matrix. B. Osteoblastic osteosarcoma composed of large, hyperchromatic cells with angular borders that produce and entrap themselves in irregular islands of os-

seous matrix. C. Productive osteosarcoma fills marrow spaces of spongiosa with sheets of tumor osteoid and bone matrix. D. Osteoblastic osteosarcoma in which a moderately productive area of tumor bone matrix (top) is being destroyed and replaced by a less differentiated, nonproductive tumor cell population (bottom).

coma, may also have areas that mimic malignant mesenchyme, hemangiosarcoma, malignant tumors of nervous tissue, and liposarcoma. Areas of malignant giant cells may be found in canine osteosarcoma; these characterized feline osteosarcoma in one study (Nielsen, 1964).

The primary benefits derived from dividing osteosarcoma into subtypes based on histomorphology are to permit the pathologist to find if there is a correlation between the structure of the tumor and its biological behavior or its susceptibility to tumor therapy and to acquaint the novice pathologist with some of the various histological patterns that osteosarcoma may take in animals. No two osteosarcomas are identical. One report indicates that it is impossible to offer a histological description that is characteristic of osteosarcoma (Nielsen *et al.*, 1954). These authors could find no basis for histological classification of these canine bone tumors because of variations in histomorphology in different tumors and within different areas of the same tumor. To date there is only one published report attempting to correlate tissue morphology of osteosarcoma in animals with clinical behavior or response to therapy (Misdorp and Hart, 1979). In that study dogs with fibroblastic osteosarcoma had a more favorable prognosis than dogs affected by other subtypes of osteosarcoma. A major difficulty one encounters in trying to subclassify osteosarcomas is the realization that often more than one histological pattern is present in a particular bone tumor, and a subdominant tissue pattern may appear to be more malignant than the principal pattern. Radiologists (Ling *et al.*, 1974) have appreciated that the radiographic pattern of a canine osteosarcoma can sometimes change rapidly as a lytic tumor acquires a mixed or productive type of pattern or vice versa. These radiographic changes are an indication of alterations in histomorphology of the tumor matrix as tumor osteoid mineralizes to form tumor bone or as tumor bone is destroyed and replaced by a more anaplastic, nonproductive tumor cell population (fig. 5.20D).

Bearing in mind the difficulties inherent in devising a classification scheme for bone sarcomas in animals, the author offers the system shown in table 5.2 as one that is useful for categorizing most canine bone sarcomas. This scheme is a modified version of one developed by Dahlin (Dahlin, 1967; Dahlin and Unni, 1977) for osteosarcoma in hu-

mans. The author has found it a useful way to correlate the morphological varieties of cell and matrix patterns with radiographic changes for teaching professional students and residents. The seven subtypes were determined by making radiographic, gross, and microscopic examinations of several hundred bone tumors of dogs presented to the University of California veterinary pathology service over a 15-year period. In most cases clinical radiographs were used to determine the plane of section through the affected bone. The bones were then sectioned lengthwise and grossly evaluated. Thin, parallel sections were made and were often radiographed on high detail film. These films were used to select representative tissues for histological examination. When one of the first six microscopic subtypes of osteosarcoma listed in table 5.2 was the predominant tissue pattern in the bone tumor, a diagnosis of that subtype was made. When no one pattern predominated and when the osteosarcoma was formed by two or more patterns of nearly equal amounts, a diagnosis of combined type of osteosarcoma was made. While this classification scheme was developed primarily for canine primary bone sarcomas, it could also apply to bone sarcomas of other domestic animals.

*Poorly Differentiated Osteosarcoma*—This primary bone tumor is produced by malignant cells that form at least small amounts of unequivocal tumor osteoid and sometimes spicules of tumor bone. The malignant mesenchymal cells may vary in appearance from small cells resembling the reticular cells of bone marrow stroma (fig. 5.20A) to large, pleomorphic cells of undifferentiated sarcoma. Most are highly aggressive bone tumors that form lytic bone lesions. Pathological fracture may occur early in the clinical course.

*Osteoblastic Osteosarcoma*—Tumors of this subtype are formed by anaplastic osteoblasts and plump to spindle-shaped osteogenic precursor cells (fig. 5.20B). Cells have hyperchromatic nuclei that are eccentrically positioned in dark-staining cytoplasm. Often the cells have angular borders. On the basis of the amount of tumor bone matrix that is produced by these tumors, they are further subcategorized as follows:

1. Nonproductive osteoblastic osteosarcomas. These usually aggressive bone tumors form lytic bone lesions and tend to provoke little periosteal

response. Pathological fracture may occur soon after onset of clinical signs.

2. Moderately productive osteoblastic osteosarcoma. Mixed pattern of destruction and production characterizes the radiographic appearance of this subtype. Lytic areas may appear radiographically in areas previously radiodense a few days earlier because of replacement of a productive area by a less differentiated population of tumor cells that form little or no mineralized matrix (fig. 5.20D). In dogs more osteosarcomas belong to this subtype than to any other.

3. Productive osteoblastic osteosarcoma. In this lesion tumor cells produce abundant tumor matrix (fig. 5.20C) inside the bone organ as well as on its surface. Tumor bone formed on the cortical surface can be so regular in structure and arrangement and the tumor cells so well differentiated that the neoplastic tissue can microscopically mimic a reactive periosteal response.

*Chondroblastic Osteosarcoma*—Malignant mesenchyme in these tumors directly produces both tumor bone matrix and neoplastic cartilage matrix. In most cases there is an intermingling of the malignant bone and cartilage elements (fig. 5.15B), but in a few lesions (fig. 5.12) the two matrix patterns may be separate. In the latter case a biopsy taken from the cartilaginous part of the tumor would be given a diagnosis of chondrosarcoma. Examination of the clinical radiograph of the tumor, however, would cast some doubt on the diagnosis since the tumor would most likely have a more aggressive, mixed pattern than would be common for most chondrosarcomas.

*Fibroblastic Osteosarcoma*—These tumors usually begin as lytic bone lesions and about half will progress to the mixed pattern when the neoplastic spindled cells in this tumor increase their capacity to form mineralized bone matrix. In early lesions (fig. 5.16B) a spindle cell population resembling that of central fibrosarcoma will predominate, and areas of unequivocal bone formation by tumor cells may be difficult to find. Advanced lesions (fig. 5.16C) may have large areas of bone matrix formation by the spindle cell population. The amount and degree of mineralization of the spicules of neoplastic osteoid will determine the radiographic appearance of the tumor. Misdorp and Hart (1979)

found that dogs with this subtype of osteosarcoma had a favorable prognosis.

*Telangiectatic Osteosarcoma*—This tumor subtype characteristically produces an aggressive, osteolytic radiographic lesion, and the bloody, cystic lesions found on gross examination (fig. 5.17A) cannot be distinguished from primary or metastatic hemangiosarcoma of bone. Microscopically, the malignant cells resemble pleomorphic and spindle-shaped osteogenic mesenchyme. Only small inconspicuous spicules of osteoid are formed in the primary and secondary tumors of this subtype. Large, blood-filled spaces in the tumor are lined by tumor cells and not by endothelium (fig. 5.17B). Metastases shed by these tumors also tend to be very bloody and cystic. In humans the telangiectatic osteosarcoma accounts for 40 of 1,000 cases of osteosarcoma, and this subtype is associated with less favorable prognosis than any other subtype of osteosarcoma (Dahlin and Unni, 1977; Matsuno *et al.*, 1976). This subtype is recognized in dogs (Gleiser *et al.*, 1981; Price and Summer-Smith, 1966; Theilen *et al.*, 1977) and also appears to be highly fatal.

*Giant Cell Type Osteosarcoma*—This variant usually produces an expansile, lytic bone lesion (fig. 5.18A). Microscopically, the tumor resembles nonproductive osteoblastic osteosarcoma except for large areas in which tumor giant cells predominate (fig. 5.18B). The tumor must be differentiated from malignant giant cell tumor of bone.

*Combined Type Osteosarcoma*—This subtype includes those tumors that do not have a dominant matrix pattern composed of one of the first six subtypes of osteosarcoma. These tumors contain two or more matrix patterns of osteosarcoma. While some of these tumors produce lytic bone lesions, most of them form a mixed radiographic pattern.

**Growth and Metastasis.** Hematogenous metastasis to the lungs is a common occurrence in osteosarcoma. Most central osteosarcomas originate in the metaphyseal spongiosa of long bones and other sites with red bone marrow. Perhaps early in the evolution of the neoplasm malignant cells gain access to the blood through the loose endothelial junctions of bone marrow sinusoids. Metastatic lung disease is found in about 10% of canine osteosarcoma patients on initial radiographic examination (Ling *et al.*, 1974). On the basis of autopsy records of the dog, the frequency of metastatic lung disease was reported to range from about 45% to more than 60% (Nielsen *et al.*, 1954; Owen, 1969). High resolution radiography of lungs removed at autopsy combined with examination of multiple tissue sections will increase the percentage of positive cases by approximately 15%. It has been suggested that if the disease were allowed to run its natural course, the figure would approach 100% (Owen, 1969). Those dogs whose lives were prolonged by surgical treatment nearly always have extensive lung metastasis at necropsy (Brodey *et al.*, 1963). A small number of dogs with lung involvement will also develop metastatic tumors in a variety of tissues supplied by the systemic circulation (Brodey *et al.*, 1963).

Osteosarcoma of the canine skull, especially those osteoblastic tumors of the paranasal sinuses and calvarium, generally results in a longer clinical course than osteosarcoma of the limbs. Death often results from local disease, but pulmonary metastasis may occur. In one group of 33 dogs with skull osteosarcoma (Hardy *et al.*, 1967), less than 31% of the cases developed metastatic disease, suggesting that the metastatic potential of skull tumors is less than that of appendicular skeletal tumors.

If the regional lymph nodes are routinely sectioned and examined microscopically, the pathologist will find tumor tissue in the nodes of about 5% of the dogs with large osteosarcomas extending into soft tissue. Invasion of the lymphoid system appears to be a late event and probably does not influence the clinical course of the disease. Turrel and Pool (1982) found that the incidence of metastatic disease in cats with osteosarcoma was much lower (less than 10%) than in dogs.

More than half of the lung metastases in dogs will reflect the appearance of the primary tumor. Metastases from simple nonproductive osteosarcomas tend to be firm to soft and fleshy but without calcified matrix. Telangiectatic primary osteosarcomas usually shed cystic, soft, bloody secondary tumors. The larger metastatic foci from productive simple and compound osteosarcomas tend to be firm to hard and bony, while the small developing lesions resemble those from the simple nonproductive osteosarcoma. Exceptions to these findings are not infrequently encountered.

Metastases were observed in 4 of 11 cats with osteosarcoma (Engle and Brodey, 1969). Lungs were involved in 3 of the cats and 1 cat also had metastases in the brain and kidneys. In the fourth cat metastatic disease was found only in the liver. This phenomenon has also been found in dogs, where there were metastases to viscera from a primary osteosarcoma of a limb, but without demonstrable secondary tumors in the lung. This suggests that the search for pulmonary lesions was either inadequate or that tumor cells passed through the pulmonary vascular bed without becoming localized in that organ.

## Chondrosarcoma

**Classification.** A chondrosarcoma is a malignant neoplasm in which tumor cells produce varying amounts of neoplastic chondroid and fibrillar matrix. However, the sarcomatous cells must never directly produce neoplastic osteoid or bone since this is a characteristic only of osteosarcoma (see Chondroblastic Osteosarcoma). A primary chondrosarcoma of bone is a malignant cartilaginous tumor that arises *de novo* within a bone organ (central or medullary chondrosarcoma) or from the periosteum (peripheral chondrosarcoma). In animals most chondrosarcomas are thought to be primary bone tumors of medullary origin, and these are the subject of the present discussion. Primary chondrosarcomas of periosteal origin are rare in animals (see Sarcomas of the Periosteum). Secondary chondrosarcomas of bone, by contrast, arise by malignant change in an antecedent lesion of bone (note that the term *secondary tumor* is sometimes used to indicate a metastatic tumor of bone). It has not yet been determined if malignant transformation in enchondroma (see Enchondroma) occurs in animals and, if so, what percentage of medullary chondrosarcomas have their origin in this lesion. However, secondary chondrosarcomas of the periosteum occasionally arise by malignant change in osteochondromas of animals (see Osteochondroma). Currently, the best clinicopathological report of chondrosarcoma in animals is a study of 35 cases in the dog (Brodey *et al.*, 1974).

**Incidence, Age, Breed, and Sex.** Chondrosarcoma of bone is a relatively rare tumor that has been found mostly in mature animals in all domestic species (Jacobson, 1971), but so few cases have been reported that little is known of the clinicopathological features of this tumor in most species of domestic animals. It is the second most common bone sarcoma in domestic species, except for sheep where this tumor probably occurs more frequently than osteosarcoma. The largest number of cases has been studied in the dog where chondrosarcoma of bone accounts for slightly less than 10% of all bone sarcomas (Brodey and Riser, 1969). This tumor affects primarily dogs of large but not giant breeds, shows no sex predilection, and occurs mostly in dogs between 5 and 9 years of age (median age 6 years) (Brodey *et al.*, 1974). Boxers and German shepherd dogs were the most commonly affected breeds in this study. In sheep most tumors are found in adult and aged ewes (Sullivan, 1960). The sex predilection in sheep is not considered to be significant because it reflects husbandry practices.

**Sites.** Flat bones are more commonly involved than long bones. Most of the few chondrosarcomas reported in cattle and horses were found in flat bones (Jacobson, 1971; Sullivan, 1960). In sheep the cartilages of the sternocostal complex were the most common site for chondrosarcoma, and the scapular cartilage and tuber coxae were mentioned frequently (Sullivan, 1960). The long bones of sheep may also bear tumors (Jacobson, 1971). In the cat the scapulae, vertebrae, and limbs appear to be the most common sites, followed by tumors of the head (Cotchin, 1957; Engle and Brodey, 1969; Jacobson, 1971; Liu *et al.*, 1974; Nielsen, 1964; Turrel and Pool, 1982). The ribs and sternum are generally spared. In dogs tumors of the ribs, turbinates, and pelvis made up 69% of 35 chondrosarcomas of bone in one study (Brodey *et al.*, 1974). The nasal region was the second most common site with 34% of the cases. In this report boxers showed a breed-associated predilection for tumors of the rib and pelvis but an absence of nasal chondrosarcomas.

**Gross Morphology.** Chondrosarcomas typically form large masses when the tumors are allowed to pursue a full clinical course without surgical intervention. Most chondrosarcomas have a convoluted surface with relatively distinct borders. On cut section tumor tissue of many chondrosarcomas will resemble hyaline cartilage (fig. 5.21A). The tumor mass is composed of multiple small nodules of soft to moderately firm tissue that ranges from translucent to milky white, grayish white, or bluish white. Often there are areas in the central region of the tu-

mor that are gray to rust colored and have a slimy consistency. This mucoid character is a major gross feature of some nasal chondrosarcomas. Irregular, chalky white foci of calcified tumor matrix are sometimes found. In some chondrosarcomas the tumor tissue is pale ivory, very firm, and tough (fig. 5.21C); it resembles fibrocartilage more than hyaline cartilage. Instead of multiple small nodules the tumor consists of several large, irregularly sized coalescing masses of tumor tissue, all of which typically have a regularly contoured external surface.

Central chondrosarcomas of long bones usually demonstrate symmetric expansile growth until the tumor penetrates the cortex and supporting layers of reactive bone (figs. 5.21B and 5.22). The tumor may extend into the parosteal connective tissues through a rather small embrasure in the cortical surface. During cortical destruction, the periosteum may lay down a smoothly contoured periosteal collar of reactive bone several millimeters thick, which may eventually be penetrated at multiple sites by tumor tissue. Reactive bone can be very dense and is ivory colored. The tumor may extend for a variable distance through the medullary cavity of the diaphysis. In some cases the limit of tumor invasion is marked by a transverse ridge of reactive bone that can be observed on clinical radiographs, but more often the tumor extends several centimeters beyond the limits observed in the radiograph. Chondrosarcomas of flat bones often demonstrate an eccentric manner of growth with costal and pelvic tumor masses tending to protrude into body cavities, whereas scapular tumors are directed primarily in a dorsolateral direction. The central and basal areas of these tumors may contain bony tissue.

**Clinical Characteristics.** Clinical signs vary with the site of skeletal involvement. Tumors of the nasal cavity cause sneezing, unilateral and sometimes bilateral purulent to bloody discharges, and nasal obstruction sometimes followed by bone destruction. Bone deformity may occur but it is uncommon. Chondrosarcomas of the cranium may produce a palpable mass in the absence of neurologic signs, but as with tumors of the vertebrae, continuous growth of the tumor often leads to compression of nervous tissue and to development of attendant clinical signs. Rib tumors tend to cause the animal little pain unless there is a pathological frac-

areas were present. Mitotic figures occurred in moderate numbers. Three of the neoplasms produced metastatic disease. Only four tumors were classified as Grade III chondrosarcomas. These tumors contained areas of undifferentiated sarcoma. Nuclear pleomorphism was marked and mitotic figures were numerous. One of the tumors produced pulmonary metastasis. The degree of differentiation of chondrosarcoma is an important indicator of prognosis in humans (Spjut *et al.*, 1971) and may prove to be of similar value in animal chondrosarcomas as more cases are studied.

Microscopic diagnosis of chondrosarcoma is based on the presence of abnormal cartilage cells with plump, atypical, hyperchromatic nuclei. Proliferation in low-grade tumors may be so slow that the only morphological indication of cell division is the presence of binucleate or multinucleated cells or the presence of lacunae containing more than one cartilage cell. Mitotic figures are a feature of more malignant tumors. There are marked variations in cell density between different chondrosarcomas and to a lesser extent within an individual neoplasm. Tumor cells typically display a variation in size and shape in a malignant cartilage tumor. Cells may mimic the mesenchymal precursors of cartilage, embryonic cartilage of the developing bone model, or cells of mature hyaline cartilage. At times tumor cells acquire the spindle cell morphology of chondroblasts located in the chondrogenic layer of the fetal perichondrium, a feature also seen in some osteosarcomas and fibrosarcomas of bone. The presence of a poorly differentiated spindle cell component at the periphery of an otherwise well-differentiated chondrosarcoma has been called "dedifferentiation" of the tumor (Dahlin and Beabout, 1971), and this finding considerably worsens the prognosis of such a tumor in humans. A spindle cell tumor margin is a fairly common feature of animal chondrosarcomas, especially tumors of the nasal cavity. After incomplete surgical removal of nasal chondrosarcoma, recurrent tumor tissue often acquires a predominant spindle cell pattern. Such tumors usually have a high mitotic index. However, dogs usually die of local disease in nasal chondrosarcoma without developing metastatic disease. Figures 5.23A–D illustrate many of the cellular features of chondrosarcoma discussed here.

There is considerable variation in the amount of chondroid matrix produced by different chondrosarcomas, but the amount or quality of matrix is of little value in prognosis. However, when the malignant cartilage cells produce matrix that secondarily becomes fibrillar and hyalinized (fig. 5.24A) so that the matrix acquires the microscopic properties of osteoid, or when chondroid matrix undergoes resorption and endochondral ossification (fig. 5.24B), the pathologist may find it extremely difficult to decide whether he is dealing with chondrosarcoma or osteosarcoma, particularly if he is asked to make this determination from a small biopsy specimen. One investigation (Brodey *et al.*, 1974) suggests that Alcian blue stain may be helpful in making this distinction. Areas of ossification in canine chondrosarcoma stain in a particular manner. Faintly staining areas of osteoid are surrounded by contiguous areas of staining chondroid matrix, a pattern not seen in canine osteosarcoma. Differentiation between chondrosarcoma and osteosarcoma is often a problem in large tumors of the ribs of dogs in which a considerable amount of cartilage and bone is produced. While these tumors have areas within them that microscopically resemble osteosarcoma, their biological behaior is more compatible with chondrosarcoma.

In making a microscopic diagnosis of chondrosarcoma the pathologist should always determine if the morphological diagnosis is compatible with the clinical and radiographic findings in the case. It is important to remember that some of the cytological features of malignancy in chondrosarcoma may be found in chondroblastic osteosarcomas, actively growing or traumatized osteochondromas, and a variety of nonmalignant responses of the periosteum and synovium to injury. Atypical chondrocytes can be found in a callus, some exostoses, traumatized ligament insertions, and in sites of chondroosseous metaplasia in the linings of joints, tendon sheaths, and bursae. These present diagnostic problems primarily when the results of the clinical and radiographic studies are unavailable or inadequate and when the pathologist is presented with a tissue specimen which cannot be oriented to the lesion.

**Growth and Metastasis.** Chondrosarcoma in the dog (Brodey *et al.*, 1974), cat (Turrel and Pool, 1982), and sheep (Sullivan, 1960) tends to grow more slowly, pursue a longer clinical course, and develop hematogenous metastasis later and with

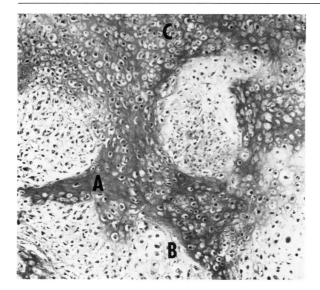

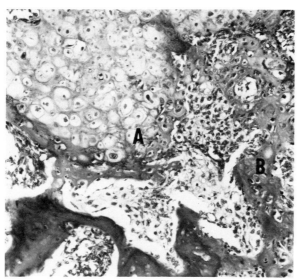

A
B    **FIGURE 5.24.** Changes in the matrix of a chondro-sarcoma. A. Hyalinized chondroid matrix (A) in a chondrosarcoma may be mistaken for osteoid. However, observe that the trabecular structures arise within a sheet of chondroid tissue and are not lined by osteoblasts (B). Cells within these trabeculae resemble chondrocytes and not osteocytes. B. Endochondral ossification occurs in many lower-grade chondrosarcomas with replacement of neoplastic cartilage (A) by nonneoplastic bone tissue (B).

much less frequency than osteosarcoma in these species. This is probably true for the other domestic species, but so few chondrosarcomas have been reported that little is known of their clinicopathological features.

## Fibrosarcoma

**Classification.** A central (medullary) fibrosarcoma of bone is a malignant neoplasm of fibrous connective tissue originating from stromal elements in the medullary cavity. Tumor cells produce varying amounts of collagenous matrix but no neoplastic bone or cartilage. This tumor should be differentiated from peripheral fibrosarcomas of bone and fibroblastic osteosarcomas of low osteogenic potential.

**Incidence, Age, Breed, and Sex.** The real incidence of central fibrosarcoma of bone in animals is undetermined. This tumor is seen less often than periosteal fibrosarcoma. Hemangiosarcoma and fibrosarcoma (peripheral and central) of bone together account for approximately 7% of the primary bone sarcomas of the dog. Central fibrosarcomas are seen primarily in mature (1 year 6 months to 12 years) male dogs of large and medium breeds (Brodey *et al.*, 1963; Jacobson, 1971; Ling *et al.*, 1974; Owen, 1962, 1969; Tjalma, 1966). They are rarely reported in other domestic animals (Jacobson, 1971).

**Clinical Characteristics.** Central fibrosarcomas of bone fall into two general groups. The most common tumors produce bone destruction over a period of several months to a year and are generally slower to metastasize than primary osteosarcomas of bone. Amputation may be curative, but recurrence at the amputation stump can occur (Brodey *et al.*, 1963). Less often the pathologist will encounter aggressive, highly anaplastic fibrosarcomas that cause rapid and massive destruction of the affected bone. Evidence of metastatic disease is not invariably present at necropsy of these animals.

**Sites.** Too few cases are recorded in the veterinary literature to provide a skeletal pattern of site predilection for the tumor. In dogs the metaphyses of long bones appear to be the most commonly affected skeletal sites (Brodey *et al.*, 1963; Jacobson, 1971; Ling *et al.*, 1974; Owen, 1962, 1969).

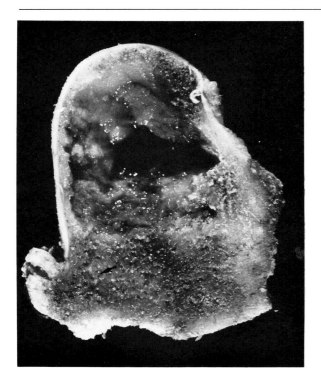

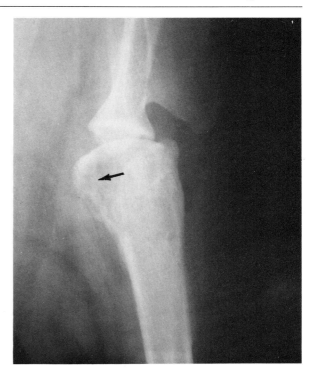

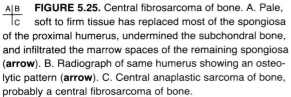

A|B
—
C    **FIGURE 5.25.** Central fibrosarcoma of bone. A. Pale, soft to firm tissue has replaced most of the spongiosa of the proximal humerus, undermined the subchondral bone, and infiltrated the marrow spaces of the remaining spongiosa (**arrow**). B. Radiograph of same humerus showing an osteolytic pattern (**arrow**). C. Central anaplastic sarcoma of bone, probably a central fibrosarcoma of bone.

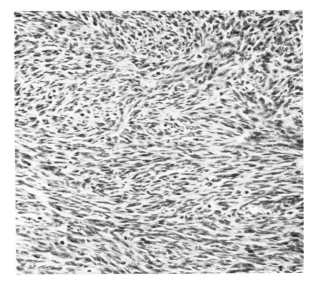

One dog had multicentric primary tumors (Owen, 1969). Tumors have also been found in the mandible and vertebral column of dogs (Jacobson, 1971; Morgan *et al.*, 1980).

**Gross Morphology.** In early or less aggressive lesions the metaphyseal spongiosa may remain partially intact and grayish white fibrous tissue fills the marrow spaces. In more aggressive tumors the bone is destroyed and replaced by soft to firm tumor tissue (fig. 5.25A). Destruction of the subchondral bone leads to extension of the neoplasm into the joint cavity through fractures in the unsupported articular cartilage. Tumor tissue may also invade the fibrous layer of the joint capsule and involve the next bone without involving the joint cavity. The tumor is partially restrained from invasion of adjacent soft tissues by the fibrous periosteum. A bony periosteal response, if present, is usually meager and tends to be evenly contoured. Soft tissue swelling, however, may be marked.

**Radiographic Appearance.** Early lesions of fibrosarcoma produce the radiographic changes of cortical destruction and periosteal response found in primary osteosarcomas and chondrosarcomas of bone (Ling *et al.*, 1974). In many cases it may be impossible on the basis of radiographic appearance alone to differentiate between central fibrosarcoma of bone and one of several bone tumors including poorly differentiated osteosarcoma, nonproductive osteoblastic osteosarcoma, anaplastic chondrosarcoma, and hemangiosarcoma of bone since all of these tumors tend to produce a lytic radiographic lesion. Progressive radiographic studies of a bone lesion produced by fibrosarcoma usually show a slower rate of bone destruction than would be found with the other more highly malignant bone tumors. Fibrosarcomas are primarily destructive tumors (fig. 5.25B). They produce a smaller tumor mass and evoke a less remarkable periosteal response than typical osteosarcomas (Ling *et al.*, 1974; Morgan, 1972).

**Histological Features.** Most central fibrosarcomas of dogs have the moderate to well-differentiated appearance of fibrosarcomas in soft tissue. In some fibrosarcomas the pathologist will encounter focal areas of dense collagen that closely resemble osteoid formation. In these instances the distinction from fibroblastic osteosarcoma may be arbi-

trary if the decision is based solely on microscopic interpretation of a small biopsy specimen. Similar diagnostic difficulties are encountered in fibrosarcomas of human bone (Dahlin and Coventry, 1967; Spjut *et al.*, 1971). Less commonly, fibrosarcomas are more anaplastic, highly cellular tumors composed of large, plump spindle cells with large hyperchromatic nuclei (fig. 5.25C). Mitotic figures are numerous. At times, it may be impossible to distinguish these highly malignant tumors from other anaplastic sarcomas including rhabdomyosarcomas and highly anaplastic osteosarcomas of low osteoblastic potential. Using special staining techniques neither cross striations in the cytoplasm nor evidence of alkaline phosphatase activity in the cells are found in this neoplasm. Histological grading of primary fibrosarcomas of bone has proven to be a useful indicator of prognosis for humans (Spjut *et al.*, 1971) and needs to be evaluated in fibrosarcomas of animal bone.

**Growth and Metastasis.** Most central fibrosarcomas of animal bone tend to cause bone lysis with local extension into soft tissue following destruction of the cortex. Well-differentiated fibrosarcomas usually do not produce metastatic disease even when present for several months, and animals with these neoplasms are good candidates for ablative surgery. Less well-differentiated fibrosarcomas may, in time, produce hematogenous metastasis. Highly anaplastic fibrosarcomas tend to pursue a rapid clinical course with respect to the site of local bone involvement. Often, dogs with highly malignant fibrosarcomas are destroyed because of the poor prognosis that is given for all anaplastic sarcomas of bone. At necropsy, however, metastatic disease is not invariably present. Perhaps amputation should be considered for highly malignant fibrosarcomas until statistical evidence is present that the survival rate of such operated animals is unacceptably low.

## Hemangiosarcoma

**Classification.** Primary hemangiosarcoma (angiosarcoma) of bone is a malignant neoplasm arising from precursor cells of endothelium in the vasculature of a bone organ.

**Incidence, Age, Breed, and Sex.** This is a relatively rare primary bone tumor in animals. It is seen mostly in dogs (Bingle *et al.*, 1974; Brodey *et al.*, 1963; Jacobson, 1971; Ling *et al.*, 1974; Morgan, 1972; Morgan *et al.*, 1980; Owen, 1969), but has been found in horses and cattle (Jacobson, 1971). Primary hemangiosarcoma of bone is slightly less common than primary fibrosarcoma of bone (peripheral and central), and together these two neoplasms constitute approximately 7% of the primary bone sarcomas of the dog. Most tumors we have seen occurred in young adult dogs (3 to 4 years old with a range from 2 to 16 years). However, Alexander and Patton (1983) reported a median age of 6 years. The disease is found in dogs of large and medium breeds with both sexes being equally represented (Ling *et al.*, 1974). The three breeds most commonly affected are boxers, Great Danes, and German shepherds (Alexander and Patton, 1983). One survey of 152 cases of primary bone sarcoma in dogs found 4 hemangiosarcomas in slightly older dogs (6 to 9 years) (Brodey *et al.*, 1963).

**Clinical Characteristics.** The tumor behaves like most aggressive primary sarcomas of bone. It causes pain, lameness, soft tissue swelling, and bone destruction. However, the tumor tends to remain confined to the medullary cavity and involves a relatively large area of bone before signs of pain become sufficiently obvious that the owner consults a veterinarian. Often a pathological fracture through the tumor site is the first clinical sign of disease.

**Sites and Gross Morphology.** The proximal and distal one-thirds of long bones are the most common sites of involvement followed by tumors of the pelvic bones, sternum, ribs, maxilla, and vertebral column (Bingle *et al.*, 1974; Brodey *et al.*, 1963; Jacobson, 1971; Ling *et al.*, 1974; Morgan, 1972; Morgan *et al.*, 1980; Owen, 1969).

On cut section the neoplasm is typically composed of dark, bloody, spongy tissue (fig. 5.26A). There may be gray to tan areas that have a rubbery consistency. Several different tumors of bone may have a similar gross appearance, including telangiectatic osteosarcoma and aneurysmal bone cyst or tumors metastatic to bone, such as osteosarcoma and hemangiosarcoma of soft tissue origin. At necropsy one must carefully examine the carcass for evidence of a primary hemangiosarcoma of soft tissue. When metastatic disease is present it may be

difficult or impossible to determine whether the skeletal lesion is a primary or secondary (metastatic) hemangiosarcoma.

Primary hemangiosarcoma of bone destroys extensive areas of normal bone architecture including metaphyseal spongiosa and cortex, but most of these tumors provoke only a modest, smoothly contoured collar of periosteal new bone. Soft tissue swelling is often not as remarkable as that seen in most osteosarcomas.

**Radiographic Appearance.** The tumor produces a highly destructive lesion often accompanied by pathological fracture. Hemangiosarcomas of long bones extend along the marrow cavity and destroy the cortical bone, but tend not to extend into the soft tissue as is the case with most primary sarcomas of bone (fig. 5.26B). Usually the amount of extracortical reactive bone surrounding the lesion is minimal (Ling *et al.*, 1974; Morgan, 1972).

**Histological Features.** Tumor tissue resembles hemangiosarcoma of soft tissue. While much of the tumor may be composed of a poorly differentiated sarcoma, areas are found in which the neoplasm attempts to form vascular channels (fig. 5.26C). Vascular spaces lined by atypical endothelial cells may form irregular clefts or more cavernous structures. The fibrous stroma supporting the vascular structures may, in some focal areas, become impregnated with blood proteins and cursorily resemble osteoid. The stroma of hemangiosarcoma does not form a calcifiable matrix. Telangiectatic osteosarcomas that have low osteoplastic potential are sometimes incorrectly diagnosed as hemangiosarcoma (fig. 5.17B). This distinction may be extremely difficult in a biopsy taken from the site of a pathological fracture caused by osteosarcoma as well as other primary and metastatic sarcomas of bone.

**Growth and Metastasis.** Hemangiosarcomas typically destroy an extensive area of bone before producing clinical signs. By this time most tumors have shed hematogenous metastases. While amputation may be curative in a few cases, there is no information currently available to suggest that an animal with an advanced primary tumor should be considered as a good candidate for ablative surgery.

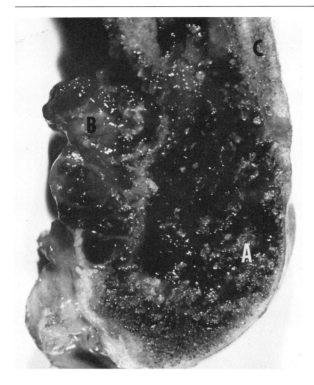

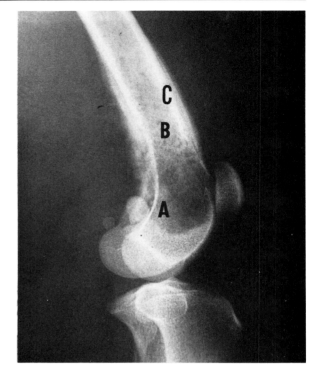

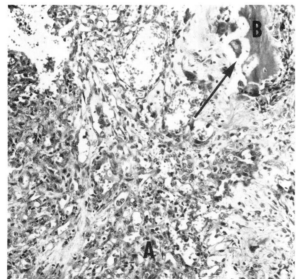

**FIGURE 5.26.** Central hemangiosarcoma of bone. A. Spongy, dark, bloody tissue replaces the spongiosa of the distal femur (A) and extends through the cortex onto the caudal surface of the bone (B). Observe the smoothly contoured periosteal response (C). B. Radiograph of the tumor showing marked osteolysis in the distal femur (A) accompanied by a permeative pattern of bone destruction in the distal shaft (B). Note the evenly contoured collar of periosteal new bone (C). C. Tumor is composed of an irregular bed of proliferating neoplastic angioblasts (A). Bone (B) is destroyed by osteoclastic resorption (**arrow**).

## Giant Cell Tumor of Bone

Giant cell tumors of bone appear to arise from primitive stromal cells of the bone marrow and produce expansile osteolytic lesions (fig. 5.27A) primarily in the ends of long bones of the appendicular skeleton, although cranial, vertebral, costal, and metacarpal lesions have been described. This is a rare primary bone tumor of animals, and most cases are reported in dogs (Crow *et al.*, 1979; Garman *et al.*, 1977; Jacobson, 1971; LeCoteur *et al.*, 1978; Pavey and Riser, 1963; Trigo *et al.*, 1983) and cats (Cotchin, 1956; Howard and Kenyon, 1967; McClelland, 1941; Pool, 1978; Popp and Simpson, 1976; Thornburg, 1979; Turrel and Pool, 1982; Whitehead, 1967). Jacobson (1971) found only one giant cell tumor in his series of 403 primary bone tumors of the dog, and he expressed skepticism regarding most cases that are in the veterinary literature. More well-documented cases are needed before this entity can be properly characterized in animals. It is mentioned here to acquaint the pathology resident with some of the features of giant cell tumor of bone so that this neoplasm will be considered in a differential diagnosis of an expansile, lytic lesion of bone.

The histogenesis of this tumor is uncertain (Dahlin, 1967). The multinucleated giant cells that are the hallmark of this distinctive neoplasm arise by fusion of proliferating, plump, ovoid to spindle-shaped neoplastic cells forming the bulk of the tumor mass. There is a marked similarity of nuclei in both mononuclear and multinucleated cells, and the borders of the giant cells are often indistinct (fig. 5.27B). Because the giant cells have the same enzyme histochemical properties as osteoclasts, these tumors were sometimes called osteoclastomas, a term that is no longer in use. Ultrastructural and histochemical studies indicate that the tumor cells arise from bone marrow stromal cells (Hanaoka *et al.*, 1970; Johnston, 1977; Schajowicz, 1961; Steiner *et al.*, 1972).

The neoplasm is highly vascular, and there is an indication that some aneurysmal bone cysts may have their origin in giant cell tumor of bone (Ackerman and Rosai, 1968). Tumor cells typically form little or no recognizable matrix. However, in humans osteoid and bone have been seen in about one-third of the tumors (Goldenberg *et al.*, 1970;

Spjut *et al.*, 1971), especially in areas of pathological fracture or following unsuccessful therapy. In these cases some tumor cells undergo metaplasia to form collagenous matrix and bone (Dahlin, 1967). Collagenous trabeculae (fig. 5.27C) and structures suggestive of osteoid spicules were present in two of the giant cell tumors examined by the author. In these cases, which were cats, tumor cells in the pulmonary metastases formed no obvious matrix and generally resembled the cells of the primary tumor mass.

Both benign and malignant variants of giant cell tumors of bone have been reported in animals with benign variants apparently being more common than malignant (Jubb *et al.*, 1985). In humans about 30% of the tumors locally recur and approximately 6% metastasize (Goldenberg *et al.*, 1970; McGrath, 1972). Limitations and exceptions are a recognized problem in the grading of giant cell tumors of human bone (Johnston, 1977; Spjut *et al.*, 1971). On occasion, a cytologically benign giant cell tumor will produce metastatic disease (Dahlin, 1967). The veterinary pathologist should be aware of these problems if confronted with tissues from one of these tumors. Diagnosis of giant cell tumor should not be based on tiny fragments of tissue from a bone lesion or an aspiration biopsy (Dahlin, 1967). In the author's experience with only six of these tumors, those that produced metastatic disease were ones that also had radiographically aggressive bone lesions; however, not all of the animals with aggressive lesions developed metastases. Giant cells may be encountered in a variety of bone lesions of animals including bone cysts, aneurysmal bone cysts, osteodystrophy fibrosa of secondary hyperparathyroidism, fibrous dysplasia, and giant cell variants of osteosarcoma (fig. 5.18B). Trigo *et al.* (1983) presented criteria for distinguishing giant cell tumor of bone from reparative granuloma in bone.

## Multilobular Tumor of Bone

**Classification.** Multilobular tumors of bone are evenly contoured, solitary, cartilaginous, osseous, or osteocartilaginous tumors of distinctive microscopic structure that undergo progressive malignant degeneration and cause the death of the animal un-

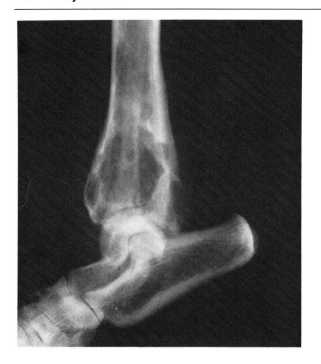

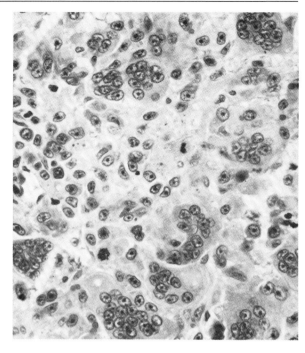

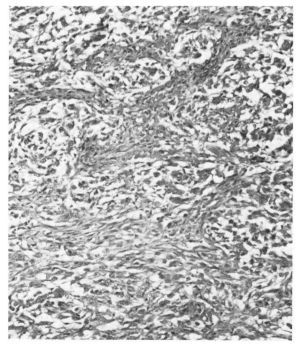

A | B    **FIGURE 5.27.** Giant cell tumor of bone. A. Radio-
C |      graph of an expansile, osteolytic lesion in the distal
tibia of a dog. B. Tissues from a malignant giant cell tumor of
the tibia. Tumor giant cells arise by fusion of rapidly proliferating neoplastic mononuclear cells. Note the similarity of
nuclei in both cell populations and the indistinct borders of
the giant cells. Lung metastases had a similar appearance.
C. Less well-differentiated area in same primary tumor but
with smaller and less characteristic giant cells. Observe that
small spindle cells form anastomotic septa of collagenous
tissue that sometimes contain spicules of bone matrix.

less complete surgical extirpation is accomplished.

This tumor was initially called "chondroma rodens" by Jacobson (1971) who examined lower-grade cartilaginous variants of this lesion in several dogs and a cat. Because the tumors had stromal features seen in chondrosarcoma and osteosarcoma but cytological and behavioral characteristics of neither, Jacobson regarded this lesion as a new type of tumor with marked similarity to human parosteal osteosarcoma.

Liu and Dorfman (1974) used the complex terminology "cartilage analog of fibromatosis" (or "juvenile aponeurotic fibroma") to identify four canine cases of multilobular tumor occurring in the skulls of dogs. These authors thought that they were dealing with soft tissue tumors arising in the dense fascia in the frontooccipital and temporal regions of the skull. They also believed that these canine skull tumors resembled a calcifying variant of juvenile aponeurotic fibroma of children known as the cartilage analog of fibromatosis, juvenile calcifying fibroma, or calcifying fibroma (Allen, 1977; Goldman, 1970; Keasbey, 1953; Lichtenstein and Goldman, 1964). However, lesions typically develop in the aponeurotic tissue on the volar sides of the hands and feet of children and do not involve the head. Histologically, the lesion is primarily composed of immature fibroblasts that infiltrate adipose tissue and muscle. Areas of calcification are common and a few random foci of disorganized chondroid tissue may be present (Lattes, 1982). In humans these lesions do not undergo malignant transformation, do not invade adjacent bone organs, and do not produce metastatic disease (Allen, 1977).

On the basis of his findings in necropsy and biopsy specimens from 10 dogs, Pool (1978) recognized that these bony growths were a unique primary bone tumor of the canine skull and were unlike other bone tumors of the skull and remaining skeleton of the dog (Ling et al., 1974). He made serial sections of the skull tumors, radiographed them on high detail film, and used the radiographs to select areas of the tumor for histological examination. Using this procedure he determined that these lesions were primary bone tumors. He found no evidence to suggest that the tumors had originated in the extraskeletal connective tissue of the head and secondarily invaded bones of the skull. One of his cases had arisen within the diploë of a skull bone and had not extended through the outer cortical plate. Pool also recognized that the lobular arrangement in histological sections was an integral feature of this bone tumor, and he found the same multilobular pattern within pulmonary metastases of one of the dogs in his study. In this case material there was a variation among the several tumors with regard to the orderliness of the lobular pattern and the nature of the matrix filling the centers of the lobules. Orderly tumors with lobules filled primarily with crude bone tissue were called multilobular osteomas, while those filled primarily with cartilage tissue were called multilobular chondromas. Examples were encountered in which many of the chondromatous nodules were undergoing endochondral ossification and had acquired an osteomatous appearance. These orderly tumors were called multilobular osteoma or chondroma based on the major type of tissue present. A third group of tumors had a disorderly lobular arrangement. Large, elongated lobules crowded out the more orderly lobules. The centers of these lobules mostly contained crude cartilage or bone matrix. However, there were other areas in these tumors where the lobular architecture had completely broken down and where malignant change had occurred in the cartilaginous, bony, or fibrous tissue elements of the tumor. These lesions were called multilobular sarcomas, and demonstrated malignant behavior by infiltrative growth into adjacent soft tissues and by metastatic disease in one case.

Initially, the author had experience mainly with the more benign end of the spectrum of these tumors. This is why he proposed the term *multilobular osteoma and/or multilobular chondroma of the canine skull* for these tumors in the previous edition of this book (Pool, 1978). Since that time the author has had experience with additional cases including two more that developed metastatic disease. He has also examined tissue from a tumor in the skull of a cat and two vertebral tumors of dogs. A tumor has since been identified as having arisen from the hard palate of a dog (Diamond et al., 1980), and another dog with a long-standing tumor developed metastatic disease (McLain et al., 1983). Recently, a multilobular tumor was reported involving the zygomatic process of a horse (Richardson and Acland, 1983). Because these tumors undergo progressive malignant degeneration, eventually acquire metastatic potential, are not limited in occurrence to the skull, and can arise in the skeleton of cats and horses as well as dogs, the author has chosen to include this tumor with primary sarcomas of bone. He proposes a slight modification in the name of this tumor and now prefers *multilobular tumor of bone*. This term avoids the more confusing terminology of Jacobson (1971) and Liu and Dorfman (1974). By eliminating the terms *osteoma* and *chondroma* from the name and by not using the term *sarcoma*, the benignity of the lesion is deemphasized while not denying the possibility that completely benign variants of this tumor may one day be recognized.

**Incidence, Age, Breed, and Sex.** The multilobular tumor of bone is the most common primary bone tumor of the dog's skull. It is much more common than the osteoma. Dogs with tumors located in the skull have an average age of 9 years (ranging from 3 to 12 years). Most dogs are of medium and large breeds, but rarely of giant breeds. No breed or sex predilection is indicated.

Too few of these tumors have been found in noncranial sites of the canine skeleton or in the heads of cats and horses to know if age, breed, and sex are significant factors in these cases. The two cats with tumors reported in the literature were a 9-month-old neutered female (Jacobson, 1971) and a castrated male of unknown age (Morton, 1985). The cat in the author's collection was 8 years old; the sex was not known. The horse was a 12-year-old thoroughbred mare (Richardson and Acland, 1983).

**Clinical Characteristics.** The dogs are usually presented because of a palpable, firm, unmovable mass arising from the surface of the bones of the skull. Less frequently, the owner's concern is directed toward a change in the dog's normal pattern of behavior. Signs are related to the degree that the tumor mass compresses and perturbs the function of adjacent structures. Some tumors may cause exophthalmia, sinus obstruction, interference with mastication, or loosening of teeth. A few tumors compress the brain and cranial nerves. These tumors may cause neurological signs that mimic those of brain tumors. Tumors occurring in accessible sites have been removed successfully (Liu and Dorfman, 1974), but local recurrence should be anticipated

(McLain *et al.*, 1983). The lesion in the zygomatic process of the horse was also successfully removed without local recurrence (Richardson and Acland, 1983).

**Sites and Gross Morphology.** The areas of the canine skull most commonly involved are the parietal crest, the temporooccipital region, including the area around the external opening of the ear canal, and the base of the zygomatic process. The frontal bone and wall of the orbit are also commonly affected sites. One dog had two separate skull tumors. Diamond *et al.* (1980) reported a lesion in the hard palate, and the author has found three tumors arising from the palate.

The tumor is a hard, nodular mass with a discrete border (fig. 5.28A). It is covered by a tough fibrous membrane when it projects into the soft tissues of the skull or by a thinner layer of intact epithelium or meninges when the tumor protrudes into the nasal sinuses or the cranial vault. Tumors ranging in size from 2 to more than 10 cm in diameter have produced clinical signs. On cut surface the tumor is composed of numerous tiny, gray, gritty nodules and a few intersecting bands of fibrous tissue containing blood vessels. A lesion is typically centered in one of the flat bones of the skull and may exhibit symmetric or eccentric enlargement. Consequently, expansile growth directed primarily into a cavity (e.g., frontal sinus, orbit, or cranial vault) would not be palpable early in the course of the disease. Tumors protruding into cavities are covered by intact membranes, and they compress the brain without invading the meninges or nervous tissue (fig. 5.28A).

**Radiographic Appearance.** Tumors are solitary nodular lesions that have smoothly contoured, sharply demarcated borders (fig. 5.29A). Normal bone structure in the affected area may be replaced by an amorphous pattern of increased radiodensity containing areas of granularity. A nodular to stippled pattern may be seen in tumors protruding into cavities or into the soft tissues of the head. The occurrence of large areas of lysis within the tumor or the development of a brush pattern along the borders of a tumor would suggest malignant change.

**Histological Features.** A typical tumor is composed of numerous contiguous lobules (fig. 5.28B and C). In well-differentiated tumors each lobule is bordered by thin septa of spindle cell mesen-

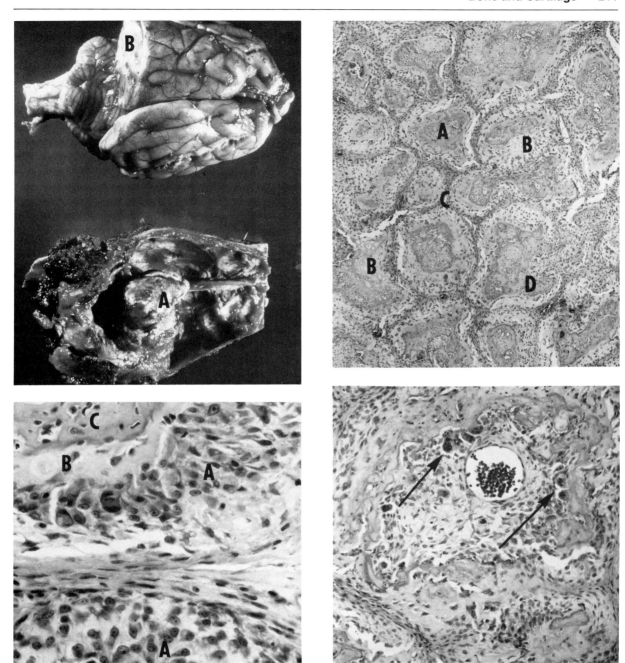

**FIGURE 5.28.** Multilobular tumor of bone (chondroma rodens). A. Smoothly contoured intracranial mass (A) covered by an intact dura mater has compressed the caudal pole (B) of the left cerebral hemisphere. B. Multilobular pattern characteristic of this tumor. Crude bone (A) and/or cartilage (B) in the center of lobules, which are bounded by thin fibrous septa (C). Blood vessels (D) in interstices between lobules. C. Plump cells resembling fetal osteoblasts (A) rim centrilobular islands of chondroid (B) and/or osseous matrix (C). D. Remodeling of lobule with vascular invasion and osteoclastic resorption (**arrows**).

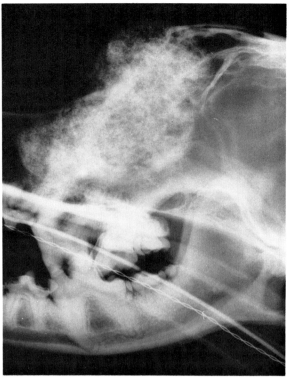

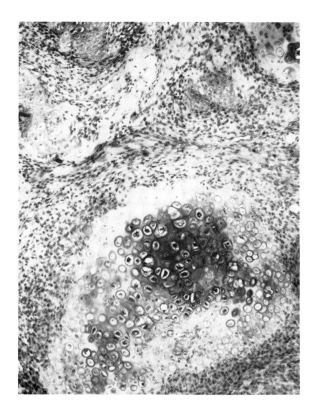

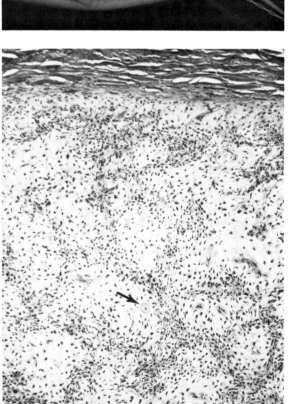

A | B
C |  **FIGURE 5.29.** Multilobular tumor of bone. A. Radio-graph of large, productive, radiodense lesion having a smoothly contoured border and composed of multinodular densities. B. Disruption of nodular pattern (top) in some tumors of the cartilaginous type, as seen here, leads to confusion with chondrosarcoma. C. Multilobular pattern is difficult to recognize in some less well-differentiated multilobular tumors. Note, however, the pattern formed by the septa and the presence of a chondrocyte (**arrow**).

chyme. Vessels travel in interstices between adjacent lobules. Vessels may penetrate the centers of lobules undergoing endochondral ossification (fig. 5.28D). The central two-thirds of a lobule may contain hyaline cartilage, tissue with matrix properties intermediate between bone and cartilage, or immature bone. The central island is typically surrounded by a zone of plump to ovoid cells that merge with fusiform septal cells. Hyperchromatic cells resembling primitive osteoblasts often form cellular palisades around the central islands of matrix. Mitotic figures are uncommon in most cases. When they are present, they suggest that malignant transformation has occurred, and a more rapid and aggressive clinical course is expected. While all of these tumors have the characteristic lobular pattern, they may vary in the amounts of cartilage and bone matrix found in the lobules. Some of the cartilaginous variants are so well-differentiated that they may be mistaken for primary chondrosarcoma of the skull (fig. 5.29B) unless adequate tumor tissue is available for inspection. Conversely, a few skull tumors will be so poorly differentiated that the lobular pattern and chondroid nature of the matrix may be overlooked (fig. 5.29C).

In the author's experience spindle cell mesenchyme never forms a major part of the skull tumor proper. None of the tumors have areas with an interwoven or herringbone pattern of fibrosarcoma. In some tumors, however, dedifferentiated spindled cells arising from the septal cells at the periphery of a tumor invade the soft tissue along muscle insertion lines.

Microscopic indicators of aggressive and malignant behavior include mitotic activity, loss of orderly lobular architecture, necrosis, hemorrhage, and overgrowth by one of the mesenchymal elements forming the lobular structure. The dedifferentiated cartilaginous element was the neoplastic component in three malignant tumors producing metastatic disease in the author's collection and in the one case reported in the literature with pulmonary metastasis (McLain *et al.,* 1983). On the basis of the tissue elements present, it appears that this tumor could also give rise to the osteoblastic osteosarcoma of the skull reported by Hardy *et al.* (1967). Chondrosarcoma reportedly arose from a tumor in a cat (Morton, 1985).

**Growth and Metastasis.** These tumors demonstrate slow but progressive growth. Because of their strategic location in the skull, the tumors usually cause death because of local disease unless removed. Local recurrence is anticipated unless the tumor and the affected bone are completely removed; however, surgical resection has been curative in the case of two dogs (Liu and Dorfman, 1974) and a horse (Richardson and Acland, 1983). The author has observed metastatic disease in three dogs with tumors present for more than 6 months. McLain *et al.* (1983) reported metastatic lung disease in a dog in which a skull tumor had been present for more than 22 months.

## Liposarcoma

Liposarcoma of bone is a primary bone tumor arising from malignant fat cell precursors in the marrow cavity. Liposarcomas of bone are very rare in animals. A central (medullary) liposarcoma (Brodey and Riser, 1966) in an 18-month-old male Labrador retriever produced an osteolytic lesion in the distal two-thirds of the left humerus with marked production of periosteal new bone and a firm, painless soft tissue swelling. The tumor, consisting of gray fatty tissue, replaced bone marrow and eroded cortical and trabecular bone. The dog showed progressive lameness in the left forelimb for approximately 1 month before diagnosis. At necropsy 2 weeks later there was no evidence of tumor beyond the primary site. Another report (Levene and Butt, 1969) described a liposarcoma that originated in the distal left tibia of an 18-month-old male miniature poodle. The animal succumbed to metastatic disease in the liver and lymph nodes 2 months following amputation of the limb.

Liposarcoma of bone resembles its soft tissue counterpart. While much of the tumor tissue may be composed of well-differentiated signet ring cells and multivesicular cells, there may be foci of fibrosarcomatous differentiation or areas of undifferentiated spindle cell sarcoma. Fat stains may be used to demonstrate the presence of fat within tumor cells. Central fibrosarcoma of bone should be differentiated from central lipoma of bone (Morgan, 1972), periosteal liposarcoma of bone (Jacobson, 1971), liposarcoma of soft tissues which secondarily involves bone (Brodey *et al.*, 1963), and tumors metastatic to bone which mimic liposarcoma (Spjut *et al.*, 1971).

## Lymphoid and Myelomatous Tumors of Bone

Lymphoma, reticulum cell sarcoma (large cell or histiocytic lymphoma), and plasma cell myeloma (multiple myeloma) are tumors that may involve bone marrow and therefore involve bone organs themselves. (Detailed descriptions of these diseases, including the histological appearance of tumor tissue, are presented in chap. 6.) These three neoplastic diseases are discussed together since they may produce similar, nonspecific, destructive radiographic lesions characteristic only of a malignant disease or, at times, a hematogenous osteomyelitis. Therefore, the final diagnosis of the bone lesions is usually based on microscopic interpretation of biopsy or necropsy tissue specimens. Impression smears are also recommended and may be essential for the diagnosis.

The former two tumors often localize in bone marrow as part of a widespread multicentric involvement of lymphohematopoietic tissues of the body. Lymphoma tends to replace bone marrow, but rarely produces sufficient bone destruction to be seen on the clinical radiograph or to cause clinical signs related to bone disease. When bone lesions do occur in lymphoma, they often involve the vertebrae and predispose them to pathological fracture (Jacobson, 1971; Owen, 1969; Squire, 1969; Staub *et al.*, 1960). However, lymphoma may produce lesions in the distal metaphyses of the long bones of dogs. The lesions are characterized radiographically by osteolysis, but without production of periosteal new bone or much soft tissue swelling (Brodey *et al.*, 1963; Morgan, 1972). Tissue sections taken from bone affected by lymphoma (fig. 5.30A) show loss of spongiosa, infiltration of marrow spaces by neoplastic lymphocytes, and extension of tumor cells into soft tissue adjacent to the bone.

Primary histiocytic lymphoma of bone occurs in humans (Spjut *et al.*, 1971) and probably occurs in animals as well (fig. 5.30B) (Brodey *et al.*, 1963;

Wilson, 1973). Highly destructive lesions are produced in the metaphyses of long bones of dogs (Brodey *et al.*, 1963; Morgan, 1972) and cats (Wilson, 1973). Destruction of articular cartilage was a feature of the lesions in the cats with this disease. Metastasis to the lungs and other organs occurs in most cases.

Plasma cell myeloma (multiple myeloma) is a malignant neoplasm of proliferating plasma cells of bone marrow. The tumor manifests itself by forming multicentric lytic lesions in the most hematopoietically active bones of the skeleton and by producing a monoclonal gammopathy. The tumor is uncommon in domestic animals. It is found more often in dogs (Bartels *et al.*, 1972; Braund *et al.*, 1979; Cordy, 1957; Lester and Mesfin, 1980; Liu, 1981; Liu *et al.*, 1977; Oduye and Losos, 1972; Orr *et al.*, 1981; Osborne *et al.*, 1968; Pennock *et al.*, 1966; Schalm, 1974; Shull *et al.*, 1978; Van Bree *et al.*, 1983; Walton and Gopinath, 1972) than in cats (Liu, 1981) or horses (Cornelius *et al.*, 1959). In one report of 40 cases in animals, 38 cases involved mostly male dogs having a mean age of 9.5 years (ranging from 2.5 to 15 years); the two cats in this report were middle aged (Liu, 1981).

In dogs the usual presenting signs include lameness, ill-defined pain, and lethargy (Osborne *et al.*, 1968; Van Bree *et al.*, 1983), but paraplegia may follow direct spinal cord compression by protrusion of tumor masses into the vertebral canal (Braund *et al.*, 1979; Van Bree *et al.*, 1983) or be secondary to pathological fracture (Braund *et al.*, 1979; Osborne *et al.*, 1968). In one report a homogenous protein, M-component, was found on serum electrophoresis in all 14 dogs that were examined (Liu *et al.*, 1977). The M-components of 12 of the dogs were IgG (5), IgA (6), and L-chain (1). Bence Jones protein was present in the urine of all 12 dogs and the 2 cats that were tested (Liu, 1981); however, we find Bence–Jones protein in the urine in less than one-fourth of our canine patients with plasma cell myeloma.

Only about two-thirds of plasma cell myeloma cases reported in dogs had radiographic signs of skeletal involvement (Van Bree *et al.*, 1983). In a group of 36 canine cases the sites of primary skeletal involvement included vertebrae (21), humerus (15), ribs (11), femur (9), pelvis (8), scapula (4), tibia (2), skull (2), and ilium (2). The two cats in

to a series of biopsy procedures because the pathologist is unaware of the radiographic and clinical findings in the case and has underdiagnosed the lesion as fibroma or scar tissue.

## Maxillary Fibrosarcoma of the Dog

These are typically low-grade fibrosarcomas that arise on the outer surface of the maxilla and slowly disfigure the dog's face. They are characterized in most instances by having an innocuous histological appearance that belies their destructive nature. The author has chosen to separate this tumor from the main group of periosteal fibrosarcomas for two reasons. First, this canine neoplasm is by far the most commonly encountered example of this rare group of neoplasms. Second, the maxillary fibrosarcoma is an important tumor of dogs that is not widely recognized but is one that apparently responds to combined radiation–hyperthermia treatments (Brewer and Turrel, 1982). Currently, the author is considering these tumors of the maxilla as being low-grade fibrosarcomas more on the basis of their behavior than on their histological appearance. These tumors are not as cellular as most canine fibrosarcomas, and they do not produce the interwoven pattern characteristic of most of those sarcomas. In fact, studies may one day show that they represent a variant of fibromatosis. However, it is difficult at this time to explain to clinicians that such a destructive tumor that eventually kills the dog is not a sarcoma.

Examples of these tumors seen by the author occurred primarily in middle-aged dogs with most dogs being around 7 years old. The three most commonly affected breeds were the golden retriever, Doberman pinscher, and German shepherd. Both sexes were represented. Although Liu *et al.* (1977) did not attempt to distinguish between periosteal and central fibrosarcomas in their 31 cases of fibrosarcoma in dogs in which bones were involved, they found that fibrosarcomas affected the maxilla of 10 dogs.

Clinically, maxillary fibrosarcomas grow slowly and are initially recognized because of a firm swelling on the side of the face. In time the tumors cause gross distortion of the face, loosening of teeth, and erosion of the maxilla. In advanced cases tumor tis-

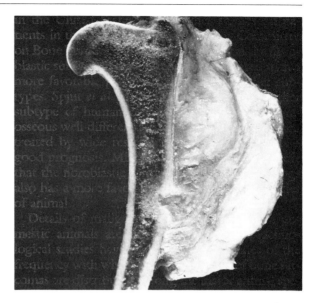

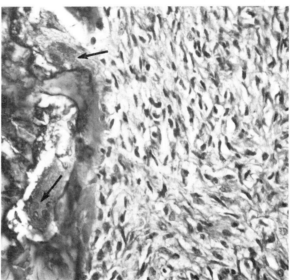

A
B
**FIGURE 5.33.** Periosteal fibrosarcoma of bone. A. Slowly growing tumor firmly attached to the cranial surface of the humerus has invaded the cortex at mid-diaphysis. B. Undemineralized tissue section of moderately well-differentiated fibrosarcoma beginning to invade the cortical surface as it follows resorption cavities cut by osteoclasts (**arrows**).

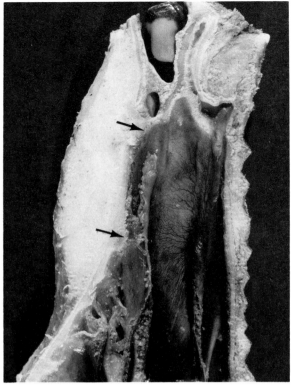

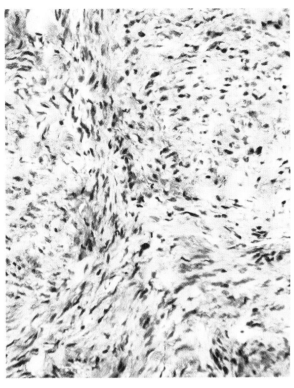

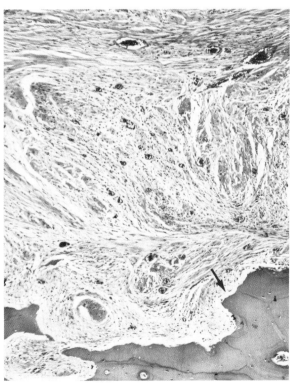

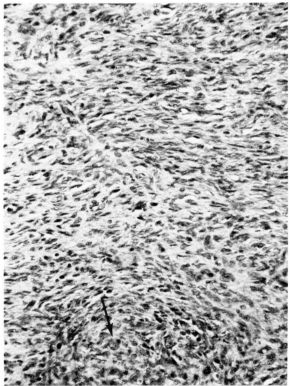

A | B
C | D

**FIGURE 5.34.** Maxillary fibrosarcoma of the dog. A. Sagittal section showing intimate association of tumor mass with external surface of maxilla and nasal bones. Note areas of cortical destruction (**arrows**). B. Well-differentiated area of tumor is easily mistaken for reactive fi-

brosis. C. Note destruction of cortical bone (**arrow**) by well-differentiated fibrosarcoma. D. Anaplastic areas (**arrow**) may be found in some tumors producing very aggressive clinical lesions.

sue may invade the nasal bone, nasal cavity, hard palate, and orbit. Disfigurement and local recurrence after surgery are the usual reasons for euthanasia.

At necropsy, after the skin and soft tissues are removed, the tumor mass remains tightly adhered to the surface of the maxilla (fig. 5.34A). Transverse serial sections through the head also show that the bulk of the tumor mass lies on the external surface of the maxilla, although tumor tissue may invade the nasal passages at multiple sites and partially compress the turbinates.

The histological appearance of these tumors is often deceiving, especially when one is examining small biopsy specimens. Most tumors are well-differentiated fibroblastic growths (fig. 5.34B) that are not encapsulated. Tumor tissue slowly infiltrates the adjacent soft tissue and destroys the underlying maxillary bone (fig. 5.34C). Biopsies of superficial tumor tissue are even more confusing since a mononuclear inflammatory cell infiltrate is often present, and there is fibrous tissue organization of edematous soft tissue in some tumors. In most tumors, areas of higher-grade malignancy (fig. 5.34D) can be found by sampling broadly. Highly malignant tumor tissue was a substantial part of only one tumor, and this tumor had been treated by radiation therapy a few months earlier. This tumor was also the only one in which metastatic disease was found at necropsy.

## Periosteal Osteosarcoma

These are osteosarcomas that arise on the surface of a bone presumably from malignant tissue in the periosteum and initially extend outward into the soft tissue. Later, the tumor may invade the underlying cortex and extend into the medullary cavity.

In humans periosteal osteosarcomas account for less than 1% of osteosarcomas (Spjut *et al.,* 1981). These tumors tend to arise more often on the surface of the diaphysis than the metaphysis of long bones. The histological pattern contains variable amounts of malignant osteoid, bone, cartilage, and fibrous tissue elements. In general, the neoplastic tissue in the periosteal osteosarcoma is intermediate in differentiation between the more malignant tissue of central osteosarcoma and the well-differentiated tissue of parosteal osteosarcoma. However, areas

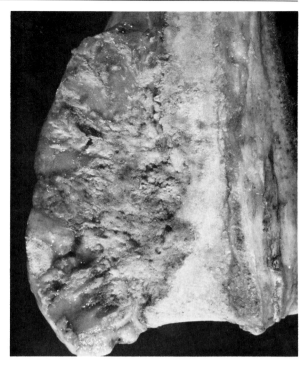

**FIGURE 5.35.** Periosteal osteosarcoma of the distal radius. Rapidly growing, highly malignant osteosarcoma appears to originate in the periosteum, invade the radius, and extend into the soft tissue.

can be selected from periosteal osteosarcoma that cannot be distinguished from microscopic fields of central osteosarcoma. Periosteal osteosarcomas are not so well-differentiated that tissue sections should be mistaken for reactive bone. In humans periosteal osteosarcoma is distinguished from central osteosarcoma because the former appears to offer a better prognosis. In a continuing study of humans described by Spjut *et al.* (1981), 11 of 36 patients had died with pulmonary metastatic disease, but 10 people had lived 5 years or longer since diagnosis.

It is the author's experience that periosteal osteosarcoma is rare in dogs, although the authors of a major textbook of veterinary pathology once indicated that most osteosarcomas of domestic animals are of periosteal origin (Smith *et al.,* 1972). The author recognizes two different types of periosteal osteosarcomas in dogs. The first type (fig. 5.35) is a highly aggressive tumor and has the same histological features and high metastatic potential as central osteosarcoma. Such tumors may actually be central osteosarcomas that have arisen in the outer spongiosa of the metaphysis of a long bone and for some undetermined reason developed an eccentric growth pattern. The author has examined radiographs of bone tumors that were thought to be periosteal osteosarcomas. On examination of the bone specimen, however, these tumors were found to be central osteosarcomas that had infarcted the medullary cavity and cortical bone. Viable tumor remained primarily along the surface and produced a bony matrix in the periosteal tissues (fig. 5.19D).

The second type of canine periosteal osteosarcoma more closely fits the description of this entity in humans, with the exception that both cases seen by the author arose on the metaphyseal surfaces rather than on the diaphyseal surfaces. Both tumors produced a dense bony matrix, and neither dog developed metastasis following limb amputation.

## Parosteal Osteosarcoma

**Classification.** Parosteal osteosarcoma (juxtacortical osteosarcoma or parosteal sarcoma) is a sarcoma on the surface of a bone and is composed typically of well-differentiated but malignant fibrous, osseous, and in some cases cartilaginous, tissues. The term *parosteal sarcoma* is preferred by some pathologists (Aegerter and Kirkpatrick, 1968) because all three mesenchymal tissue types may be present in a tumor. The neoplasm arises in bone-forming periosteal connective tissue and not in extraskeletal tissues beside the bone as the name implies. In humans these tumors are distinguished from the more common central or intramedullary osteosarcomas of bone by a longer clinical course and a higher survival rate, especially for patients receiving proper surgical care (Ackerman and Rosai, 1968). Four reports (Banks, 1971; Jacobson, 1971; Liu *et al.*, 1974; Turrel and Pool, 1982) have indicated that a similar tumor exists in animals. One of these authors (Jacobson, 1971) refers to this neoplasm as parosteal osteoma since these tumors are not as frankly malignant as typical cases of osteosarcoma. Currently, parosteal osteosarcoma is a poorly defined entity in domestic animals, and further

study is necessary to determine whether this parosteal tumor of animals is analogous to human parosteal osteosarcoma in clinical behavior and in radiographic and histomorphological appearance.

**Incidence, Age, Breed, and Sex.** Although this is a well-recognized entity in humans and represents approximately 2% of all human primary bone tumors (Ackerman and Rosai, 1968), parosteal osteosarcomas have only recently been described in animals (Banks, 1971; Jacobson, 1971; Liu *et al.*, 1974; Turrel and Pool, 1982). Since these tumors have not been previously reported in the veterinary literature, even in the more extensive reviews of canine (Brodey and Riser, 1969; Brodey *et al.*, 1963; Ling *et al.*, 1974; Owen, 1969) and feline (Cotchin, 1957; Engle and Brodey, 1969; Nielsen, 1964) bone tumors, they are either very uncommon or they may have gone unrecognized. One report (Jacobson, 1971) on the comparative pathology of bone tumors included 31 animal bone tumors fitting this category. (Jacobson used the term *parosteal osteoma* to designate this neoplasm, a term considered by some bone tumor pathologists [Spjut *et al.*, 1971] as inappropriate and misleading, at least for the behavior of the tumor as it occurs in humans.) There were 14 cases in dogs ranging in age from 6 months to 13 years with a mean age of 7 years. The dogs were mostly of the large and giant breeds with about twice as many males as females represented. Eleven cases were found in cats ranging in age from 1 to 13 years with a mean age of 7 years. Three tumors were found in horses and one each in a pig and a cow. It remains unclear how closely the animal tumors of this report resemble parosteal osteosarcoma of humans.

In a second report (Banks, 1971) parosteal osteosarcoma was diagnosed in a 10-year-old male German shepherd and a 14-year-old domestic short-haired cat. Liu *et al.* (1974) found this tumor in three male and one female domestic cats with an average age of 7 years 8 months (range 4 to 10 years). Turrel and Pool (1982) found this tumor in two cats of ages 10 and 14 years, respectively.

**Clinical Characteristics.** In humans parosteal osteosarcoma has a duration of months to years. The tumor produces a slowly expanding lesion that may or may not be painful and tender. Swelling and interference with locomotion can be the major complaints. The tumor tends to recur locally following surgical excision (Scaglietti and Calandriello, 1962), but these patients may have a life expectancy of several years. Invasion of the medullary cavity is thought to adversely affect the prognosis (Spjut *et al.*, 1971). Death from pulmonary metastasis indicates the unequivocal malignant behavior of this tumor.

In animals with tumors diagnosed as parosteal osteosarcoma the clinical course is of longer duration than that for central osteosarcoma of bone. In the feline subject of one report (Banks, 1971) the lesion was present for slightly more than 1 year after diagnosis and for more than 2 years in the canine patient. In the dog the tumor eventually metastasized to the lung, and these secondary tumors had the microscopic features of chondrosarcoma. The usual clinical finding in parosteal osteosarcoma of animals is the presence of a firm, slowly enlarging mass located on the surface of a bone. The lesion may not be painful initially, but eventually it produces disfiguration, interferes with function, and may cause lameness. In the horse (Jacobson, 1971) a tumor of the cervical vertebrae caused staggering and partial paralysis.

**Sites.** In one study (Jacobson, 1971) specific tumor sites were not indicated; however, Jacobson (1969) reported elsewhere the regional locations of several tumors as follows: for the dog there were three tumors in the head, four in the foreleg, and four in the hindleg; for the cat there were two tumors each in the foreleg, hindleg, ribs, and pelvis; for the horse the maxilla, metacarpus, and cervical vertebra had one tumor each. In the second report (Banks, 1971) the lesion in the cat involved the shaft of the right humerus, whereas in the dog the tumor was found on the distal one-third of the left radius. Liu *et al.* (1974) reported three tumors of the frontal bone and one in the right ramus of the mandible, all in cats. The two cats examined by Turrel and Pool (1982) had diaphyseal lesions of a humerus and a femur. In humans tumors typically are located on the metaphyseal surfaces of long tubular bones of an extremity. Lesions of similar radiographic and microscopic morphology have also been seen on the mandible (Aegerter and Kirkpatrick, 1968).

**Gross Morphology.** The surface of the tumor is generally smooth, but it may be multinodular with a dense fibrous capsule. Tumor tissue is firm to hard

and gritty. The tumor arises on the cortical surface from either a sessile or pedunculated base. Initially, the cortex is undisturbed. Cortical destruction with invasion of the marrow cavity is a late event.

**Radiographic Appearance.** The tumor is located on the surface of the bone (fig. 5.36A). It has an evenly contoured border and the underlying cortex and metaphyseal spongiosa remain intact for a long time. Tumor matrix typically makes an amorphous pattern with variations in radiodensity. The base of some tumors may be pedunculated or sessile after the manner of an osteochondroma. A radiolucent line separating a portion of the tumor from the underlying cortex, while considered to be of diagnostic importance when present in the tumors of humans (Copeland and Geschickter, 1959), has not been seen in the tumors of animals (Jacobson, 1971).

**Histological Features.** In humans (Spjut *et al.*, 1971) many parosteal osteosarcomas, especially early lesions, have an innocent histological character. The fibroosseous and occasionally the cartilaginous stromal elements more closely resemble reactive tissue than a neoplastic proliferation. Cellularity is generally low, but areas of moderate cell density are not uncommon. There may be little or no pleomorphism of tumor cells and typically no mitotic figures are found. Diagnosis is based in large part on the characteristic radiographic appearance of the lesion and appropriate clinical findings. Other human parosteal osteosarcomas are less inscrutable and the malignant character of the stroma is more obvious with multiple areas of malignant fibrous stroma, osteoid, bone, and cartilage.

The microscopic appearance of parosteal osteosarcomas in animals needs further clarification. The diagnostic criterion in one study (Jacobson, 1971) was the finding of a periosteal tumor with a neoplastic stroma in which the cells were too pleomorphic for a benign tumor, yet lacked the marked pleomorphism, cellular density, and mitotic activity of a frankly malignant tumor. More advanced lesions approximated the gross and microscopic appearance of osteosarcoma. Jacobson stated that these parosteal tumors may crudely mimic the structure of an osteochondroma. Chondrocyes with malignant features, however, were present in the fibrocartilaginous and osseous tissues that made up the apical tissue, whereas the marrow spaces of

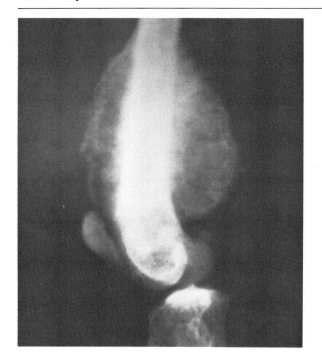

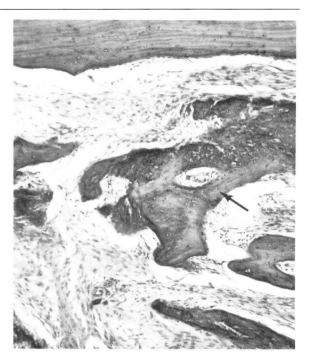

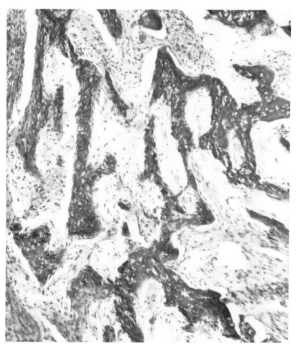

A|B
C| **FIGURE 5.36.** Parosteal osteosarcoma. A. Radiograph of tumor arising from the cortical surface of the distal femur. Note evenly contoured surface of tumor. B. Tumor lying adjacent to the cortical surface (top) is a low-grade spindle cell tumor that produces crude spicules of woven bone, some of which has been remodeled and partially replaced by lamellar bone tissue (**arrow**). C. Tissue from periphery of tumor is composed of a haphazard pattern of woven bone spicules formed by fusiform tumor cells without anaplastic features.

the bony stalk contained fibrous tissue instead of fatty and hematopoietic marrow.

The histomorphology of the primary tumors of the feline and canine patients in another report (Banks, 1971) resembled central osteosarcoma. A biopsy of the lesion in the dog taken early in the course of the disease suggested osteosarcoma; however, at death the pulmonary metastases were those of chondrosarcoma. Liu *et al.* (1974) illustrated one of four cases of parosteal osteosarcoma of the domestic cat.

In the parosteal osteosarcomas examined by the author (figs. 5.36B and C), the tumor tissue was a haphazard fibroosseous tissue centered on the cortical surface. Bony trabeculae formed by the fibrous tissue had no consistent pattern of orientation. Tumor cells resembled fibroblasts and had no anaplastic features.

**Growth and Metastasis.** Parosteal osteosarcomas demonstrate slow but continuous growth on the surface of a bone. In time the tumor may acquire a more aggressive clinical behavior and will invade the cortex and extend into a medullary cavity. Pulmonary metastasis may occur, but only many months after the clinical disease first becomes apparent.

## SECONDARY TUMORS OF BONE

Malignant neoplasms originating in soft tissues or in the skeleton itself may secondarily involve bones by direct extension or by hematogenous metastasis. The subject is discussed in many articles (Brodey *et al.*, 1966; Kas *et al.*, 1970; Liu and Harvey, 1981; Liu *et al.*, 1974; Morgan *et al.*, 1980; Owen, 1969; Russell and Walker, 1983). Secondary bone tumor may also refer to a bone tumor that has arisen in a preexisting lesion, for example, malignant transformation of an osteochondroma to a chondrosarcoma (Banks and Bridges, 1956) or to an osteosarcoma (Owen and Bostock, 1971).

Local bone destruction is a feature of many infiltrating neoplasms, especially tumors arising in mucous membranes of the heads of animals. Familiar examples are malignant melanoma, carcinoma, and fibrosarcoma of the oral cavity and carcinoma of the nasal cavity and conjunctiva. Soft tissue tumors that are less common causes of local bone destruction include carcinoma of the nail bed of dogs and cats, fibrosarcoma, hemangiosarcoma, rhabdomyosarcoma, and synovial sarcoma. These tumors are centered on soft tissue and tend to produce bone destruction late in the course of the disease. With the possible exception of certain nasal tumors, the clinician can usually distinguish between invasive tumors of soft tissue and primary bone tumor.

Metastatic bone disease in animals, however, particularly in the early stages of development, can mimic the radiographic appearance of a primary bone sarcoma, osteomyelitis, and fungal infection of bone (Morgan, 1972). In one report of 20 metastatic bone tumors in dogs, the radiographic diagnosis with one exception was primary malignant bone tumor (Kas *et al.*, 1970). In most of the dogs in this study the secondary bone tumors produced osteolytic lesions with extensive periosteal new bone formation. Metastatic lesions may be osteolytic, osteoblastic, or mixed. Occasionally all three radiographic patterns can be seen in an animal with multiple metastatic foci (figs. 5.37A, B, and C) (Pool *et al.*, 1974). At times the reactive bone produced in response to metastatic carcinoma can be so primitive that it may resemble tumor bone of osteosarcoma (fig. 5.37D). A review of the clinical and radiographic findings with particular attention to the history, age, breed, and sex of the animal and a knowledge of the number and precise skeletal locations of the bone lesion(s) enables one to greatly narrow the range of possible causes of the bone disease. A biopsy is generally necessary for the definitive diagnosis.

Tumor metastases tend to localize in skeletal sites with high vascularity such as bones with abundant red marrow. The author has seen tumor metastases localize within the periosteal new bone of hypertrophic pulmonary osteoarthropathy in 2 dogs with osteosarcoma and in 1 dog with transitional cell carcinoma. In one study of 24 dogs with metastatic bone disease, 80% of the secondary tumors involved four skeletal sites: ribs, 11 cases; vertebrae, 9; humeri, 7; and femurs, 4 (Brodey *et al.*, 1966). Tumors involved rib shafts, the large proximal metaphysis of the humerus (6 of 7 cases), and both metaphyses of the femur in equal numbers. In our diagnostic service we have seen metastatic involvement of the scapula in several cases. All carci-

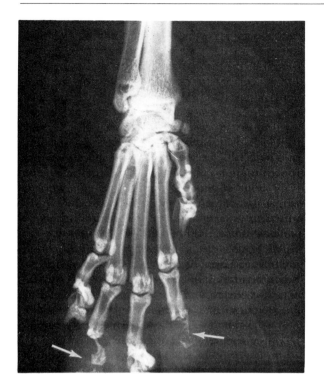

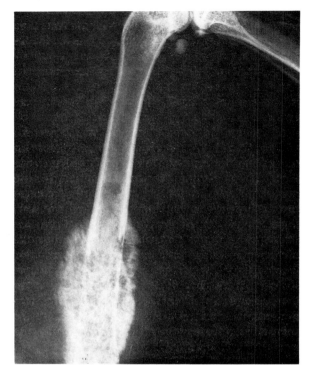

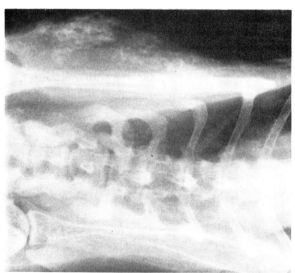

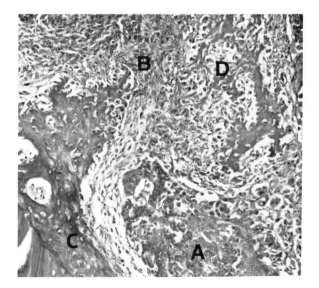

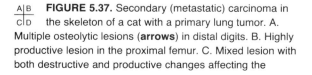

**FIGURE 5.37.** Secondary (metastatic) carcinoma in the skeleton of a cat with a primary lung tumor. A. Multiple osteolytic lesions (**arrows**) in distal digits. B. Highly productive lesion in the proximal femur. C. Mixed lesion with both destructive and productive changes affecting the scapula. D. Metastatic carcinoma (A) has provoked a pronounced proliferation of collagenous stroma (B) and reactive bone (C). At times the reactive bone may be so immature as to resemble tumor bone matrix (D).

nomas and sarcomas from most organ systems have produced metastatic disease on rare occasion in the canine skeleton (Brodey *et al.,* 1966; Jacobson, 1971; Kas *et al.,* 1970; Owen, 1969), but none of these tumors produces a pathognomonic radiographic appearance. It is generally recognized that in dogs there is a relative scarcity of tumors metastatic to bone compared with humans, but the reason for this is unclear (Brodey *et al.,* 1966; Owen, 1969).

# REFERENCES

Ackerman, L. V., and Rosai, J. (1968) *Surgical Pathology.* 4th ed. The C.V. Mosby Company (Saint Louis).

Aegerter, E., and Kirkpatrick, J. A. (1968) *Orthopedic Diseases.* 3d ed. W. B. Saunders Company (Philadelphia).

Alexander, J. W., and Patton, C. S. (1983) Primary Tumors of the Skeletal System. *Vet. Clin. N. Amer. Small Anim. Pract.* 13, 181–195.

Allen, P. W. (1977) The Fibromatoses: A Clinicopathologic Classification Based on 140 Cases, Part 2. *Amer. J. Surg. Path.* 1, 305–321.

Banks, W. C. (1971) Parosteal Osteosarcoma in a Dog and a Cat. *J. Amer. Vet. Med. Assoc.* 158, 1412–1415.

Banks, W. C., and Bridges, C. H. (1956) Multiple Cartilaginous Exostosis in a Dog. *J. Amer. Vet. Med. Assoc.* 129, 131–135.

Banks, W. C., Morris, E., Herron, M. R., and Green, R. W. (1975) Osteogenic Sarcoma Associated with Internal Fixation in Two Dogs. *J. Amer. Vet. Med. Assoc.* 167, 166–167.

Bartels, J. E., Cawley, A. J., McSherry, B. J., and Percy, D. H. (1972) Multiple Myeloma (Plasmacytoma) in a Dog. *J. Amer. Vet. Radiol. Soc.* 13, 36–42.

Bingle, S. A., Brodey, R. S., Allen, H. L., and Riser, W. H. (1974) Haemangiosarcoma of Bone in the Dog. *J. Small Anim. Pract.* 15, 303–322.

Boever, W. J., Kennedy, S., and Kane, K. K. (1977) Ossifying Fibroma in a Greater Kudu. *Vet. Med. Small Anim. Clin.* 72, 1483–1486.

Braund, K. G., Everett, R. M., Bartels, J. E., and De-Buysscher, E. (1979) Neurologic Complications of IgA Multiple Myeloma Associated with Cryoglobulinemia in a Dog. *J. Amer. Vet. Med. Assoc.* 174, 1321–1325.

Brewer, W. G., and Turrel, J. M. (1982) Radiotherapy and Hyperthermia in the Treatment of Fibrosarcomas in the Dog. *J. Amer. Vet. Med. Assoc.* 181, 146–150.

Brodey, R. S. (1960) A Clinical and Pathologic Study of 130 Neoplasms of the Mouth and Pharynx in the Dog. *Amer. J. Vet. Res.* 31, 787–812.

Brodey, R. S., and Riser, W. H. (1966) Liposarcoma of Bone: Case Report. *J. Amer. Vet. Radiol. Soc.* 7, 27–33.

———. (1969) Canine Osteosarcoma: A Clinico-pathologic Study of 194 Cases. *Clin. Orthop.* 62, 54–64.

Brodey, R. S., McGrath, J. T., and Reynolds, H. A. (1959) A Clinical and Radiological Study of Canine Bone Neoplasms. Part I. *J. Amer. Vet. Med. Assoc.* 134, 53–71.

Brodey, R. S., Reid, C. F., and Sauer, R. M. (1966) Metastatic Bone Neoplasms in the Dog. *J. Amer. Vet. Med. Assoc.* 148, 29–48.

Brodey, R. S., Riser, W. H., and Van der Heul, R. O. (1974) Canine Skeletal Chondrosarcoma: A Clinicopathologic Study of 35 Cases. *J. Amer. Vet. Med. Assoc.* 165, 68–78.

Brodey, R. S., Sauer, R. M., and Medway, W. (1963) Canine Bone Neoplasms. *J. Amer. Vet. Med. Assoc.* 143, 471–495.

Brown, R. J., Trevethan, W. P., and Henry, V. L. (1972) Multiple Osteochondroma in a Siamese Cat. *J. Amer. Vet. Med. Assoc.* 160, 433–435.

Carrig, C. B., and Seawright, A. A. (1969) A Familial Canine Polyostotic Fibrous Dysplasia with Subperiosteal Cortical Defects. *J. Small Anim. Pract.* 10, 397–405.

Copeland, M. M., and Geschickter, C. F. (1959) The Treatment of Parosteal Osteoma of Bone. *Surg. Gynec. Obstet.* 108, 537–548.

Cordy, D. R. (1957) Plasma Cell Myeloma in a Dog. *Cornell Vet.* 47, 498–502.

Cornelius, C. E., Goodbarry, R. F., and Kennedy, P. C. (1959) Plasma Cell Myelomatosis in a Horse. *Cornell Vet.* 49, 478–493.

Cotchin, E. (1956) Further Examples of Spontaneous Neoplasms in the Domestic Cat. *Brit. Vet. J.* 112, 263–272.

———. (1957). Neoplasia in the Cat. *Vet. Rec.* 69, 425–434.

Crow, S. E., Hall, A. D., Walshaw, R., and Wortman, J. A. (1979) Giant Cell Tumor (Osteoclastoma) in a Dog. *J. Amer. Anim. Hosp. Assoc.* 15, 473–476.

Dahlin, D. C. (1967) *Bone Tumors.* 2d ed. Charles C. Thomas (Springfield, Illinois).

Dahlin, D. C., and Beabout, J. W. (1971) Dedifferentiation of Low-Grade Chondrosarcomas. *Cancer* 28, 461–466.

Dahlin, D. C., and Coventry, M. B. (1967) Osteogenic Sarcoma: A Study of Six Hundred Cases. *J. Bone Joint Surg.* 49A, 101–110.

Dahlin, D. C., and Unni, K. K. (1977) Osteosarcoma of Bone and Its Important Recognizable Varieties. *Amer. J. Surg. Path.* 1, 61–72.

Diamond, S. S., Raflo, C. P., and Anderson, M. P. (1980) Multilobular Osteosarcoma in the Dog. *Vet. Path.* 17, 749–763.

Dorn, C. R., Taylor, D. O. N., Schneider, R., Hibbard, H. H., and Klauber, M. R. (1968) Survey of Animal Neoplasms in Alameda and Contra Costa Counties, California. II. Cancer Morbidity in Dogs and Cats from Alameda County. *J. Nat. Cancer Inst.* 40, 307–318.

Engle, G. C., and Brodey, R. S. (1969) A Retrospective Study of 395 Feline Neoplasms. *J. Amer. Hosp. Assoc.* 5, 21–31.

Enneking, W. F., and Kagan, A. (1975) "Skip" Metastases in Osteosarcoma. *Cancer* 36, 2192–2205.

Fölger, A. F. (1917) Geschwulste bei Tieren. *Ergebn. Allg. Path. Path. Anat.* 18, 372–676.

Gambardella, P. C., Osborne, C. A., and Stevens, J. B. (1975) Multiple Cartilaginous Exostoses in the Dog. *J. Amer. Vet. Med. Assoc.* 166, 761–768.

Garman, R. H., Powel, F. R., and Tompsett, J. W. (1977) Malignant Giant Cell Tumor in a Dog. *J. Amer. Vet. Med. Assoc.* 171, 546–548.

Gleiser, C. A., Raulston, G. L., Jardine, J. H., Carpenter, R. H., and Gray, K. N. (1981) Telangiectatic Osteosarcoma in the Dog. *Vet. Path.* 18, 396–398.

Goldenberg, R. R., Campbell, C. J., and Bonfiglio, M. (1970) Giant Cell Tumor of Bone. An Analysis of Two Hundred and Eighteen Cases. *J. Bone Joint Surg.* 52, 619–633.

Goldman, R. L. (1970) The Cartilage Analogue of Fibromatosis (Aponeurotic Fibroma). Further Observations Based on Seven New Cases. *Cancer* 26, 1325–1331.

Gourley, I. M. G., Morgan, J. P., and Gould, D. H. (1970) Tracheal Osteochondroma in a Dog: A Case Report. *J. Small Anim. Pract.* 11, 327–335.

Hanaoka, H., Friedman, B., and Mack, R. P. (1970) Ultrastructure and Histogenesis of Giant-Cell Tumor of Bone. *Cancer* 25, 1408–1423.

Hardy, W. D., Jr., Brodey, R. S., and Riser, W. H. (1967) Osteosarcoma of the Canine Skull. *J. Amer. Vet. Radiol. Soc.* 8, 5–16.

Howard, E. B., and Kenyon, A. J. (1967) Malignant Osteoclastoma (Giant Cell Tumor) in a Cat with Associated Mast Cell Response. *Cornell Vet.* 57, 398–409.

Jacobson, S. A. (1969) Parosteal Osteoma (Juxtacortical Osteogenic Sarcoma) in Animals. *Amer. J. Path.* 58, 85a.

———. (1971) *The Comparative Pathology of the Tumors of Bone.* Charles C. Thomas (Springfield, Illinois).

Johnson, L. C. (1953) A General Theory of Bone Tumors. *Bull. N.Y. Acad. Med.* 29, 164–171.

Johnston, J. (1977) Giant Cell Tumor of Bone. *Ortho. Clin. N. Amer.* 8, 751–770.

Jubb, K. V. F., Kennedy, P. C., and Palmer, N. (1985) *Pathology of Domestic Animals.* 3d ed. Academic Press (New York).

Kas, N. P., Van der Heul, R. O., and Misdorp, W. (1970) Metastatic Bone Neoplasms. *Zbl. Vet. Med.* A17, 909–919.

Keasbey, L. E. (1953) Juvenile Aponeurotic Fibroma (Calcifying Fibroma). A Distinctive Tumor Arising in the Palms and Soles of Young Children. *Cancer* 6, 338–346.

Lattes, R. (1982) Tumors of the Soft Tissues. In: *Atlas of Tumor Pathology.* 2d series, fascicle 1/revised. Armed Forces Institute of Pathology (Washington, D.C.).

LeCoteur, R. A., Nimmo, J. S., Price, S. M., and Pennock, P. W. (1978) A Case of Giant Cell Tumor of Bone (Osteoclastoma) in a Dog. *J. Amer. Anim. Hosp. Assoc.* 14, 356–362.

Lester, S. J., and Mesfin, G. M. (1980) A Solitary Plasmacytoma in a Dog with Progression to a Disseminated Myeloma. *Can. Vet. J.* 21, 284–286.

Levene, A., and Butt, K. (1969) Personal communication. In: Owen, L. N., *Bone Tumors in Man and Animals.* Butterworth & Co. (London).

Lichtenstein, L. (1972) *Bone Tumors.* 4th ed. The C.V. Mosby Co. (Saint Louis).

Lichtenstein, L., and Goldman, R. L. (1964) The Cartilage Analogue of Fibromatosis. A Reinterpretation of the Condition Called "Juvenile Aponeurotic Fibroma." *Cancer* 17, 810–816.

Lichtenstein, L., and Jaffe, H. L. (1943) Chondrosarcoma of Bone. *Amer. J. Path.* 19, 553–589.

Ling, G. V., Morgan, J. P., and Pool, R. R. (1974) Primary Bone Tumors in the Dog: A Combined Clinical, Radiographic, and Histologic Approach to Early Diagnosis. *J. Amer. Vet. Med. Assoc.* 165, 55–67.

Liu, S. K. (1981) Tumors of Bone and Cartilage. In: Bojrab, M. T., ed., *Pathophysiology in Small Animal Surgery.* Lea and Febiger (Philadelphia).

Liu, S. K., and Dorfman, H. D. (1974) The Cartilage Analogue of Fibromatosis (Juvenile Aponeurotic Fibroma) in Dogs. *Vet. Path.* 11, 60–67.

Liu, S. K., and Harvey, H. J. (1981) Metastatic Bone Neoplasms in the Dog. In: Bojrab, M. T., ed. *Pathophysiology in Small Animal Surgery.* Lea and Febiger (Philadelphia).

Liu, S. K., Dorfman, H. D., Hurvitz, A. L., and Patnaik, A. K. (1977) Primary and Secondary Bone Tumors in the Dog. *J. Small Anim. Pract.* 18, 313–326.

Liu S. K., Dorfman, H. D., and Patnaik, A. K. (1974) Primary and Secondary Bone Tumors in the Cat. *J. Small Anim. Pract.* 15, 144–156.

Livesey, M. A., Keane, D. P., and Sarmiento, J. (1984) Epistaxis in a Standardbred Weanling Caused by Fibrous Dysplasia. *Equine Vet J.* 16, 144–146.

Matsuno, T., Unni, K. K., McLeod, R. A., and Dahlin, D. C. (1976) Telangiectatic Osteogenic Sarcoma. *Cancer* 38, 2538–2547.

McClelland, R. B. (1941) A Giant-Cell Tumor in the Tibia in a Cat. *Cornell Vet.* 31, 86–87.

McGrath, J. T. (1960) *Neurologic Examination of the Dog.* 2d ed. Kimpton (London).

McGrath, P. J. (1972) Giant Cell Tumor of Bone. An Analysis of Fifty-Two Cases. *J. Bone Joint Surg.* 54, 216–229.

McLain, D. L., Hill, J. R., and Pulley, L. T. (1983) Multilobular Osteoma and Chondroma (Chondroma Rodens) with Pulmonary Metastasis in a Dog. *J. Amer. Anim. Hosp. Assoc.* 19, 359–362.

Misdorp, W., and Hart, A. A. M. (1979) Some Prognostic and Epidemiologic Factors in Canine Osteosarcoma. *J. Nat. Cancer Inst.* 62, 537–545.

Morgan, J. P. (1972) *Radiology of Veterinary Orthopedics.* Lea and Febiger (Philadelphia).

———. (1974) Systematic Radiographic Interpretation of Skeletal Diseases in Small Animals. *Vet. Clin. N. Amer.* 4, 611–625.

Morgan, J. P., Ackerman, N., Bailey, C. S., and Pool, R. R. (1980) Vertebral Tumors in the Dog: A Clinical, Radiologic, and Pathologic Study of 61 Primary and Secondary Lesions. *Vet. Radiol.* 21, 197–212.

Morgan, J. P., Carlson, W. D., and Adams, O. R. (1962) Hereditary Multiple Exostoses in the Horse. *J. Amer. Vet. Med. Assoc.* 140, 1320–1322.

Morton, D. (1985) Chondrosarcoma Arising in a Multilobular Chondroma in a Cat. *J. Amer. Vet. Med. Assoc.* 186, 804–806.

Mundy, G. R., Luben, R. A., Raisz, L. G., Oppenheim, J. J., and Buell, D. N. (1974) Bone-resorbing Activity in Supernatants from Lymphoid Cell Lines. *N. Engl. J. Med.* 290, 867–871.

Netherlands Committee on Bone Tumors. (1966) Radiological Atlas of Bone Tumors I. (The Hague and Paris).

Nieberle, K., and Cohrs, P. (1967) *Textbook of Special Pathological Anatomy of Domestic Animals.* Pergamon Press (Oxford).

Nielsen, S. W. (1964) Neoplastic Diseases. In: Catcott, E. J., ed., *Feline Medicine and Surgery.* American Veterinary Publications (Wheaton, Illinois, and Santa Barbara, California)

Nielsen, S. W., Schroder, J. D., and Smith, D. L. T. (1954) The Pathology of Osteogenic Sarcoma in Dogs. *J. Amer. Vet. Med. Assoc.* 124, 28–35.

Oduye, O. O., and Losos, G. J. (1972) Multiple Myeloma in a Dog. *J. Small Anim. Pract.* 22, 31–37.

Orr, C. M., Higginson, J., Baker, J. R., and Jones, D. R. E. (1981) Plasma Cell Myeloma with IgG Paraproteinaemia in a Bitch. *J. Small Anim. Pract.* 22, 31–37.

Osborne, C. A., Perman, V., and Sautter, J. H. (1968) Multiple Myeloma in the Dog. *J. Amer. Vet. Med. Assoc.* 153, 1300–1319.

Owen, L. N. (1962) The Differential Diagnosis of Bone Tumors in the Dog. *Vet. Rec.* 74, 439–446.

———. (1969) *Bone Tumors in Man and Animals.* Butterworth & Co. (London).

Owen, L. N., and Bostock, D. E. (1971) Multiple Cartilaginous Exostoses with Development of a Metastasizing Osteosarcoma in a Shetland Sheepdog. *J. Small Anim. Pract.* 12, 507–512.

Owen, L. N., and Stevenson, D. E. (1961) Observations on Canine Osteosarcoma. *Res. Vet. Sci.* 2, 117–129.

Pavey, J. J., and Riser, W. H. (1963) What's Your Diagnosis? *J. Amer. Vet. Med. Assoc.* 142, 51–52.

Pennock, P., Jonsson, L., and Olsson, S. E. (1966) Multiple Myeloma: Case Report. *J. Small Anim. Pract.* 7, 343–349.

Pool, R. R. (1978) Tumors of Bone and Cartilage. In: Moulton, J. E., ed., *Tumors of Domestic Animals.* 2d ed. University of California Press (Berkeley).

———. (1981) Osteochondromatosis. In: Bojrab, M. T., ed., *Pathophysiology in Small Animal Surgery.* Lea and Febiger (Philadelphia).

Pool, R. R., and Carrig, C. B. (1972) Multiple Cartilaginous Exostoses in a Cat. *Vet. Path.* 9, 350–359.

Pool, R. R., and Harris, J. M. (1975) Feline Osteochondromatosis. *Feline Pract.* 5, 24–30.

Pool, R. R., Bodle, J. F., Mantos, J. J., and Ticer, J. W. (1974) Primary Lung Carcinoma with Skeletal Metastases in the Cat. *Feline Pract.* 4, 36–41.

Pool, R. R., Morgan, J. P., Parks, N. J., Farnham, J. E., and Littman, M. S. (1983) Comparative Pathogenesis of Radium-induced Intracortical Bone Lesions in Humans and Beagles. *Health Physics* 44, Suppl. 1, 155–177.

Popp, J. A., and Simpson, C. F. (1976) Feline Malignant Giant Cell Tumor of Bone Associated with C Type Virus Particles. *Cornell Vet.* 66, 529–535.

Prata, R. G., Stoll, S. G., and Zaki, F. A. (1975) Spinal Cord Compression Caused by Osteocartilaginous Exostoses of the Spine in Two Dogs. *J. Amer. Vet. Med. Assoc.* 166, 371–375.

Price, C. H. G., and Summer-Smith, G. (1966) Malignant Bone Aneurysm in a Dog. An Unusual Example of Osteosarcoma. *Brit. Vet. J.* 122, 51–54.

Priester, W. A., and Mantel, N. (1971) Occurrence of Tumors in Domestic Animals: Data for 12 United States and Canadian Colleges of Veterinary Medicine. *J. Nat. Cancer Inst.* 47, 1333–1344.

Pritchard, D. J., Finkel, M. P., and Reilly, C. A. (1975) The Etiology of Osteosarcoma. *Clin. Orthop.* 111, 14–22.

Richardson, D. W., and Acland, H. M. (1983) Multilobular Osteoma (Chondroma Rodens) in a Horse. *J. Amer. Vet. Med. Assoc.* 182, 289–291.

Riddle, W. E., and Leighton, R. L. (1970) Osteochondromatosis in a Cat. *J. Amer. Vet. Med. Assoc.* 156, 1428–1430.

Rumbaugh, G. D., Pool, R. R., and Wheat, J. D. (1978) Atypical Osteoma of the Nasal Passage and Paranasal Sinus in a Bull. *Cornell Vet.* 68, 544–554.

Russell, R. G., and Walker, M. (1983) Metastatic and Invasive Tumors of Bone in Dogs and Cats. *Vet. Clin. N. Amer. Small Anim. Pract.* 13, 163–180.

Scaglietti, O., and Calandriello, B. (1962) Ossifying Parosteal Sarcoma. *J. Bone Joint Surg.* 44, 635–647.

Schajowicz, F. (1961) Giant-Cell Tumors of Bone (Osteoclastoma). *J. Bone Joint Surg.* 43, 1–29.

Schalm, O. W. (1974) Multiple Myeloma in a Dog. *Calif. Vet.* 28, 30–33.

Schneider, R. (1978) General Considerations. In: Moulton, J. E., ed., *Tumors in Domestic Animals.* 2d ed. University of California Press (Berkeley).

Shull, R. M., Osborne, C. A., and Barret, R. E. (1978) Serum Hyperviscosity Syndrome Associated with IgA Multiple Myeloma in Two Dogs. *J. Amer. Anim. Hosp. Assoc.* 14, 58–70.

Shupe, J. L., Olson, A. E., Sharma, R. R., and Van Kampen, K. R. (1970). Multiple Exostoses in Horses. *Mod. Vet. Pract.* 51, 34–36.

Smith, H. A., Jones, T. C., and Hunt, R. D. (1972) *Veterinary Pathology.* 4th ed. Lea and Febiger (Philadelphia).

Spjut, H. J., Dorfman, H. D., Fechner, R. E., and Ackerman, L. V. (1971) Tumors of Bone and Cartilage. In: *Atlas of Tumor Pathology.* 2d series, fascicle 5. Armed Forces Institute of Pathology (Washington, D.C.).

Spjut, H. J., Fechner, R. E., and Ackerman, L. V. (1981) Tumors of Bone and Cartilage. In: *Atlas of Tumor Pathology.* 2d series, fascicle 5/supplement. Armed Forces Institute of Pathology (Washington, D.C.)

Squire, R. A. (1969) Spontaneous Hemopoietic Tumors of Dogs. In: Lingeman, C. H., and Garner, F. M., eds., *Comparative Morphology of Hematopoietic Neoplasms.* National Cancer Institute Monograph 32, U.S. Government Printing Office (Washington, D.C.), 97–109.

Staub, O. C., Olander, H. F., and Theilen, G. H. (1960) A Case Report of Lymphosarcoma in a Cow. *Cornell Vet.* 50, 251–258.

Steiner, G. J., Ghosh, L., and Dorfman, H. D. (1972) Ultrastructure of Giant Tumors of Bone. *Human Path.* 3, 569–586.

Stevenson, S., Hohn, R. B., Pohler, O. E. M., Fetter, A. W., Olmstead, M. L., and Wind, A. P. (1982) Fracture-associated Sarcoma in the Dog. *J. Amer. Vet. Med. Assoc.* 180, 1189–1196.

Stout, A. P., and Lattes, R. (1967) Tumors of the Soft Tissues. In: *Atlas of Tumor Pathology.* 2d series, fascicle 1. Armed Forces Institute of Pathology (Washington, D.C.).

Sullivan, D. J. (1960) Cartilaginous Tumors (Chondroma and Chondrosarcoma) in Animals. *Amer. J. Vet. Res.* 21, 531–535.

Theilen, G. H., and Madewell, B. R. (1979) Tumors of the Skeleton. In: Theilen, G. H., and Madewell, B. R., eds., *Veterinary Cancer Medicine.* Lea and Febiger (Philadelphia)

Theilen, G. H., Leighton, R., Pool, R., and Park, R. D. (1977) Treatment of Canine Osteosarcoma for Limb Preservation Using Osteotomy, Adjuvant Radiotherapy, and Chemotherapy (A Case Report). *Vet. Med. Small Anim. Clin.* 72, 179–183.

Thornburg, L. P. (1979) Giant Cell Tumor of Bone in a Cat. *Vet. Path.* 16, 255–257.

Tjalma, R. A. (1966) Canine Bone Sarcoma: Estimation of Relative Risk as a Function of Body Size. *J. Nat. Cancer. Inst.* 36, 1137–1150.

Trigo, F. J., Leathers, C. W., and Brobst, D. F. (1983) A Comparison of Canine Giant Cell Tumor and Giant Cell Reparative Granuloma of Bone. *Vet. Path.* 20, 215–222.

Turrel, J. M., and Pool, R. R. (1982) Primary Bone Tumors in the Cat: A Retrospective Study of 15 Cats and a Literature Review. *Vet. Radiol.* 23, 152–166.

Van Bree, H., Pollet, L., Cousemont, W., Van Der Stock, J., and Mattheeuws, D. (1983) Cervical Cord Compression as a Neurologic Complication in an IgG Multiple Myeloma in a Dog. *J. Amer. Anim. Hosp. Assoc.* 19, 317–323.

Walker, M. A., Duncan, J. R., Shaw, J. W., and Chapman, W. W. (1975) Aneurysmal Bone Cyst in a Cat. *J. Amer. Vet. Med. Assoc.* 167, 933–934.

Walton, G. S., and Gopinath, C. (1972) Multiple Myeloma in a Dog with Some Unusual Features. *J. Small Anim. Pract.* 13, 703–708.

Whitehead, J. E. (1967) Neoplasia in the Cat. *Vet. Med. Small Anim. Clin.* 62, 357–358.

Wilson, J. W. (1973) Reticulum Cell Sarcoma of Long Bone Terminating as Respiratory Distress. *Vet. Med. Small Anim. Clin.* 68, 1398–1401.

Wolke, R. E., and Nielsen, S. W. (1966) Site Incidence of Canine Osteosarcoma. *J. Small Anim. Pract.* 7, 484–492.

Wykes, P. M., Withrow, S. J., Powers, B. E., and Park, R. D. (1985) Closed Biopsy for Diagnosis of Long Bone Tumors: Accuracy and Results. *J. Amer. Anim. Hosp. Assoc.* 21, 489–494.

# 6

*Jack E. Moulton and John W. Harvey*

# Tumors of the Lymphoid and Hematopoietic Tissues

## LYMPHOID TUMORS

Lymphoid tumors comprise one of the most common groups of tumors in domestic animals, and there is considerable confusion with regard to their nomenclature and classification. This arises not only because of the multiplicity of terms that have been applied to the various manifestations of lymphoid tumors but also because of inherent complexities in the biology of lymphoid cells that are only now being unraveled.

It is often useful to use terms from human medicine when classifying these tumors in animals because much is known about the tumors in humans that can be applied to animals. Furthermore, use of established terms highlights similarities and avoids the introduction of additional terms into the literature. Unfortunately, this practice can lead to confusion when conditions in humans and animals differ in some significant features or when it is not known for certain that the neoplasms in the two species are similar. It is also important to avoid using outdated or inappropriate terms from human medicine for animal tumors.

Human lymphomas were traditionally divided into four distinct types: lymphoma (lymphosarcoma), giant follicular lymphoma, reticulum cell sarcoma, and Hodgkin's disease. Extensive confusion developed from use of these four terms since it was impossible to classify the tumors that had varying degrees of differentiation or an admixture of lymphocytes or reticulum cells. Also, there was confusion about what constituted a reticulum cell type of lymphoma. Thus, it was necessary to develop a new classification based more on cytology, and the classification of Rappaport and Braylan (1975) for non-Hodgkin's lymphomas came into wide use. When this classification was used for humans, prognosis for the patient and the regimen of therapy could be determined.

The classification we have outlined for use in domestic animals (table 6.1) was adapted from the scheme of Rappaport and Braylan (1975) and is similar to the one proposed for animals by Jarrett and Mackey (1974). Our classification also includes division of the tumors into immunological types similar to the ones proposed by Lukes and Collins (1974) and Mann *et al.* (1979). Commonly used equivalents are placed in parentheses. It is important to note that the terms *lymphoma, malignant lymphoma,* and *lymphosarcoma* are used synonymously. The term *lymphosarcoma* is an old one and is not used much in human medicine. It has been used in the past to describe some well-differentiated and poorly differentiated diffuse lymphomas. It is not used to describe nodular lymphoma, histiocytic lymphoma, Burkitt's lymphoma, Hodgkin's disease, or mycosis fungoides.

An anatomical and age classification is also included since the anatomical location of the lymphoma and the age of the host clearly have a relationship with the growth characteristics of the neoplasm and its effect on the host. For example, in the bovine species, the lymphoma may be divided

**TABLE 6.1. Classification of Lymphoid Tumors in Domestic Animals**

Lymphoma (lymphosarcoma)
    Cytological classification
        Well-differentiated (lymphocytic)
        Intermediate differentiation (prolymphocytic)
        Poorly differentiated (lymphoblastic)
        Large cell or "histiocytic"
    Pattern classification
        Follicular (nodular)
        Diffuse
    Anatomical classification
        Multicentric
        Thymic
        Alimentary
        Cutaneous
        Solitary
    Immunomorphological classification
        B-cell type
        T-cell type
        Null-cell type

Mycosis fungoides

Lymphocytic leukemia, acute and chronic

Plasma cell tumors, multiple myeloma and extramedullary
    plasmacytoma

Thymoma, predominantly epithelial or lymphocytic

Hodgkin's-like disease

---

therapy. In domestic animals, however, this classification fails to point out significant clinical or therapeutic differences (Crow *et al.*, 1977; Madewell, 1975; Weller *et al.*, 1980).

Results in humans indicate that a classification that combines immunological and cytochemical markers with histology and cytology gives the best prediction of survival or response to therapy. Use of these identification techniques in domestic animals is just beginning, so the feasibility of this concept in veterinary medicine has not been thoroughly tested.

In the classification scheme used here, we avoid use of the antiquated term *reticulum cell sarcoma*. The term *reticulum cell* has been used to describe a variety of cell types, none of which are believed to be lymphocytes. In most instances, cells classified as reticulum cells have been either large mononuclear phagocytes (macrophages) or large, branched fibroblastic cells (reticular cells) that together with associated reticular fibers, make up the stromal meshwork of hematopoietic organs. Large reticulum cells were once considered to be hematopoietic stem cells. These stem cells are now recognized to be morphologically indistinguishable from small lymphocytes. The term *histiocytic lymphoma* is also a misnomer since lymphomas arise from the transformation of lymphocytes and not from histiocytes (macrophages of the mononuclear phagocyte system). The term is still widely used, but *large cell lymphoma* is preferred. In addition, there is a tendency now to substitute *follicular* for *nodular* lymphoma since it has been shown in humans and domestic animals that most of these tumors arise from the B-lymphocytes in the lymphocytic follicle.

Lymphoid tumors in humans and animals have also been divided on the basis of the tumor cells having nuclear cleavage. The cleaved cells are believed to have their origin in the germinal centers. Using this criterion, Valli *et al.* (1981) reported that cleaved cell lymphomas were rare in the dog but represented approximately one-fourth of the lymphomas in the cat and cow. Animals with cleaved neoplastic cells are usually older than those without cleaved cells. This is particularly true in the cow. This older age incidence may be related to lower malignancy and longer clinical course in the host with neoplasms arising from the lymphocytic follicles.

into calfhood, juvenile/thymic, enzootic/adult, and skin types, each of which has different epidemiological or biological consequences. The tumors in dogs are also divided into anatomic types, such as multicentric, alimentary, thymic, and skin types. Epidemiological differences are best established in the bovine. It should also be pointed out that the classification methods used here are largely independent of one another. As in all classifications, tumors will be found that fall in between the designated categories. The etiological implications of the various manifestations of lymphoid neoplasia have been well worked out in the feline and bovine species, but are largely unknown in the other domestic species.

The Rappaport classification is based on the architectural arrangement of the neoplastic cells and their cytological identification by light and/or electron microscopic methods. In humans this classification identifies tumor types that have a different clinical course in the host or respond differently to

Some claim that this neoplasm is more common in Scottish terriers than can be accounted for by the population proportion of this breed (Bloom and Meyer, 1945; Mulligan, 1949; White, 1946). This claim, however, was not confirmed in a large series of these tumors studied by Schneider at the University of California. Priester (1967) found the relative risk to be significantly higher for boxers than for any other purebred dog. The incidence is about the same in male dogs as in females.

**Clinical Characteristics.** Life expectancy in dogs with the multicentric form of lymphoma averages 10 weeks after diagnosis of the tumor, but many dogs die sooner. A few live 6 months to 1 year. The duration is shorter for the alimentary form than for the multicentric form, averaging 8 weeks; dogs seldom live more than 6 months from first recognition of the disease. This probably reflects the ease of diagnosis and extent of clinical complications more than differences in the time course of the two forms. Dogs with the longest life expectancy after diagnosis of lymphoma are often 12 years old or more. The estimated survival times average less than 6 months after disease onset in untreated middle-aged dogs and often less than 2 months in dogs younger than 2 years (Squire, 1969a).

The initial clinical signs of lymphoma are often vague and nonspecific. In the multicentric form the first sign is usually rapid enlargement of the lymph nodes. The superficial and visceral nodes are bilaterally and symmetrically enlarged (3 to 10 times), readily palpable, smooth, well defined, painless, rubbery, mobile, and rarely adherent to the skin or adjacent tissue. The neoplastic lymph nodes may display periodic reductions in size even without therapy, but growth recurs. The spleen is enlarged and palpable as a well-defined painless mass in half of the cases; the liver may be enlarged with the edges palpable behind the costal arch. Tonsils, when involved, are usually large, pale, nonulcerated, and they protrude from the crypts. Subcutaneous edema is highly characteristic in one or more sites such as the hindlimb, external genitalia, lower jaw, and ventral sternum. The mucous membranes are pale if anemia exists, and some dogs with severe liver involvement have icterus. Occasionally a thymic mass is palpable in the posterior cervical region.

In the alimentary form of lymphoma, signs are associated with alimentary obstruction. Diarrhea is found in about 80% of affected dogs, and some have blood in their feces. Thirst is related to the degree of diarrhea or vomiting.

Over 90% of dogs with lymphoma are either normal hematologically or have a modest leukocytosis resulting from an increase in circulating neutrophils. Lymphocytic leukemia without solid tumor growth occurs in less than 10% of dogs with lymphoma and is a separate disease (Hodgkins et al., 1980). Dogs may have impaired immunological response to heterologous antigens, but cell-mediated immunity is unaffected (Onions et al., 1978). Hypercalcemia is one of the more common paraneoplastic conditions associated with lymphoma, but the pathogenesis of this condition is not fully understood. Possible causes are a parathormonelike substance produced by the neoplastic cells, prostaglandin, an osteoclast-activating factor, or vitamin D-like steroid production. There is no evidence of primary parathyroid hyperplasia, hypervitaminosis D, or osseous breakdown from metastasis of the neoplasm to the skeletal system. Hypercalcemia in these dogs causes atony of cardiac and skeletal muscles, depression of the nervous system, and hypercalcemic nephropathy.

**Sites.** Two anatomical forms predominate: the multicentric and the alimentary (Jarrett et al., 1966; Weipers et al., 1964). The former is more common in our material. Thymic, skin, and leukemic forms are uncommon. In the multicentric type, there is bilateral involvement of almost every superficial lymph node and most deep lymph nodes and involvement of the liver and spleen. Other sites that may be affected are the alimentary tract, kidney, heart, tonsil, pancreas, and bone marrow. Occasionally involved are the eye, skin, and skeletal muscle and rarely the central nervous system. Paralysis is caused by metastasis to the spinal cord or epidural space.

The earliest neoplastic change in the multicentric form is reported to be the lymph nodes of the throat and the neck (Cotchin, 1954), but these locations might make them merely the first affected lymph nodes to be noticed. The lymph nodes that become neoplastic are, in descending order of frequency, the mandibular, cervical, precapsular, retropharyngeal, mediastinal, mesenteric, popliteal, sublumbar, tracheal, bronchial, peripenile, iliac, axillary, and inguinal. The largest visceral lymph

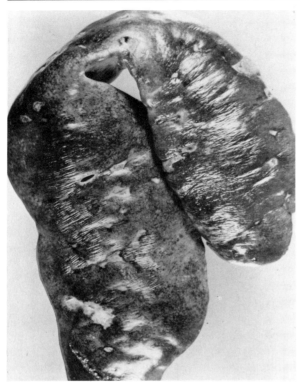

**FIGURE 6.2.** Lymphoma of the dog showing greatly enlarged spleen.

nodes with lymphoma are often the mesenteric and sublumbar. The thymus is affected less often.

In the alimentary form of the neoplasm the superficial lymph nodes and spleen are seldom neoplastic, whereas in the multicentric form these organs are almost always involved. Any part of the gastrointestinal tract or any of the mesenteric lymph nodes may be involved, and frequently both are affected. Less often affected are other abdominal and thoracic organs and other visceral lymph nodes, such as the anterior sternal nodes.

The thymic form of lymphoma occasionally occurs, and resembles the tumor in the cat. Skin involvement with single or multiple dermal plaques is sometimes the main presenting sign, and there is subsequent recognition of multicentric involvement.

**Gross Morphology.** The enlarged neoplastic lymph nodes vary in diameter from 1 to 9 cm. They are freely movable and nonadherent, although some, particularly the mesenteric nodes, are often fused. The nodes are moderately firm, although a few are centrally necrotic and soft or partly liquefied; the capsule of the node is tense. The demarcation between the cortex and medulla is usually lost, and the tissue is homogeneous, smooth, and glistening on cut surface. The color is pinkish gray, cream, or light tan.

The spleen has multiple small nodular masses resembling enlarged lymphocytic follicles or occasionally shows diffuse involvement with marked enlargement (fig. 6.2). The enlarged spleen is turgid and friable. Infarcts are occasionally observed.

The affected liver is uniformly enlarged and has disseminated small pale foci with accentuation of peripheral lobular pattern, or it may contain multiple large, pale, homogeneous tumor nodules.

When the neoplasm metastasizes to the bone, it replaces the marrow which appears homogeneous, soft, and whitish. The kidney usually exhibits multiple white to cream-colored nodules in the cortex, or it may be diffusely enlarged and pale.

Nodular and diffuse growths also appear in the gastrointestinal tract. In the stomach and intestine the neoplasm may diffusely invade throughout the wall. The intestinal solitary lymphocytic follicles are almost always enlarged.

**Histological Features.** Of the different cytological forms of lymphoma in the dog, the intermediate, poorly differentiated, and large cell (histiocytic) types are most common. The well-differentiated form of lymphoma is less often seen.

The architecture of the lymph node is usually completely effaced by neoplastic cells. Capsular and perinodal invasion are also common. With lesser involvement, early in the neoplastic process there can be invasion of the nodal cortex with the medulla unaffected. Nodular aggregations of tumor cells are often detected in the cortex (fig. 6.3A). Holmberg *et al.* (1976*a*) observed that nodular involvement was particularly associated with the alimentary form of lymphoma in the dog, although it is also seen in some of the multicentric forms of the tumor.

The tumor cells have somewhat characteristic morphology as seen by electron microscopy, with variations occurring dependent upon the degree of usually limited to the cortex, although in advanced cases they may coalesce and extend into the medulla. The kidney then becomes diffusely enlarged. The capsule may be thickly infiltrated with neoplastic tissue and strips with difficulty.

Splenic enlargement varies from slight to massive. There can be discretely enlarged lymphocytic follicles in less involved spleens and more homogeneous thickening in severely affected spleens.

The liver, like the spleen, is involved to varying degrees. It is sometimes considerably enlarged and has an accentuated lobular pattern caused by pale tumor infiltrates in the portal and periacinar regions. Reddish speckling of the surviving lobular parenchyma adds contrast to the pale neoplastic areas. Sometimes, as in the spleen, involvement of the liver is detected only microscopically. Other organs occasionally involved are the heart, nasal passages, larynx, skin, salivary glands, tongue, esophagus, uterus, brain, spinal cord, pancreas, adrenals, thyroid glands, and tonsils.

**Histological Features.** According to Mackey and Jarrett (1972), alimentary lymphomas in the cat are of any of the four major cytological types: stem cell, "histiocytic," lymphoblastic, or prolymphocytic. The lymphoblastic type predominated in their material. A similar pattern was obtained for the leukemic form. They found that multicentric lymphomas in the cat were prolymphocytic, histiocytic, or mixed lymphocytic–histiocytic. The thymic lymphomas were lymphoblastic or prolymphocytic. Mackey and Jarrett (1972) speculated on the pathogenesis of lymphoid neoplasia in the cat on the basis of anatomical type and histological pattern of involvement in affected lymphoid organs. They found experimentally induced (by FeLV) neoplasia to be particularly useful because earlier stages in tumor development were available for study. That is, the total obliteration of architectural landmarks commonly encountered in advanced spontaneous cases had not yet occurred. Their conclusions were as follows. Early intestinal lymphoid neoplasia in the alimentary form was detected in germinal centers of Peyer's patches. Lesions became confluent as they enlarged and more generalized infiltrations occurred (Fig. 6.4B). The early involvement in mesenteric and other lymph nodes was also within germinal centers. In the spleen, proliferation of neoplastic lymphoid cells began either in the germinal centers or at the margins of lymphocytic follicles. Neoplastic cells in the liver were usually limited to the portal and periacinar areas.

Mackey and Jarrett (1972) suggested that alimentary lymphomas are thymus independent and possibly marrow derived. As mentioned above, the histological pattern of development of the alimentary form of lymphoma in the cat conforms to the nodular (follicular) pattern in humans. By analogy, this would strengthen the likelihood that alimentary lymphoma is of B-lymphocyte origin. Mackey and Jarrett found that in contrast to the alimentary form of lymphoma, nodal involvement in the thymic and multicentric forms begins with infiltration and proliferation of neoplastic cells in paracortical zones of the lymph nodes. This was taken to indicate thymus dependence (i.e., T-cell neoplasia). Whether B-cell or T-cell histogenesis of alimentary and multicentric lymphomas exists in the cat remains to be determined.

The massive replacement of bone marrow by neoplastic cells in leukemia is characteristic and is accompanied by extramedullary dissemination of neoplastic cells along hematopoietic pathways. In contrast, the involvement of bone marrow in the various anatomical forms of lymphoma is inconstant and not extensive. It is not necessarily associated with the presence of neoplastic cells in the bloodstream.

Feline lymphoma is sometimes associated with membranous glomerulonephritis similar to that found in mice and humans with lymphoid malignancies (Anderson and Jarrett, 1971; Glick *et al.*, 1978). An immune complex origin for this change is likely.

**Hematology.** A leukemic blood picture is not characteristic of lymphoid neoplasia in the cat, only occurring in about 12% of cases, although careful examination reveals lymphoblasts or prolymphocytes in about 40% of cases (Schalm *et al.*, 1975). The probability of finding abnormalities of the blood increases with duration of the disease. An absolute lymphopenia occurs in as many as 50% of cases, and there is a neutrophilia in approximately 25% of them. Neutropenia may also occur. The most frequent hematological abnormality is a normocytic or macrocytic anemia that is found in about 50% of cases (Crighton, 1968; Meincke *et al.*, 1972; Nielsen, 1969). This is probably caused by one or more of the following factors: (1) action of FeLV on hematopoietic stem cells; (2) increased erythrophagocytosis in spleen and lymph nodes, possibly because of an altered immune response or concurrent hemobartonellosis; (3) anemia of chronic disease; and (4) invasion of bone marrow by neoplastic lymphoid cells.

**Etiology and Transmission.** The general epidemiology of FeLV was reviewed by Hardy (1981*a,b,c*) and Hardy *et al.* (1977). For years veterinarians had noticed a clustering in the occurrence of cases of feline lymphoma. In 1964 Jarrett *et al.* (1964*a,b*) discovered that the neoplasm was caused by a type C oncornavirus (henceforth referred to as retrovirus or reverse transcriptase-containing RNA virus) and that the virus was transmitted horizontally (nongenetically). The contagiousness of FeLV for cats was shown clearly by indirect fluorescent antibody testing of a large number of cats in household environments. After discovery of the contagious nature of the virus, a test and removal program was devised to prevent the spread of the disease in the pet cat population. There has never been any evidence that humans living with infected cats can become infected with the virus.

It is now known that FeLV also causes a number of nonneoplastic diseases such as anemia (which is often nonresponsive), leukopenia, and thymic atrophy. It is also believed to be the etiological agent for fetal abortions or resorptions in cats. Other diseases, such as feline infectious peritonitis and chronic infections of viral or bacterial origin, are more common in cats that carry FeLV, although the virus is not known to be the direct cause of these diseases. Most likely the related diseases occur because cats infected with FeLV are immunosuppressed and more susceptible to other disease agents (Bech-Nielsen *et al.*, 1981).

The pathogenesis of FeLV replication in the cat has been reviewed by Rojko and Olsen (1984). Following adsorption and penetration of cells, FeLV is uncoated and the RNA is copied into a single strand of complementary DNA using virion reverse transcriptase. This DNA serves as a template for the formation of the double-stranded DNA provirus that integrates to become part of the cat genome. The synthesis and integration of provirus can only occur in proliferating cells (cells that undergo DNA synthesis).

Viral RNA is transcribed from the integrated provirus by DNA-dependent RNA polymerases and translated on host ribosomes to generate precursor structural and envelope proteins and reverse transcriptase. Eventually, intact virus particles bud from the cell surface (fig. 6.4C). The occurrence of productive or partially productive FeLV infection of cells is correlated with the expression of envelope protein and core protein at the cell surface.

In addition to virus production, integrated DNA provirus can, at times, induce neoplastic transformation of infected cells. A common tumor-specific antigen called feline oncornavirus-associated cell membrane antigen (FOCMA) occurs on the surface of FeLV infected neoplastic lymphoid and myeloid cells. It now appears that FOCMA also appears on the surface of nonneoplastic cells infected with virus.

Seroepidemiological studies have shown that FeLV is contagious and transmitted from cat to cat in the natural environment. This horizontal transmission differs from the vertical type transmission found with some other oncornaviruses in which genetic information of the virus, incorporated into the host cell genome, is transmitted from parent to offspring via the gametes. The virus may be found in any of the tissues or secretions of infected cats. The usual means of transmission are by respiratory secretions, saliva, or urine, since cats lick or groom one another, sneeze on one another, and often use communal litter or feeding pans. The virus may also be transmitted to the fetus through the placenta or to the kitten in the mother's milk.

The presumed site of entry of the virus following contact in nature is the nasal cavity or oropharynx. Initial replication of the virus occurs in the tonsils or pharyngeal lymph nodes and is followed by amplification of viral multiplication in other lymph nodes in the region. Infected lymphocytes are carried by lymphatics or blood, and infected monocytes carried by blood are transported to secondary sites such as the bone marrow and lymph nodes throughout the body (especially the lymph nodes of the intestinal tract) where massive viral replication occurs. Following viral replication in lymphoid cells, viremia occurs and can be recognized in blood lymphocytes and monocytes by immunofluorescence. Concomitant infection also occurs in the glandular epithelial cells that line the crypts of the solitary lymphocytic follicles in the intestinal tract. Unless viral multiplication is halted at this time by the development of a specific antiviral immunological response, virus infection may extend to the mucosal and glandular epithelium throughout the body with resultant release of infectious virus into respiratory and salivary secretions and into the urine.

Most adult cats infected with FeLV under natural conditions are protected from the development of a persistent viremia by the production of virus-neutralizing antibodies and are protected from developing neoplastic cells by formation of complement-dependent antibody to FOCMA (cell membrane antigens). Once established, however, the viremia may persist for a long period of time, although some cats are capable of mounting sufficient immunological response to permanently eliminate the virus-infected cells from the bloodstream. Recent studies, however, indicate that cats with self-limiting infections have not eliminated all the cells with integrated provirus, but rather have a persistent nonproductive (latent) infection that may or may not be reactivated at a later date (Rojko *et al.*, 1982). This phenomenon probably accounts for lymphoma cases that are FeLV negative but FOCMA positive.

More cats with FeLV infection die as a result of nonneoplastic diseases (a variety of infections associated with immunosuppression, anemia, and leukopenia) than from lymphoma. Also, the relative risk for the development of a lymphoma or myeloproliferative disease is increased with the duration of the viremia.

A positive immunofluorescence test for viral antigen in the cytoplasm of circulating neutrophils and platelets is usually indicative of a viremia originating from bone marrow infection. A sensitive enzyme-linked immunosorbent assay (ELISA) has been developed that can measure viral antigen in the serum of cats. This test can detect viremia prior to significant virus replication in the bone marrow.

## Transmissible Feline Fibrosarcoma

In 1969 Snyder and Theilen described a fibrosarcoma in the skin of a cat that developed multicentrically and, after a period of growth, showed regression. Microscopically, the neoplasm appeared as sheets of fusiform cells arranged in whorled patterns. The cells had abundant cytoplasm and numerous mitotic figures, and lymphocytes were often present in neoplasms undergoing regression. Injection of cell-free extracts from this neoplasm into kittens and puppies resulted in similar tumors at the inoculation sites. By electron microscopy the cytoplasm of the tumor cells revealed virus particles that were morphologically indistinguishable from those in feline lymphoma or myeloproliferative disease. The latent period after injection of virus was shorter in kittens than in older cats, and the kittens developed larger neoplasms (Snyder and Dungworth, 1973). In cats and puppies regression of the neoplasm following a period of growth was associated with an increased level of antibody directed toward the virus-associated cell surface membrane (Essex and Snyder, 1973).

The feline fibrosarcoma virus is defective, and the virogene (provirus) may remain in the cell without producing infectious virus or without causing neoplastic transformation of the fibroblasts. The infective virus, however, can be "rescued" by coinfection with FeLV; the FeLV supplies the missing envelope protein for the sarcoma virus to multiply. Thus, transmissible fibrosarcoma can be seen in any cat with FeLV. There is also a relationship between the level of FOCMA in cats and their susceptibility to transmissible fibrosarcoma virus. For example, cats with high levels of FOCMA either never develop the sarcoma, or if the tumor is present, it undergoes regression.

In addition to producing sarcoma in cats, this virus can cause neoplastic transformation of cells *in vitro* from different species, including the dog, sheep, and subhuman primates (Sarma *et al.*, 1978). The virus in cell culture loses none of its infectiousness for the cat.

## Lymphoid Neoplasia of Cattle

**General Considerations.** Lymphoma (lymphosarcoma or leukosis) in cattle can occur in any of the cytological forms listed in table 6.1 and in any of the anatomical forms except for a clearly separable alimentary one. There are correlations between anatomical forms and epidemiological features of the disease that have not been found in other species. Calves up to about 6 months of age have a specific multicentric form of the disease. Young (adolescent) cattle between the approximate ages of 6 and 30 months predominantly have the thymic form. In both calves and adolescent cattle the skin form of lymphoma occurs in sporadic fashion, that is, as isolated random cases in herds of cattle. The multicentric form in adult cattle is often found to be enzootic, that is, as multiple cases within an individual herd.

**Incidence.** Lymphoma of cattle occurs worldwide but has a greater incidence in some countries. Statistics from the United States Federal Meat Inspection Service on the prevalence of the neoplasm in cattle show average annual rates of 18 per 100,000 cattle slaughtered, and of 2 per 100,000 calves slaughtered (Migaki, 1969). The disease may have typical enzootic occurrence in multiple case herds as in countries such as Germany, Denmark, Sweden, and the United States (Bendixen, 1957; Dobberstein and Paarmann, 1934; Lübke, 1944; Niepage, 1953; Theilen et al., 1964), or the condition may occur sporadically as in Great Britain and the Netherlands (Anderson and Jarrett, 1968; Anderson et al., 1969b; Misdorp and Dodd, 1968; Weipers et al., 1964).

In previous years the incidence of lymphoma showed increase in some countries. The neoplasm in cattle was originally reported as being more common in eastern than in western Germany (Fortner, 1944), but the incidence in western Germany doubled in a 10-year period, probably related to the movement of cattle from the east to the west. The incidence in Sweden changed in 5 years from 0.25% to 0.54%. Lymphoma in cattle was found to be more common in certain districts or even on some farms than in the general population (Bendixen, 1960). One farm in Germany had 12 cases in 70 cattle during one winter, and another had 9 cases in 60 cattle during a 5-month period (Schöttler and Schöttler, 1934).

**Age, Breed, and Sex.** The average age of cattle with lymphoma is 5 to 8 years, but all age groups are affected. It appears in animals more than 8 years of age and in calves 3 months old or less (Stasney and Feldman, 1938; Udall and Olafson, 1930). The tumor has also been found in fetuses (Bolle, 1950; Hatziolos, 1960; Katzke, 1935; Macklin and Miller, 1971; Misdorp, 1965). The incidence of tumors shows a consistent increase as age advances (Conner et al., 1966; Sorenson et al., 1964).

In Minnesota it was found that dairy cattle 6 to 7 years old are twice as likely to get the disease as dairy cattle 2 to 5 years old (Anderson et al., 1971). In Michigan the incidence for Holstein cattle is 32 per 100,000 animals that are 7 years and older, compared with 3 per 100,000 animals younger than 1 year of age (Conner et al., 1966). A sharp difference exists in Great Britain, where 35% of the cases are in cattle less than 2 years old and 61% in cattle less than 4 years old (Anderson and Jarrett, 1968).

There is no known breed of cattle that is genetically more or less susceptible to this neoplasm. It is accepted that the greater prevalence of the disease in dairy breeds compared with beef breeds is related to differing epidemiological factors and not to genetic susceptibility. It is seen more in female than in male cattle, probably because of the preponderance of females at risk.

**Clinical Characteristics.** In the multicentric form of lymphoma the main clinical feature is enlargement of the superficial lymph nodes. The most prominent lymph nodes are the prescapular, precrural, and supramammary, but nearly all nodes may be affected, although the extent to which individual nodes are involved may vary. Massive involvement of iliac lymph nodes can frequently be detected by rectal palpation. Cattle with lymphoma can exhibit posterior paralysis, which is usually caused by compression of the spinal cord from the tumor growing within the spinal epidural space. Orbital invasion by tumor cells or pressure from enlarged lymph nodes often causes protrusion of the eyeball or eversion of the conjunctiva. Abomasal thickening by tumor growth can result in pyloric stenosis and subsequent tympanism. Secondary ulceration of the abomasal mucosa causes hemorrhage. Cardiac involvement often results in a rapid irregular pulse and signs similar to those of traumatic pericarditis. Distension and pulsation of the jugular vein, chronic general passive hyperemia, and edema are common. Splenic engorgement by tumor cells is occasionally associated with splenic rupture and early death of the host. Pressure from enlarged lymph nodes may cause vulvar prolapse.

In the skin form, there is widespread nodularity

and often hair loss due to dermal infiltration of neoplastic cells.

The thymic form of lymphoma in young cattle was described by Dungworth *et al.* (1964). This form of the neoplasm results in a prominent swelling in the lower neck, just cranial to the thoracic inlet, and a large mass in the anterior mediastinum causing signs of respiratory difficulty. The thymic enlargement is often accompanied by subcutaneous edema and jugular distension. Enlargement of the thoracic part of the thymus presents a difficult diagnostic problem because signs are similar to those produced by other space-occupying lesions in the thoracic cavity including pleural or pericardial effusions and pneumonia. Enlargement of lymph nodes is not a significant feature of this lymphoma.

**Sites.** The distribution of lymphomas of different types generally varies with the age of the affected animal. In calves there is uniform neoplastic enlargement of all lymph nodes, extensive bone marrow infiltration with extension to the subperiosteum, and major involvement of the liver and spleen (Hugoson, 1967; Theilen and Dungworth, 1965). The thymus, heart, kidneys, and uterus are also affected in more than 50% of affected calves. This is a multicentric anatomical form, but it is a special one by virtue of the predominant involvement of hematopoietic tissues. In its distribution pattern in bone marrow, spleen, liver, and lymph nodes, it closely resembles the leukemic form of lymphoid neoplasia.

In adolescent cattle approximately 6 to 30 months of age, the thymic form is the usual one encountered. There is massive enlargement of the cervical or thoracic parts of the thymus and frequent involvement of the bone marrow in the younger animals. Lymph nodes adjacent to the thymus are commonly affected but to a minor degree. Involvement of distant nodes and other organs can be found but is not a significant gross feature.

Adult cattle have a multicentric form of the disease. Statistical compilations indicate that the lymph nodes, heart, abomasum, kidneys and ureters, uterus, spinal epidural fat, and intestine are (in decreasing order) the sites most often affected (Dungworth *et al.*, 1968; Lübke, 1944; Marshak *et al.*, 1962), but there is considerable variation in specific organ involvement from one animal to another. The liver and spleen are affected in about one-third of the cases. Other organs and tissues are involved less often. The iliac, supramammary, and mesenteric lymph nodes are more consistently affected than other nodes.

There is an alimentary form of lymphoma in the bovine, but it is less common than in the dog and cat.

The skin form of lymphoma as described by Bendixen and Friis (1965) affects mostly young adult cattle on a sporadic basis. The characteristic lesions are multiple nodular swellings in the dermis, particularly on the dorsal and lateral surfaces of the head, neck, body, and perineal region. Frequently there may be one or more periods of regression and recurrence of dermal nodules, eventually with accompanying distribution of lesions as in the multicentric form. As with other forms, the distinction between the multicentric and skin forms is not always clear (Marshak *et al.*, 1966).

The leukemic form of lymphoid neoplasia as specifically defined in the classification is rare in cattle. The resemblance of leukemia to the calfhood pattern of lymphoma is discussed above.

**Gross Morphology.** Involved lymph nodes are increased in size many times and sometimes fused (figs. 6.5A–C). The consistency of the affected node is firm, fleshy, or friable; the color is grayish white, pale yellow, or pale pink. Of importance in gross identification of a neoplastic node is the homogeneous amorphous appearance on cut section, with lack of distinction between cortex and medulla. The lymph nodes in early cases can be mistaken for hyperplasia or lymphadenitis, which also cause an increase in size, but (with few exceptions) a distinction can be made between the cortex and medulla in these nodes. Lymph nodes with lymphoma often have areas of hyperemia or hemorrhage, and sometimes necrosis and softening. At other times in rapidly enlarging nodes there are discrete, yellow necrotic foci. Hemolymph node involvement is inconsistent, but may be severe when the disease is widespread. Hemolymph nodes may become neoplastic when the neighboring lymph nodes are normal; the reverse situation is also encountered.

In the adult multicentric form of lymphoma, cardiac lesions are usually found in the right atrium. They also occur in other chambers of the heart. They appear as nodular or diffuse, pale, fleshy

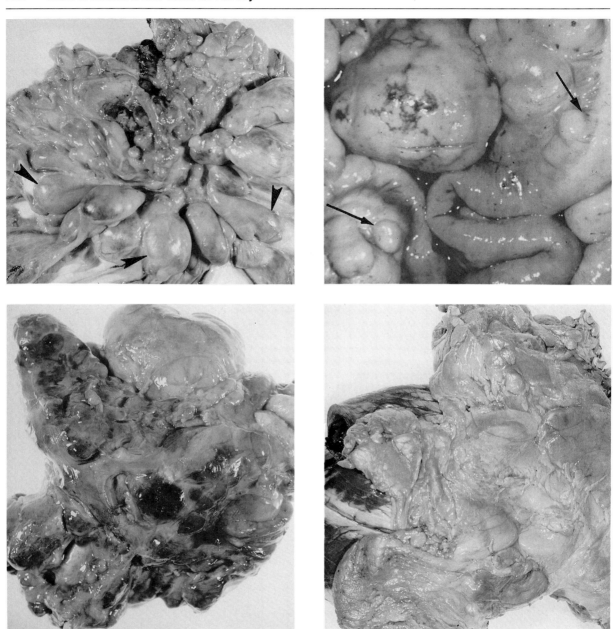

A|B  **FIGURE 6.5.** Lymphoma in the cow. A. Massive lymph
C|D  node enlargements (**arrowheads**) in the mesentery.
B. Enlarged mesenteric lymph nodes (**arrows**). C. Fusion of
ileocecal lymph nodes. D. Involvement of myocardium.

masses (Järplid, 1964) (fig. 6.5D). In the calfhood and adolescent forms of lymphoma, cardiac lesions are more randomly distributed than in the adult form of lymphoma.

In the adult multicentric form of lymphoma in the bovine, the walls of the abomasum and, to a lesser extent, the first part of the duodenum are greatly thickened by tumor growth and sometimes as thick as 5 cm (fig. 6.6A). The infiltrations of neoplastic lymphocytes are usually diffuse. Usually the submucosa is involved most severely. In cut section the wall of the abomasum is white or pale cream in color and resembles a thick, homogeneous mass of fat. Some lymphomas extend into the adjacent omasum or reticulum. The surface of the abomasal mucosa is usually atrophied and often ulcerated because of ischemia resulting from displacement of submucosal blood vessels by infiltrating tumor cells. When only minor abomasal involvement is present, there may be only one or several small areas of fleshy thickening in the submucosa. When large masses are present, however, they may extend around the entire circumference of the abomasum and encroach on the intestinal lumen.

Other organs such as the kidneys, uterus, liver, and spleen have discrete pale neoplastic nodules or more diffuse infiltrations. Spinal involvement usually consists of discrete or fused, pale neoplastic nodules lying in the epidural space. They are most often found in the lumbar region adjacent to intervertebral foramens. They can easily be missed if epidural fat is plentiful.

With thymic involvement either the cervical or thoracic parts of the thymus are affected. Typically the cervical mass is shaped like a truncated cone with the base at the thoracic inlet and the apex extending a variable distance up the neck toward the thyroid isthmus. The dorsal surfaces of large tumors are grooved for the passage of the trachea and esophagus. These structures may be compressed. The carotid arteries and jugular veins are embedded in the dorsal parts of large neoplasms. Some masses are encapsulated, whereas others show peripheral invasion into neighboring structures. Thymic structure can be recognized only in the smallest tumors. On cut surface, the tumors often have lobules of various sizes separated by fibrous septa. The neoplastic tissue is homogeneous, firm, and white or

pale grayish yellow. Hemorrhages and necrotic foci may be seen.

The massive infiltration of bone marrow by lymphoma cells characteristically observed in calves often results in necrosis and infarction of marrow in the shafts of long bones and, to a lesser extent, in the cancellous bone of vertebral bodies and epiphyses of long bones. Necrotic marrow is mottled gray to yellowish green and is caseous or friable. There is rarefaction of cancellous bone and thinning of cortices of ribs, sternum, pelvis, and bones of the axial skeleton. Subperiosteal neoplastic accumulations are usually present in the ribs and vertebral bodies. The sternum, pelvis, and cranial bones are affected less often.

**Histological Features.** All cytological types of lymphoma appear in cattle: well-differentiated to poorly differentiated types. Depending on cell type, small cell lymphocytic, prolymphocytic, lymphoblastic, and large cell tumors occur (in order of decreasing frequency). Tumors with intermixed cell types are fairly common, however, and even where bulky lesions of uniform cell type appear, there can be foci of early involvement where a more varied and less differentiated population of cells can be seen.

General hallmarks of lymphoid neoplasia in cattle such as partial or complete obliteration of lymph node architecture and invasive destruction of other tissues and organs are the same as in lymphomas of other species. The detection of early lesions in adult cattle requires a detailed gross and microscopic examination of the heart, abomasum, and uterus and of the iliac, supramammary, mesenteric, prescapular, precrural, popliteal, and thoracic lymph nodes. Histologically, neoplastic cells in lymph nodes are often found initially in medullary sinuses. The other two organs of major importance in the adult multicentric form are the heart (fig. 6.6B) and abomasum; the initial site in the heart is often the subepicardial tissue of the right atrium and the initial site in the abomasum is within the submucosal layer.

In the thymic lesion large tumor nodules may be found. These are separated completely or partially by fibrous tissue septa of variable thickness. Within each lobule there is further subdivision by slender vascular connective tissue trabeculae. Diffuse masses of neoplastic cells appear in various degrees of com-

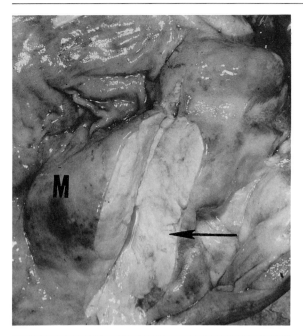

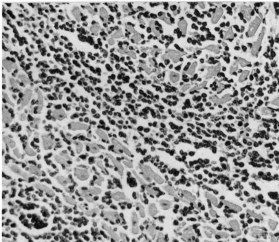

A    **FIGURE 6.6.** Lymphoma of the cow. A. Thickening
B    of wall of abomasum from tumor cell invasion. The
mucosa (M) has been incised (**arrow**). B. Diffuse infiltration
of tumor cells in the myocardium.

pactness, and the cells tend to form in groups or strands, separated by a delicate network of fibrovascular stroma. The firmness of the tumor is related to the density of the fibrous tissue. A widespread distribution of reticulum fibers is a prominent feature of this lymphoma.

The ultrastructure of neoplastic cells in bovine lymphoma has been described in a number of reports (Fujimoto *et al.*, 1969; Knocke, 1964; Ueberschär, 1968; Weber *et al.*, 1969). A notable ultrastructural feature in the neoplastic lymphoid cells is the presence of fingerlike projections or loops of nuclear membrane (Olson *et al.*, 1970, 1973). This may occur in lymphocytes in solid tissue or blood. The frequency of this change is 2 to 5% of tumor cells. There is good correlation between this nuclear abnormality and the presence of C type retrovirus in lymphocytes.

Chromosomal studies of neoplastic lymphocytes have not revealed any abnormalities. The modal chromosome number is either diploid ($2n = 60$) or hyperdiploid (Hare *et al.*, 1964; Weinhold and Müller, 1971; Weipers *et al.*, 1964).

**Hematology.** A significant number of clinically normal adult cattle from herds with multiple case incidence of lymphoma have a persistent elevation of lymphocytes in their blood, with or without the presence of atypical cells. Recognition of this persistent lymphocytosis in association with what is referred to in the European literature as enzootic leukosis led to the development of "keys" (Götze *et al.*, 1953) for early diagnosis of lymphoma. According to the degree of elevation of the blood lymphocyte count, an animal is considered to be suspect or positive for the pretumorous phase of lymphoma. The presence of immature or atypical lymphocytes in the bloodstream places the cow in the suspicious or positive category. A similar key was developed by Theilen *et al.* (1964). They defined lymphocytosis as being when the lymphocyte number was greater than the mean number of lymphocytes plus three standard deviations for the appropriate age group. Although there generally is a good correlation between the occurrence of multiple cases of lymphoma in a herd and a well-defined pattern of persistent lymphocytosis in adult animals within the herd, the association is not invariable (Marshak *et al.*, 1963; Olson and Simon, 1967). On an indi-

mans, but most patients eventually develop extra-cutaneous lesions in various organs.

Histological lesions are characterized by epidermal infiltrates of atypical lymphocytes, either singly or in clusters, called Pautrier's microabscesses. Lymphocytes vary in size and generally have hyper-convoluted vesicular to hyperchromatic nuclei. In advanced stages lymphoid cells may appear blastic with large vesicular rounded nuclei and prominent nucleoli (Bunn and Poiesz, 1983).

The epidermotropism of the cells helps to differentiate this neoplasm from a lymphoma arising in a lymphoid organ with metastasis to the skin. The epidermis over the neoplasm is flattened, lacking in rete pegs, and shows slight hyperkeratosis. Sheets of epidermis may be detached.

In early stages the upper dermis contains a polymorphic infiltrate of atypical lymphocytes, neutrophils, eosinophils, plasma cells, and mast cells. In more advanced stages, the infiltrate becomes more monomorphous and extends deeper into the dermis and around hair follicles.

Lymphoproliferative diseases resembling mycosis fungoides (cutaneous T-cell lymphomas) in humans are uncommon in dogs (Brown *et al.*, 1980; Kelly *et al.*, 1972; McKeever *et al.*, 1982; Shadduck *et al.*, 1978), and only one case has been described in a cat (Caciolo *et al.*, 1983). Alopecia, pruritis, erythema, and scaling of skin are common. Progression of disease from epidermal infiltrates to tumor stages and metastasis to internal organs appears to occur more rapidly in animals than in humans. A case of thymoma in a dog had metastasis to the paracortical (T-cell) zone of the regional lymph nodes, but absence of metastasis in other sites.

Cases in dogs may not be adequately evaluated until late in the disease because they are frequently misdiagnosed as atopic dermatitis, seborrhea, pyoderma, hypothyroidism, etc. Multiple biopsies are often required to demonstrate the epidermotrophic nature of the disease in cases with extensive tumor development, secondary inflammation, or ulcerations.

Nuclear indention or lobulation is generally less dramatic than in humans and is not usually appreciated by light microscopy. Cerebriform nuclei were demonstrated by electron microscopy in a dog that had a leukemic form of cutaneous lymphoma resembling Sezary syndrome (Thrall *et al.*, 1984).

Lymphoid cells in the single feline case of mycosis fungoides (Caciolo *et al.*, 1983) had round nuclei.

At this writing the T-lymphocyte origin of this disorder has not been documented in dogs. The feline case of mycosis fungoides was shown to involve T-lymphocytes.

## Lymphocytic Leukemia

The tendency for a lymphoid neoplasm to manifest leukemia is dependent on the site of origin and type and stage of development of the neoplastic cells. Neoplastic cells often retain the migratory patterns of their normal counterparts (Berard *et al.*, 1981). As a result, neoplasms arising from bone marrow lymphoid cells (lymphoid stem cells, pre-B-cells, B-cells, and pre-T-cells) generally have a leukemic manifestation. Thymic lymphomas may, at times, have an associated leukemic manifestation because thymocytes normally enter the blood en route to peripheral tissues. In contrast, plasma cell neoplasms rarely become leukemic because plasma cells do not normally circulate. Similarly, tumors involving germinal center cells generally do not manifest leukemia until late in the disease.

In human medicine, the term *lymphocytic leukemia* is used to describe lymphoproliferative disorders that appear to originate in bone marrow and are generally apparent in the circulation. Lymphoid leukemias in humans are classified into well-differentiated and poorly differentiated types. The well-differentiated type, called chronic lymphocytic leukemia, is characterized by mature lymphocytes that predominate in blood and bone marrow (Sweet *et al.*, 1977). The poorly differentiated type, called acute lymphocytic or lymphoblastic leukemia, is characterized by a large number of prolymphocytes and/or lymphoblasts in bone marrow. Immature lymphoid cells are usually, but not invariably, observed in blood. Terms such as *malignant lymphoma* or *lymphosarcoma* are used for lymphoid neoplasms originating in lymphoid tissues other than bone marrow (Necheles, 1979). When patients with lymphoma develop a leukemic blood picture, the terms *leukemic lymphoma* or *lymphoma with leukemia* may be applied.

Unfortunately the terminology used for lymphoid neoplasia in domestic animals has not been consistent. Terms such as leukemia, leukosis, lymphoma, and lymphosarcoma have been employed without regard to the nature of the neoplasm. Animals with solid lymphoid tumors have been classified as having leukemia, even in the absence of recognizable neoplastic cells in the circulation or bone marrow. In other cases, animals with bone marrow and blood involvement (without tumor formation) have been classified as having multicentric (Hardy, 1981*b*) or unclassified lymphoma (Meincke *et al.*, 1972).

Although it is clear that "true" lymphoid leukemia is much less common than lymphoma in domestic animals (Anderson *et al.*, 1969*a;* Jarrett *et al.*, 1966), accurate determination of its frequency is not available because examinations of blood and bone marrow are not always done and because specific efforts have usually not been made to differentiate leukemia from lymphoma.

Animals with lymphoid leukemia have pronounced bone marrow involvement and usually blood involvement, with variable organ infiltrates similar to those in myeloproliferative disorders. Secondary neoplastic infiltrates are most commonly observed in spleen, liver, and lymph nodes.

## Acute Lymphocytic Leukemia

**Humans.** Acute lymphocytic leukemia (ALL) is characterized by an increase in immature lymphoctyes (lymphoblasts and prolymphocytes) in bone marrow and usually in blood. Although ALL occurs in humans of any age, it is predominantly a disease of children. Through use of cytochemistry and immunological and biochemical surface markers, it is becoming increasingly apparent that ALL in humans is a mixed group of disorders. Approximately 70 to 80% of cases in humans lack conventional surface markers for either B- or T-lymphocytes (Chessells, 1982; Thiel *et al.*, 1980).

Non-T- and non-B-cell ALL appear to originate in bone marrow and have been referred to as null-cell ALL. Many of these cases have a glycoprotein surface antigen referred to as the common-ALL antigen (Chessells, 1982). The common-ALL antigen is not leukemia specific; it is also present on normal lymphopoietic blast cells (Bernard *et al.*, 1981). The null-cell classification is determined primarily by exclusion. The percentages of cases classified as null-cell type by conventional means (e.g., E rosettes, heteroantisera, complement, $F_c$ receptors, and surface immunoglobulin) have decreased. They will decrease further as cells are classified as T- and B-cell progenitors with the aid of new enzyme markers and monoclonal antibodies to various surface antigens (Gaedicke and Drexler, 1982; Nadler *et al.*, 1981; Thiel *et al.*, 1980).

Approximately 20% of cases of ALL in humans are recognized to have T-cell markers (Chessells, 1982; Gaedicke and Drexler, 1982). Because T-cell ALL in children is frequently associated with a mediastinal mass, it has been suggested that it might develop rapidly following the dissemination of neoplastic cells originating in the thymus or lymph nodes and that it might therefore be considered a leukemic stage of a T-cell lymphoblastic lymphoma (Chessells, 1982). Marked phenotypic differences were found, however, when T-cell lymphoblastic lymphoma, without blood or marrow involvement, was compared to T-cell ALL (Bernard *et al.*, 1981). Therefore, it seems unlikely that these two conditions represent different clinical stages of a single neoplastic process (Nadler *et al.*, 1981). In humans, the earliest lymphoid precursors in the thymus bear antigens shared by a fraction of bone marrow lymphocytes, but they lack antigens expressed on mature T-cells. It appears likely that many cases of T-cell ALL result from a proliferation of prothymocytes in the bone marrow (Bernard *et al.*, 1981; Nadler *et al.*, 1981).

Very few cases of ALL in humans have B-lymphocyte markers. Cases in children have most often been seen in association with diffuse intraabdominal lymphoma and probably represent a disseminated lymphoma rather than a true leukemia.

Most disseminated lymphomas in adult humans are of the B-lymphocyte type. Consequently, the application of "surface marker" analysis has facilitated the differentiation of ALL and leukemic lymphoma in adults (Aisenberg and Wilkes, 1976).

The total leukocyte count in ALL in humans is higher than normal in slightly more than one-half of the cases. When the total count is normal or low, however, blasts can usually be demonstrated in blood and can always be demonstrated in bone marrow. Most cases have nonregenerative anemia, thrombocytopenia, and neutropenia at the time the disease is recognized. Common symptoms such as fatigue, purpura, and infections are attributable to these cytopenias. Common physical findings, including splenomegaly, hepatomegaly, and lymphadenopathy, are attributable to leukemic infiltrates (Necheles, 1979).

**Cats.** Acute lymphocytic leukemia has been recognized in animals, but in general has not been well characterized. Lymphocytic leukemia without solid tumor formation accounts for 7 to 46% of cats with lymphoid neoplasia, depending on geographic location (Cotter and Essex, 1977; Theilen and Madewell, 1979). Most lymphoid leukemias in cats appear to be of the acute lymphocytic type (Mackey and Jarrett, 1972). Although lymphocyte maturation in the circulation may vary from relatively mature-appearing lymphocytes to lymphoblasts, prolymphocytes and lymphoblasts dominate the bone marrow (figs. 6.8A and B). Cotter and Essex (1977) reported similarities in clinical signs and laboratory findings between acute lymphocytic leukemia in cats and humans. In cats the history and clinical signs are usually vague and limited to pallor, lethargy, weakness, anorexia, and weight loss. Often there is a history of fever and prior antibiotic therapy for bacterial infection. A moderate to marked anemia is consistently present. Total leukocyte counts are most often normal or low, but markedly high counts may occasionally occur. Immature lymphoid cells can generally be recognized in blood, but a bone marrow examination is required to reach a diagnosis in some cases. Severe thrombocytopenia and associated bleeding tendencies occur in cats, but less frequently than recognized in humans (Cotter and Essex, 1977). Splenomegaly, hepatomegaly, and variable lymphadenopathy may be present in association with diffuse organ infiltrates.

Approximately two-thirds of all cases of feline ALL are FeLV positive. Detailed studies of lymphocyte types present in feline ALL have not been reported, but Essex (1982) has stated that most are of the T-lymphocyte type.

**Dogs.** It has been estimated that ALL may account for 5 to 10% of lymphoid neoplasms in the dog (MacEwen *et al.*, 1977*b*). It is usually seen as a rapidly developing disorder of dogs, with a median age of 5.5 years reported by Matus *et al.* (1983). Hematological studies generally reveal anemia with many lymphoblasts and/or prolymphocytes in the

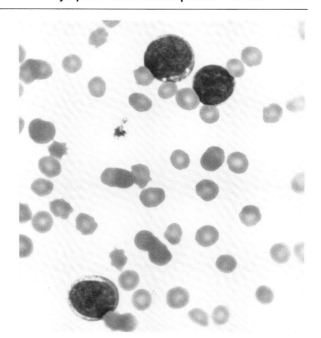

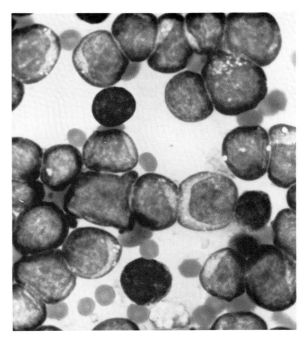

A
B
**FIGURE 6.8.** Acute lymphocytic leukemia of the cat. Blood (A) and bone marrow (B) aspirate. Observe that lymphoid cells in bone marrow are large with fine chromatin and obvious nucleoli. Giemsa stain.

circulation (De Schepper *et al.*, 1974; MacEwen *et al.*, 1977*b*), although occasional cases may have hypercellular bone marrow dominated by lymphoid cells, including lymphoblasts, with few abnormal cells in the circulation (MacEwen *et al.*, 1981; Schalm, 1980). Dogs with ALL are often neutropenic, but neutrophilia may also occur (Matus *et al.*, 1983). Mild to moderate thrombocytopenia is common, but hemorrhage is seldom a problem. Hepatosplenomegaly, with or without peripheral lymphadenopathy, is often observed. Two cases of ALL have been examined using conventional surface markers (Onions, 1977). One was associated with a thymic mass, but the second did not have an associated thymic enlargement. Both leukemias were devoid of conventional surface markers. Other investigators have compared ultrastructural characteristics of lymphoid cells from dogs with lymphoma to dogs with lymphoid leukemia (Chapman *et al.*, 1981). Insufficient information was given to determine whether the leukemic cases represented true ALL or leukemic lymphoma. Lymphoblasts from cases with leukemia were smaller than those with lymphoma without leukemia. Minor differences in ultrastructural morphology were also reported.

**Cattle.** Sporadic cases of lymphoid neoplasia that do not appear to be caused by BLV occur in young cattle. A calf form occurring primarily in dairy calves less than 6 months of age is characterized by generalized lymphoblastic infiltrates in various tissues, with the most dramatic involvements in bone marrow, lymph nodes, liver, and spleen (Hugoson, 1967; Theilen and Dungworth, 1965). This lymphoid malignancy has been classified as a multicentric lymphoma, but should perhaps be considered as an ALL (Muscoplat *et al.*, 1974). In addition to massive bone marrow involvement, one-half of the cases reported had overt leukemia. Not surprisingly, thrombocytopenia and severe anemia are often present. Common clinical findings include a sudden weight loss, weakness, and generalized lymphadenopathy, followed by a short clinical course and death. Lymphocytes from a limited number of calves with ALL have been devoid of conventional surface markers (Raich *et al.*, 1983; Takashima *et al.*, 1977).

**Horses.** Lymphoid neoplasia is much less common in the horse than in cats, dogs, or cattle (Neu-

feld, 1973*a,b*; Schalm and Carlson, 1982; Theilen and Fowler, 1962). Most cases occur as lymphoma without leukemia, but cases of leukemic lymphoma have been reported (Madewell *et al.*, 1982; Neufeld, 1973*b*). One clearly described case of ALL has been reported in a 7-year-old thoroughbred horse (Roberts, 1977). A second probable case was classified as a lymphoma (Green and Donovan, 1977). The horse described by Roberts (1977) had severe anemia, neutropenia, and thrombocytopenia as a result of almost complete replacement of normal bone marrow elements by immature lymphoid cells. Extensive neoplastic infiltrates were seen in other hematopoietic organs, but no solid tumors were present.

### Chronic Lymphocytic Leukemia

Chronic lymphocytic leukemia (CLL) or well-differentiated lymphocytic leukemia is characterized by an increased number of mature lymphocytes in both blood and bone marrow. This form of leukemia in humans is reported almost exclusively in people over 50 years of age. In addition to blood and bone marrow involvement, common clinical and laboratory findings include peripheral lymphadenopathy, hepatosplenomegaly, anemia, and thrombocytopenia (Sweet *et al.*, 1977).

In domestic animals, well-differentiated lymphocytic leukemia similar to CLL in humans has been reported primarily in dogs (Braund *et al.*, 1978; Harvey *et al.*, 1981; Hodgkins *et al.*, 1980; MacEwen *et al.*, 1977*a*; Pfeiffer *et al.*, 1976; Thrall, 1981). Chronic lymphocytic leukemia in dogs is primarily a disease of middle to old age. A lymphocytosis has always been recognized, with cell counts generally in excess of 20,000/$\mu$l. The highest total lymphocyte count reported was nearly 500,000/$\mu$l (Thrall, 1981). Most involved lymphocytes appear small and mature (figs. 6.9A–D), but low percentages of immature lymphocytes may also be seen. Absolute neutrophil counts are normal or increased. Platelet counts are normal to slightly decreased and most cases have slight to moderate anemia. Severe neutropenia, thrombocytopenia, and anemia were recognized in one case with marked organ infiltration (Pfeiffer *et al.*, 1976). Concomitant hyperglobulinemia appears to occur with greater frequency in dogs than in humans. Four cases have

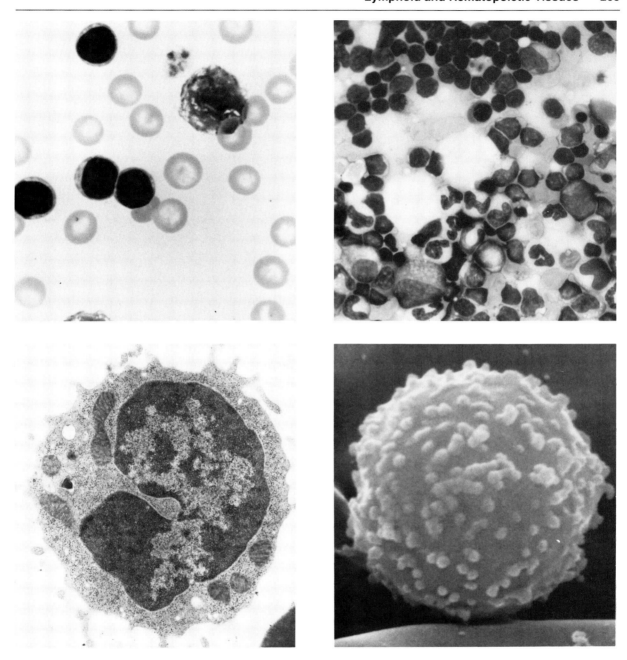

A|B
C|D    **FIGURE 6.9.** Chronic lymphocytic leukemia of the dog. A. Blood film with small mature lymphocytes and a leukocyte that is broken apart (basket cell). B. Bone marrow touch impression with more than 50% small lymphocytes present. C. Transmission electron micrograph with typical blood lymphocyte. The nucleus has abundant heterochromatin. D. Scanning electron micrograph of typical peripheral blood lymphocyte with short surface microvilli.

been described with monoclonal hyperglobulinemia (three with IgM and one with IgA) and associated hyperviscosity syndromes (Braund *et al.*, 1978; MacEwen *et al.*, 1977*a*). The number of lymphocytes in bone marrow varies from 25 to nearly 100% of the total nucleated cells present. Most lymphocytes in bone marrow aspirates are mature (fig. 6.9B), but small percentages of immature lymphoid cells have also been recognized.

Common clinical findings include lethargy, anorexia, and splenomegaly or hepatosplenomegaly. Peripheral lymphadenopathy is generally not seen. Diffuse infiltrates of predominant small lymphocytes have been observed in various organs, but solid lymphoid tumors have not been described. Although rapid death may occur in severely affected animals, others may survive several years, even without specific therapy (Harvey *et al.*, 1981). Attempts to evaluate cell surface markers have been made in two animals. In one case, the lymphocytes were shown to be of the B-cell type (Harvey *et al.*, 1981); in the other, the percentages of B- and T-lymphocytes were considered to be normal (Hodgkins *et al.*, 1980). It is assumed that the four cases reported with monoclonal hyperglobulinemia were also of the B-lymphocyte type.

Chronic lymphocytic leukemia occurs in cats (Holzworth, 1963; Thrall, 1981), but it appears to be a rare disorder that has not been well defined. One must differentiate lymphocytic leukemia from other causes of lymphocytosis besides leukemic lymphoma. Physiologic lymphocytosis commonly occurs in fearful, excited kittens as a result of epinephrine release. Lymphocytosis may also be observed in patients with adrenal insufficiency or illness characterized by prolonged antigenic stimulation. Lymphocytosis with atypical lymphocytes may be seen after vaccination.

## Leukemic Lymphoma

Animals with lymphomas may develop a terminal leukemic phase as a result of metastasis of neoplastic cells to blood and bone marrow. Cells may be numerous enough in blood to cause increased total lymphocyte counts. It is proposed that this condition be referred to as "leukemic lymphoma" or "lymphoma with leukemia" to distinguish it from true lymphocytic leukemia. The frequency of

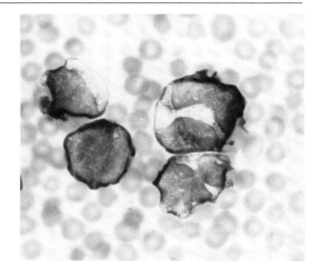

**FIGURE 6.10.** Blood film from a Holstein cow with leukemic lymphoma. Observe exceptionally large lymphoid cells with pleomorphic, monocytoid nuclei. Giemsa stain.

occurrence of the leukemic phase of lymphoma in animals is not well defined because of the lack of antemortem examination of blood in some cases and early euthanasia in other cases that might have eventually become leukemic. Less than one-third of dogs, cats, and cattle with lymphoma have substantial numbers of neoplastic lymphocytes in their circulation prior to death or euthanasia (Hardy, 1981*b*; Ferrer *et al.*, 1979; Squire *et al.*, 1973). Leukemic lymphoma has also been recognized in horses (Madewell *et al.*, 1982; Neufeld, 1973*b*; Schalm and Carlson, 1982).

In cattle, it is important to differentiate two BLV-induced disorders, namely, persistent lymphocytosis and leukemic lymphoma (Ferrer *et al.*, 1979). Persistent lymphocytosis results from a benign proliferation of B-lymphocytes. Some lymphocytes with atypical morphology may occur in persistent lymphocytosis, but no tumors or other evidence of illness are present. The leukemic phase of lymphoma develops late in the disease when tumors and/or clinical illness are apparent. Neoplastic cells in the circulation are generally bizarre with marked variation in size and nuclear pleomorphism (fig. 6.10). Persistent lymphocytosis is neither a disease nor a subclinical form of lymphoma. Although some cattle with persistent lymphocytosis develop lymphoma, most do not, and lymphoma may develop without a preleukemic persistent lymphocytosis phase (Ferrer *et al.*, 1979).

It is difficult at times to differentiate true leukemia from leukemic lymphoma in animals examined for the first time in terminal stages of disease. Both conditions can have peripheral lymphoid tumors and leukemic blood picture late in the disease. These conditions are more easily separated early when lymphoma is present without neoplastic cells in blood or bone marrow, and when leukemia shows no evidence of tumor formation.

## Plasma Cell Tumor (Multiple Myeloma or Plasmacytoma)

The term *multiple myeloma* is used in human medicine for systemic proliferations of malignant plasma cells or their recognizable precursors, usually with involvement of bone marrow. Localized and initially benign-seeming proliferations of mature plasma cells, sometimes in extraskeletal locations, have been designated as solitary plasmacytomas. Solitary plasmacytomas in humans have a benign course that may last for several years, but most terminate in a malignant phase. Two cases with solitary plasmacytomas have been reported in dogs (MacEwen *et al.*, 1984*b*).

**Incidence, Age, Breed, and Sex.** Multiple myeloma is rare in animals. Cases have been recorded in the dog, horse, cat, pig, and cow. The animals involved are generally adult or aged, although a plasma cell tumor has been reported in a calf (Pedini and Romanelli, 1955). In a series of 22 cases in dogs reviewed by Osborne *et al.* (1968), the mean age was 9 years (ranging from 30 months to 16 years). Similarly, MacEwen and Hurvitz (1977) reported a mean age of 8.3 years for both dogs and cats with multiple myeloma. No definite breed or sex predisposition has been recognized.

**Clinical Characteristics.** Where sufficient cases in dogs have been reported for a pattern to emerge, lameness, evidence of pain associated with one or more regions of the skeleton, and pathological fractures are the most common clinical signs. Anemia, hemorrhagic diathesis, depression, weight loss,

renal dysfunction, and palpable tumor masses are less consistently observed. Although multiple punctate areas of radiolucency (so-called punched-out areas) in radiographs of the skeleton are not as constant a feature in animals as they are in humans, there are usually osteoporotic or osteolytic lesions detectable by radiography. These are associated with diffuse or localized neoplastic accumulations.

Abnormal immunoglobulins (usually β- or γ-globulins) or their light or heavy chain components can be produced by neoplastic proliferations of lymphocytes or plasma cells. Because of their lower molecular weight, light chain components (Bence–Jones protein) are primarily detected in urine, and the remainder of the abnormal immunoglobulins are detected in blood. The abnormal proteins have been collectively called paraproteins. The majority of plasma cell tumors in humans produce IgA and IgG classes of immunoglobulin, although occasionally they are associated with an IgM monoclonal gammopathy (Rappaport and Braylan, 1975). Bence–Jones proteins are frequently found in the urine of humans with multiple myeloma. They are less commonly reported in animals with multiple myeloma probably because the abnormal proteins associated with the condition have not been sought. In 22 cases of multiple myeloma in dogs (including 2 of their own), Osborne *et al.* (1968) found that hyperglobulinemia was present in all dogs for which the information was available and that Bence–Jones proteinuria was present in 4 of 8 dogs for which the test was mentioned. Specific characterization of Bence–Jones proteinemia and proteinuria in a dog with multiple myeloma was reported by Hurvitz *et al.* (1971). Canine cases with IgA and IgG myeloma proteins have been reported (MacEwen and Hurvitz, 1977; Medway *et al.*, 1967; Rockey and Schwartzman, 1967). In addition, two rare cases of nonsecretory multiple myeloma have been reported in dogs (MacEwen *et al.*, 1984*a*). Cats with multiple myeloma have had elevated γ-globulin in serum (Farrow and Penney, 1971; Holzworth, 1960*a*; Holzworth and Meier, 1957; MacEwen and Hurvitz, 1977). Cats examined by MacEwen and Hurvitz (1977) had IgG myeloma proteins; they were negative for FeLV. Cornelius *et al.* (1959) demonstrated elevated β-globulin in the blood and urine of a horse with multiple myeloma. The animal also had low

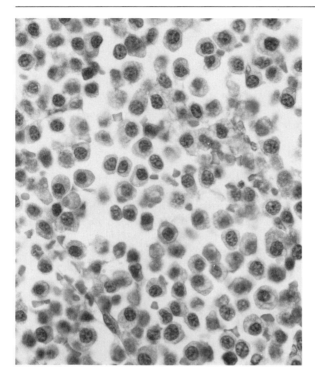

FIGURE 6.11. Plasma cell myeloma in the vertebra of a dog showing cells with hyperchromatic, eccentrically placed nuclei.

serum albumin and cholesterol concentrations and a high level of albumin in the urine.

**Sites.** Multiple myelomas characteristically affect bone marrow and thus the bones themselves. Marrow involvement is focal or diffuse, and there may or may not be involvement of extraskeletal sites. The latter are most commonly lymph nodes, spleen, liver, and kidney, but a variety of other organs such as the lungs, adrenals, pancreas, and prostate can be involved to a lesser degree. Lesions are often found in bones most active in hematopoiesis. The tibia, rib, humerus, and pelvis are commonly affected in most species, but in the dog the vertebrae are most often involved. The tumor is rarely seen distal to the elbow and stifle joints in the dog.

**Gross Morphology.** The bone marrow cavity containing the neoplastic tissue is focally or diffusely expanded, gelatinous, soft, and reddish gray. The bone cortex may be thin, and some tumors contain remnants of bone spicules that remain after os-

teolysis. The periosteum is occasionally thickened (Bloom, 1946). Sometimes there is complete destruction of cortical bone with extension of the neoplastic tissue into adjacent fascia and muscle. The lymph nodes and spleen may be slightly to moderately enlarged, and the liver may contain multiple pale spherical foci of various sizes. Renal involvement is evidenced by spherical or radially elongated cortical foci.

**Histological Features.** In severe cases, plasma cells constitute as much as 99% of the marrow cells. Precursor cells of the granulocytic-erythroid series are deficient in number because of displacement by plasma cells. In a few cases neoplastic plasma cells have been found in the peripheral blood (Holzworth and Meier, 1957; Pedini and Romanelli, 1955).

The neoplastic cells grade from imperfectly differentiated to fairly typical plasma cells (fig. 6.11). Considerable variation is present, even in the same tumor. In the undifferentiated tumors, detection of characteristic plasma cell forms can be difficult. The differentiated neoplastic cells may be of uniform or variable size, but they are usually larger than normal plasma cells. Their nuclei are hyperchromatic and are placed eccentrically or centrally in the cell. The nuclear chromatin is more homogeneous than the clumped type of chromatin found at the periphery of the nucleus of normal plasma cells. The cytoplasm is usually basophilic and might be vacuolated. In some tumors a number of the cells are distended by a crystalline or homogeneous acidophilic proteinaceous secretion. The more undifferentiated cells are large and contain one or often two or more nuclei with finely dispersed chromatin and one or more prominent nucleoli. Bizarre giant cell forms may be present. Mitotic figures are either uncommon or plentiful.

In the bones, the neoplastic plasma cells are distributed in a sparse, delicate stroma that contains many immature blood vessels that consist only of cavities lined by endothelium. Foci of osteolysis usually show no osteoblastic activity at the margins. Focal hemorrhages and necrosis are common. Primary amyloidosis is frequent in human cases of myeloma, but has been reported in only 2 of 22 cases in dogs (Osborne *et al.,* 1968); the kidney was involved in 1 of these 2 cases. Protein casts are commonly seen in the kidneys, and the associated renal

less frequent than in the hyperplastic germinal center. The medullary cords of the hyperplastic lymph nodes are usually thickened and filled with small lymphocytes and varying numbers of mature plasma cells. Often the medullary cords are completely replaced by plasma cells. Plasmablasts and preplasmacytes are also present but are difficult to identify by light microscopy alone. The medullary cord change is usually accompanied by germinal center hyperplasia. Sometimes in the hyperplastic lymph node, however, the germinal centers are blastic, but mature plasma cells are absent in the medullary cords. The follicles may also appear in a regressive phase or even as primary follicles, although the cords may contain many plasma cells. Thus, the two changes may not always be synchronous.

Careful histological observation is needed to differentiate between hyperplasia and early neoplasia originating in paracortical or corticomedullary regions. Features indicative of diffuse hyperplasia in these regions, whether or not accompanied by follicular hyperplasia, are uniformly sized lobules of the paracortex (the T-lymphocyte zone) which may have a mottled appearance due to admixture of numerous small, dark-staining lymphocytes (T-cells) and large, sparsely scattered histiocytes with clear or light-staining cytoplasm (the so-called starry sky cells). Hyperplasia and hypertrophy of the endothelium of the postcapillary venules also occur in the paracortex and are useful indicators of reactive hyperplasia. The medullary sinus structure is preserved in the hyperplastic node, and the sinuses often contain increased numbers of histiocytes. Finally, it should be noted that spillover of lymphoid cells into the capsule of lymph nodes and into perinodal fat is not an indicator of neoplasia unless the intranodal picture is also indicative of neoplasia. Such spillover can be found, if sought, in nodes reacting to profound antigenic stimulation.

## Histiocytic Lymphadenopathy of the Cat

One entity or, more likely, a group of entities deserving of specific mention is what we are temporarily calling histiocytic lymphadenopathy (lymphadenitis) in cats. Cats are presented with malaise and generalized lymphadenopathy and possibly with fever or anemia or both. The characteristic appearance of a biopsied lymph node is of widespread filling of the sinuses by mature-appearing histiocytic cells with plentiful acidophilic cytoplasm. Sometimes the cells accumulate in such numbers as to encroach severely on the normal architectural components of the node. In some cats the condition resolves, but in others it blends into a myeloproliferative disorder. Further study is needed for precise delineation of this entity.

## MYELOPROLIFERATIVE DISORDERS

The term *myeloproliferative disorders* (or myeloproliferative diseases) was introduced by Dameshek (1951) to designate a group of bone marrow cell disorders that had previously been considered separate entities. Myeloproliferative disorders are characterized by the purposeless proliferation of one, several, or all of the nonlymphoid marrow cell lines: granulocytic, monocytic, erythrocytic, or megakaryocytic. Myeloproliferative disorders are generally considered to be neoplastic, either malignant or benign. The extent to which the various myeloproliferative disorders (by the degree and nature of their proliferation) fulfill the criteria for malignant neoplasia depends on the particular entity and to some extent on the viewpoint of the observer. A number of hematologists also classify preleukemic syndromes (hematopoietic dysplasia) as myeloproliferative disorders (Linman and Bagby, 1976).

The concept of myeloproliferative disorders was developed for a number of reasons. First, although the proliferation of one marrow cell type may predominate, a marrow cell line is almost never singly affected. Morphological or functional disorders of other cell lines can usually be detected (Quesenberry and Levitt, 1979). Second, many of these disorders appear to evolve into one another. For instance, in humans various combinations among chronic granulocytic leukemia, polycythemia vera, hemorrhagic thrombocythemia, and myelofibrosis with myeloid metaplasia are found, and acute granulocytic leukemia is a possible termination in all of them (Silverstein, 1968). Changing manifestations of myeloproliferative disease have also been recognized in animals. In cats, for example, chronic erythremic myelosis (excessive proliferation of nu-

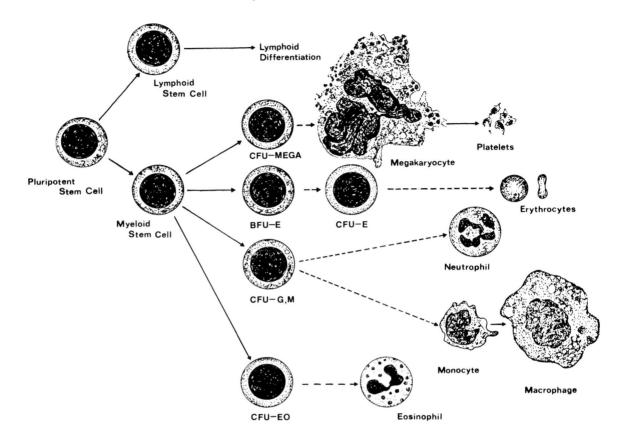

**FIGURE 6.16.** Proposed scheme of blood cell production. BFU-E denotes erythrocyte burst-forming unit; CFU-E, erythrocyte colony-forming unit; CFU-Mega, megakaryocyte colony-forming unit; CFU-G,M, granulocyte (neutrophil) and monocyte colony-forming unit; CFU-EO, eosinophil colony-forming unit.

cleated erythroid cells, with mature stages predominating) may evolve into erythroleukemia and eventually, acute granulocytic leukemia (Harvey, 1981; Harvey *et al.*, 1978; Schalm *et al.*, 1975).

A third justification for the unitary concept of myeloproliferative disorders is that blood cell lines are derived from common pluripotential stem cells (Quesenberry and Levitt, 1979). This fact probably accounts for the other two points discussed above. A conceptual outline of hematopoiesis based on information principally derived from *in vivo* spleen assay and *in vitro* cell culture techniques is given in fig. 6.16.

Both humoral (e.g., erythropoietin) and microenvironmental factors are important in regulating proliferation, differentiation, and maturation of the various bone marrow cell lines. Cells recognized to be important in the local control of hematopoiesis include reticular stromal cells (fibroblasts), T-lymphocytes, macrophages, and endothelial cells (Quesenberry and Levitt, 1979).

## Etiologies of Myeloproliferative Disorders

There is convincing evidence that myeloproliferative disorders in humans are primarily neoplastic disorders involving pluripotential myeloid stem cells responsible for granulocyte, monocyte, erythrocyte, and platelet production. In some cases of chronic granulocytic leukemia (CGL), an earlier stem cell (common also to the lymphoid system) may be involved because a substantial percentage of people with CGL undergo blast transformation to blasts with lymphoid characteristics (Quesenberry and Levitt, 1979). In some cases of myelomonocytic leukemia, the affected stem cell may be a more differentiated one, common to the granulocytic and monocytic cell line (see fig. 6.1). Evidence for the clonal nature of myeloproliferative disorders in humans has been obtained primarily by studying chromosomal abnormalities and X-linked glucose-6-phosphate dehydrogenase isoenzymes in various marrow cell lines (Fialkow, 1982).

Current investigations into the etiological basis of leukemia involve four major, possibly interrelated areas: genetic susceptibility, somatic mutation, viral infection, and immunological dysfunction (Necheles, 1979; Williams *et al.*, 1977). Feline leukemia virus has clearly been shown to cause lymphoid tumors and leukemia in cats (Jarrett *et al.*, 1964*a, b*). These malignancies may result not only from the viral induction of a mutant cell line but also because the virus is immunosuppressive and can depress the immunological surveillance system, thus allowing neoplastic clones to proliferate freely.

A large percentage of cats with myeloproliferative disease are FeLV positive (Hardy, 1981*b*). The existence of FeLV infections in cats probably accounts for the higher frequency of myeloproliferative disorders in cats than in other domestic animal species. Two explanations for the paucity of experimental cases of myeloproliferative disease in cats have been suggested. Some authors have suggested that other factors, such as the increased marrow proliferation that occurs in cats recovering from feline panleukopenia or hemobartonellosis, may increase the likelihood that a mutant cell line will be induced by FeLV (Schalm *et al.*, 1975). Others have suggested that a virus strain(s) with a propensity to produce myeloproliferative disease probably exists, but has not been isolated and used experimentally (Theilen and Madewell, 1979).

Myeloproliferative disorders are common in cats, uncommon in dogs, and rare in other animal species. The natural etiology or, more likely, etiologies of myeloproliferative disorders in species other than the cat is unknown. Irradiation has been experimentally shown to be a potent leukemogenic agent in dogs (Dungworth *et al.*, 1969; Seed *et al.*, 1977;

Tolle *et al.*, 1979) and pigs (Howard and Clarke, 1970), resulting in several myeloproliferative disease syndromes.

## Natural Course of Myeloproliferative Disorders

It has been recognized for many years that the development of overt myeloproliferative neoplasia in humans may be preceded for months to years by a phase of hematological abnormalities, during which blood and bone marrow examinations are not diagnostic of leukemia. Although the term *preleukemia* is frequently used, the term *hematopoietic dysplasia* is preferred because overt leukemia does not always develop in people with dysplastic hematological abnormalities (Linman and Bagby, 1976). The conclusion that a condition is truly preleukemic can only be made in retrospect.

### Hematopoietic Dysplasia

Cytopenias dominate the early phase of this syndrome in humans. A refractory anemia (either sideroblastic or megaloblastic) is the most consistent finding. Leukopenia, thrombocytopenia, or both often occur. Anisocytosis and poikilocytosis of erythrocytes are frequently observed. Other noteworthy findings in the peripheral blood include nucleated red blood cells out of proportion to the degree of polychromasia, large bizarre platelets, immature granulocytes, abnormal granulocyte morphology (large size, hypersegmentation, hyposegmentation, etc.), and monocytosis (Linman and Bagby, 1976).

The bone marrow may be normocellular, but is more frequently hypercellular with maturation defects in erythrocytic, granulocytic, and megakaryocytic cell lines. Erythrocyte hyperplasia may occur, and megaloblastoid erythrocyte precursors or ringed sideroblasts may be present. Disordered granulopoiesis is often present in leukopenic patients with an "arrest" or "bulge" at the myelocyte–metamyelocyte stage. Megakaryocyte hyperplasia is sometimes present. Megakaryocytes often have abnormal nuclear and/or cytoplasmic morphology. Dwarf megakaryocytes may be present. The terms *dyserythropoiesis* and *ineffective erythro-*

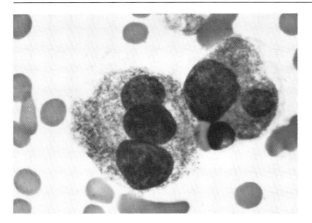

**FIGURE 6.17.** Two dwarf megakaryocytes in a bone marrow aspirate from a cat with hematopoietic dysplasia. Observe small size, discrete nuclear lobes, and mature granular cytoplasm. Wright–Giemsa stain.

*poiesis* have been used to describe anemic people when bone marrow erythroid abnormalities are present; the term *ineffective granulopoiesis* is used when myeloid abnormalities are prominent in leukopenic patients.

Clinical signs, frequently reported in hematopoietic dysplasia in humans, include lethargy, intermittent fever, recurrent infections, slow-healing lesions of the skin and mucous membrane, and petechial or ecchymotic hemorrhages. Splenomegaly and hepatomegaly are rare (Linman and Bagby, 1976).

Hematopoietic dysplasia, having many of the clinical and laboratory findings discussed above, is relatively common in cats (Harvey, 1981). Cats with hematopoietic dysplasia are leukopenic and/or anemic. Platelet counts may be low, normal, or high. Large bizarre platelets are commonly observed. Although a slight to moderate reticulocytosis may be present at times, most cases appear to be nonregenerative. Some cases exhibit marked anisocytosis of erythrocytes. The mean cell volume is increased above normal with surprising frequency. Nucleated erythrocytes out of proportion to the degree of polychromasia may be present, and occasional immature neutrophils or hypersegmented neutrophils are seen.

Bone marrow generally has normal to increased cellularity. A "maturation arrest" in the granulocyte series with increased immature stages, and a markedly decreased number of mature neutrophils is often seen in neutropenic cats. Unfortunately, without repeated blood examination it is not always possible to differentiate transient marrow leukocyte abnormalities in cats recovering from acute leukopenia from those with prolonged ineffective granulopoiesis. Erythroid abnormalities that may be present in hematopoietic dysplasia include increased immaturity of erythroid precursors, megaloblastoid erythroid precursors, and rarely, erythroid precursors containing multiple siderotic cytoplasmic inclusions. Abnormal dwarf megakaryocytes (fig. 6.17) are often present (J. W. Harvey, unpublished data).

Many, but not all, cats with hematopoietic dysplasia are FeLV positive. A few affected cats given supportive therapy have eventually developed myeloid leukemia (Madewell *et al.*, 1979; Maggio *et al.*, 1978). Most, however, have been euthanized when it was determined that the cat had refractory anemia or leukopenia (particularly if they were FeLV positive). Cats may die from complications such as bacterial infection or hemorrhage. If cats were given the long-term supportive care given to human patients, a high percentage of cases with hematopoietic dysplasia might prove to be preleukemic phases of myeloproliferative disease and eventually develop overt leukemia. The term *hematopoietic dysplasia* is preferable to the term *preleukemic syndrome* because a rare case may spontaneously recover (Lester and Searcy, 1981). In addition to three cases that developed myeloproliferative disease, Maggio *et al.* (1978) described nine FeLV positive cats with unexplained cytopenias and/or refractory anemias that subsequently developed lymphoblastic leukemia. Information given concerning bone marrow morphology was not sufficient to determine whether or not any of these cases would be classified as hematopoietic dysplasia by the criteria given above. Findings of marrow hypoplasia in three of these cases and increased lymphocytes in four cases are not generally considered to be criteria for hematopoietic dysplasia.

In addition to producing dysplastic and neoplastic conditions, FeLV can also produce anemias and cytopenias as a result of damage produced by, or in response to, viral replication in marrow elements (Mackey *et al.*, 1975*a*; Onions *et al.*, 1982; Pedersen *et al.*, 1977). Hardy (1981*a*) classified

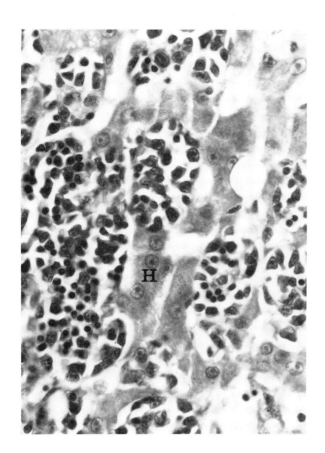

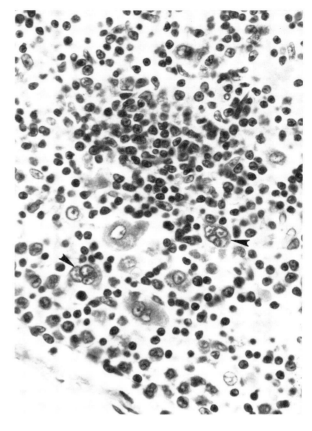

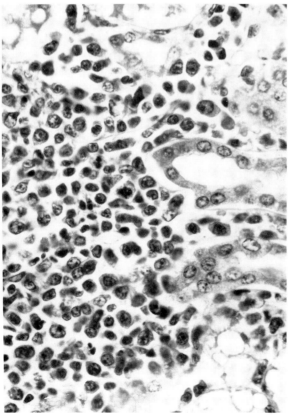

**FIGURE 6.19.** Erythroleukemic form of myeloproliferative disease in the cat. A. Cellular invasion in the hepatic sinusoids. The hepatic cord cells (H) are distorted by infiltrating cells. B. Peripheral splenic tissue. Observe megakaryocytes (**arrowheads**). C. Invasion of interstitial tissue of kidney.

fication of disorders into general categories can still be useful in estimating life expectancy, in predicting the likelihood that therapy can be effective in inducing a remission, and in selecting the most useful therapeutic approach.

Unfortunately, there is no uniform system for consistently classifying these disorders, owing to the variability of morphological features of the disease. Criteria used for classification include the predominant cell type(s) involved in the manifestation of disease, whether the disorder appears acute (characterized by the proliferation of blast and other immature cells) or chronic (characterized by the predominance of more mature cell types), and whether or not neoplastic cells are present in the bloodstream (Williams *et al.*, 1977).

The term *leukemia* was originally used to describe an abnormal proliferation of leukocytes in blood-forming organs (bone marrow, spleen, and lymph nodes), resulting in the presence of immature leukocytes in blood. When it became apparent that a large number of neoplastic cells were not always present in the circulation, the original meaning of the term was modified by adding adjectives such as aleukemic or subleukemic. Leukemia is now used to described the neoplastic proliferation of leukocytes in bone marrow whether or not the disease is overt (neoplastic cells in the circulation). Disorders without circulating neoplastic cells are frequently referred to as smoldering leukemias.

The classification of a disorder as acute or chronic is useful. These terms describe the degree of immaturity of the proliferating cells. In general, acute myeloproliferative disorders are less likely to respond to therapy and patients tend to have shorter survival rates than those with chronic disorders (Gale, 1979; Williams *et al.*, 1977).

Various manifestations of disease that are classified as acute myeloproliferative disorders are given in table 6.3. Unfortunately, acute myeloproliferative disorders do not always fit clearly into one of these categories. It is unclear where the acute myeloproliferative disorder in cats, sometimes referred to as reticuloendotheliosis, should be placed in this scheme. The term *reticuloendotheliosis* is inappropriate and is not used to describe myeloproliferative disease in humans. Although this manifestation could be placed in the undifferentiated or unclassified category, most of the immature cells morphologically appear to be abnormal erythroid cells, making a classification of acute erythremic myelosis or erythroleukemia (if myeloblasts are also present) a reasonable choice. Chronic myeloproliferative disease syndromes are generally more clearly defined (table 6.4), but considerable overlap exists.

**Special Stains and Procedures.** In routinely stained blood films, identification of primitive cells as belonging to a particular maturation series is difficult because of the absence of reliable distinguishing cellular characteristics. A variety of special

### TABLE 6.3. Classification of Acute Myeloproliferative Disorders

| Terminology | Predominant cell type(s) |
| --- | --- |
| Undifferentiated (unclassified) leukemia | Unknown |
| Acute granulocytic leukemia | Granulocytic |
| Progranulocytic leukemia[a] | Granulocytic |
| Myelomonocytic leukemia | Granulocytic, monocytic |
| Monocytic leukemia | Monocytic |
| Erythroleukemia[b] | Erythroid, granulocytic |
| Acute erythremic myelosis[b] | Erythroid |
| Megakaryocytic myelosis | Megakaryocytic |

[a] Generally considered to be a variant of acute granulocytic leukemia.
[b] Considered to be part of the erythroleukemia complex. The most undifferentiated of these types have previously been called reticuloendotheliosis.

### TABLE 6.4. Classification of Chronic Myeloproliferative Disorders

| Terminology | Predominant cell type(s) |
| --- | --- |
| Chronic granulocytic leukemia | Neutrophilic granulocytes |
| Eosinophilic leukemia[a] | Eosinophilic granulocytes |
| Basophilic leukemia[a] | Basophilic granulocytes |
| Chronic erythremic myelosis[b] | Erythroid cells |
| Polycythemia vera | Erythrocytes |
| Thrombocythemia | Platelets |
| Myelofibrosis with myeloid metaplasia | Megakaryocytes, granulocytes, erythroid cells |
| Malignant histiocytosis | Macrophages |

[a] Generally considered variants of chronic granulocytic leukemia.
[b] Considered to be part of the erythroleukemia complex.

stains may be used to aid in the diagnosis and classification of myeloproliferative disorders. Only those showing the most promise at this time are discussed. One of the most useful, as well as easiest to perform, is the peroxidase stain. Neutrophilic granulocytes and their precursors (except the most primitive myeloblasts) are peroxidase positive in all species. Monocytes are negative or only slightly positive, and lymphocytes are always negative (Jain, 1970). The Sudan black B stain gives similar results. The alkaline phosphatase stain has been recommended as an aid in differentiating acute granulocytic leukemia from acute lymphocytic leukemia and monocytic leukemia in dogs and cats (Jain *et al.*, 1981; Schalm *et al.*, 1975). Immature neutrophilic stages are reported positive, with lymphoblasts and monoblasts being negative. In contrast to humans, however, the alkaline phosphatase stain cannot be used in differentiating chronic granulocytic leukemia from leukemoid reactions in dogs and cats because cells in the late stages of neutrophilic maturation (metamyelocytes, bands, and mature neutrophils) are usually negative (Jain, 1971). The reported finding of alkaline phosphatase positive myeloblasts needs further verification because this enzyme is reported to develop in humans in neutrophilic myelocytes with the formation of the specific granules. If it occurs in primary granules in dogs and cats, one would expect later granulocyte stages to be positive as well. Nonspecific esterase (α-napthyl acetate esterase and α-napthyl butyrate esterase) staining procedures have been recommended for the identification of monocytes (Jain *et al.*, 1981). Megakaryocyte precursors are also reported to be strongly positive, and lymphocytes are at times positive for α-napthyl acetate esterase staining (Holscher *et al.*, 1978; Innes *et al.*, 1982; Li *et al.*, 1973; Osbaldiston *et al.*, 1978). Esterase staining properties of various leukocytes are dependent on species as well as technique (substrate, pH, and staining time) (Osbaldiston *et al.*, 1978). Consequently, the techniques used and interpretation of results may vary slightly with the species studied.

The measurement of serum lysozyme activity (muramidase) is useful as a diagnostic aid in animals. This bacteriolytic enzyme is synthesized in granulocytes and monocytes and stored in lysosomes. Serum lysozyme concentrations have been highest and most consistently elevated in humans in association with monocytic and myelomonocytic leukemias, but it may also be increased in other myeloproliferative disorders and in diseases with increased granulocyte and/or monocyte turnover (Atwater and Erslev, 1977).

Markedly increased serum lysozyme activity has been reported in dogs with acute granulocytic and myelomonocytic leukemia (Shifrine *et al.*, 1973). Lesser increases in activity (above normal) have been reported in dogs in association with various other types of neoplasia (Feldman *et al.*, 1981) and inflammatory conditions (Shifrine *et al.*, 1973). A case of myelomonocytic leukemia in a horse was reported to have serum lysozyme activity above that in normal horses and horses with inflammatory conditions (Brumbaugh *et al.*, 1982).

The development of monoclonal antibodies to antigens on the surface of blood cells, bone marrow cells, and lymphoid cells at various stages of differentiation and maturation shows great promise in the diagnosis (and possibly treatment) of leukemia and lymphoma in humans (Nadler *et al.*, 1981). The development of similar immunological markers for cells in domestic animals would allow more accurate classification of myeloproliferative and lymphoproliferative disorders.

## Acute Granulocytic Leukemia (Acute Myeloblastic Leukemia)

Acute granulocytic leukemia (AGL) is characterized by the presence of a large percentage of myeloblasts and/or progranulocytes in the peripheral blood and/or bone marrow. When progranulocytes predominate, the term *progranulocytic* (promyelocytic) *leukemia* is used in humans. Disseminated intravascular coagulation (DIC) occurs frequently with this form of leukemia in humans (Gale, 1979). Progranulocytic leukemia is rare in cats (Fraser *et al.*, 1974; Schalm *et al.*, 1975) and has not been reported in other domestic animals.

Although some cases of granulocytic leukemia exhibit sufficient cellular maturation for a diagnosis to be made on routinely stained blood or bone marrow smears, other cases have few, if any, neoplastic granulocytes that are more mature than myeloblasts (Fraser *et al.*, 1974). In these cases it is difficult to be certain that the immature cells are in fact of granulocytic origin. Morphological criteria that help differentiate acute granulocytic leukemia from acute lymphocytic leukemia include larger size, more abundant cytoplasm, greater separation of nuclear chromatin, and greater prominence of nucleoli in myeloblasts compared with lymphoblasts. Peroxidase and alkaline phosphatase stains are useful in differentiating acute granulocytic leukemia from other acute leukemias.

Total leukocyte counts are low, normal, or high. Most of the early cases of acute granulocytic leukemia reported in cats had increased leukocyte counts and many neoplastic granulocytes in the blood circulation (Fraser *et al.*, 1974; Holzworth, 1960*b*; Schalm *et al.*, 1975). As a result of increased use of bone marrow aspiration in the examination of cats with cytopenia and refractory anemia, it now appears that a substantial number of cats with acute granulocytic leukemia have few or no recognizable neoplastic cells in the circulation (Duncan and Prasse, 1976; Harvey, 1981; Madewell *et al.*, 1979). Acute granulocytic leukemia is a rare malignancy in dogs (Theilen and Madewell, 1979). It is primarily a disease of young to middle-aged dogs (Schalm *et al.*, 1975). Myeloblasts, progranulocytes, and neutrophilic myelocytes have usually been recognized in blood in association with high total leukocyte counts (Meier, 1957; Nielsen, 1970; Schalm *et al.*, 1975), but occult granulocytic leukemia can occur (Sutton and Wilkins, 1981). Although early stages of neutrophilic development may also occur in the circulation in chronic granulocytic leukemia, they generally occur with disproportionately increased frequency (relative to later stages of development) in acute granulocytic leukemia. Myeloblasts, progranulocytes, and myelocytes are the predominant cell types found in the bone marrow.

A single case of acute granulocytic leukemia was reported in the horse (Lewis and Leitch, 1975). Naturally occurring cases of granulocytic leukemia in cattle and swine have been diagnosed only at necropsy (Nielsen, 1970). Only one case reported in a calf had sufficient hematological information to permit an accurate diagnosis of acute granulocytic leukemia (Hyde *et al.*, 1958). A variety of myeloproliferative disorders, including acute granulocytic leukemia, have been produced experimentally in dogs and miniature swine exposed to radioactive elements (Dungworth *et al.*, 1969; Howard and Clarke, 1970; Tolle *et al.*, 1979).

## Neoplasms of the Mononuclear Phagocyte System

Cells of the mononuclear phagocyte system, including promonocytes, monocytes, and macrophages (tissue histiocytes), are derived from a bone marrow stem cell. Promonocytes in the marrow give rise to monocytes that circulate in the blood for a short time and then enter the tissues where they become macrophages of all types. Although a majority of tissue macrophages are derived from blood monocytes under normal conditions, reactive proliferations of macrophages occur in the tissue in response to various inciting agents.

Neoplastic disorders involving mononuclear phagocytes include monocytic leukemia, myelomonocytic leukemia, and malignant histiocytosis (Groopman and Golde, 1981). A variety of other histiocytoses have been described in humans that are proposed to be reactions to unknown inciting agents rather than being neoplastic.

### Myelomonocytic Leukemia

Myelomonocytic leukemia is often considered to be a variant of acute granulocytic leukemia. It is characterized by the occurrence of primitive cells of both the granulocytic and monocytic series in the bloodstream (fig. 6.20). Some cells have round nuclei and resemble myeloblasts, and others appear monocytoid and are characterized by prominent nuclear pleomorphism. It is not surprising that this manifestation occurs since these cell types share a common stem cell (fig. 6.1). Naturally occurring cases of myelomonocytic leukemia have been reported in dogs (Jain *et al.*, 1981; Linnabary *et al.*, 1978; Ragan *et al.*, 1976), cats (Loeb *et al.*, 1975; Stann, 1979), and a horse (Brumbaugh *et al.*, 1982). A diagnosis of myelomonocytic leukemia may be substantiated by the use of special stains (see previous discussion). The spectrum in this disorder can range from almost pure acute granulocytic leukemia with a small percentage of monocytoid cells to al-

1971; Hendrick, 1981; Schalm, 1980; Silverman, 1971; Simon and Holzworth, 1967). Two cases in dogs and one in a pig have been diagnosed at necropsy (Nielsen, 1970).

Total leukocyte counts have been markedly increased, with a predominance of mature eosinophils and their precursors. Mature eosinophils outnumbered the immature stages that were also present in the circulation. Surprisingly, the cats were either not anemic or only moderately anemic, although eosinophils and their precursors dominated the bone marrow and infiltrated many body tissues. The diagnosis of eosinophilic leukemia should be made cautiously after the elimination of other causes of eosinophilia, such as parasitism, allergic disorders, and eosinophilic enteritis.

Eosinophilic leukemia in cats is unique since it is the only myeloproliferative disorder that is not caused by FeLV (Hardy, 1981*b*). Eosinophilic leukemia is a part of a feline hypereosinophilic syndrome that also includes eosinophilic enteritis and disseminated eosinophilic disease (Hendrick, 1981). Most cases diagnosed as having eosinophilic leukemia in cats have had eosinophilic enteritis and diarrhea in addition to marked eosinophilia with eosinophilic infiltrates in liver, spleen, and other organs. There are no clearly established criteria to differentiate disseminated eosinophilic disease from eosinophilic leukemia. The idea that rampant visceral infiltration of eosinophils need not be considered leukemia (Bengtsson, 1968) is itself controversial in both human and veterinary medicine.

## Basophilic Leukemia

Basophilic leukemia is a variant of chronic granulocytic leukemia. Basophilic leukemia has been rarely reported in the dog (MacEwen *et al.*, 1975; Nielsen, 1970). One well-documented case in a dog was characterized by leukocytosis (50,800 leukocytes per μl), moderate anemia, and marked thrombocytosis (MacEwen *et al.*, 1975). Eighty-eight percent of the leukocytes were of the basophilic series. Most basophilic cells were mature, but a significant left shift was present. There was also an absolute eosinophilia (3,556 cells per μl).

One likely case of basophilic leukemia was reported in a cat (Henness and Crow, 1977). All early

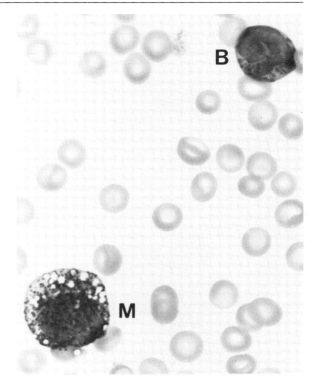

**FIGURE 6.24.** Mast cell (M) and basophil (B) in blood from a dog with noncutaneous systemic mastocytosis. Wright– Giema stain. (Courtesy of *Vet. Clin. N. Amer. Small Anim. Pract.*)

case reports of basophilic leukemia in cats and some in dogs (Alroy, 1972) appear to have been cases of systemic mastocytosis (Nielsen, 1970; Schalm *et al.*, 1975). Mast cells have numerous purplish cytoplasmic granules and round nuclei (fig. 6.24 and 6.25A). Basophils have segmented nuclei. Canine basophils have bluish cytoplasm and granulation is scant. Feline basophils have many round, pale lavender cytoplasmic granules, some of which superimpose on the nucleus giving it a "moth-eaten" appearance (fig. 6.25B).

## Myeloproliferative Diseases with Megakaryocytic Predominance

Abnormal megakaryocytic hyperplasia has been observed in humans with myeloproliferative disease syndromes such as chronic granulocytic leukemia,

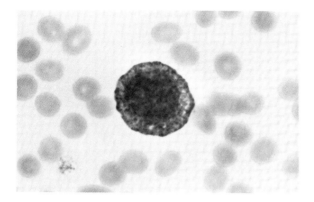

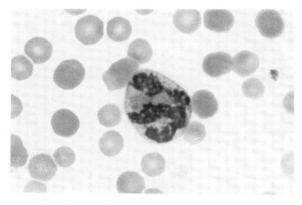

**FIGURE 6.25.** Feline mast cell and basophil morphology. A. Mast cell in blood of a cat with noncutaneous mastocytosis. Observe round nucleus and numerous dark granules. B. Feline basophil. Observe segmented nucleus. Numerous pale granules in cytoplasm overlying the nucleus give it a "moth-eaten" appearance. Wright–Giemsa stain.

myelofibrosis with myeloid metaplasia, and polycythemia vera. In rare cases of myeloproliferative disease, abnormal megakaryocytic proliferation is the primary or dominant finding in the bone marrow and other organs of the mononuclear phagocyte system. Two syndromes have been described in humans: megakaryocytic myelosis, which mainly involves the proliferation of abnormal megakaryocytes, and thrombocythemia, which is mainly the uncontrolled production of platelets (Williams *et al.*, 1977).

### Megakaryocytic Myelosis (Megakaryocytic Leukemia or Malignant Megakaryocytosis)

This disorder is characterized by abnormal megakaryocytic hyperplasia in the bone marrow (fig. 6.26) and other organs of the hematopoietic system. Megakaryocytes are morphologically abnormal. Some are small (dwarf megakaryocytes) and have few or no nuclear lobulations. In some instances there are two separate nuclei. Dwarf megakaryocytes or undifferentiated blast cells may be present in the circulation. A thrombocytopenia exists in some cases, whereas platelet counts in excess of $1 \times 10^6$ per μl occur in others. A progressive refractory anemia is consistently present, and leukocyte counts are variable. Splenomegaly resulting from the infiltration of megakaryocytes is usually present. Rare cases of megakaryocytic myelosis have been reported in dogs (Harvey *et al.*, 1982; Holscher *et al.*, 1978; Rudolph and Hubner, 1972) and cats (Michel *et al.*, 1976; Saar, 1970).

### Thrombocythemia (Essential, Primary, Idiopathic, or Hemorrhagic)

Thrombocythemia in humans is characterized by hyperplasia of megakaryocytic cells in marrow and persistently elevated platelet counts in excess of $1 \times 10^6$ per μl in blood. Many megakaryocytes in the marrow are bizarre in appearance. Some are gigantic with multiple lobulations or voluminous cytoplasm. Giant platelets and platelets with abnormal morphology may be seen in the circulation. The disorder is characterized by spontaneous or excessive posttraumatic hemorrhage. Most patients are not anemic unless hemorrhage is substantial. A neutrophilia is usually present, and moderate eosinophilia and platelets with abnormal morphology may be seen in the circulation. Splenomegaly may occur due to "congestion." Infiltration of tissues by marrow elements usually does not occur (Williams *et al.*, 1977). Obviously, there is an overlap between this syndrome and megakaryocytic myelosis. It is important to differentiate transient thrombocytosis from thrombocythemia, where platelet counts are persistently increased. No cases of primary thrombocythemia have been reported in animals.

## Myelofibrosis with Myeloid Metaplasia

Myelofibrosis with myeloid metaplasia is a chronic myeloproliferative disorder characterized by abnormal growth of erythroid, myeloid, and megakaryocytic cell types, as well as varying degrees of marrow fibrosis and myeloid metaplasia in the spleen and liver (Burkhardt *et al.*, 1975). It is a neoplastic disorder involving the pluripotential hematopoietic stem cell (Quesenberry and Levitt, 1979). The myeloid metaplasia in spleen and liver should not be viewed as a normal extramedullary hematopoiesis secondary to marrow destruction. Cellular infiltrates represent abnormal marrow elements that replicate in these organs even when marrow fibrosis is minimal. The myelofibrosis and osteosclerosis occur secondary to marrow damage (Burkhardt *et al.*, 1975).

The onset of disease in bone is nearly always insidious. Anemia is present in a majority of people when first examined. Splenomegaly is nearly always present, and hepatomegaly occurs in 75% of cases. Infarction of the spleen is common. Osteosclerosis is generally patchy and occurs in less than half of the

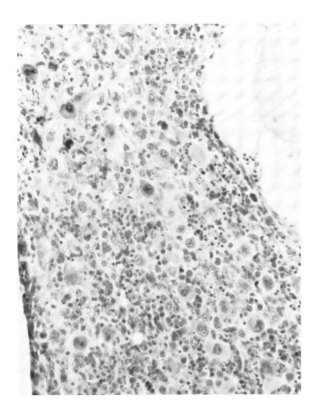

**FIGURE 6.26.** Abnormal megakaryocytic hyperplasia in a bone marrow core biopsy from a dog with myeloproliferative disease. Hematoxylin and eosin stain. (Courtesy of *Vet. Clin. N. Amer. Small Anim. Pract.*)

cases (Williams *et al.*, 1977). A leukocytosis with left shift is usually present, as are nucleated erythroid cells of varying degrees of maturity. The presence of an excessive number of immature leukocytes and nucleated erythroid cells in the blood has been termed *leukoerythroblastic reaction*. Platelets are morphologically and functionally abnormal. Platelet counts are increased early in the disorder in one-third of the cases, but thrombocytopenia may be present as the disease progresses (Williams *et al.*, 1977).

Bone marrow is usually not obtainable by means of needle aspiration because of the fibrosis. When marrow core biopsies are obtained, megakaryocytes are nearly always preserved and often are increased in number, even in fibrotic areas. Megakaryocytes may also be prominent in other hematopoietic organs.

This syndrome is not well documented in animals. Patchy to diffuse myelofibrosis has been recognized in cats with myeloproliferative disease (Hardy, 1981*b*; Harvey *et al.*, 1978; Herz *et al.*, 1969; Ward *et al.*, 1969). Myelofibrosis probably occurs late in the course of the disease. A specific isolate of FeLV has been used to experimentally produce osteosclerosis and erythroid hypoplasia in kittens (Hoover and Kociba, 1974), and osteosclerosis and myelofibrosis have been reported clinically in a cat infected with FeLV (Flecknell *et al.*, 1978). In these instances the marrow lesions were apparently induced directly by the virus rather than occurring secondary to myeloproliferative disease. One case of osteosclerosis has been reported in a cat with myeloproliferative disease (Zenoble and Rowland, 1979); this animal was hypercalcemic. The osteosclerotic changes were different from those of other cats with osteosclerosis and were believed to have resulted from pseudohyperparathyroidism secondary to myeloproliferative disease.

Myelofibrosis and osteosclerosis have been reported in a dog with a myeloproliferative disease classified as megakaryocytic leukemia (Rudolph and Hubner, 1972). This case fulfilled many of the criteria of the myelofibrosis and myeloid metaplasia syndrome in humans. In addition to patchy myelofibrosis and osteosclerosis, the dog had marked splenic enlargement, massive infiltrates of abnormal megakaryocytes in organs of the mononuclear phagocyte system, extramedullary hematopoiesis in the spleen, splenic infarcts, substantial anemia with occasional nucleated erythrocytes in the circulation, and neutropenia with a slight left shift. Dungworth *et al.* (1969) reported variable myelofibrosis in some dogs with smoldering granulocytic leukemias induced by $^{90}$Sr. Pathological findings were similar to the myelofibrosis with myeloid metaplasia syndrome described for humans, although megakaryocytes were rare or absent from the marrow.

Myelofibrosis may also be secondary to marrow damage other than that associated with myeloproliferative disease. Myelofibrosis occurs after irradiation or the use of myelotoxic drugs, or it may be idiopathic. Myelofibrosis has been reported as a terminal event in dogs with hereditary deficiency of erythrocyte pyruvate kinase (Prasse, 1977).

## Polycythemia Vera

Polycythemia vera is a chronic myeloproliferative disease in humans and is characterized by a striking absolute increase in the number of erythrocytes and total blood volume. At least two-thirds of the cases have leukocytosis (with left shift), thrombocytosis, and splenomegaly. The bone marrow is hyperplastic, with a normal myeloid to erythroid ratio (M:E ratio) and normal cellular morphology. The skin has a peculiar reddish purple color, and a variety of vasomotor and neurological symptoms may be present. Signs of disease are generally attributed to the expanded blood volume and its increased viscosity and to vascular thrombosis. The abnormal cellular proliferation appears to originate as pluripotential hematopoietic stem cell defects (Quesenberry and Levitt, 1979).

Polycythemia vera is rare in dogs (McGrath, 1974; Peterson and Randolph, 1982) and one case has been reported in a cat (Reed *et al.*, 1970) and one in a Hereford steer (Fowler *et al.*, 1964). A familial polycythemia (erythrocytosis) has been described in a family of highly inbred Jersey calves (Tennant *et al.*, 1967). This condition in Jersey cattle does not appear to be a myeloproliferative disease because animals that reached adulthood spontaneously recovered and an erythropoietin-enhancing factor was found in the serum (Van Dyke *et al.*, 1968).

Animals with polycythemia vera have dark red mucous membranes. Other clinical findings that oc-

curred singly or together in approximately one-half of the cases in dogs included polyuria and polydipsia, neurological or neuromuscular disorder, and hemorrhage. The packed cell volume in polycythemia vera was always increased (65 to 82%), but leukocytosis occurred in no more than half of the cases and thrombocytosis was not reported. Thrombosis was reported once and splenomegaly twice in dogs with the disease (McGrath, 1974).

A diagnosis of polycythemia vera is made by eliminating other possible causes of increased erythrocyte-packed cell volume. To make a diagnosis, one must first determine that an absolute increase in erythrocyte mass exists. This is done most accurately by radioactive labeling of erythrocytes. A relative erythrocytosis resulting from splenic contraction or dehydration is generally transient and easily recognized.

It is more difficult to differentiate primary polycythemia (polycythemia vera) from secondary polycythemia, which may occur as a result of chronic lung disease, renal tumors, hydronephrosis, renal vascular impairment, right-to-left cardiac shunts, and tumors that produce erythropoietinlike substances. One diagnostic procedure that is useful is a thorough physical examination, including palpation, cardiac auscultation, arterial $PO_2$ measurements, radiography, and serum erythropoietin concentration (Peterson and Randolph, 1982). If the animal is young, a congenital high oxygen affinity hemoglobinopathy should be considered, although this has not yet been documented in animals. Finally, one should remember that normal greyhound dogs often have packed cell volumes of slightly more than 60%.

Animals with polycythemia vera do not have marked thrombocytoses or splenomegaly, do not consistently have leukocytoses, and do not terminate with acute leukemias or other forms of myeloproliferative disease. Consequently, some question remains whether these disorders in animals are truly part of the myeloproliferative disease complex. Terms such as *erythremia* or *primary erythrocytosis* may be more appropriate.

## NONCUTANEOUS SYSTEMIC MASTOCYTOSIS AND MAST CELL LEUKEMIA

Malignant mast cell proliferations with systemic distribution of the neoplastic cells in the pattern common to leukemia are discussed here. Noncutaneous systemic mastocytosis in animals is primarily recognized in cats, but rare cases have been observed in dogs.

The origin of mast cells is controversial. They have been reported to be derived from undifferentiated mesenchymal cells of connective tissue (Coombs *et al.*, 1965), from thymus cells (Ishizaka *et al.*, 1976), and from mononuclear phagocytes or a common precursor cell (Sterry and Czarnetzki, 1982). It is suggested that mast cell precursors originate in bone marrow (Hatanaka *et al.*, 1979), circulate in blood in the mononuclear leukocyte fraction (Zucker-Franklin *et al.*, 1981), and develop (following appropriate peripheral stimulation) into mature mast cells in tissue sites (Hatanaka *et al.*, 1979). Although biochemical and functional characteristics of mast cells and basophils are similar, morphological differences between mature mast cells and basophils can be demonstrated by light microscopy (figs. 6.23 and 6.24) and electron microscopy in the dog and cat (Schalm *et al.*, 1975; Shively *et al.*, 1969; Ward and Hurvitz, 1972; Ward *et al.*, 1972; Weiss *et al.*, 1968).

Most cases of mass cell neoplasia in dogs occur in old animals and begin as single or multiple well-circumscribed tumor nodules in the skin. Tumor metastasis is commonly recognized at necropsy (Hottendorf and Nielsen, 1968). Most cases have mast cell accumulations in regional lymph nodes and one-half or more have evidence of metastasis to the spleen and liver. Other organs commonly involved include lung, kidney, heart, and bone marrow. Although the hematogenous transport of neoplastic cells is common, prominent mastocytemia has rarely been reported (Davis *et al.*, 1981; Fowler *et al.*, 1966). Mast cells, however, may be found in low numbers in blood in a substantial number of cases by the examination of multiple buffy coat smears. Noncutaneous systemic mastocytosis with mastocytemia is extremely rare in the dog (Davies *et al.*, 1981). Lombard *et al.* (1963) reported that canine mast cell tumors are caused by a virus, and

Rickard and Post (1968) reported a transmissible mast cell leukemia.

In contrast to the dog, a majority of cases of mast cell neoplasia in cats do not have skin involvement. Noncutaneous systemic mastocytosis is primarily a disease of old cats (Garner and Lingeman, 1970; Liska *et al.*, 1979). It is not caused by FeLV (Liska *et al.*, 1979). Common presenting complaints include emesis, abdominal distention, and anorexia. Abdominal distention occurs primarily as a result of splenomegaly. Splenic involvement is so consistent and often so dramatic that the term *splenic mastocytosis* has been used in the past to describe this feline disease (Nielsen, 1969). Mast cell infiltrates may also be recognized in liver, lymph nodes, and bone marrow; approximately one-half of the cats have mastocytemia (Nielsen, 1969). This peripheral blood involvement has been confused with basophilic leukemia. Although extensive, the disease in cats may progress slowly. Long-term survival (2 years or more) has been reported in some cats with systemic mastocytosis, even following splenectomy (Confer *et al.*, 1978; Liska *et al.*, 1979).

A diagnosis of mast cell neoplasia is made by demonstrating a large number of mast cells in affected organs using fine needle aspirates, fresh imprints, or histological sections of surgically excised tissue. Mast cell granules are identified in exfoliative cytological preparations following staining with new methylene blue in physiological saline (Schalm *et al.*, 1975) or with routine Romanowsky type blood stains (e.g., Wright–Giemsa). Some caution is needed in interpreting exfoliative cytological preparations because a small number of mast cells are normally encountered in tissues such as skin, bone marrow, and liver. Also, a slight to moderately increased number may be seen in response to various parasitic and chronic inflammatory conditions. Rare circulating mast cells have even been observed in the blood of dogs without mast cell neoplasia.

Organ infiltrates are often similar to those seen with myeloid or lymphoid leukemias, but they form discrete spherical foci more readily than the leukemias. Special stains such as Giemsa or toluidine blue are needed to demonstrate mast cell granules in histological sections because the granules do not stain with hematoxylin and eosin. Mast cell morphology varies in cases of systematic mastocytosis.

When stained by Wright or Giemsa stain or by other modifications of the Romanowsky stains, mature mast cells are globular, approximately 20 μm in diameter, and have a round centrally or eccentrically placed nucleus. The cytoplasm is packed with small, uniform, purple granules that can be so numerous as to partially obscure the nucleus. Anaplastic mast cells may have cytoplasmic vacuoles and fewer recognizable granules. Recently, a case of disseminated mast cell neoplasm with terminal mastocytemia was reported in a dog (Lester *et al.*, 1981) in which the circulating neoplastic cells lacked metachromatic granules and resembled abnormal vacuolated monoctyes or lymphocytes. Additional special stains and electron microscopy were utilized to make the diagnosis.

Eosinophilic infiltrates in mast cell tumors are common in dogs. An associated eosinophilia may also be present, and unexplained basophilias have been recognized in several canine cases of systemic mastocytosis (Allan *et al.*, 1974; Davies *et al.*, 1981). Neither eosinophilia nor eosinophilic infiltrates are common in cats with systemic mastocytosis (Liska *et al.*, 1979; Nielsen, 1969).

Gastric and duodenal ulcers are frequently observed in association with systemic mastocytosis in both dogs and cats (Davies *et al.*, 1981; Liska *et al.*, 1979). Lesions vary from pinpoint erosions to perforating ulcers. The pathogenesis of this ulceration is not fully understood. Induction of hyperacidity, hypermotility, and vascular damage by histamine have been considered to be potential ulcerogenic mechanisms (Fishman *et al.*, 1979; Howard *et al.*, 1969).

## REFERENCES

Aisenberg, A. C. (1981) Cell-Surface Markers in Lymphoproliferative Disease. *N. Engl. J. Med.* 304, 331–336.

Aisenberg, A. C., and Wilkes, B. (1976) Lymphosarcoma Cell Leukemia: The Contribution of Cell Surface Study to Diagnosis. *Blood* 48, 707–715.

Allan, G. S., Watson, A. D. J., Duff, B. C., and Howlett, C. R. (1974) Disseminated Mastocytoma and Mastocytemia in a Dog. *J. Amer. Vet. Med. Assoc.* 165, 346–359.

Alroy, J. (1972) Basophilic Leukemia in a Dog. *Vet. Path.* 9, 90–95.

Al-Zubaidy, A. J. (1981) Malignant Thymoma with Metastases in a Dog. *Vet. Rec.* 109, 490–492.

Anderson, L. J., and Jarrett, W. F. H. (1968) Lymphosarcoma (Leukemia) in Cattle, Sheep and Pigs in Great Britain. *Cancer* 22, 398–405.

————. (1971) Membranous Glomerulonephritis Associated with Leukemia in Cats. *Res. Vet. Sci.* 12, 179–180.

Anderson, L. J., Jarrett, W. F. H., and Crighton, G. W. (1969a) A Classification of Lymphoid Neoplasms of Domestic Mammals. In: Lingeman, C. H., and Garner, F. M., eds., *Comparative Morphology of Hematopoietic Neoplasms*. National Cancer Institute Monograph 32. U.S. Government Printing Office (Washington, D.C.), 343–353.

Anderson, L. J., Sandison, A. T., and Jarrett, W. F. H. (1969b) A British Abattoir Survey of Tumours in Cattle, Sheep and Pigs. *Vet. Rec.* 84, 547–551.

Anderson, R. K., Sorensen, D. K., Perman, V., Dirks, V. A., Snyder, M. M., and Bearman, J. E. (1971) Selected Epizootiologic Aspects of Bovine Leukemia in Minnesota (1961–1965). *Amer. J. Vet. Res.* 32, 563–577.

Armstrong, S. J., Souza, P. N. de, Wreghitt, T. G., Nagington, J., Mahy, B. W. J., and Owen, L. N. (1978) Studies on a Possible Viral Aetiology of Canine Lymphosarcoma and Mammary Tumours. *Brit. J. Cancer* 38, 175.

Atwater, J., and Erslev, A. J. (1977) Assay of Serum and Urine Lysozyme (Muramidase). In: Williams, W. J., Beutler, E., Erslev, A. J., and Rundles, R. W., eds., *Hematology*. 2d ed. McGraw-Hill (New York), 1636–1638.

Bäckgren, A. W. (1965) Lymphatic Leukosis in Dogs: An Epizootological, Clinical and Haematological Study. *Acta Vet. Scand.* 6, suppl. 1, 80.

Baumgartener, L. E., Olson, C., Miller, J. M., and Van der Maaten, M. J. (1975) Survey for Antibodies of Leukemia (C-Type) Virus in Cattle. *J. Amer. Vet. Med. Assoc.* 166, 249–251.

Bech-Nielsen, S., Fulton, R. W., Downing, M. M., and Hardy, W. D., Jr. (1981) Feline Infectious Peritonitis and Viral Respiratory Diseases in Feline Leukemia Virus Infected Cats. *J. Amer. Anim. Hosp. Assoc.* 17, 759–765.

Bendixen, H. J. (1957) Undersøgelser over kvaegets leukose. I. Kvaegleukosens forekomst og udbredelse i Danmark. *Nord. Vet. Med.* 9, 1–33.

————. (1960) Untersuchunger über die Rinderleukose in Dänemark. II. Pathogenese und Enzootologie der übertragbaren Rinderleukose. *Dtsch. Tierärztl. Wschr.* 67, 57–63.

Bendixen, H. J., and Friis, N. F. (1965) Die Hautleukose bei Rindern in Dänemark. *Wien. Tierärztl. Mschr.* 52, 496–505.

Bengtsson, E. (1968) Eosinophilic Leukemia—An Immunopathological Reaction? *Acta Paediat. Scand.* 57, 245–249.

Benjamin, S. A., and Noronha, F. (1967) Cytogenetic Studies in Canine Lymphosarcoma. *Cornell Vet.* 57, 526–542.

Berard, C. W., and Dorfman, R. F. (1974) Histopathology of Malignant Lymphomas. In: Rosenberg, S. A., ed., *Clinics in Haematology.* Vol. 3, no. 1. W. B. Saunders (London), 39–76.

Berard, C. W., Greene, M. H., Jaffe, E. S., Magrath, I., and Ziegler, J. (1981) A Multi-disciplinary Approach to Non-Hodgkins Lymphomas. *Ann. Intern. Med.* 94, 218–235.

Bernard, A., Boumsell, L., Reinherz, E. L., Nadler, L. M., Ritz, J., Coppin, H., Richard, Y., Valensi, F., Dausset, J., Flandrin, G., Lemerle, J., and Schlossman, S. F. (1981) Cell Surface Characterization of Malignant T Cells from Lymphoblastic Lymphoma Using Monoclonal Antibodies: Evidence of Phenotypic Differences Between Malignant T Cells from Patients with Acute Lymphoblastic Leukemia and Lymphoblastic Lymphoma. *Blood* 57, 1105–1110.

Bessis, M. (1973) *Living Blood Cells and Their Ultrastructure.* Springer-Verlag (New York), 767.

Biester, H. E., and McNutt, S. H. (1926) A Case of Lymphoid Leukemia in the Pig. *J. Amer. Vet. Med. Assoc.* 69, 762–768.

Blanchard, L., Poisson, J., and Drieux, H. (1939) Pathologie comparée des tumeurs du thymus. Son intérêt pour l'Histogénèse. *Rec. Méd. Vét.* 115, 129–153.

Bloom, F. (1946) Intramedullary Plasma Cell Myeloma Occurring Spontaneously in a Dog. *Cancer Res.* 6, 718–722.

Bloom, F., and Meyer, L. M. (1945) Malignant Lymphoma (So-Called Leukemia) in Dogs. *Amer. J. Path.* 21, 683–715.

Bolle, W. (1950) Zur Pathologie des tierischen Fetus. *Berl. Münch. Tierärztl. Wschr.* 1, 14–15.

Bostock, D. E., and Owen, L. N. (1973) Porcine and Ovine Lymphosarcoma: A Review. *J. Nat. Cancer Inst.* 50, 933–939.

Bowler, G. E. (1948) Malignant Neoplasm (Lymphoblastoma) of the Liver in a Hog. *J. Amer. Vet. Med. Assoc.* 113, 557–558.

Bowles, C. A., White, G. S., and Lucas, D. (1975) Rosette Formation by Canine Peripheral Blood Lymphocytes. *J. Immunol.* 144, 399–402.

Braund, K. G., Everett, R. M., and Albert, R. A. (1978) Neurological Manifestations of Monoclonal IgM Gammopathy Associated with Lymphocytic Leukemia in a Dog. *J. Amer. Vet. Med. Assoc.* 172, 1407–1410.

Brown, N. O., Nesbitt, G. H., Patnaik, A. K., and MacEwen, E. G. (1980) Cutaneous Lymphosarcoma in the Dog: A Disease with Variable Clinical and Histologic Manifestations. *J. Amer. Anim. Hosp. Assoc.* 16, 565–572.

Broxmeyer, H. E., Grossbard, E., Jacobsen, N., and Moore, M. A. S. (1979) Persistence of Inhibiting Activity Against Normal Bone-Marrow Cells During Remission of Acute Leukemia. *N. Engl. J. Med.* 301, 346–351.

Brumbaugh, G. W., Stitzel, K. A., Zinkl, J. G., and Feldman, B. F. (1982) Myelomonocytic Myeloproliferative Disease in a Horse. *J. Amer. Vet. Med. Assoc.* 180, 313–316.

Bunn, P. A., and Poiesz, B. J. (1983) Cutaneous T-Cell Lymphomas (Mycosis Fungoides and Sézary Syndrome). In: Williams, W. J., Beutler, E., Erslev, A. J., and Lichtman, M. A., eds. *Hematology.* 3d ed. McGraw-Hill (New York), 1056–1066.

Burkhardt, R., Alder, S. S., Conley, C. L., Pincus, T., Lennert, K., and Till, J. E. (1975) *Dahlem Workshop on Myelofibrosis–Osteosclerosis Syndrome.* Vieweg (Braunschweig), 1–330.

Burny, A., Bruck, C., Chantrenne, H., Cleuter, Y., Dekegel, D., Ghysdael, J., Kettman, R., Leclercq, M., Leunen, J., Mammerickx, M., and Portetelle, D. (1980) Bovine Leukemia Virus: Molecular Biology and Epidemiology. In: Klein, G., ed., *Viral Oncology.* Raven Press (New York), 231–289.

Burridge, M. J., Puhr, D. M., and Hennemann, J. M. (1982) Epidemiological Study of Bovine Leukaemia Virus Infection in Florida. In: Straub, O. C., ed., *Fourth International Symposium on Bovine Leukosis.* Martinus Nijhoff Publishers (The Hague, Boston, London), 373–380.

Butler, J. J. (1975) The Natural History of Hodgkin's Disease and its Classification. In: Rebuck, J. W., Berard, C. W., and Abell, M. R., eds., *The Reticuloendothelial System.* International Academy Pathology Monograph. Williams and Wilkins (Baltimore), 184–212.

Caciolo, P. L., Hayes, A. A., Patnaik, A. K., Nesbitt, G. H., and Pack, F. D. (1983) A Case of Mycosis Fungoides in a Cat and Literature Review. *J. Amer. Anim. Hosp. Assoc.* 19, 505–512.

Cello, R. M., and Hutcherson, B. (1962) Ocular Changes in Malignant Lymphoma of Dogs. *Cornell Vet.* 52, 492–523.

Chapman, A. L., Bopp, W. J., Torres, J., and Cohen, H. (1981) An Electron Microscopic Study of the Cell Types in Canine Lymphoma and Leukaemia. *J. Comp. Path.* 91, 331–340.

Chessells, J. M. (1982) Acute Lymphoblastic Leukemia. *Sem. Hemat.* 19, 155–171.

Chevrel, M. L., Rénier, F., Richier, M. E., Ramée, M. P., and Tréguer, F. (1969) Le Lymphosarcome porcin. *Rec. Méd. Vét.* 145, 135–147.

Cohen, H., Chapman, A. L., Eberg, J. W., Bopp, W. J., and Gravelle, C. R. (1970). Cellular Transmission of Canine Lymphoma and Leukemia in Beagles. *J. Nat. Cancer Inst.* 45, 1013–1023.

Confer, A. W., Langloss, J. M., and Cashell, I. G. (1978) Long-Term Survival of Two Cats with Mastocytosis. *J. Amer. Vet. Med. Assoc.* 172, 160–161.

Conner, G. H., LaBelle, J. A., Langham, R. F., and Crittenden, M. (1966) Studies on the Epidemiology of Bovine Leukemia. *J. Nat. Cancer Inst.* 36, 383–388.

Coombs, J. W., Lagunoff, D., and Benditt, E. P. (1965) Differentiation and Proliferation of Embryonic Mast Cells of the Rat. *J. Cell Biol.* 25, 577–597.

Coons, F. H., George, J. W., and Appel, G. O. (1976) Reticuloendotheliosis in a Dog. *Cornell Vet.* 66, 249–257.

Cooper, B. J., and Watson, A. D. J. (1975) Myeloid Neoplasia in a Dog. *Aust. Vet. J.* 51, 150–154.

Cordes, D. O., and Shortridge, E. H. (1971) Neoplasms of Sheep: A Survey of 256 Cases Recorded at Ruakura Animal Health Laboratory. *N.Z. Vet. J.* 19, 55–64.

Cornelius, C. E., Goodbary, R. F., and Kennedy, P. C. (1959) Plasma Cell Myelomatosis in a Horse. *Cornell Vet.* 49, 478–493.

Cotchin, E. (1954) Further Observations on Neoplasms in Dogs, with Particular Reference to Site of Origin and Malignancy. I. Cutaneous, Female Genital and Alimentary Systems. II. Male Genital, Skeletal, Lymphatic and Other Systems. *Brit. Vet. J.* 110, 218–232, 274–286.

———. (1956) Further Examples of Spontaneous Neoplasms in the Domestic Cat. *Brit. Vet. J.* 112, 263–272.

Cotter, S. M. (1979) Anemia Associated with Feline Leukemia Virus Infection. *J. Amer. Vet. Med. Assoc.* 175, 1191–1194.

Cotter, S. M., and Essex, M. (1977) Animal Model: Feline Acute Lymphoblastic Leukemia and Aplastic Anemia. *Amer. J. Path.* 87, 265–268.

Crighton, G. W. (1968) The Haematology of Lymphosarcoma in the Cat. *Vet. Rec.* 82, 155–157.

Crow, S. E., Theilen, G. H., Benjamini, E., Torten, M., Henness, A. M., and Buhles, W. C. (1977) Chemoimmunotherapy for Canine Lymphosarcoma. *Cancer* 40(5), 2102–2108.

Dameshek, W. (1951) Some Speculations on the Myeloproliferative Syndromes. *Blood* 6, 372–375.

———. (1969) The DiGuglielmo Syndrome Revisited. *Blood* 34, 567–572.

Danelius, G. (1941) Leukosis in a Horse. *Cornell Vet.* 31, 314.

Davies, A. P., Hayden, D. W., Klausner, J. S., and Perman, V. (1981) Noncutaneous Systemic Mastocytosis and Mast Cell Leukemia in a Dog: Case Report and Literature Review. *J. Amer. Anim. Hosp. Assoc.* 17, 361–368.

De Schepper, J., Van Der Stock, J., and De Rick, A. (1974) Hypercalcaemia and Hypoglycaemia in a Case of Lymphatic Leukaemia in a Dog. *Vet. Rec.* 94, 602–603.

Dixon, R. J., and Moriarty, K. M. (1983) Alpha Napthyl Acetate Esterase Activity is Not a Specific Marker for Ovine T Lymphocytes. *Vet. Immun. Immunopath.* 4, 505–512.

Dobberstein, J., and Paarmann, E., (1934) Die Sogen. Lymphadenose des Rindes (Rinderleukose). *Z. Infekt.-Kr. Haust.* 46, 65–109.

Dockrell, H. M., Seymour, G. J., Playfair, J. H. L., and Greenspan, J. S. (1978) Cytochemical Identification of T and B Cells *in situ* in Mouse Lymphoid Tissue and Lymph Nodes from the Rat, Gerbil and Cat. *Ann. Immun. (Inst. Pasteur)* 129, 617–633.

Dorfman, R. F., and Warnke, R. (1974) Lymphadenopathy Simulating the Malignant Lymphomas. *Human Path.* 5, 519–550.

Dorn, C. R., Taylor, D. O. N., and Hibbard, H. H. (1967) Epizootiologic Characteristics of Canine and Feline Leukemia and Lymphoma. *Amer. J. Vet. Res.* 28, 993–1001.

Drieux, H., and Priouzeau, M. (1945) Les tumeurs du thymus chez les bovidés. *Bull. Acad. Vét. Fr.* 18, 137–153.

Duncan, J. R., and Prasse, K. W. (1976) Clinical Examination of Bone Marrow. *Vet. Clin. N. Amer.* 6, 597–608.

Dungworth, D. L., Goldman, M., Switzer, J. W., and McKelvie, D. H. (1969) Development of a Myeloproliferative Disorder in Beagles Continuously Exposed to $^{90}$Sr. *Blood* 34, 610–632.

Dungworth, D. L., Theilen, G. H., and Lengyel, J. (1964) Bovine Lymphosarcoma in California. II. The Thymic Form. *Path. Vet.* 1, 323–350.

Dungworth, D. L., Theilen, G. H., and Ward, J. M. (1968) Early Detection of the Lesions of Bovine Lymphosarcoma. In: Bendixen, H. J., ed., *Leukemia in Animals and Man.* Proceedings of the Third International Symposium on Comparative Leukemia Research, 1967. *Bibl. Haemat.* 30, 206–211.

Engelbreth-Holm, J. (1942) *Spontaneous and Experimental Leukemia in Animals.* Oliver and Boyd (Edinburgh and London).

Enke, K.-H., Jungnitz, M., and Rössger, M. (1961) Ein kasuisticher Beitrag zur lymphatischen Leukose des Schafes. *Dtsch. Tierärztl. Wschr.* 68, 359–364.

Essex, M. E. (1982) Feline Leukemia: Naturally Occurring Cancer of Infectious Origin. *Epidem. Rev.* 4, 189–203.

Essex, M. E., and Snyder, S. P. (1973) Feline Oncornavirus-Associated Cell Membrane Antigen. I. Serologic Studies with Kittens Exposed to Cell-free Materials from Various Feline Fibrosarcomas. *J. Nat. Cancer Inst.* 51, 1007–1012.

Farrow, B. R. H., and Penney, R. (1971) Multiple Myeloma in a Cat. *J. Amer. Vet. Med. Assoc.* 158, 606–613.

Feldman, B. F., Madewell, B. R., and Miller, R. B. (1981) Serum Lysozyme (Muramidase) Activity in Dogs with Neoplastic Disease. *Amer. J. Vet. Res.* 42, 1319–1321.

Ferrer, J. F., Marshak, R. R., Abt, D. A., and Kenyon, S. J. (1979) Relationship Between Lymphosarcoma and Persistent Lymphocytosis in Cattle: A Review. *J. Amer. Vet. Med. Assoc.* 175, 705–708.

Fialkow, P. J. (1982) Cell Lineages in Hematopoietic Neoplasia Studied with Glucose-6-Phosphate Dehydrogenase Cell Markers. *J. Cell. Phys. Suppl.* 1, 37–43.

Fishman, R. S., Fleming, R. C., and Li, C. Y. (1979) Systemic Mastocytosis with Review of Gastrointestinal Manifestations. *Mayo Clin. Proc.* 54, 51–54.

Flecknell, P. A., Gibbs, C., and Kelly, D. F. (1978) Myelosclerosis in a Cat. *J. Comp. Path.* 88, 627–631.

Forbus, W. D., and Davis, C. L. (1946) A Chronic Granulomatous Disease of Swine with Striking Resemblance to Hodgkin's Disease. *Amer. J. Path.* 22, 35–37.

Fortner, J. (1944) Untersuchungen uber die Rinderleukose. *Z. Infekt.-Kr. Haust.* 60, 215–233.

Fowler, E. H., Wilson, G. P., Roengk, W. J., and Koestner, A. (1966) Mast Cell Leukemia in Three Dogs. *J. Amer. Vet. Med. Assoc.* 149, 281–285.

Fowler, M. E., Cornelius, C. E., and Baker, N. F. (1964) Clinical and Erythrokinetic Studies on a Case of Bovine Polycythemia Vera. *Cornell Vet.* 54, 153–160.

Fraser, C. J., Joiner, G. N., Jardine, J. H., and Gleiser, C. A. (1974) Acute Granulocytic Leukemia in Cats. *J. Amer. Vet. Med. Assoc.* 165, 355–359.

Frazier, M. E., Ushijima, R. N., and Pratt, J. R. (1972) Characterization of C Type Virus Isolated from Leukemic Swine. In: *Abstracts of the Annual Meeting of the American Society for Microbiology.* 72d Annual Meeting, Philadelphia. American Society of Microbiology (Washington, D.C.).

Fujimoto, Y., Miller, J., and Olson, C. (1969) The Fine Structure of Lymphosarcoma in Cattle. *Path. Vet.* 6, 15–29.

Gaedicke, G., and Drexler, H. G. (1982) The Use of Enzyme Marker Analysis for Subclassification of Acute Lymphoblastic Leukemia in Childhood. *Leuk. Res.* 6, 437–448.

Gale, R. P. (1979) Advances in the Treatment of Acute Myelogenous Leukemia. *N. Engl. J. Med.* 300, 1189–1199.

Garner, F. M., and Lingeman, C. H. (1970) Mast Cell Neoplasms of the Domestic Cat. *Path. Vet.* 7, 517–530.

Gaus, O. (1939) Leukose des Gesäuges beim Schwein. *Dtsch. Tierärztl. Wschr.* 47, 340–342.

Gilmore, C. E., and Holzworth, J. (1971) Naturally Occurring Feline Leukemia: Clinical, Pathologic, and Differential Diagnostic Features. *J. Amer. Vet. Med. Assoc.* 158, 1013–1025.

Gilmore, C. E., Gilmore, V. H., and Jones, T. C. (1964) Reticuloendotheliosis, a Myeloproliferative Disorder of Cats: A Comparison with Lymphocytic Leukemia. *Path. Vet.* 1, 161–183.

Glick, A. D., Horn, R. G., and Holscher, M. (1978) Characterization of Feline Glomerulonephritis Associated with Viral-induced Hematopoietic Neoplasms. *Amer. J. Path.* 92, 321–332.

Götze, R., Ziegenhagen, G., and Merkt, H. (1953) Zur Diagnose der Leukose des Rindes. *Mh. Tierheilk,* 5, 201–211.

Green, P. D., and Donovan, L. A. (1977) Lymphosarcoma in a Horse. *Can. Vet. J.* 18, 257–258.

Grewal, A. S., Rouse, B. T., and Babiak, L. A. (1976) Erythrocyte Rosettes—A Marker for Bovine T Cells. *Can. J. Comp. Med.* 40, 298–304.

Groopman, J. E., and Golde, D. W. (1981) The Histiocytic Disorders: A Pathophysiologic Analysis. *Ann. Intern Med.* 94, 95–107.

Grüttner, F. (1927) Lymphomatose beim Schwein. *Z. Fleish-U. Milchhyg.* 37, 154–155.

Hadlow, W. J. (1978) High Prevalence of Thymoma in the Dairy Goat. *Vet. Path.* 15, 153–169.

Hall, G. A., Howell, J. M., and Lewis, D. G. (1972) Thymoma with Myasthenia Gravis in a Dog. *J. Path.* 108, 177–180.

Hardy, W. D., Jr. (1981a) Feline Leukemia Virus Nonneoplastic Diseases. *J. Amer. Anim. Hosp. Assoc.* 17, 941–949.

———. (1981b) Hematopoietic Tumors of Cats. *J. Amer. Anim. Hosp. Assoc.* 17, 921–940.

———. (1981c) The Feline Leukemia Virus. *J. Amer. Anim. Hosp. Assoc.* 17, 951–980.

Hardy, W. D., Jr., McLelland, A. J., MacEwen, E. G., Hess, P. W., Hayes, A. A., and Zuckerman, E. E. (1977) The Epidemiology of the Feline Leukemia Virus. *Cancer* 39, Supplement, 1850–1855.

Hare, W. C. D., McFeely, R. A., Abt, D. A., and Feierman, J. R. (1964) Chromosomal Studies in Bovine Lymphosarcoma. *J. Nat. Cancer Inst.* 33, 105–118.

Hartsock, R. J. (1975) Reactive Lesions in Lymph Nodes. In: Rebuck, J. W., Berard, C. W., and Abell, M. R., eds., *The Reticuloendothelial System.* International Academy Pathology Monograph. Williams and Wilkins (Baltimore), 152–183.

Harvey, J. W. (1981) Myeloproliferative Disorders in Dogs and Cats. *Vet. Clin. N. Amer. Small Anim. Pract.* 11, 349–381.

Harvey, J. W., Henderson, C. W., French, T. W., and Meyer, D. J. (1982) Myeloproliferative Disease with Megakaryocytic Predominance in a Dog with Occult Dirofilariasis. *Vet. Clin. Path.* 11, 5–11.

Harvey, J. W., Shields, R. P., and Gaskin, J. M. (1978) Feline Myeloproliferative Disease: Changing Manifestations in the Peripheral Blood. *Vet. Path.* 15, 437–448.

Harvey, J. W., Terrell, T. G., Hyde, D. M., and Jackson, R. I. (1981) Well-Differentiated Lymphocytic Leukemia in a Dog: Long-Term Survival Without Therapy. *Vet. Path.* 18, 37–47.

Hatanaka, K., Kitamura, Y., and Nishimune, Y. (1979) Local Development of Mast Cells from Bone Marrow in the Skin of Mice. *Blood* 53, 142–147.

Hatziolos, B. C. (1960) Lymphoblastic Lymphoma in a Bovine Fetus. *J. Amer. Vet. Med. Assoc.* 136, 368–375.

Hendrick, M. (1981) A Spectrum of Hypereosinophilic Syndromes Exemplified by Six Cats with Eosinophilic Enteritis. *Vet. Path.* 18, 188–200.

Henness, A. M., and Crow, S. E. (1977) Treatment of Feline Myelogenous Leukemia: Four Case Reports. *J. Amer. Vet. Med. Assoc.* 171, 263–266.

Henness, A. M., Crow, S. E., and Anderson, B. C. (1977) Monocytic Leukemia in Three Cats. *J. Amer. Vet. Med. Assoc.* 170, 1325–1328.

Herz, A., Theilen, G. H., Schalm, O. W., and Munn, R. J. (1969) C-Type Virus Particles Demonstrated in Bone Marrow Cells of the Cat with Myeloproliferative Disease. *Calif. Vet.* 23(4), 16–19.

Hill, R. R. H., and Clatworthy, R. H. (1971) Macroglobulinaemia in the Dog, the Canine Analogue of Gamma M Monoclonal Gammopathy, *J. S. Afr. Vet. Med. Assoc.* 42, 309–313.

Hirsch, V. M., Searcy, G. P., and Bellamy, J. E. C. (1982) Comparison of ELISA and Immunofluorescent Antigens in Blood of Cats. *J. Amer. Anim. Hosp. Assoc.* 18, 933–938.

Hodgkins, E. M., Zinkl, J. G., and Madewell, B. R. (1980) Chronic Lymphocytic Leukemia in the Dog. *J. Amer. Vet. Med. Assoc.* 177, 704–707.

Hoerni, B., Legrand, E., and Chauvergne, J. (1970) Les Réticulopathies. Animales de type hodgkinien. *Bull. Cancer* 57, 37–54.

Holmberg, C. A., Manning, J. S., and Osburn, B. I. (1976a) Canine Malignant Lymphomas: Comparison of Morphologic and Immunologic Parameters. *J. Natl. Cancer Inst.* 56, 125–135.

———. (1976b) Feline Malignant Lymphomas: Comparison of Morphologic and Immunologic Characteristics. *Amer. J. Vet. Res.* 37, 1455–1460.

Holmes, D. D., Brock, W. E., Tennille, N. B., and Rice, W. M. (1964) Myelosarcoma (Plasma-Cell Type) in a Dog. *J. Amer. Vet. Med. Assoc.* 145, 234–240.

Holscher, M. A., Collins, R. D., Glick, A. D., and Griffith, B. O. (1978) Megakaryocytic Leukemia in a Dog. *Vet. Path.* 15, 562–565.

Holzworth, J. (1960a) Leukemia and Related Neoplasms in the Cat. I. Lymphoid Malignancies. *J. Amer. Vet. Med. Assoc.* 136, 47–69.

———. (1960b) Leukemia and Related Neoplasms in the Cat. II. Malignancies Other Than Lymphoid. *J. Amer. Vet. Med. Assoc.* 136, 107–121.

———. (1963) Neoplasia of Blood-Forming Organs in Cats. *Ann. N.Y. Acad. Sci.* 108, 691–701.

Holzworth, J., and Meier, H. (1957) Reticulum Cell Myeloma in a Cat. *Cornell Vet.* 47, 302–316.

Holzworth, J., and Nielsen, S. W. (1955) Visceral Lymphosarcoma of the Cat. II. *J. Amer. Vet. Med. Assoc.* 126, 26–36.

Hoover, E. A., and Kociba, G. J. (1974) Bone Lesions in Cats with Anemia Induced by Feline Leukemia Virus. *J. Natl. Cancer Inst.* 53, 1277–1284.

Hottendorf, G. H., and Nielsen, S. W. (1968) Pathologic Report of 29 Necropsies on Dogs with Mastocytoma. *Path. Vet.* 5, 102–121.

Howard, E. B., and Clarke, W. J. (1970) Strontium-90-Induced Hematopoietic Neoplasms in Miniature Swine. In: Clarke, W. J., Howard, E. B., and Hackett, P. L., eds., *Myeloproliferative Disorders of Animals and Man.* Proceedings of the Eighth Annual Hanford Biology Symposium, Richland, Washington, 1968. U.S. Atomic Energy Commission, Division of Technical Information, U.S.A., 379–401.

Howard, E. B., Sawa, T. R., Neilsen, S. W., and Kenyon, A. J. (1969) Mastocytoma and Gastrointestinal Ulceration. *Path. Vet.* 6, 146–158.

Hugoson, G. (1967) Juvenile Bovine Leukosis: An Epizootiological, Clinical, Patho-Anatomical and Experimental Study. *Acta Vet. Scand. Suppl.* 22, 1–108.

Hurvitz, A. I. (1970) Fine Structure of Cells from a Cat with Myeloproliferative Disorder. *Amer. J. Vet. Res.* 31, 747–753.

Hurvitz, A. I., Haskins, S. C., and Fischer, C. A. (1970) Macroglobulinemia with Hyperviscosity Syndrome in a Dog. *J. Amer. Vet. Med. Assoc.* 157, 455–460.

Hurvitz, A. I., Kehoe, J. M., Capra, J. D., and Prata, R. (1971) Bence–Jones Proteinemia and Proteinuria in a Dog. *J. Amer. Vet. Med. Assoc.* 159, 1112–1116.

Hyde, J. L., King, J. M., and Bentinck-Smith, J. (1958) A Case of Bovine Myelogenous Leukemia. *Cornell Vet.* 48, 269–276.

Innes, D. J., Mills, S. E., and Walker, G. K. (1982) Megakaryocytic Leukemia. Identification Utilizing Anti-Factor VIII Immunoperoxidase. *Amer. J. Clin. Path.* 77, 107–110.

Ishizaka, T., Okudaira, H., Mauser, L. E., and Ishizaka, K. (1976) Development of Rat Mast Cells *in Vitro.* Differentiation of Mast Cells from Thymus Cells. *J. Immunol.* 116, 747–754.

Jain, N. C. (1970) A Comparative Study of Leukocytes of Some Animal Species. *Folia Hemat.* 94, 49–63.

———. (1971) Alkaline Phosphatase Activity in Leukocytes of Dogs and Cats. *Blut* 22, 133–143.

Jain, N. C., Madewell, B. R., Weller, R. E., and Geissler, M. C. (1981) Clinical-Pathological Findings and Cytochemical Characterization of Myelomonocytic Leukemia. *J. Comp. Path.* 91, 17–31.

Järplid, B. (1964) Studies on the Site of Leukotic and Preleukotic Changes in the Bovine Heart. *Path. Vet.* 1, 366–408.

Jarrett, W. F. H., and Mackey, L. J. (1974) Neoplastic Diseases of the Haematopoietic and Lymphoid Tissues. *Bull. Wld. Hlth. Org.* 50, 21–34.

Jarrett, W. F. H., Anderson, L. J., Jarrett, O., Laird, H. M., and Stewart, M. F. (1971) Myeloid Leukaemia in a Cat Produced by Feline Leukaemia Virus. *Res. Vet. Sci.* 12, 385–387.

Jarrett, W. F. H., Crawford, E. M., Martin, W. B., and Davie, F. (1964a) Leukaemia in the Cat: A Virus-like Particle Associated with Leukaemia (Lymphosarcoma). *Nature* 202, 567–568.

Jarrett, W. F. H., Crighton, G. W., and Dalton, R. G. (1966) Leukaemia and Lymphosarcoma in Animals and Man. I. Lymphosarcoma or Leukaemia in the Domestic Animals. *Vet. Rec.* 79, 693–699.

Jarrett, W. F. H., Martin, W. B., Crighton, G. W., Dalton, R. G., and Stewart, M. F. (1964b) Leukaemia in the Cat: Transmission Experiments with Leukaemia (Lymphosarcoma). *Nature* 202, 566–567.

Jennings, A. R. (1953) Blood and Visceral Changes in Canine Leukaemia (Lymphadenosis). *J. Comp. Path.* 63, 85–92.

Johnstone, A. C. (1974) *Malignant Lymphomas in Sheep.* Ph.D. Thesis, Massey University. Palmerston, North, New Zealand.

Joiner, G. N., Fraser, C. J., Jardine, J. H., and Trujillo, J. M. (1976) A Case of Chronic Granulocytic Leukemia in a Dog. *Can. J. Comp. Med.* 40, 153–160.

Jolly, R. D. (1967) Nodular Hyperplasia of the Ovine Spleen, *N.Z. Vet. J.* 15, 91–94.

Kadin, M. E., Kamoun, M., and Lamberg, J. (1981) Erythrophagocytic Tγ Lymphoma: A Clinicopathologic Entity Resembling Malignant Histiocytosis. *N. Engl. J. Med.* 304, 648–653.

Kajikawa, O., Koyama, H., Yoshikawa, T., Tsubaki, S., and Saito, H. (1983) Use of Alpha Napthyl Acetate Esterase Staining to Identify T Lymphocytes in Cattle. *Amer. J. Vet. Res.* 44, 1549–1552.

Kakuk, T. J., Hinz, R. W., Langham, R. F., and Conner, G. H. (1968) Experimental Transmission of Canine Malignant Lymphoma to the Beagle Neonate. *Cancer Res.* 28, 716–723.

Kammermann, B., Pflugshaupt, R., and Stunzi, H. (1969) Beobachtungen am Plasmozytom des Hundes (Plasmacytoma in the Dog). *Schweiz. Arch. Tierheilk.* 111, 555–586.

Katzke, D. (1935) Die fetale Leukämie des Rindes. *Z. Infekt.-Kr. Haust.* 47, 161–165.

Kelly, D. F., Halliwell, R. E. W., and Schwartzman, R. M. (1972) Generalized Cutaneous Eruption in a Dog, with Histologic Similarity to Human Mycosis Fungoides. *Brit. J. Dermatol.* 86, 164–171.

Kettmann, R., Portetelle, D., Mammerickx, M., Cleuter, Y., Dekegel, D., Galoux, M., Ghysdael, J., Burny, A., and Chantrenne, H. (1976) Bovine Leukemia Virus: An Exogenous RNA Oncogenic Virus. *Proc. Nat. Acad. Sci.* 73, 1014–1018.

Knocke, K.-W. (1964) Elektronenmikroskopische Befunde an Lymphknoten und Lymphoidzellen des peripherischen Blutes bei der Leukose des Rindes. *Zbl. Vet. Med.* 11B, 1–10.

Koeffler, H. P., and Golde, D. W. (1981) Chronic Myelogenous Leukemia. New Concepts. *N. Eng. J. Med.* 304, 1201–1209.

Larson, V. L., Sorensen, D. K., and Perman, V. (1970) Epizootiologic Studies on the Natural Transmission of Bovine Leukemia. *Amer. J. Vet. Res.* 31, 1533–1538.

Lattes, R. (1962) Thymoma and Other Tumors of the Thymus: An Analysis of 107 Cases. *Cancer* 15, 1224–1260.

Legendre, A. M., and Becker, P. U. (1979) Feline Skin Lymphoma: Characterization of Tumor and Identification of Tumor-stimulating Serum Factor(s). *Amer. J. Vet. Res.* 40, 1805–1807.

Leifer, C. E., Matus, R. E., Patnaik, A. K., and MacEwen, E. G. (1983) Chronic Myelogenous Leukemia in the Dog. *J. Amer. Vet. Med. Assoc.* 183, 686–689.

Lester, S. J., and Searcy, G. P. (1981) Hematologic Abnormalities Preceding Apparent Recovery from Feline Leukemia Virus Infection. *J. Amer. Vet. Med. Assoc.* 178, 471–474.

Lester, S. J., McGonigle, L. F., and McDonald, G. K. (1981) Disseminated Anaplastic Mastocytoma with

Terminal Mastocythemia in a Dog. *J. Amer. Anim. Hosp. Assoc.* 17, 355–360.

Lewis, H. B., and Leitch, M. (1975) A Case of Granulocytic Leukemia in a Horse. In: Kitchen, H., and Krehbiel, J. D., eds., *Proceedings of the First International Symposium on Equine Hematology.* American Association of Equine Practitioners (Golden, Colorado), 141–143.

Li, C. Y., Lam, K. W., and Yam, L. T. (1973) Esterases in Human Leukocytes. *J. Histochem. Cytochem.* 22, 1–12.

Linman, J. W., and Bagby, G. C. (1976) The Preleukemic Syndrome: Clinical and Laboratory Features, Natural Course, and Management. *Blood Cells* 2, 11–31.

Linnabary, R. D., Holscher, M. A., Glick, A. D., Powell, H. S., and McCollum, H. M. (1978) Acute Myelomonocytic Leukemia in a Dog. *J. Amer. Anim. Hosp. Assoc.* 14, 71–75.

Liska, W. D., MacEwen, E. G., Zaki, F. A., and Garvey, M. (1979) Feline Systemic Mastocytosis: A Review and Results of Splenectomy in Seven Cats. *J. Amer. Anim. Hosp. Assoc.* 15, 589–597.

Liu, S., and Carb, A. V. (1968) Erythroblastic Leukemia in a Dog. *J. Amer. Vet. Med. Assoc.* 152, 1511–1516.

Loeb, W. F., Lamont, P. H., and Capen, C. C. (1970) Monocytic Leukemia in a Dog. In: Clarke, W. J., Howard, E. B., and Hackett, P. L., eds., *Myeloproliferative Disorders of Animals and Man.* Proceedings of the Eighth Annual Hanford Biology Symposium, Richland, Washington, 1968. U.S. Atomic Energy Commission, Division of Technical Information, U.S.A., 687–702.

Loeb, W. F., Rininger, B., Montgomery, C. A., and Jenkins, S. (1975) Myelomonocytic Leukemia in a Cat. *Vet. Path.* 12, 464–467.

Lombard, L. S., Moloney, J. B., and Rickard, C. G. (1963) The Transmission of Canine Mastocytoma. *Ann. N.Y. Acad. Sci.* 108, 1086–1105.

Lübke, A. (1944) Zur Pathologie der Rinderleukose. Ihre Stellung als Geschwulstkrankheit des Reticuloendothelialen Gewebes. *Virchows Arch.* 312, 190–229.

Lukes, R. J., and Collins, R. D. (1974) Immunologic Characterization of Human Malignant Lymphomas. *Cancer* 34, 1488–1503.

Lund, L. (1924) Die lymphatische Leukämie des Schweines. *Dtsch. Tierärztl. Wschr.* 32, 368–373.

MacEwen, E. G., and Hurvitz, A. I. (1977) Diagnosis and Management of Monoclonal Gammopathies. *Vet. Clin. N. Amer.* 7, 119–132.

MacEwen, E. G., Drazner, F. H., McClelland, A. J., and Wilkins, R. J. (1975) Treatment of Basophilic Leukemia in a Dog. *J. Amer. Vet. Med. Assoc.* 166, 376–380.

MacEwen, E. G., Hurvitz, A. I., and Hayes, A. (1977a) Hyperviscosity Syndrome Associated with Lymphocytic Leukemia in Three Dogs. *J. Amer. Vet. Med. Assoc.* 170, 1309–1312.

MacEwen, E. G., Patnaik, A. K., Hayes, A. A., Wilkins, R. J., Hardy, W. D., Kassel, R. L., and Old, L. J. (1981)

Temporary Plasma-induced Remission of Lymphoblastic Leukemia in a Dog. *Amer. J. Vet. Res.* 42, 1450–1452.

MacEwen, E. G., Patnaik, A. K., Hurvitz, A. I., Bradley, R., Claypoole, T. F., Withrow, S. J., Erlandson, R. A., and Lieberman, P. H. (1984a) Nonsecretory Multiple Myeloma in Two Dogs. *J. Amer. Vet. Med. Assoc.* 184, 1283–1286.

MacEwen, E. G., Patnaik, A. K., Johnson, G. F., Hurvitz, A. I., Erlandson, R. A., and Lieberman, P. H. (1984b) Extramedullary Plasmacytoma of the Gastrointestinal Tract in Two Dogs. *J. Amer. Vet. Med. Assoc.* 184, 1396–1398.

MacEwen, E. G., Patnaik, A. K., and Wilkins, R. J. (1977b) Diagnosis and Treatment of Canine Hematopoietic Neoplasms. *Vet. Clin. N. Amer.* 7, 105–132.

Mackey, L. J., and Jarrett, W. F. H. (1972) Pathogenesis of Lymphoid Neoplasis in Cats and Its Relationship to Immunologic Cell Pathways. I. Morphologic Aspects. *J. Nat. Cancer Inst.* 49, 853–865.

———. (1975) Two Populations of Lymphocytes in the Cat. *Vet. Rec.* 96, 41.

Mackey, L., Jarrett, W., Jarrett, O., and Laird, H. (1975a) Anemia Associated with Feline Leukemia Virus Infection in Cats. *J. Natl. Cancer Inst.* 54, 209–217.

Mackey, L. J., Jarrett, W. F. H., and Lauder, I. M. (1975b) Monocytic Leukaemia in the Dog. *Vet. Rec.* 96, 27–30.

Macklin, A. W., and Miller, L. D. (1971) Disseminated Malignant Lymphoma in a Bovine Fetus. *Cornell Vet.* 61, 310–319.

Madewell, B. R. (1975) Chemotherapy for Canine Lymphosarcoma. *Amer. J. Vet. Res.* 36, 1525–1528.

Madewell, B. R., and Feldman, B. F. (1980) Characterization of Anemias Associated with Neoplasia in Small Animals. *J. Amer. Vet. Med. Assoc.* 176, 419–425.

Madewell, B. R., Carlson, G. P., MacLachlan, N. J., and Feldman, B. F. (1982) Lymphosarcoma with Leukemia in a Horse. *Amer. J. Vet. Res.* 43, 807–812.

Madewell, B. R., Jain, N. C., and Weller, R. E. (1979) Hematologic Abnormalities Preceding Myeloid Leukemia in Three Cats. *Vet. Path.* 16, 510–519.

Maggio, L., Hoffman, R., Cotter, S. M., Dainiak, N., Mooney, S., and Maffei, L. A. (1978) Feline Preleukemia: An Animal Model of Human Disease. *Yale J. Biol. Med.* 51, 469–476.

Mammerickx, M. (1970) Sur l'utilisation du mouton pour les expériences sur la leucose bovine. *Exp. Anim.* 3, 285–293.

Mann, R. B., Jaffe, E. S., and Berard, C. W. (1979) Malignant Lymphomas—A Conceptual Understanding of Morphologic Diversity. *Amer. J. Path.* 94, 105–192.

Mantovani, M. (1951) I Cancri del timo in patologia comparata. *Profilassi* 24, 85–91.

Marshak, R. R., Coriell, L. L., Lawrence, W. C., Croshaw, J. E., Jr., Schryver, H. F., Altera, K. P., and Nichols, W. W. (1962) Studies on Bovine Lymphosarcoma. I. Clinical Aspects, Pathological Alterations, and Herd Studies. *Cancer Res.* 22, 202–217.

Marshak, R. R., Hare, W. C. D., Abt, D. A., Croshaw, J. E., Jr., Switzer, J. W., Ipsen, I., Dutcher, R. M., and Martin, J. E. (1963) Occurrence of Lymphocytosis in Dairy Cattle Herds with High Incidence of Lymphosarcoma. *Ann. New York Acad. Sci.* 108, 1284–1301.

Marshak, R. R., Hare, W. C. D., Dutcher, R. M., Schwartzman, R. M., Switzer, J. W., and Hubben, K. (1966) Observations on a Heifer with Cutaneous Lymphosarcoma. *Cancer* 19, 724–734.

Matus, R. E., Leifer, C. E., and MacEwen, E. G. (1983) Acute Lymphoblastic Leukemia in a Dog: A Review of 30 Cases. *J. Amer. Vet. Med. Assoc.* 183, 859–862.

McGrath, C. J. (1974) Polycythemia Vera in Dogs. *J. Amer. Vet. Med. Assoc.* 164, 1117–1122.

McKeever, P. J., Grindem, C. B., Steven, J. B., and Osborne, C. A. (1982) Canine Cutaneous Lymphoma. *J. Amer. Vet. Med. Assoc.* 180, 531–536.

McTaggart, H. S., Head, K. W., and Laing, A. H. (1971) Evidence for a Genetic Factor in the Transmission of Spontaneous Lymphosarcoma (Leukaemia) of Young Pigs. *Nature* 232, 557–558.

Medway, W., and Rapp, J. P. (1962) A Case of Chronic Granulocytic Leukemia with Thrombocytopenia in a Dog. *Cornell Vet.* 52, 247–260.

Medway, W., Weber, W. T., O'Brien, J. A., and Krawitz, L. (1967) Multiple Myeloma in a Dog. *J. Amer. Vet. Med. Assoc.* 150, 386–395.

Meier, H. (1957) Neoplastic Diseases of the Hematopoietic System (So-Called Leukosis Complex) in the Dog. *Zbl. Vet. Med.* 4, 633–688.

Meincke, J. E., Hobbie, W. V., and Hardy, W. D. (1972) Lymphoreticular Malignancies in the Cat. *J. Amer. Vet. Med. Assoc.* 160, 1093–1100.

Mettam, A. E. (1915) A Case of Lymphosarcoma in the Horse: Arteriosclerotic Changes in Heart and Lungs. *J. Comp. Path.* 28, 36–43.

Michel, R. L., O'Handley, P., and Dade, A. W. (1976) Megakaryocytic Myelosis in a Cat. *J. Amer. Vet. Med. Assoc.* 168, 1021–1025.

Migaki, G. (1969) Hematopoietic Neoplasms of Slaughter Animals. In: Lingeman, C. H., and Garner, F. M., eds., *Comparative Morphology of Hematopoietic Neoplasms*. National Cancer Institute Monograph 32. U.S. Government Printing Office (Washington, D.C.), 121–151.

Miles, C. P., Moldovanu, G., Miller, D. G., and Moore, A. (1970) Chromosome Analysis of Canine Lymphosarcoma: Two Cases Involving Probable Centric Fusion. *Amer. J. Vet. Res.* 31, 783–790.

Miller, J. M., and Olson, C. (1972) Precipitating Antibody to an Internal Antigen of the C-Type Virus Associated with Bovine Lymphosarcoma. *J. Nat. Cancer Inst.* 49, 1459–1461.

Miller, J. M., and Van der Maaten, M. J. (1979) Infectivity Test of Secretions and Excretions from Cattle Infected with Bovine Leukemia Virus. *J. Nat. Cancer Inst.* 62, 425–428.

Misdorp, W. (1965) Tumors in Newborn Animals. *Path. Vet.* 2, 328–343.

Misdorp, W., and Dodd, D. C. (1968) Lymfatische Leucose bij Runderen in Nederland: Een Histopathologische Studie [Bovine lymphatic leukosis in the Netherlands; a histopathological study]. *T. Diergeneesk.* 93, 943–952.

Miura, S., and Ohshima, K. (1967) Monocytic Leukemia in Cattle I. Cytologic Observations in Two Cases. *Jpn. J. Vet. Sci.* 29, 141–150.

Moldovanu, G., Moore, A. E., Friedman, M., and Miller, D. G. (1966) Cellular Transmission of Lymphosarcoma in Dogs. *Nature* 210, 1342–1343.

Monlux, A. W., Anderson, W. A., and Davis, C. L. (1956) A Survey of Tumors Occurring in Cattle, Sheep, and Swine. *Amer. J. Vet. Res.* 17, 646–677.

Mori, Y., and Lennert, K. (1969) *Electron Microscopic Atlas of Lymph Node Cytology and Pathology.* Springer-Verlag (New York), 309.

Moulton, J. E., and Bostick, W. L. (1958) Canine Malignant Lymphoma Simulating Hodgkin's Disease in Man. *J. Amer. Vet. Med. Assoc.* 132, 204–209.

Mueller, J., Brun del Re, G., Buerki, H., Keller, H. U., Hess, M. W., and Cottier, H. (1975) Nonspecific Acid Esterase Activity: A Criterion for Differentiation of T and B Lymphocytes in Mouse Lymph Nodes. *Eur. J. Immun.* 5, 270–274.

Mulligan, R. M. (1949) *Neoplasms of the Dog.* Williams and Wilkins (Baltimore).

Muscoplat, C. C., Johnson, D. W., Pomeroy, K. A., Olson, J. M., Larson, V. L., Stevens, J. B., and Sorenson, D. K. (1974) Lymphocyte Subpopulations and Immunodeficiency in Calves with Acute Lymphocytic Leukemia. *Amer. J. Vet. Res.* 35, 1571–1573.

Nadler, L. M., Ritz, J., Griffin, J. D., Todd, R. F., Reinherz, E. L., and Schlossman, S. F. (1981) Diagnosis and Treatment of Human Leukemias and Lymphomas Utilizing Monoclonal Antibodies. *Prog. Hemat.* 12, 187–255.

Necheles, T. F. (1979) *The Acute Leukemias.* Stratton Intercontinental Medical Book Corporation (New York), 1–70.

Neufeld, J. L. (1973a) Lymphosarcoma in a Mare and Review of Cases at the Ontario Veterinary College, *Can. Vet. J.* 14, 149–153.

———. (1973b) Lymphosarcoma in the Horse: A Review. *Can. Vet. J.* 14, 129–135.

Nielsen, S. B., Piper, C. E., and Ferrer, J. F. (1978) Natural Mode of Transmission of the Bovine Leukemia Virus: Role of Blood-Sucking Insects. *Amer. J. Vet. Res.* 39, 1089–1092.

Nielsen, S. W. (1969) Spontaneous Hematopoietic Neoplasms of the Domestic Cat. In: Lingeman, C. H., and Garner, F. M., eds., *Comparative Morphology of Hematopoietic Neoplasms.* National Cancer Institute Monograph 32. U.S. Government Printing Office (Washington, D.C.), 73–94.

Nielsen, S. W. (1970) Myeloproliferative Disorders in Animals. In: Clarke, W. J., Howard, E. B., and Hackett, P. L., eds., *Myeloproliferative Disorders of Animals and Man.* Proceedings of the Eighth Annual Hanford Biology Symposium, Richland, Washington, 1968. U.S. Atomic Energy Commission, Division of Technical Information, U.S.A., 297–313.

Nielsen, S. W., and Holzworth, J. (1953) Visceral Lymphosarcoma of the Cat. *J. Amer. Vet. Med. Assoc.* 122, 189–197.

Niepage, H. (1953) Erhebungen über die Rinderleukose und Untersuchungen des Blutbildes. *Mh. Vet. Med.* 8, 21–25.

Olson, C., Hoss, H. E., Miller, J. M., and Baumgartener, L. E. (1973) Evidence of Bovine C-Type (Leukemia) Virus in Dairy Cattle. *J. Amer. Vet. Med. Assoc.* 163, 355–357.

Olson, C., Miller, J. M., Miller, L. D., and Gillette, K. G. (1970) C-Type Virus and Lymphocytic Nuclear Projections in Bovine Lymphosarcoma. *J. Amer. Vet. Med. Assoc.* 156, 1880–1883.

Olson, C., Miller, L. D., Miller, J. M., and Hoss, H. E. (1972) Transmission of Lymphosarcoma from Cattle to Sheep. *J. Nat. Cancer Inst.* 49, 1463–1467.

Olson, R. E., and Simon, J. (1967) Lymphocyte Counts of Lymphosarcoma-Free Hereford Cattle. *J. Amer. Vet. Med. Assoc.* 151, 1430–1434.

Onions, D. (1977) B- and T-Cell Markers on Canine Lymphosarcoma Cells. *J. Natl. Cancer Inst.* 59, 1001–1006.

———. (1980) RNA-Dependent DNA Polymerase Activity in Canine Lymphosarcoma. *Eur. J. Cancer* 16, 345–349.

Onions, D., Jarrett, O., Testa, N., Frassoni, F., and Toth, S. (1982) Selective Effect of Feline Leukaemia Virus on Early Erythroid Precursors. *Nature* 296, 156–158.

Onions, D. E., Owen, L. N., and Bostock, D. E. (1978) Leukocyte Migration Inhibition Responses in Canine Lymphosarcoma. *Int. J. Cancer* 22, 503–507.

Onuma, M., Ishihara, K., Ohtani, T., Honma, T., Mikami, T., and Izawa, H. (1979) Seroepizootiological Survey on Antibodies Against Bovine Leukemia Virus in Japanese Black Cattle. *Jpn. J. Vet. Sci.* 41, 601–605.

Onuma, M., Okada, K., Yamazaki, I., Fujinaga, K., Fujimoto, Y., and Mikami, T. (1978) Induction of C-Type Virus in Cell Lines Derived from Calf Form Bovine Lymphosarcoma. *Microbiol. Immunol.* 22, 683–691.

Osbaldiston, G. W., Sullivan, R. J., and Fox, A. (1978) Cytochemical Demonstration of Esterases in Peripheral Blood Leukocytes. *Amer. J. Vet. Res.* 39, 683–685.

Osborne, C. A., Perman, V., Sautter, J. H., Stevens, J. B., and Hanlon, G. F. (1968) Multiple Myeloma in the Dog. *J. Amer. Vet. Med. Assoc.* 153, 1300–1319.

Owen, L. N. (1971) Serial Transplantation of Canine Lymphocytic Leukaemia. *Europ. J. Cancer* 7, 525–528.

Pangalis, G. A., Waldman, S. R., and Rappaport, H. (1978) Cytochemical Finding in Human Nonneoplastic Blood and Tonsillar B and T Lymphocytes. *Amer. J. Clin. Path.* 69, 314–318.

Paulsen, J., Best, E., Frese, K., and Rudolph R., (1971) Enzootische lymphatische Leukose bei Schafen-Lymphozytose, pathologische Anatomie und Histologie. *Zbl. Vet. Med.* 18B, 33–43.

Paulsen, J., Rudolph, R., Hoffman, R., Weiss, E., and Schliesser, Th. (1972) C-Type Virus Particles in Phytohemagglutinin-Stimulated Lymphocyte Cultures with Reference to Enzootic Lymphatic Leukosis in Sheep. *Med. Microbiol. Immunol.* 158, 105–112.

Pedersen, N. C., Theilen, G., Keane, M. A., Fairbanks, L., Mason, T., Orser, B., Chen, C. H., and Allison, C. (1977) Studies of Naturally Transmitted Feline Leukemia Virus Infection. *Amer. J. Vet. Res.* 38, 1523–1531.

Pedini, B., and Romanelli, V. (1955) Il plasmocitoma negli animali domestici. Osservazioni e considerazioni su di un caso riscontrato nel vitello. *Arch. Vet. Ital.* 6, 193–214.

Peterson, M. E., and Randolph, J. F. (1982) Diagnosis of Canine Primary Polycythemia and Management with Hydroxyurea. *J. Amer. Vet. Med. Assoc.* 180, 415–418.

Pfeiffer, R. L., Jeraj, K., Mehlhoff, T., and O'Leary, T. P. (1976) Lymphosarcoma: Small Cell Type With Ocular Manifestations in a Dog. *Canine Pract.* 3, 50–54.

Pollet, L., Van Hove, W., and Mattheeuws, D. (1978) Blastic Crisis in Chronic Myelogenous Leukaemia in a Dog. *J. Small Anim. Pract.* 19, 469–475.

Prasse, K. W. (1977) Pyruvate Kinase Deficiency. In: Kirk, R. W., ed., *Current Veterinary Therapy VI. Small Animal Practice.* W. B. Saunders (Philadelphia), 434–435.

———. (1980) Clinical, Hematological and Postmorterm Findings in Feline Leukovirus Infected Cats: A Retrospective Study of 95 Naturally Occurring Cases. 31st Annual Meeting of American College of Veterinary Pathologists, New Orleans.

Presentey, B., Jerushalmy, Z., and Mintz, U. (1979) Eosinophilic Leukemia: Morphological, Cytological, and Electron Microscopic Studies. *J. Clin. Path.* 32, 261–271.

Priester, W. A. (1967) Canine Lymphoma: Relative Risk in the Boxer Breed. *J. Nat. Cancer Inst.* 39, 833–845.

Quesenberry, P., and Levitt, L. (1979) Hematopoietic Stem Cells. *New Eng. J. Med.* 301, 755–763, 819–823, 868–872.

Ragan, H. A., Hackett, P. L., and Dagle, G. E. (1976) Acute Myelomonocytic Leukemia Manifested as Myelophthisic Anemia in a Dog. *J. Amer. Vet. Med. Assoc.* 169, 421–425.

Raich, P. C., Takashima, I., and Olson, C. (1983) Cytochemical Reactions in Bovine and Ovine Lymphosarcoma. *Vet. Path.* 20, 322–329.

Rappaport, H., and Braylan, R. C. (1975) Changing Concepts in the Classification of Malignant Neoplasms of the Hematopoietic System. In: Rebuck, J. W., Berard, C. W., and Abell, M. R., eds., *The Reticuloendothelial System.* International Academy Pathology Monograph. Williams and Wilkins (Baltimore), 1–19.

Rebhun, W. C., and Bertone, A. (1984) Equine Lymphosarcoma. *J. Amer. Vet. Med. Assoc.* 184, 720–721.

Reed, C., Ling, G. V., Gould, D., and Kaneko, J. J. (1970) Polycythemia Vera in a Cat. *J. Amer. Vet. Med. Assoc.* 157, 85–91.

Ressang, A. A., Baars, J. C., Calafat, J., Mastenbroek, N., and Quak, J. (1976) Studies on Bovine Leukaemia. III. The Hematological and Serological Response of Sheep and Goats to Infection with Whole Blood from Leukaemic Cattle. *Zbl. Vet. Med.* 23, 662–668.

Rickard, C. G., and Post, J. E. (1968) Cellular and Cell-Free Transmission of a Canine Mast Cell Leukemia. In: Bendixen, H. J., ed., *Leukemia in Animals and Man.* Karger (Basel), 279–281.

Rigal, D., Bendali-Ahcène, S., Monier, J. C., Mohana, K., and Fournel, C. (1983) Identification of Canine T Lymphocytes by Membrane Receptor to Peanut Agglutinin: T-Lymphocyte Identification in Dogs with Lupus-like Syndrome. *Amer. J. Vet. Res.* 44, 1782–1788.

Roberts, M. C. (1977) A Case of Primary Lymphoid Leukaemia in a Horse. *Equine Vet. J.* 9, 216–219.

Robinson, M. (1974) Malignant Thymoma with Metastases in a Dog. *Vet. Path.* 11, 172–180.

Rockey, J. H., and Schwartzman, R. M. (1967) Skin Sensitizing Antibodies: A Comparative Study of Canine and Human PK and PCA Antibodies and a Canine Myeloma Protein. *J. Immunol.* 98, 1143–1151.

Rojko, J. L., and Olsen, R. G. (1984) The Immunobiology of Feline Leukemia Virus. *Vet. Immunol. Immunopath.* 6, 107–165.

Rojko, J. L., Hoover, E. A., Quackenbush, S. L., and Olsen, R. G. (1982) Reactivation of Latent Feline Leukemia Virus Infection. *Nature* 298, 385–388.

Rudolph, R., and Hubner, C. (1972) Megakaryozytenleukose beim Hund. *Kleintier-Praxis.* 17, 9–13.

Rudolph, R., and Paulsen, J. (1972) Ultrastruktur lymphatischer Zellen bei Leukose des Schafes. *Berl. Münch. Tierärztl. Wschr.* 85, 85–87.

Saar, C. (1970) Erythro-Megakaryozythaemia bei einer Katze. *Berl. Münch. Tierärztl. Wschr.* 83, 70–74.

Saar, C., Opitz, M., Barten, U., and Burow, H. (1970) Lymphoide Retikulose mit Makroglobulinämie (Makroglobulinämie Waldenström) bei einem Hund. *Berl. Münch. Tierärztl. Wschr.* 83, 168–172.

Samagh, B. S., and Kellar, J. A. (1982) Seroepidemiological Survey of Bovine Leukaemia Virus Infection in Canadian Cattle. In: Straub, O. C., ed., *Fourth International Symposium on Bovine Leukosis.* Martinus Nijhoff Publishers (The Hague, Boston, London), 614.

Sandison, A. T., and Anderson, L. J. (1969) Tumours of the Thymus in Cattle, Sheep, and Pigs. *Cancer Res.* 29, 1146–1150.

Sarma, P. S., Log, T., Skuntz, S., Krishnan, S., and Burkley, K. (1978) Experimental Horizontal Transmission of Feline Leukemia Viruses of Subgroups A, B, and C. *J. Nat. Cancer Inst.* 60, 871–874.

Schalm, O. W. (1976) Myeloproliferative Disorders in the Cat. *Calif. Vet.* 30(6), 32–37.

———. (1980) *Manual of Feline and Canine Hematology.* Veterinary Practice Publishing Co. (Santa Barbara, California), 59–98, 205–223.

Schalm, O. W., and Carlson, G. P. (1982) Blood and Blood Forming Organs. In: Mansman, R. A., and McAllister, E. S., eds., *Equine Medicine and Surgery.* 3d ed. American Veterinary Publications (Santa Barbara, California), 377–414.

Schalm, O. W., and Theilen, G. H. (1970) Myeloproliferative Disease in the Cat Associated with C-type Leukovirus Particles in Bone Marrow. *J. Amer. Vet. Med. Assoc.* 157, 1686–1696.

Schalm, O. W., Jain, N. C., and Carroll, E. J. (1975) *Veterinary Hematology.* 3d ed. Lea and Febiger (Philadelphia), 807.

Schappert, H. R., and Geib, L. W. (1967) Reticuloendothelial Neoplasms Involving the Spinal Canal of Cats. *J. Amer. Vet. Med. Assoc.* 150, 753–757.

Schechter, G. P., Guccion, J., Matthews, M., Fischmann, B., and Bunn, P. A. (1981) Erythrophagocytic Tγ Lymphoma. *N. Engl. J. Med.* 305, 103.

Schöttler, F., and Schöttler, H. (1934) Ueber Aetiologie und Therapie der aleukämischen Lymphadenose des Rindes. *Berl. Tierärztl. Wschr.* 50, 497–502, 513–517.

Scott, D. W., Miller, W. H., Tasker, J. B., Schultz, R. D., and Meuten, D. J. (1979) Lymphoreticular Neoplasia in a Dog Resembling Malignant Histiocytosis (Histiocytic Medullary Reticulosis) in Man. *Cornell Vet.* 69, 176–197.

Seed, T. M., Tolle, D. V., Fritz, T. E., Devine, R. L., Poole, C. M., and Norris, W. P. (1977) Irradiation-induced Erythroleukemia and Myelogenous Leukemia in the Dog. Hematology and Ultrastructure. *Blood* 50, 1061–1079.

Shadduck, J. A., Reddy, L., Lawton, G., and Freeman, R. (1978) A Canine Cutaneous Lymphoproliferative Disease Resembling Mycosis Fungoides in Man. *Vet. Path.* 15, 716–724.

Shifrine, M., Chrisp, C. E., Wilson, F. D., and Heffernon, U. (1973) Lysozyme (Muramidase) Activity in Canine Myelogenous Leukemia. *Amer. J. Vet. Res.* 34, 695–696.

Shimizu, M., Pan, I. C., and Hess, W. R. (1976) T and B Lymphocytes in Porcine Blood. *Amer. J. Vet. Res.* 37, 309–317.

Shively, J. W., Feldt, C., and Davis, D. (1969) Fine Structure of Formed Elements in Canine Blood. *Amer. J. Vet. Res.* 30, 893–905.

Silberberg-Sinakin, I., Gigli, I., Baer, R. L., and Thorbecke, G. J. (1980) Langerhans Cells: Role in Contact Hypersensitivity and Relationship to Lymphoid Dendritic Cells and to Macrophages. *Immun. Rev.* 53, 203–232.

Silverman, J. (1971) Eosinophilic Leukemia. *J. Amer. Vet. Med. Assoc.* 158, 199.

Silverstein, M. N. (1968) Myeloproliferative Diseases: Their Shifting Spectrums. *Postgrad. Med.* 43, 167–171.

Simon, N., and Holzworth, J. (1967) Eosiniphilic Leukemia in a Cat. *Cornell Vet.* 57, 579–597.

Snyder, S. P., and Dungworth, D. L., (1973) Pathogenesis of Feline Viral Fibrosarcomas: Dose and Age Effects. *J. Nat. Cancer Inst.* 51, 793–798.

Snyder, S. P., and Theilen, G. H. (1969) Transmissible Feline Fibrosarcoma. *Nature* 221, 1074–1075.

Sorenson, D. K., Anderson, R. K., Perman, V., and Sautter, J. H. (1964) Studies of Bovine Leukemia in Minnesota. Presented at Third International Meeting on Diseases of Cattle, Copenhagen, Denmark, August 20–22. *Nord. Vet. Med.* 16, suppl. 1, 562–572.

Squire, R. (1969a) Spontaneous Hematopoietic Tumours of Dogs. In: Lingeman, C. H., and Garner, F. M., eds. *Comparative Morphology of Hematopoietic Neoplasms.* National Cancer Institute Monograph 32. U.S. Government Printing Office (Washington, D.C.), 97–116.

———. (1969b) Non-neoplastic Hyperplasia of Lymph Nodes of Animals. In: Lingeman, C. H., and Garner, F. M., eds., *Comparative Morphology of Hematopoietic Neoplasms.* National Cancer Institute Monograph 32. U.S. Government Printing Office (Washington, D.C.), 257–266.

Squire, R. A., Bush, M., Melby, E. C., Neeley, L. M., and Yarbrough, B. (1973) Clinical and Pathological Study of Canine Lymphoma: Clinical Staging, Cell Classification, and Therapy. *J. Natl. Cancer Inst.* 51, 565–574.

Stann, S. E. (1979) Myelomonocytic Leukemia in a Cat. *J. Amer. Vet. Med. Assoc.* 174, 722–723.

Stasney, J., and Feldman, W. H. (1938) Leukemic Lymphoblastoma in a Calf: A Hematologic and Histologic Study. *Amer. J. Cancer* 34, 240–247.

Sterry, W., and Czarnetzki, B. M. (1982) *In Vitro* Differentiation of Rat Peritoneal Macrophages into Mast Cells: An Enzymecytochemical Study. *Blut* 44, 211–220.

Strandström, H., Veijalainen, P., Moennig, V., Hunsmann, G., Schwarz, H., and Schafer, W. (1974) C-Type Particles Produced by a Permanent Cell Line from a Leukemic Pig. I. Origin and Properties of the Host-Cells and Some Evidence for the Occurrence of C-Type Like Particles. *Virology* 57, 175–178.

Sullivan, D. J., and Anderson, W. A. (1959) Embryonal Nephroma in Swine. *Amer. J. Vet. Res.* 20, 324–332.

Sutton, R. H., and Wilkins, S. (1981) A Case of Canine Myeloid Neoplasia. *J. Small Anim. Pract.* 22, 139–147.

Sweet, D. L., Golomb, H. M., and Ultman, J. E. (1977) The Clinical Features of Chronic Lymphocytic Leukemia. *Clin. Haemat.* 6, 185–202.

Takashima, I., Olson, C., Driscoll, D. M., and Baumgartener, L. E. (1977) B-Lymphocytes and T-Lymphocytes in Three Types of Bovine Lymphosarcoma. *J. Natl. Cancer Inst.* 59, 1205–1209.

Talerman, A., and Gwynn, R. (1970) Epithelial Thymoma in a Dog. *J. Path.* 101, 62–64.

Tarr, M. J., Olson, R. G., Krakowka, G. S., Cockerell, G. L., and Gabel, A. A. (1977) Erythrocyte Rosette Formation of Equine Peripheral Blood Lymphocytes. *Amer. J. Vet. Res.* 38, 1775–1779.

Taylor, D., Hokama, Y., and Perri, S. F. (1975) Differentiation of Feline T and B Lymphocytes by Rosette Formation. *J. Immun.* 115, 862–865.

Tennant, B., Asbury, A. C., Laben, R. C., Richards, W. P. C., Kaneko, J. J., and Cupps, P. T. (1967) Familial Polycythemia in Cattle. *J. Amer. Vet. Med. Assoc.* 150, 1493–1509.

Theilen, G. H., and Dungworth, D. L. (1965) Bovine Lymphosarcoma in California. III. The Calf Form. *Amer. J. Vet. Res.* 26, 696–709.

Theilen, G. H., and Fowler, M. E. (1962) Lymphosarcoma (Lymphocytic Leukemia) in the Horse. *J. Amer. Vet. Med. Assoc.* 140, 923–930.

Theilen, G. H., and Madewell, B. R. (1979) Leukemia-Sarcoma Disease Complex. In: Theilen, G. H., and Madewell, B. R., eds., *Veterinary Cancer Medicine,* Lea and Febiger (Philadelphia), 204–288.

Theilen, G. H., Dungworth, D. L., Lengyel, J., and Rosenblatt, L. S. (1964) Bovine Lymphosarcoma in California. I. Epizootiologic and Hematologic Aspects. *Hlth. Lab. Sci.* 1, 96–106.

Theilen, G. H., Schalm, O. W., and Gilmore, V. (1961) Clinical and Hematologic Studies of Lymphosarcoma in a Herd of Cattle. *Amer. J. Vet. Res.* 22, 23–31.

Thiel, E., Rodt, H., Huhn, D., Netzel, B., Grosse-Wilde, H., Ganeshaguru, K., and Thierfelder, S. (1980) Multimarker Classification of Acute Lymphoblastic Leukemia: Evidence for Further T Subgroups and Evaluation of their Clinical Significance. *Blood* 56, 759–772.

Thrall, M. A. (1981) Lymphoproliferative Disorders. Lymphocytic Leukemia and Plasma Cell Myeloma. *Vet. Clin. N. Amer. Small Anim. Pract.* 11, 321–347.

Thrall, M. A., Macy, D. W., Snyder, S. P., and Hall, R. L. (1984) Cutaneous Lymphosarcoma and Leukemia in a Dog Resembling Sézary Syndrome in Man. *Vet. Path.* 21, 182–186.

Thurmond, M. C., and Burridge, M. J. (1982) A Study of the Natural Transmission of Bovine Leukaemia Virus: Preliminary Results. In: Straub, O. C., ed., *Fourth International Symposium on Bovine Leukosis.* Martinus Nijhoff Publishers (The Hague, Boston, London), 244–250.

Tolle, D. V., Cullen, S. M., Seed, T. M., and Fritz, T. E. (1983) Circulating Micromegakaryocytes Preceding Leukemia in Three Dogs Exposed to 2.5*R*/day Gamma Radiation. *Vet. Path.* 20, 111–114.

Tolle, D. V., Seed, T. M., Fritz, T. E., and Norris, W. P. (1979) Irradiation-induced Canine Leukemia: A Proposed New Model. Incidence and Hematopathology. In: Baum, S. J., and Ledney, G. D., eds., *Experimental Hematology Today.* Springer Publishers (New York), 247–256.

Tricot, G., Broeckaert-Van Orshoven, A., Van Hoof, A., and Verwilghen, R. L. (1982) Sudan Black B. Positivity in Acute Lymphoblastic Leukaemia. *Brit. J. Haemat.* 51, 615–621.

Udall, D. H., and Olafson, P. (1930) Pseudoleukemia in a Calf. *Cornell Vet.* 20, 81–84.

Ueberschär, S. (1968) Zytologische Untersuchungen bei der Rinderleukose. *Zbl. Vet. Med.* 15B. 163–173.

Valli, V. E., McSherry, B. J., Dunham, B. M., Jacobs, R. M., and Lumsden, J. H. (1981) Histocytology of Lymphoid Tumors in the Dog, Cat and Cow. *Vet. Path.* 18, 494–512.

Van Den Hoven, R., and Franken, P. (1983) Clinical Aspects of Lymphosarcoma in the Horse: A Clinical Report of 16 Cases. *Equine Vet. J.* 15, 49–53.

Van der Maaten, M. J., and Miller, J. M. (1976) Induction of Lymphoid Tumors in Sheep with Cell-free Preparations of Bovine Leukemia Virus. *Bibl. Haemat.* 43, 377–379.

Van der Maaten, M. J., Miller, J. M., and Schmerr, M. J. F. (1982) Factors Affecting the Transmission of Bovine Leukaemia Virus from Cows to Their Offspring. In: Straub, O. C., ed., *Fourth International Symposium on Bovine Leukosis.* Martinus Nijhoff Publishers (The Hague, Boston, London), 225–240.

Van Dyke, D., Nohr, M. C., and Tennant, B. (1968) Erythropoietin Enhancing Factor in Serum of a Calf with Primary Familial Polycythaemia. *Nature* 217, 1027–1028.

Ward, J. M., and Hurvitz, A. I. (1972) Ultrastructure of Normal and Neoplastic Mast Cells of the Cat. *Vet. Path.* 9, 202–211.

Ward, J. M., Sodikoff, C. H., and Schalm, O. W. (1969) Myeloproliferative Disease and Abnormal Erythrogenesis in the Cat. *J. Amer. Vet. Med. Assoc.* 155, 879–888.

Ward, J. M., Wright, J. F., and Wharran, G. H. (1972) Ultrastructure of Granulocytes in the Peripheral Blood of the Cat. *J. Ultrastruct. Res.* 39, 389–396.

Weber, A., Andrews, J., Dickinson, B., Larson, V., Hammer, R., Dirks, V., Sorensen, D., and Frommes, S. (1969) Occurrence of Nuclear Pockets in Lymphocytes of Normal, Persistent Lymphocytotic and Leukemic Adult Cattle. *J. Nat. Cancer Inst.* 43, 1307–1315.

Webster, W. M. (1966) Neoplasia in Food Animals with Special Reference to High Incidence in Sheep. *N.Z. Vet. J.* 14, 203–214.

Weinhold, E., and Müller, A. (1971) Untersuchungen über Chromosomenanomalien bei der Rinderleukose. *Berl. Münch. Tierärztl. Wschr.* 84, 146–149.

Weipers, W. L., Jarrett, W. F. H., Martin, W. B., Crighton, G. W., and Stewart, M. F. (1964) Lymphosarcoma in Domestic Animals. *Ann. Rep. Br. Emp. Cancer Campaign* 42, 682–685.

Weischer, F. (1944) Erbbedingtheit und Bekämpfung der Rinderleukose. *Dtsch. Tierärzt. Wschr.* 52/50, 83–84.

Weiss, E., Rudolph, R., and Deutschländer, N. (1968) Untersuchungen zur Ultrastruktur und Ätiologie der Mastzellentumoren des Hundes. *Path. Vet.* 5, 199–211.

Weller, R. E., Holmberg, C. A., Theilen, G. H., and Madewell, B. R. (1980) Histologic Classification as a Prognostic Criterion for Canine Lymphosarcoma. *Amer. J. Vet. Res.* 41, 1310–1314.

Wells, G. A. H. (1974) Hodgkin's Disease-like Lesions in the Dog. *J. Path.* 112, 5–10.

Wheeler, M. S., Wilson, E. C., and Stass, S. A. (1981) Erythroleukophagocytosis by Leukemic Cells—A Nonspecific Finding. *Amer. J. Clin. Path.* 75, 266–267.

White, E. G. (1946) Discussion on Leukaemia and Leukosis in Man and Animals. *Proc. R. Soc. Med.* 39, 735–740.

Williams, W. J., Beutler, E., Erslev, A. J., and Rundles, R. W. (1977) *Hematology.* 2d ed. McGraw-Hill (New York), 770–850.

Wittmann, W., and Urbaneck, D. (1969) Untersuchungen zur Ätiologie der Rinderleukose 8. Übertragungsversuche mit Blut leukosekranker Rinder auf Schaflämmer. *Arch. Exp. Vet. Med.* 23, 709–713.

Yam, L. T., Li, C. Y., and Crosby, W. H. (1971) Cytochemical Identification of Monoctyes and Granulocytes. *Amer. J. Clin. Path.* 55, 283–290.

Yang, T. J., Jantzen, P. A. and Williams, L. F. (1979) Acid α-Napthyl Acetate Esterase: Presence of Activity in Bovine and Human T and B Lymphocytes. *Immunology* 38, 85–93.

Yoshiki, T., Mellors, R. C., and Hardy, W. D. (1973) Common Cell Surface Antigens Associated with Murine and Feline C-type RNA Leukemia Viruses. *Proc. Nat. Acad. Sci.* 70, 1878–1882.

Zawidzka, Z. Z., Janzen, E., and Grice, H. C. (1964) Erythremic Myelosis in a Cat: A Case Resembling Di-Guglielmo's Syndrome in Man. *Path. Vet.* 1, 530–541.

Zenoble, R. D., and Rowland, G. N. (1979) Hypercalcemia and Proliferative, Myelosclerotic Bone Reaction Associated with Feline Leukovirus Infection in a Cat. *J. Amer. Vet. Med. Assoc.* 175, 591–595.

Zucker-Franklin, D., Hirayama, N., and Schnipper, E. (1981) The Presence of Mast Cell Precursors in Rat Peripheral Blood. *Blood* 58, 544–551.

## 7

*Jack E. Moulton*
# Tumors of the Respiratory System

## TUMORS OF THE UPPER RESPIRATORY TRACT

### Nasal Cavity and Paranasal Sinus Tumors of the Dog

**Classification.** There are many different types of tissue in the walls of the nasal cavities and paranasal sinuses, including bone, cartilage, fibrous connective tissue, blood vessels, lining epithelium, and glandular epithelium. These tissues can provide origin for a wide variety of tumors that are found at these sites. A classification of various neoplasms of the nasal cavity and paranasal sinuses is shown in table 7.1.

**Incidence.** In the dog, adenomas and papillomas are much less frequently diagnosed than malignant neoplasms. In 3,000 cases of neoplasms surveyed by Brodey (1970), nasal or paranasal carcinomas occurred in slightly over 1% of dogs. The incidence rate for upper respiratory neoplasms as determined by Dr. R. Schneider (Animal Neoplasm Registry, University of California) for Alameda and Contra Costa counties in the San Francisco Bay area is 2.5 tumors per 100,000 dogs. This compares with an incidence of 8.2 per 100,000 dogs for all types of respiratory tumors. In a study by Dr. C. von Tscharner and the author at the University of California of 81 upper respiratory tumors in dogs (1968 to 1978), 64 tumors were of epithelial origin and 16 of nonepithelial origin.

Among 153 cases of carcinoma of the nasal cavities and paranasal sinuses in dogs reported since 1950 (Bedford, 1959; Berkelhammer, 1949; Bradley and Harvey, 1973; Cotchin, 1967) plus 64 studied by the author, there was a total of 73 squamous cell carcinomas, 91 adenocarcinomas (including 6 mucinous carcinomas), and 53 undifferentiated carcinomas.

Zaki and Liu (1974) reported 5 adenocarcinomas originating in the olfactory glands of dogs. These are the only ones recorded in the literature. These tumors had large sheets of epithelial cells and abundant stromal fibrosis. The tumor cells invaded the adjacent olfactory and prefrontal areas and the cerebral hemispheres.

Nonepithelial nasal and sinus tumors of dogs include chondrosarcoma, fibrosarcoma, osteosarcoma, mast cell sarcoma, undifferentiated sarcoma (of uncertain origin), angiosarcoma, and leiomyosarcoma (in descending order of frequency). Fibroma, chondroma, and osteoma have also been identified. Since the nonepithelial neoplasms are similar to their counterparts at other sites, they are not considered in detail in this section.

**Age, Breed, and Sex.** The average age of onset for nasal and sinus epithelial neoplasms in dogs is 9 years (ranging from 18 months to 18 years); however, when age-related incidence rates are calculated per 100,000 dogs, the average morbidity rate occurs at an age several years older than this. The morbidity rate is much lower below 6 years of age. The average age of onset for sarcoma of the nasal

**TABLE 7.1. Tumors of the Nasal Cavities and Paranasal Sinuses**

Epithelial origin

    Papilloma

    Adenoma

    Carcinoma

        Squamous cell (epidermoid) carcinoma

        Adenocarcinoma

        Undifferentiated carcinoma (includes transitional
            carcinoma)

Nonepithelial (mesodermal) origin

    Fibroma and fibrosarcoma

    Chondroma and chondrosarcoma

    Osteoma and osteosarcoma

    Myxoma and myxosarcoma

    Miscellaneous: undifferentiated sarcoma, mastocytoma,
        angiosarcoma, leiomyosarcoma, and lipoma

cavity and paranasal sinuses in dogs is approximately 7 years 4 months (ranging from 18 months to 17 years). This is considerably younger than for carcinoma at this site but not as young as for lymphoma that appears in young dogs.

Carcinoma of the nasal cavity and sinuses is reported as occurring more in long-nosed than in short-nosed (brachycephalic) breeds of dogs and in medium-sized or large breeds such as the collie, German shepherd, and spaniel. Approximately one-third of the neoplasms are found in these breeds. According to Cook (1964), these breeds, particularly the collie, are also prone to other diseases of the upper respiratory tract, such as idiopathic ulceration of the anterior nares, "mucocutaneous disease," and "collie nose" (a symmetrical ulceration of the skin over the bridge of the nose associated with solar irradiation). Reif and Cohen (1971) claimed that this apparent breed susceptibility to neoplasms shows only a surface area dependency (i.e. the larger size of the nose) in which the probability of development of neoplasms at a given site is proportional to the number of cells and their potential to undergo neoplastic transformation.

The study done by von Tscharner and the author in California is in variance to these reports of a higher frequency of nasal tumors in long-nosed breeds than in short-nosed breeds. The highest incidence of nasal tumors was found in the Siberian husky, followed by the bulldog and Great Dane. After these three breeds, the collie and Shetland sheepdog, typical long-nosed breeds, had the highest incidence of tumors. The conflicting data indicate that further studies are needed before breed can be considered a predisposing factor. Apparently, the male dog is affected with these neoplasms more often than the bitch. In a collection of 61 nasal and paranasal neoplasms studied by the author, there were 46 tumors in male dogs and 15 in bitches.

**Clinical Characteristics.** In the differential diagnosis of nasal tumors in dogs, consideration must be given to rhinitis, sinusitis, osteomyelitis, foreign body lesions, trauma, and periodontal abscessation of the molars. Diagnosis between malignancy and infection in the nasal cavity may be difficult because so many of the neoplasms are secondarily infected. Early in the disease, the affected animals show nasal discharge and conjunctival hypersecretion due to obstruction of the lacrimal duct. Later, they have inspiratory difficulty, attacks of asphyxia mainly during swallowing, prolonged mucopurulent or hemorrhagic nasal discharge, exophthalmia, loss of condition, sneezing, and grunting. Tumors of the nasal cavity or sinuses often cause little or no externally observable enlargement. The clinical signs in dogs usually last for 3 months or more.

Morgan *et al.* (1972) described affected dogs radiographically as having erosion or severe destruction of the nasal turbinate bones, nasal septum, overlying cortical bone, and cribriform plate. The radiographs show filling of the nasal cavity and frontal sinus and deviation of the nasal septum. The nasal cavity has loss of the normal fine trabecular pattern because of the destruction of the turbinate bones by the expanding and invading neoplasm. External soft tissue masses are occasionally observed; these represent the extension of the neoplasms through the overlying bone. Deep biopsy and/or exfoliative cytology are needed to confirm the diagnosis, and it is important for the pathologist to receive solid pieces of tissue to differentiate the neoplasm from inflammatory exudate.

The period between onset of clinical signs and presentation for treatment in dogs is usually 2 months according to Bradley and Harvey (1973). These authors point out that prognosis is poor with these neoplasms, and dogs seldom survive more

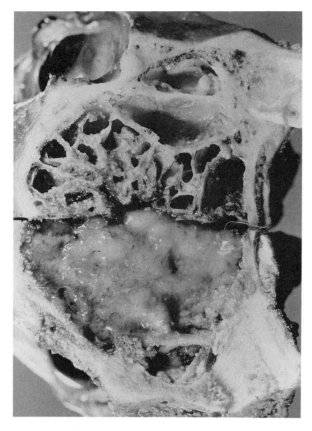

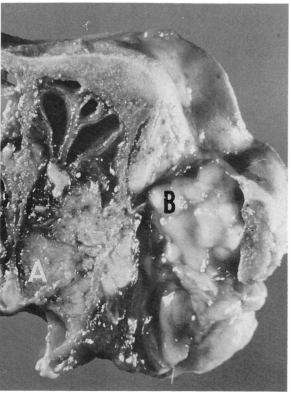

than 1 year. While it may be possible to treat cases early, the tumor is often extensive by the time diagnosis is made. Radical surgery may be successful if the tumor is confined to the turbinate system or nasal septum, but surgery is more complicated if the neoplasm involves the bone forming the nasal arch, cribriform plate, or inner plate of the frontal sinus. Radiation therapy is also employed, but survival time after radiation is often short, usually from 4 to 12 months.

**Sites.** The exact location of neoplasms in the nasal cavities of dogs is difficult to determine since the tumors can extend into surrounding areas such as the sinuses. Also, the opposite is true: neoplasms of the sinuses can extend into the nasal cavity causing signs similar to primary tumors of the nasal cavity. The three principal anatomical sites for these neoplasms are the nasal cavity, the vestibulum (located directly behind the orifice and lined by squamous epithelium), and the paranasal sinuses (usually the frontal sinus and less often the maxillary sinus).

In a group of canine neoplasms of the nasal cavity and paranasal sinuses collected from the literature (Cook, 1964; Cotchin, 1967; Morgan *et al.*, 1972) and in a large group of the tumors studied at the University of California, 170 of the neoplasms were primarily located in the nasal cavities, 38 in the paranasal sinuses, 7 in the vestibulum, and 1 in the ethmoid–cribriform region.

The epithelium of the turbinate bones is probably the cell of origin for most nasal carcinomas in dogs; the tumors arise here and spread to other areas. Unless the vestibulum is involved, the neoplasms are not necessarily seen during anterior rhinoscopy.

**Gross Morphology.** Papillomas of the nasal or sinus cavities may be solitary or multiple, have a verrucous or papillary pattern, and grow out from the surface membrane. Adenoma is usually a well-circumscribed lesion and is often quite small. By

**FIGURE 7.1.** Carcinoma in the nasal cavity of the dog. A. Cross section through nasal cavity (rostral) showing carcinoma occupying one side. B. Cross section of nasal cavity, more caudal than section in A, showing carcinoma in ventral half of nasal cavity (A) and growth into maxillary sinus (B).

and 5 experimental nasal papillary adenomas of sheep in Germany. These tumors were solitary or multiple, unilateral or bilateral, and they first appeared as nodules in the nasal mucosa. The neoplasms enlarged and involved the posterior parts of the nasal cavity and pharynx, and reached into the larynx during the later stages of growth. The tumors also grew into the frontal and maxillary sinuses causing erosion of the cranial bones, and some invaded the gingiva and orbit. Metastasis was never found.

In the earliest stages of growth the neoplasms reported by Cohrs (1952, 1953) had focal proliferations of nasal glandular elements. About half of the tumors had papillary growth pattern, although solid masses of tumor cells were also seen. In the larger growths some of the cells had mucin secretion and cysts were sometimes formed. Stromal fibrosis was variable though extensive in some masses, and metaplastic chondroid and osteoid elements were occasionally observed.

Cohrs (1953) reviewed the history of these neoplasms in sheep. In the early 1940s multiple cases of these tumors were reported in three widely separated areas of Germany. The disease continued to spread, but only a small number of sheep became affected in each flock. In one flock, six sheep were killed because of the neoplasms in 1942, eight in 1943, and nine in 1944. During the late 1940s, almost 15% of the sheep in one flock were affected. There was evidence that sheep developed the disease after being introduced into an infected flock. The neoplasms were successfully transmitted in 5 of 15 inoculated sheep, using tumor cell suspensions or bacteria-free filtrates of tumor tissue.

Gussmann (1962) in Germany also reported endemic ethmoturbinate tumors of sheep that occurred over a period of 7 years in one flock. He found six cases in four other flocks. From 1959 to 1961, tumors of this type were seen in 13 yearling and adult sheep in one flock, the youngest animal affected being 4 months old. The neoplasms developed from the nasal submucosal glands or surface epithelium and all had squamous metaplasia. Attempts at transmission were unsuccessful.

Drieux et al. (1952) described neoplasms of the nasal cavity of two sheep in the Ardennes region of France. One of these tumors was examined histologically and proved to be an adenocarcinoma. This tumor caused a swelling of the frontal region and protuberance of one of the eyes from its socket. Metastasis was not found in either of the affected animals.

An endemic rhinitis condition in sheep characterized by formation of soft vegetations of the ethmoid and turbinate epithelium was reported by Camy (1955) in France, but no histological examination was done.

Young et al. (1961) described tumors of the ethmoturbinate mucosa in two flocks of sheep in Montana in the United States. Tumors were examined in four sheep, three from one flock and one from another flock. The sheep were 3 to 7 years old and both sexes were represented. The neoplasms were of the adenocarcinoma type but of low-grade malignancy.

According to Cotchin (1967), the tumors reported by Young et al. (1961) are probably identical with those reported by Nieberle (1939) and Cohrs (1952, 1953). He believes that the principal problem in diagnosing tumors of the ethmoturbinate region of sheep and other species is determining whether the tumors are truly neoplastic or merely hyperplastic.

More recently, enzootic nasal adenocarcinomas were reported in a survey of neoplasms in veterinary diagnostic laboratories in Canada (McKinnon et al., 1982). These tumors occurred in sheep in most provinces of Canada and were found in different breeds of sheep including various crossbreeds. Over half of the neoplasms were observed in sheep less than 2 years of age. Most tumors were sporadic, but a third of the cases occurred in six related flocks, indicating that the disease could be enzootic. The tumors originated unilaterally or occasionally bilaterally in the olfactory mucosa of the ethmoid turbinates. They were expansive and sometimes locally aggressive, but metastasis was not found. Histologically, the tumors were diagnosed as adenoma or adenocarcinoma. The etiology was not established, but retroviruslike particles were observed in tumor tissue from one sheep.

### Goat

Lombard (1966) reported an outbreak of an apparently infectious papillomatosis of the nasal cavity in goats in the Seine-et-Oise area of France. The incidence of these tumors was 2.3%.

## Cow

Tumors of the mucosa of the ethmoturbinates of cattle are best known in Sweden and appear with striking frequency, apparently in endemic form. They are also seen in horses in that country, but with less frequency. Their histological type varies from undifferentiated carcinoma to adenocarcinoma; sarcomas and mixed tumors also occur. Most of the tumors on the same farm are of the same histological type.

Endemic ethmoturbinate tumors in cattle (and horses) have been known in Sweden since the latter part of the nineteenth century. The first important report was that of Stenstrom (1909), who described five cases of malignant "round cell" tumors that arose from the ethmoturbinates in cattle. The cattle were in close contact with each other and all became affected within 1 year. Stenstrom (1915) later reported ethmoturbinate neoplasms in 41 cattle and 7 horses. Of these animals, 19 cows and 7 horses were from the same farm and were in close contact. The cows were first affected in 1908, and subsequent cases occurred in each succeeding year through 1913, except in 1910 when the area where the cows were kept was disinfected. The seven equine tumors occurred between 1912 and 1913. The evidence for an infectious etiological agent in cattle was the occurrence of multiple cases in different family lines and the introduction of the infection into herds previously unaffected.

The average age of cows with endemic ethmoturbinate tumors in Stenstrom's 1915 report was 10 years (range 5 to 14 years). The tumors arose from the ethmoid region and often invaded the adjacent sinuses. Metastasis was verified histologically in the lymph nodes of six cows and in the lungs of one cow. The tumors were all classified as adenocarcinoma except for one squamous cell carcinoma.

Magnusson (1916) in Sweden described endemic neoplasia of the ethmoid bone in 20 cattle and 5 horses. Carcinoma was found in 10 animals, sarcoma in 9, and mixed epithelial and mesenchymal tumors in 6 animals. The tumors were bilateral in 7 cases and unilateral in 18 cases. Metastasis to the re-

gional lymph nodes was found in 7 of 25 animals; in 5 animals there was invasion into the cribriform plate. The carcinomas originated in the surface epithelium of the ethmoturbinates in 4 animals and the mucosal glands in 3 animals. Evidence for endemic spread of the neoplasms was that 7 affected cattle came from the same farm and 4 new cases appeared later at the same farm.

Stalfors (1917) in Sweden described neoplasms (sarcoma and adenocarcinoma) in the posterior part of the nasal cavities of four cows. An attempt to transmit these tumors by instillation of tumor material into the nasal cavity of a normal cow was unsuccessful. Another report of these neoplasms in cattle was by Plum (1934) in Denmark, who diagnosed a sarcoma originating from the posterior part of the nasal cavity.

Jackson (1936) has claimed that ethmoturbinate tumors of cattle similar to those found in Sweden also occur in South Africa. He reported a case of myxosarcoma of the paranasal sinuses in a cow and transitional cell (squamous cell or undifferentiated?) carcinoma in cattle, one in the nasopharynx and another in the ethmoid mucosa. These animals had deformity of the face due to swelling of the frontal and maxillary regions, dyspnea, discharge of blood and suppurative exudate from the nostrils, unilateral exophthalmos, and swelling of regional lymph nodes.

Damodaran et al. (1974) collected neoplasms of the ethmoturbinate region from 42 cattle and 10 buffaloes between 1956 and 1973 in Tamil Nadu State in India. The cattle were 6 to 10 years of age. The neoplasms occurred about equally in the Sindhi and exotic breeds of cattle. The animals had epistaxis, mucopurulent rhinorrhea, dyspnea, exophthalmos, blindness, swelling of the forehead, and circling. Histologically, 44 of the tumors were adenocarcinoma and 7 were squamous cell carcinoma.

An insidious epidemic of nasal adenocarcinoma occurred in a high-yielding Dutch breed of cattle and in pigs in Brazil (Amaral and Nesti, 1963). Between 1958 and 1962 in eight districts of this country, 75 cattle and 185 pigs were affected. The neoplasms tended to occur with higher incidence on certain farms; on one farm 180 sows were affected. The neoplasms occurred in the nasal cavity and infiltrated the adjacent sinuses and nasal septum. In advanced cases, the bone structure was invaded. No information was given on metastasis.

Attempts were made to detect the presence of virus by electron microscopic examination. From sections of one tumor Nair *et al.* (1981) observed the maturation and assembly of virus particles at the plasma membrane; however, they pointed out that because of the localization of the neoplasms where they were exposed to air flowing through the nasal passages, there was the possibility of a contaminate virus unrelated to the tumor.

### Horse

In addition to the ethmoturbinate neoplasms of horses reported by Stenstrom (1915) and Magnusson (1916) in Sweden, four cases of malignant neoplasms in the posterior nasal cavity and sinuses of horses were observed by Bergman in 1914 (cited by Cotchin, 1967). The tumors arose from the mucosa of the ethmoid bone, often filled the entire nasal cavity, and invaded into the paranasal sinuses and cranial cavity.

An endemic occurrence of ethmoturbinate tumors in horses was also reported in Norway (Horne and Stenersen, 1916). On one farm, 5 cases appeared among 15 horses and 1 case occurred in a cow that was in contact with the horses. The tumors in horses were diagnosed as squamous cell carcinoma and adenocarcinoma; the tumor in the cow was diagnosed as a "spindle-cell" sarcoma.

Rahko *et al.* (1972) reported three myxomas in the posterior nasal cavities of horses in Finland. Clinically, the first sign was purulent discharge, sometimes with blood, from one or both nostrils. The neoplasms destroyed the nasal concha, penetrated the right paranasal sinuses, and produced deformation of the adjacent bone.

Cotchin (1967) cited a report by Forsell (1913) who described "round-cell" sarcoma of the ethmoid bone, nasal cavity, and sinuses of five mature horses, including three animals that were from the same premises. Attempts at transmission were unsuccessful.

Rajan *et al.* (1973) collected 92 primary nasal neoplasms from various domestic animals in India. Of these tumors, 42 were in buffaloes, 30 in pigs, 18 in cattle, and 1 each in a goat and a dog.

## Nasal Polyps

**Definition.** A nasal polyp is a pedunculated growth arising from the mucous surface of the nasal cavity and resulting from hyperplasia of the mucous membrane or from exuberant proliferation of fibrous connective tissue. Nasal polyps should not be confused with pedunculated fibroma or papilloma, which are true neoplasms. Polyps are usually the result of chronic inflammation. The etiology of most polyps is unknown. The growths are usually multiple (polyposis) and sometimes recur after removal. They may give rise to complications associated with secondary infection.

**Incidence and Sites.** Nasal polyps are usually found in the horse, but they are also seen in the dog and cat. In the horse they are usually unilateral but can be bilateral and may cause respiratory distress. Nasal polyps usually occur in adult horses, but there is no particular age predisposition. No breed or sex predilection is known.

**Morphology.** Grossly, polyps are often small, approximately 2 cm in diameter, but some become large enough to occlude the nasal cavity. They are moist and glistening and round, ovoid, or pedunculated. The growths are firm or rubbery and commonly have a slimy, smooth, or roughened surface, which may be ulcerated. The color is white, pink, or red.

Histologically, polyps consist of edematous fibroblastic tissue that is suggestive of soft fibroma except for the absence of whorls. Some polyps have dense fibrous tissue that is highly vascularized and may have thrombosed blood vessels. The polyps are covered with cuboidal or columnar epithelium. The superficial part of the growth often exhibits infection and granulation tissue.

Hemorrhagic polyps of the ethmoid region in the horse have been described (Cook and Littlewort, 1974; Platt, 1975) and seem to constitute a pathological entity. The polyps appear within one nasal chamber, sometimes extending to the nostril or the choanae, and originate (at least in part) from the upper nasal passages. Except for ulceration and secondary infection, the growths have a smooth surface. On cut section some areas of the polyp appear hemorrhagic, even as hematomas, but in the extremities of the lesion the tissue is dense with brownish discoloration. Histologically, the polyps are highly vascular and have a distinctive microscopic appearance resulting from repeated hemorrhage, breakdown of hemoglobin, and organization by fibrous tissue. Marked ferruginous and calcareous encrustations of the fibrous collagenous fibers, sometimes with giant cell formation, are observed. In one case reported by Platt (1975), the lesion involved the mucous membrane of the paranasal sinus and resembled a hemangioma with extensive capillary formation.

## TUMORS OF THE NASOPHARYNX, GUTTURAL POUCHES, LARYNX, AND TRACHEA

### Nasopharynx

Tumors of the nasopharynx are rare in domestic animals with the exception of squamous cell carcinoma of the tonsil in the dog, which is described in chapter 8 (Tumors of the Alimentary Tract). Cotchin (1967) observed squamous cell carcinoma involving the mucous membrane of the pharynx and the root of the tongue in a 3-year-old dog and a squamous cell carcinoma of the pharynx with nodal metastasis in a 14-year-old female cat. The nasopharynx is not a rare location for malignant melanoma in the dog.

### Gutteral Pouches

The guttural pouches in horses are diverticulae of the eustachian tubes and lie between the pharynx and base of the skull. The epithelial lining of the pouches is stratified, ciliated, or columnar, and there are serous and mucous glands in the submucosa. A squamous cell carcinoma of the septum between the guttural pouches in an 11-year-old stallion was described by Kuscher et al. (1944).

### Larynx

Collet (1935) reviewed the early literature on neoplasms of the larynx and reported an undifferentiated carcinoma of the larynx in an 11-year-old cat. Wilmes (1938) described a squamous cell carci-

noma in the arytenoid cartilage region of an 18-year-old horse and found only two other cases in the literature.

Cotchin (1967) reported three cases of squamous cell carcinoma of the larynx in cats in London. The cats were aged 10 years, 14 years, and 6 months. Lieberman (1954) found an adenocarcinoma in the right wall of the larynx of a 10-year-old male cat. Metastasis was found in the cervical lymph nodes, lungs, spleen, adrenal glands, and liver.

### Laryngeal Oncocytoma of the Dog

**Incidence, Age, Breed, Sex, and Clinical Characteristics.** Laryngeal neoplasms are rare in dogs. Various tumor types including squamous cell carcinoma, adenocarcinoma, osteosarcoma, melanoma, mast cell tumor, and rhabdomyosarcoma are found (Wheeldon et al., 1982). Squamous cell carcinoma has been considered the most prevalent type, but oncocytoma has been found to represent a substantial proportion of canine laryngeal neoplasms, especially in younger dogs. From 1977 to 1983, this tumor accounted for 2 of 6 laryngeal tumors at the University of Florida (Calderwood-Mays, 1984). Most of the information presented here is taken from the paper of Calderwood-Mays (1984).

About half of the laryngeal oncocytomas occur in 2-year-old dogs. There is no breed or sex predisposition.

The clinical signs in dogs with this tumor are often insidious and can develop over many months. Most dogs show a history of wheezing, hoarseness, stertorous breathing, coughing, loss of bark or change of bark to a "squeak," and signs of dyspnea.

**Gross Morphology.** Oncocytoma usually appears as a well-circumscribed mass, approximately 1 cm in diameter, that projects from the lateral laryngeal ventricle and may partly obstruct it. The tumor is either soft or firm and sometimes friable. The tumor tissue is mottled tan to white or pink in color and usually contains large areas of hemorrhage. The soft texture and hemorrhage in the tumor may suggest a hemangiosarcoma.

**Histological Features.** The histological features have been similar in all oncocytomas reported to date. The growth occurs in the submucosal connective tissue between the mucosa and laryngeal cartilage, which it displaces, but the epithelium over the neoplasm is usually preserved. The neoplasm is usually well contained and often encapsulated. It is composed of sheets of large cells divided into faint lobules by a fine fibrovascular stroma. Areas of necrosis and hemorrhage are present. The hemorrhage is between cells in channels of various sizes, but there is no obvious endothelial lining in the channels.

The tumor cells are striking. They appear epithelioid, pleomorphic, and of various sizes. Many of the cells have a bulging, brightly eosinophilic, finely granular or foamy cytoplasm. Some cells have large, clear cytoplasmic vacuoles. The nuclei are round and of moderate size and contain one or occasionally several nucleoli. Cytoplasmic invagination into the nucleus is common. Mitotic figures are seldom seen. By electron microscopy (Pass *et al.*, 1980) the tumor cell cytoplasm can be seen to be filled with a large number of mitochondria that may be pleomorphic or slightly condensed. The mitochondria account for the granular appearance of the cytoplasm seen by light microscopy. The cytoplasm may also contain glycogen granules and rough endoplasmic reticulum. Cells with fewer mitochondria contain more glycogen granules. Desmosomes have been seen in some cells.

Oncocytes in humans are epithelial cells with deeply eosinophilic cytoplasm and usually contain large numbers of mitochondria. These cells occur normally in the human parathyroid glands (oxyphil cells), thyroid gland ("Hurthle" cells), salivary gland, nasopharynx, larynx, tongue, trachea, pituitary gland, and adrenal gland. The occurrence and distribution of oncocytes in domestic animals are not well known. The histogenesis of the cells is unknown.

A definite diagnosis of this unique canine tumor can be established by light microscopy. The differential diagnosis of hemangiosarcoma can be ruled out by the microscopic features of the tumor. Differential diagnosis for the large, eosinophilic granular cells may include granular cell tumor, chemodectoma, and rhabdomyosarcoma. Special stains will help to differentiate them. The granular cell tumor is strongly periodic acid–Schiff (PAS) stain positive, and chemodectoma is PAS and phosphotungstic acid–hematoxylin (PTAH) stain negative. Ap-

plication of PTAH stain to the oncocytoma will enhance the cytoplasmic granularity. Rhabdomyosarcoma is anaplastic and invasive and may contain multinucleated cells or cell cross striations.

**Growth Characteristics.** The behavior of oncocytoma cannot be predicted with certainty. Most of the published cases have been diagnosed at necropsy. The history and encapsulation of the neoplasm suggest benignancy. After fairly complete resection was accomplished in two reported cases (Calderwood-Mays, 1984), there was no tumor recurrence. The outlook for other laryngeal tumors, especially squamous cell carcinoma, is not usually so promising.

### Trachea

Ball *et al.* (1936) and Harmes (1913) described primary epithelial neoplasms of the trachea in domestic animals. Ball *et al.* (1936) described a rare adenocarcinoma of the lower trachea in a 7-year-old mongrel dog. There was no metastasis. Harmes (1913) described a "round cell" sarcoma of the trachea in a 6-year-old gelding. Cotchin (1967) reviewed the literature on these rare tumors.

## TUMORS OF THE LUNG

## General Considerations

**Incidence.** There have been many reports on lung carcinoma in the dog and cat, some citing references as far back as 1872. Lung neoplasms in these species make them interesting models for comparative studies of lung carcinoma in humans. Interest in the animal tumors is strong because of the great increase in lung carcinoma in humans during the last several decades. This increase is probably related to cigarette smoking and perhaps to atmospheric pollutants. The dog and cat breathe the same polluted air as humans, are exposed to the same irradiation, eat similar foods often containing the same additives, and are allowed to live a full lifespan.

Most of the statistics on animal tumors are limited to dogs and cats. Food animals are not usually allowed to live their whole lifespan because of economic reasons, thus they never reach the "cancer age." The slaughter of swine and ruminants in adolescence or early maturity is the reason for their scanty literature on lung and other neoplasms. There is no reported relationship between the incidence of lung carcinoma and the urban versus rural environment of the dog and cat.

In Europe and North America, lung carcinoma occurs in approximately 0.5% of dogs and cats that die from all causes and are examined at necropsy. In a survey (R. Schneider, Animal Neoplasm Registry, University of California) on neoplasms of all types affecting dogs in two counties in California, lung carcinoma was found in 4.17 dogs per 100,000. A report from the Dominican Republic (Reinoso de Columna, 1966) showed an 11% incidence of lung carcinoma among all neoplasms in dogs and cats.

Lung carcinoma in dogs and cats has increased at least twofold during the last 20 years. Most investigators believe this increase is related to the greater age reached by dogs and cats today as a result of modern vaccinations against infectious virus diseases which previously greatly limited the life span of these animals. Also, the greater number of necropsy examinations today affects the incidence data. There is no experimental evidence to relate this increase to various pollutants in the environment as suggested by Ten Thije and Ressang (1956). However, a study in Russia indicates that city dogs have a significantly higher incidence of lung carcinoma than country dogs; the difference was attributed to air pollution (Leake, 1961).

With the rise in lung carcinoma in humans, there has been a disproportionate increase in squamous cell (epidermoid) and anaplastic small cell and large cell carcinomas, but no significant increase in other carcinoma types. There has been no such disproportionate increase in these or other types of carcinomas in animals. Even with the experimental exposure of dogs to carcinogenic substances such as cigarette smoke or radioisotopes, there has been no increase in the types of carcinomas most prevalent in humans, although there has been an overall increase in carcinomas, probably associated with greater diagnostic competence among veterinarians.

The literature on lung tumors in domestic animals was reviewed by Lund (1924), Monlux (1952), Moulton *et al.* (1981), Nielsen (1970), and Nielsen and Horava (1960). Monlux (1952) found 129 cases of primary pulmonary tumors in domestic animals in the literature and described 21 cases of his own.

In domestic animals, adenocarcinoma is undoubtedly the most prevalent type of carcinoma. Squamous (epidermoid) and anaplastic small cell and large cell carcinomas are less common. Anaplastic small cell carcinoma is rarely found in the cat.

The following sections give the occurrence of lung neoplasms in different domestic animals.

*Dog*—The overall frequency of lung tumors among dogs examined at necropsy in various veterinary facilities throughout the world from 1928 to 1984 is 1.24%. This includes lung tumors reported from the United States (Brodey and Craig, 1965; Mulligan, 1949; Nielsen and Horava, 1960), Great Britain (Cotchin, 1959), Germany (Sedlmeir and Dahme, 1958; Stunzi, 1971), and France (Fontaine and Parodi, 1964). The annual incidence of lung carcinoma in Alameda and Contra Costa counties in the San Francisco Bay area was estimated in 1968 to be 4.17 per 100,000 dogs in the general canine population (Dorn *et al.*, 1968). During subsequent years this incidence has changed very little.

*Cat*—Few lung neoplasms have been reported in the cat (Jonas and Hukill, 1968). The incidence of lung tumors in cats examined at necropsy is 0.38%. The various histological types of lung carcinomas in the cat differ from the dog in that squamous cell carcinoma is far more common in the cat and outnumbers all other carcinomas combined.

*Cow*—Primary lung neoplasms are rare in cattle and are not of economic importance, but occasionally adenoma and adenocarcinoma are seen as incidental findings at slaughter. Krahnert (1954) made a survey of the literature of lung tumors in cattle and found a worldwide incidence of 2.8% among all neoplasms in this species. In the United States, Monlux *et al.* (1956) found three pulmonary neoplasms in 1.4 million cattle examined at slaughter. Migaki *et al.* (1974) found 25 lung neoplasms in 1.3 million slaughtered cattle. Brandley and Migaki (1963) reported only 21 lung tumors among 1,000 neoplasms of all types collected from cattle at slaughter. Owen (1965) collected only 50 unequivocal cases of lung neoplasms from the literature, and most of these neoplasms were incidental findings at slaughter. Anderson and Sandison (1968) in an abattoir survey in Great Britain found 19 primary lung tumors among 1 million cattle slaughtered in 1 year.

Sanford and Bundza (1982) reported a rare adenocarcinoma of differentiated type in the lung of a Hereford steer. The neoplasm consisted of multiple masses of varying size. Histologically, the tumor consisted of intraductal papillae covered by tall columnar cells resting on a basement membrane. Another carcinoma of the bovine lung was reported by Leipold *et al*. (1974). The neoplasm involved the dorsal two-thirds of the lung, and metastatic lesions were found in the bronchial and mediastinal lymph nodes, heart, spleen, rumen, small intestine, adrenal glands, and kidneys. Histologically, the neoplasm arose from the bronchial epithelium and invaded the bronchi, bronchioles, and alveoli. Intrapulmonary spread occurred via lymphatics and air spaces. Marked stromal fibrosis was present.

Adenocarcinoma of the lung is found in the water buffalo (*Bubalus bubalis*). Kharole *et al*. (1975) observed five of these tumors during a 12-month period in India. In all cases the neoplasms appeared as firm, whitish nodules oriented around the main airways. Metastasis was found in the regional lymph nodes of two animals. Histologically, the tumors consisted of irregular tubules lined by single or multiple layers of anaplastic epithelium. Abundant fibrous stroma was present.

*Goat*—There are few reports on pulmonary tumors in goats. Brandley and Migaki (1963) found one of these neoplasms in 900,000 goats in an examination of abattoir material. A report by Altman *et al*. (1970) suggested that these tumors in goats are not quite as rare as previously thought; they found an incidence of 0.5% in 2,500 castrated male white Angora goats allowed to live to old age in a research establishment. The majority of these neoplasms were subpleural and associated with the smaller bronchioles.

A type of papilloma found occasionally in the lungs of Angora goats was reported by Pearson (1961). The neoplasms appeared in the diaphragmatic lobes and were multiple in approximately half of the goats. The papillomas were light yellow to gray and embedded in the lung parenchyma. All of the papillomas were well-circumscribed.

*Other Species*—In a survey of British abattoirs by Anderson and Sandison (1968), no primary lung neoplasms were found in 4.5 million sheep and approximately 4 million pigs. Primary carcinoma of the lung is rarely reported in the horse.

## Papillary Adenoma of the Lung

**Incidence and Sites.** The few descriptions of papillary adenoma in the lung of domestic animals indicate that it is rare. The neoplasm has been reported in the ox, dog, cat, and goat (see previous section), although it undoubtedly also occurs in other domestic species. There is no known age susceptibility, although most reported cases have been in adults. There is no breed or sex prevalence.

**Gross Morphology and Histological Features.** These tumors are unicentric or multicentric, often 2 to 4 cm in diameter, and occur in one or both lungs. They originate in the bronchi and often project into the bronchus as papillary growths. The tumors arise from either the surface epithelium of the bronchi or from the bronchial mucous glands.

Histologically, the adenomas are encapsulated and have a papillary structure. The epithelial cells are cuboidal or columnar and are supported by well-vascularized connective tissue stalks. The epithelial cells often show mucin secretion, and pools of mucin may form as cysts lined by flattened epithelium.

## Carcinoma of the Lung

**Classification.** The chief obstacle in comparing data on lung carcinoma in domestic animals, especially in dogs and cats, is the lack of a simple classification. It is difficult to compare data from different laboratories because of the lack of agreement on nomenclature. One useful classification is that of the World Health Organization (Stunzi *et al*., 1974), but even this is unnecessarily complicated. Most classifications have been adapted largely from those used for human lung tumors and are based on information we often do not have in animals.

Classifications based entirely on topographical nomenclature (e.g., bronchial, bronchiolar, bronchiolar–alveolar, or alveolar carcinoma) are sometimes difficult to use in the veterinary field because the carcinomas are usually so far advanced by the

**TABLE 7.2. Histological Classification of Lung Carcinomas**

| Type of carcinoma | Synonyms |
| --- | --- |
| Bronchogenic carcinoma | Adenocarcinoma, epidermoid carcinoma |
| Bronchiolar–alveolar carcinoma | Adenocarcinoma, bronchiogenic carcinoma |
| Epidermoid carcinoma | Squamous cell carcinoma |
| Bronchial gland carcinoma | Adenocarcinoma |
| Anaplastic carcinoma | Alveolar cell carcinoma |
|    Anaplastic small cell carcinoma | "Oat" cell carcinoma, lymphocytelike carcinoma |
|    Anaplastic large cell carcinoma | Giant cell carcinoma |

time the animal is examined that it is difficult to determine the exact site of tumor origin. Most carcinomas in the dog and cat are peripheral in location and multifocal rather than hilar as in humans; these factors also complicate classification.

Too much reliance on cell type (e.g., columnar, cuboidal, or anaplastic) or on the pattern of gland formation as an indication of origin is risky because single carcinomas often show variations in morphology. Many of the specimens are from incomplete necropsies done by practicing veterinarians, so we cannot always rely on gross descriptions. With lung tumors, as with other tumors, there is always the problem of whether the piece of tissue submitted is representative of the whole mass.

Regardless of these problems, we have no alternative except to classify lung carcinomas on the basis of anatomical origin, when possible, and on the prevailing histological pattern. A histological classification is shown in table 7.2.

*Bronchogenic Carcinoma*—This type of carcinoma is uncommon in domestic animals. For example, Stunzi *et al.* (1974) did not find topographical evidence of bronchial origin (bronchogenic carcinoma, as is understood by the term in human pathology) in any of the lung carcinomas examined in dogs. Few carcinomas of bronchial origin were found in the collection of lung carcinomas studied by the author. The bronchogenic carcinoma is usually hilar in location and has a unicentric origin compared with bronchiolar–alveolar carcinoma, which is more often peripheral in location and often multifocal in origin.

*Bronchiolar–Alveolar Carcinoma*—This is the most prevalent type of lung carcinoma in the dog and cat. The frequent occurrence of bronchiolar–alveolar carcinoma in the dog and cat (77 and 72%, respectively), and the infrequency of bronchogenic carcinoma and epidermoid carcinoma, is in sharp contrast to humans.

*Epidermoid Carcinoma (Squamous Carcinoma)*—This represents about 15% of the carcinomas in dogs and cats. It usually derives from bronchial epithelium that has undergone squamous metaplasia.

*Bronchial Gland Carcinoma*—This carcinoma is considered rare, but may be more common than is appreciated, especially in the cat. Since most bronchial glands are found in the major airways in the hilus, carcinomas of these glands are situated in this region of the lung. The neoplasm is often misdiagnosed as bronchiolar–alveolar carcinoma or epidermoid carcinoma. Bronchial gland carcinoma has its origin in the serous and/or mucous glands of the bronchial mucosa.

*Anaplastic Carcinoma* (small and large cell types)—This carcinoma is extremely rare. A few acceptable cases have been found in dogs and cats (Moulton *et al.*, 1981).

One type of carcinoma not included in this classification is the endemic pulmonary carcinoma of sheep, called *jaagsiekte* or pulmonary adenomatosis. This neoplasm is of bronchiolar or alveolar origin, but is difficult to fit into the classification of carcinomas, so it is considered separately (see Jaagsiekte or Pulmonary Adenomatosis of Sheep).

**Clinical Characteristics.** The clinical characteristics of lung carcinoma have been described for dogs but rarely for other domestic species. The clinical course of invasive carcinoma of the lungs in dogs averages 9.6 weeks (ranging from 1 week to 7 months) (Brodey and Craig, 1965). Most dogs with lung carcinoma have no clinical signs in the early stages, but later may show nonproductive cough, dyspnea, cachexia, rales, cardiac insufficiency, emesis, and pericardial effusion.

Dogs with carcinomas or other primary neoplasms of the lung may get hypertrophic osteoarthropathy. Brodey (1971) reported on 60 dogs with this condition and found primary lung tumors in 18 of them. Metastatic tumors in the lungs, such as osteosarcoma, and some chronic inflammatory processes are also associated with this condition. Surgical excision of the primary neoplasm of the lung usually results in regression of the lesions of hypertrophic osteoarthropathy in a period from 2 weeks to 7 months. Recurrence of the condition is found when further metastasis occurs in the lungs.

Lung carcinoma occurs in dogs at an average age of 11 years. Anaplastic small cell carcinoma, a rare form of lung carcinoma, may occur at a younger age (average 7 to 8 years) in dogs. Lung carcinomas of all types seldom occur at less than 6 years of age in dogs. In a study of lung carcinoma in a closed beagle colony, however, the carcinoma appeared as early as 5 years of age and demonstrated an increasing occurrence thereafter as a function of age (Taylor *et al.,* 1979). Squamous cell carcinoma probably occurs in dogs older than those with bronchiolar–alveolar carcinoma, but this age incidence is not clearly established.

The average age of cats with lung carcinoma is 12 years, which is slightly older than for dogs. The average age for lung tumors in cattle is 5 years.

Most reviews indicate no breed prevalence for lung carcinoma in dogs and cats, but some workers report a higher incidence of the tumors in the boxer breed of dogs (Brodey and Craig, 1965; Nielsen, 1970). In Russia, the boxer and East European sheepdog supposedly represent almost half of the dogs with lung carcinoma. Sex predilection for carcinoma has not been found in any domestic species.

**Sites.** Most carcinomas of the lung give no indication of their site of origin, and normal lung tissue is rapidly replaced. The tumors are usually large at the time of recognition and the point of origin cannot always be determined. It is clear, however, that some carcinomas arise distal to the major bronchi and that others are oriented around the bronchi, giving an indication of origin from this site. In others, the bronchial epithelium is intact, and there is stenosis rather than dilation of the bronchi, which suggests origin from the bronchial glands. The carcinomas appear as solitary or sometimes multiple masses in the hilus of the lung or embedded within the lobes of the lung, or the neoplasms appear multiple often in peripheral sites. The tumors may involve an entire lobe or any part of a lobe or lobes in one or both lungs. The multifocal, peripherally located carcinomas are the most common in domestic animals, especially in the dog; in contrast, the hilar region is most common in hu-

mans. The right lung is involved more often than the left lung in the dog, possibly because it is larger.

Bronchiolar–alveolar carcinoma is usually found peripherally in the lung in subpleural sites and usually arises from the terminal bronchi, bronchioles, or alveoli. Squamous cell carcinoma and bronchial gland carcinoma develop in or around the larger bronchi in the hilar region of the lung. Anaplastic carcinoma, which has its origin in the alveoli or terminal bronchioles, is found in any part of the lung.

It is still debatable whether carcinoma of the lung, particularly bronchiolar–alveolar carcinoma, arises unicentrically or multicentrically. If a single nodule is removed surgically and there are no subsequent recurrences at other sites, this is good evidence for unicentric origin. Multiple lesions suggestive of multicentric origin may represent rapid dissemination from a single focus.

Monlux (1952) reported 45 primary lung carcinomas in dogs, with and without metastasis; among these, 37 were multifocal in one or more lung lobes. Multifocal origin could not be distinguished from solitary origin when intrapulmonary metastasis had occurred. In this group, 15 of the carcinomas had diffuse areas of infiltration involving one or more complete lung lobes. Of the 13 lung carcinomas described by Nielsen (1970), 4 were multifocal and the rest were solitary lesions. The multifocal tumors were often small, varying from 2 mm to 4 cm in diameter. Most lesions were 2 cm in diameter when appearing as multifocal growths and 5 cm in diameter when appearing as solitary growths. When large growths were present, several small masses were often found in the same lung.

**Gross Morphology.** Carcinomas of the lung are either expansive or infiltrative. Solitary or multiple masses may be raised above the surface of the lung. They may be diffuse and resemble lobar consolidation in pneumonia (fig. 7.4A). Diffuse involvement may occur from coalescence of multiple areas of growth, particularly in bronchiolar–alveolar carcinoma. Even in diffuse lesions, nodularity is often seen at the periphery of the growth (fig. 7.4B). These nodules are a few millimeters to several centimeters in diameter, pinkish white or light yellow, and may have irregular borders. Some neoplasms are invasive, have poorly defined margins, and blend in with fibrous stroma. Cavitation within the larger neoplasms may occur secondarily to necrosis, and

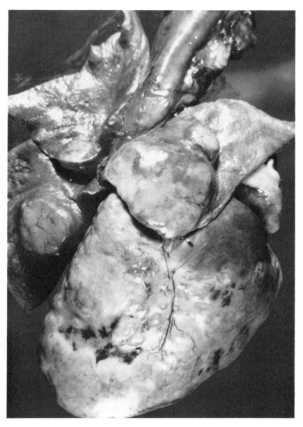

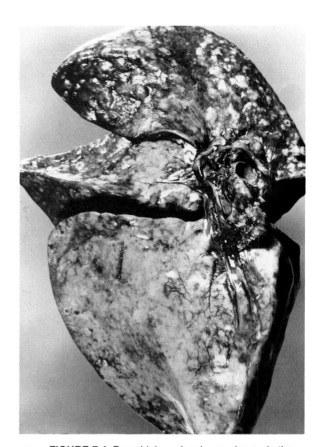

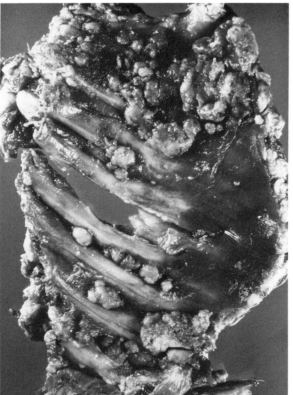

A | B
C |

**FIGURE 7.4.** Bronchiolar−alveolar carcinoma in the lung with spread to the pleura of a dog. A. Large diffuse mass involving most of the right diaphragmatic and intermediate lobules and part of the left diaphragmatic lobe. B. Multiple coalescing nodules of growth appearing as a diffuse mass in the diaphragmatic lobe. C. Spread of lung carcinoma to pleura showing multiple nodules implanted on the parietal surface.

purplish mottling from hemorrhage is common. Irregular areas of atelectasis are seen in the lung tissue immediately around the neoplastic tissue. The carcinomas do not usually adhere to the chest wall, although they invade the hilar region and mediastinum. Occasionally, there is implantation of carcinoma on the pleural surface (fig. 7.4C).

## Histological Features

*Bronchogenic Carcinoma*—This neoplasm is found topographically in relationship to a bronchus, as evidenced histologically by the presence of bronchial cartilage or smooth muscle of bronchial origin. Bronchogenic carcinoma can often be traced to bronchial surface epithelium, which is often columnar and ciliated. Care must be taken to distinguish this carcinoma from bronchial gland carcinoma; the latter carcinoma is also hilar in location and related to a bronchus, but does not arise from the surface epithelium and can be traced to the bronchial glands. In many instances the criteria for separating these two carcinomas are not found, so classification is guesswork. Also, many of the histological features for bronchiolar–alveolar carcinoma (described below) are also found in bronchogenic carcinoma, especially the more anaplastic types. Bronchogenic carcinoma usually shows a papillary or glandular type morphology. These tumors are composed of tall columnar cells, often with carrot-shaped cells with apical mucin droplets (fig. 7.5A). The epithelium is single layered and regular in formation, usually with basilar located nuclei (figs. 7.5B and C), or the epithelium is stratified when covering papillae or ductlike lumens. The tumor is more differentiated than bronchiolar–alveolar carcinoma, but may show a pleocellular pattern (fig. 7.5D) and infiltration with fibrosing stromal response. Metaplasia of epithelium to squamous type is occasionally seen.

*Bronchiolar–Alveolar Carcinoma*—It is important to distinguish between the differentiated and undifferentiated bronchiolar–alveolar carcinomas, especially in the cat, which has a high incidence of the undifferentiated type.

Undifferentiated carcinoma is far more invasive and has a greater tendency to metastasize than the differentiated type, thus the affected animal has a poorer prognosis. There are several criteria used in separating differentiated from undifferentiated carcinomas. The differentiated tumors have well-formed glandular structures, lack epithelial stratification, have uniform cell size, infrequent mitotic figures, minimal stromal fibrosis, and single-layered columnar epithelium with uniform basal nuclei. In contrast, the undifferentiated tumors have few recognizable components to indicate origin, and they have irregularly arranged stratified epithelium that lacks nuclear polarity. They also show detachment of cells, irregular cell size, frequent mitotic figures, and abundant fibrous stroma. The undifferentiated type shows extensive invasion of the fibrous stroma, lymphatics, and/or blood vessels. Both types of carcinoma grow extensively within the alveoli. Metaplasia of cuboidal or columnar cells to squamous cells is found in a few of these tumors, but keratinization is almost never seen.

One of the common histological features of the differentiated bronchiolar–alveolar carcinoma is well-formed glands that are often bronchiolar or alveolar in appearance. Epithelial cell types range from regularly spaced, tall, columnar cells to pleomorphic cuboidal cells. Terms such as "cylindrical cell," "columnar cell," or "cuboidal cell" used in classification should be avoided since it is common to have different cell types in the same neoplasm.

A papillary growth pattern is the most common form of the differentiated carcinoma in domestic carnivores and ruminants. Uniform cuboidal cells are located on delicate stromal septa with continuous infoldings, and occasional large papillae project into the lumens (fig. 7.6A). Some papillary ingrowths may be irregular in formation and project into tubulelike structures (fig. 7.6B). The papillae may be exaggerated, especially in parts of the tumor immediately beneath the pleura. Such structures may present extremely complex patterns of transverse and tangential sections of the papillary fronds. Sometimes the papillary masses disintegrate and undergo various degrees of necrosis, leaving a mass of cellular or amorphous debris with varying numbers of inflammatory cells. The stroma of the papillary growths may show metaplasia to cartilage and bone; these tissues may be abundant but are never neoplastic in nature. A true primary "mixed tumor" (containing both epithelial and connective tissue components) has not been encountered. The height

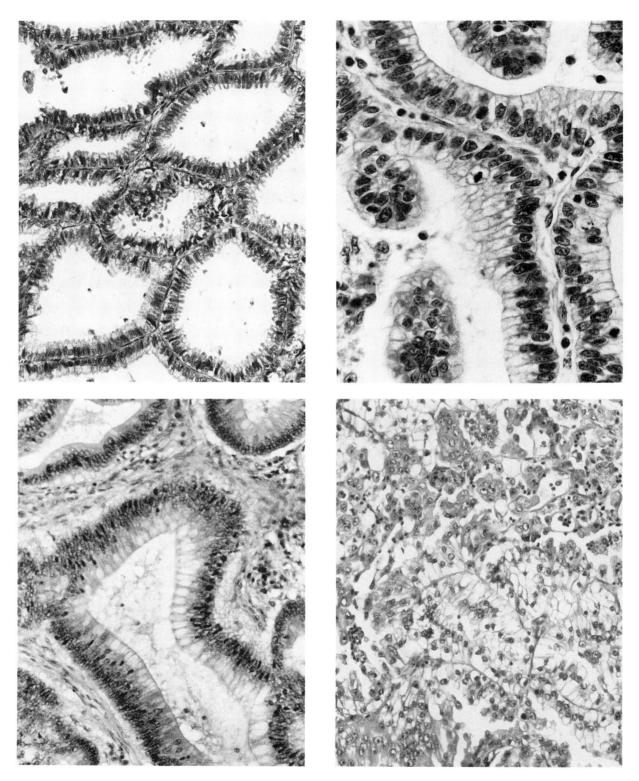

A|B
C|D

**FIGURE 7.5.** Bronchogenic carcinoma. A. Columnar cells with carrotlike shapes. Apex of each cell protrudes into gland lumen; nucleus is at the base. B. Tall columnar cells with clear mucin containing cytoplasm and basilar palisaded nuclei. C. Tall columnar ciliated epithelial cells that appear as goblet cells (large vacuoles of mucin in cytoplasm). D. Variation in pattern showing cells with clear cytoplasm (mucin secretion) intermixed with cells that are more deeply stained and probably more anaplastic.

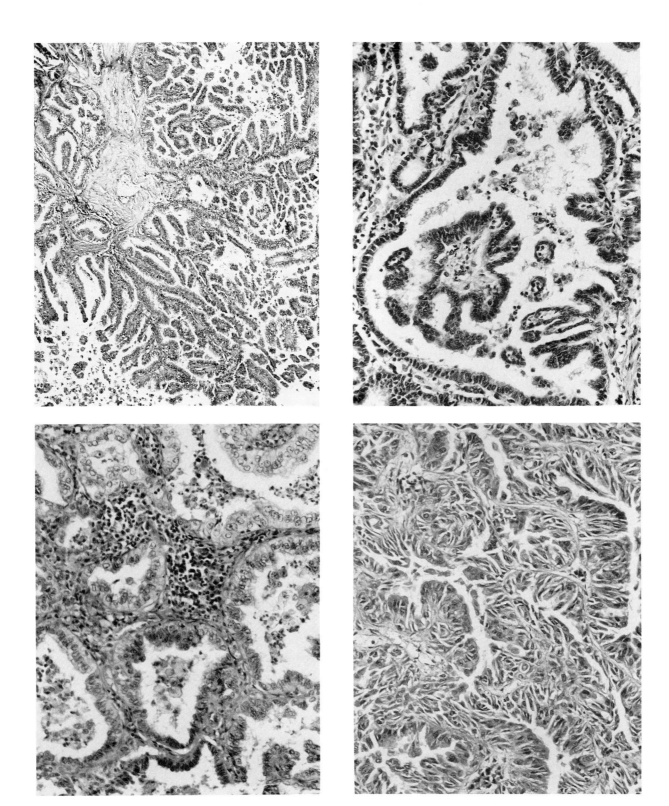

**FIGURE 7.6.** Bronchiolar−alveolar carcinoma of the dog (A, B, and D) and cat (C). A. Papillary growth of cells arranged on delicate fibrous stalks; well-differentiated neoplasm. B. Columnar cells forming irregular glandlike structure, with small, irregular papillae projecting into lumen. Papillae sectioned tangentially appear unconnected to wall.

C. Tumor with cuboidal and columnar cells that form bronchiolar or alveolarlike spaces. The neoplasm is infected and inflammatory cells are present in the interstitium and gland lumens. D. More undifferentiated carcinoma composed of tall columnar cells that are irregularly arranged.

of the papillary epithelium varies, but in most cases the cells are columnar with large, ovoid, basal nuclei. Occasionally, there are extremely tall epithelial cells with basal vacuoles that may or may not contain mucinous material. A carcinoma with mucinous material may be designated as *mucinous carcinoma*. The mucin is secreted by the tumor cells; it does not accumulate in significant amounts from adjacent normal cells. Also, the columnar cell may have a carrotlike shape, with the apex of the cell protruding into the gland lumen and the nucleus at the base of the cell. In a few of these tumors the epithelial cells have cilia, as in bronchogenic carcinoma.

Plaques of invasive tumor cells may be observed in lymphatic vessels or bronchiolar lumens, but are rare in blood vessels. In the apparently normal lung surrounding the tumor, small metastatic tumor foci are sometimes seen. Central ischemic necrosis, often with cholesterol cleft formation and with a limited amount of dystrophic calcification, is frequent. Secondary pneumonia, serofibrinous pleuritis with adhesions, and suppuration are common, especially in highly invasive carcinomas.

In some differentiated bronchiolar–alveolar carcinomas a cuboidal cell pattern, either combined with cylindrocellular areas or as a uniform cuboidal cell proliferation, is observed (fig. 7.6C). These cuboidal cells show monotonously uniform papillary tumor proliferation, or they may have a tubular or acinar type structure. Cellular growth may obliterate the lumens of these units. Cuboidal cells may also appear in a multilayered pattern and in nests and cords. Tall columnar cells in cordlike ribbons may have palisaded nuclei, often located at the basilar poles of the cells (fig. 7.6D). Sometimes tumor cells appear polygonal or spindle shaped.

Usually, there is only a limited spread of tumor cells via the alveoli. Clusters of tumor cells may be observed in lymphatic vessels and even in bronchiolar lumens, but they are rare in blood vessels. In the normal lung that surrounds tumor foci, small metastatic tumor emboli may be seen. Infiltration of the interalveolar stroma and peribronchial tissue occurs and reactive fibrosis develops. This also occurs in the central cores of papillae. Diffuse fibrosis is rare.

The undifferentiated carcinoma has a characteristic histological appearance consisting of irregular, poorly formed glands of various sizes and shapes that resemble immature bronchioles or alveoli (figs.

7.7A–D and 7.8A–C). Papillary growth may also be observed and is similar to that of the differentiated carcinoma, but the papillae are less regular. Small acinar structures with micropapillae are common. Epithelial cell stratifications lining the glandlike structures are more common in this neoplasm than in the differentiated type. The epithelial cells are cuboidal rather than columnar and they lack nuclear polarity. Detachment of neoplastic cells into gland lumens is common; some lumens are nearly filled with these cells. The tumor cells may line the inner walls of the blood vessels, and this pavementing can be mistaken for glandular formation. The typical carcinoma cells are irregular in size and shape and have large, open-faced nuclei, prominent nucleoli, and common mitotic figures.

Stromal fibrosis, often diffuse, is far more common in the undifferentiated than the differentiated carcinoma and is always accompanied by stromal invasion of carcinoma cells. Invasion is also seen in local lymphatics in most of these carcinomas.

Metaplasia of glandular epithelium to squamous cell type is common, and metaplasia of the stroma to cartilage and bone is seen occasionally.

*Epidermoid Carcinoma*—The histological origin of this neoplasm is sometimes in dispute. Most of these neoplasms arise from the lining epithelium of major bronchi, but some may arise from metaplasia of cuboidal or columnar cells in bronchiolar–alveolar carcinoma. Squamous metaplasia in a gland-forming carcinoma does not justify use of such terms as "combined carcinoma" or "composite carcinoma." Scattered throughout the nonkeratinized areas of epidermoid carcinoma may be small pseudolumens containing eosinophilic proteinaceous material. Because of these pseudolumens, the designation "adenoacanthoma" has been used.

The dominant squamous cell appearance and absence of glandular pattern are important features in this neoplasm. The carcinoma is composed of solid, often branching cords or masses of cells of irregular shape and size (fig. 7.9A). The presence of intercellular bridges and/or keratinization is essential for diagnosis, although keratinization is not always a feature of the neoplasm. Some of the squamous cells are large and polygonal and others are flattened and stratified. Occasionally, solid cords of squamous cells with central necrosis resemble glands. Epidermoid carcinoma is highly invasive and is always accompanied by plentiful fibrosis of stroma. Tumor

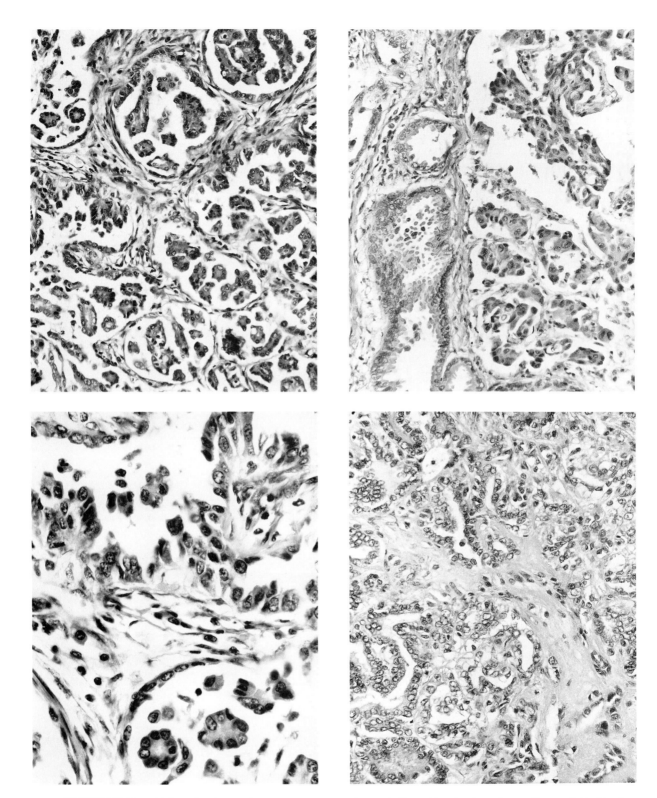

A | B
C | D

**FIGURE 7.7.** Bronchiolar–alveolar carcinoma, un-differentiated type, of the dog. A. Small acinar structures with micropapillae. B. Bronchiolarlike structure lined by columnar cells and surrounded by stromal connective tissue on left side of photograph and pleomorphic cells lacking nu-clear polarity and forming irregular papillae on right side of photograph. C. Intraglandular papillae, some cut in cross section. D. Irregular glandlike formations and stromal fibrosis. (A and D, courtesy of *Vet. Path.*)

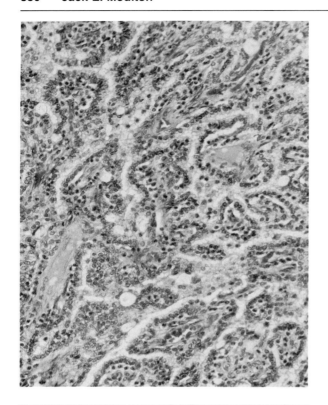

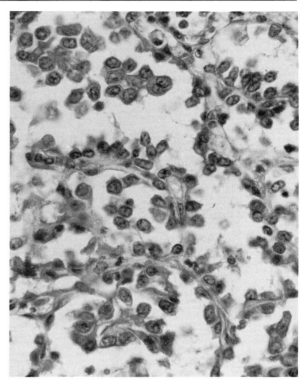

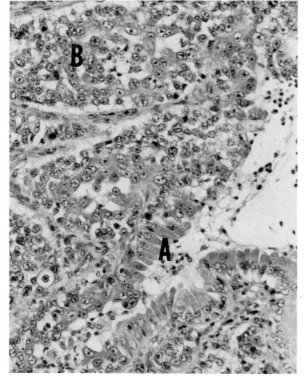

**FIGURE 7.8.** Bronchiolar–alveolar carcinoma in the lung of a dog. A. Cuboidal cells form alveolarlike structures and/or form a lining in existing alveoli and grow into the lumens. B. Anaplastic type tumor with cuboidal non-secretory cells that line up along the alveolar septa or detach and appear free in the lumens. C. Tumor showing possible origin from bronchiolar epithelium (A). There is minimal differentiation of cells (B) into glandular structures.

cells are found in lung alveoli (fig. 7.9B) and in local lymphatics in many of the carcinomas.

In humans, precancerous changes are common in the larger airways prior to the formation of epidermoid carcinoma. Changes such as cellular atypia, irregular hyperplasia, and metaplasia of columnar cells to squamous cells are encountered. Such precancerous changes are rarely described in animals, probably because the early stages are seldom seen in animals; by the time histological examination is made the carcinoma is too advanced to detect early changes.

*Bronchial Gland Carcinoma*—The difficulty in making a diagnosis of this neoplasm is tracing its origin to the bronchial glands. Lymphatic permeation along peribronchial lymphatics by metastasis of other lung carcinomas and permeation by metastasis of adenocarcinoma from nonpulmonary sites both resemble bronchial gland carcinoma. This neoplasm has a distinct histological pattern consisting of (1) a glandular type growth arising from the bronchial glands in the wall of the bronchus and extending into peribronchial tissue (fig. 7.10A), (2) squamous metaplasia of carcinoma cells in more peripheral sites (fig. 7.10B), and (3) hyperplastic thickening of bronchial epithelium overlying the neoplastic tissue. A mixture of squamous metaplasia (like epidermoid carcinoma) and tubular formation (like bronchiolar–alveolar carcinoma) often occurs in junctional sites such as between the cartilagenous plates of the bronchi.

Invasion of squamous or tubular type cells accompanied by stromal fibrosis is seen in almost all of these carcinomas. Infiltration of lymphatics by tumor cells is a consistent finding.

*Anaplastic Carcinoma*—Anaplastic carcinoma arises from the alveolar epithelial cells. These neoplasms have been subdivided extensively according to cytological type, for example, lymphocytelike, "oat," fusiform, polygonal, and giant cell types. It is

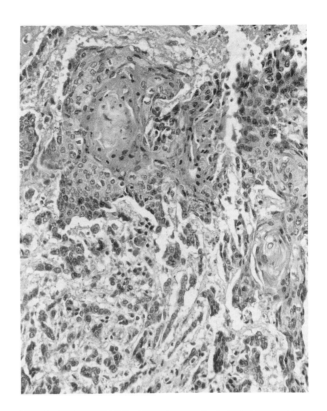

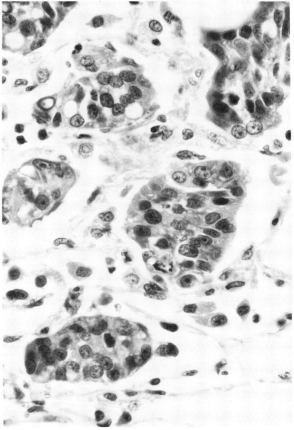

A
—
B

**FIGURE 7.9.** Epidermoid carcinoma in the lung of the dog. A. Solid, irregular trabeculae of neoplastic squamous cells that extend downward from epithelial lining of a bronchus; some keratinization is seen. B. Sectioned cords of squamous cells invading the lung alveoli.

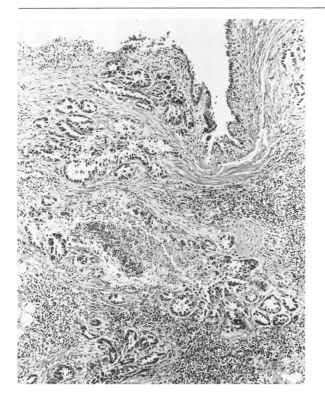

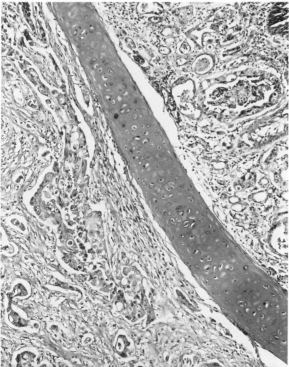

useful, at least for the present, to divide these neoplasms into anaplastic small cell and anaplastic large cell types and omit all other terminology. The small cell carcinoma usually is a distinct type, but the large cell type is a less clearly separable neoplasm and is often misdiagnosed as bronchiolar–alveolar carcinoma. The large cell carcinoma is seen in dogs but rarely if ever in other domestic species. One form of this tumor, which occurs most often in the cat, resembles pulmonary adenomatosis (jaagsiekte) of sheep. It should be noted that epithelialization of the alveoli, alveolar ducts, or terminal bronchioles occurs in certain chronic inflammatory reactions of the lung and may be confused with anaplastic carcinoma.

1. *Anaplastic small cell carcinoma.* The neoplasm may be situated in the hilus or in the central part of the lung lobe, but rarely in the periphery of the lung. The most consistent histological feature of this neoplasm is the presence of small, round, hyperchromatic cells that fill the pulmonary alveoli and may distort or obscure the alveoli (figs. 7.11A–D). A fusiform cell type that has larger cells with clearly visible cytoplasm can also be present. Large masses of tumor cells usually show central necrosis and may resemble keratinized debris, leading to a false diagnosis of squamous cell carcinoma. The surviving bronchiolar epithelium in the region of a small cell carcinoma may show hyperplasia and metaplasia. There is no clear-cut topographical evidence of bronchial, bronchiolar, or alveolar origin. Invasion into the alveoli, blood vessels, and lymphatics is occasionally seen in this neoplasm. This carcinoma metastasizes widely via the bloodstream and/or lymphatics.

The neoplastic cells are uniform in size and spherical, ovoid, or spindle shaped ("oat" cells) and they resemble blast cells. They have dark basophilic nuclei, many mitotic figures, and a thin rim of cyto-

A
B    **FIGURE 7.10.** Bronchial gland carcinoma of the cat. A. Low magnification showing lumen of bronchus at top with carcinoma arising from bronchial glands (between surface epithelium and cartilage plate at bottom). B. Peribronchial cartilage plate surrounded by infiltrative glandular and squamous neoplastic cells. (B, courtesy of *Vet. Path.*)

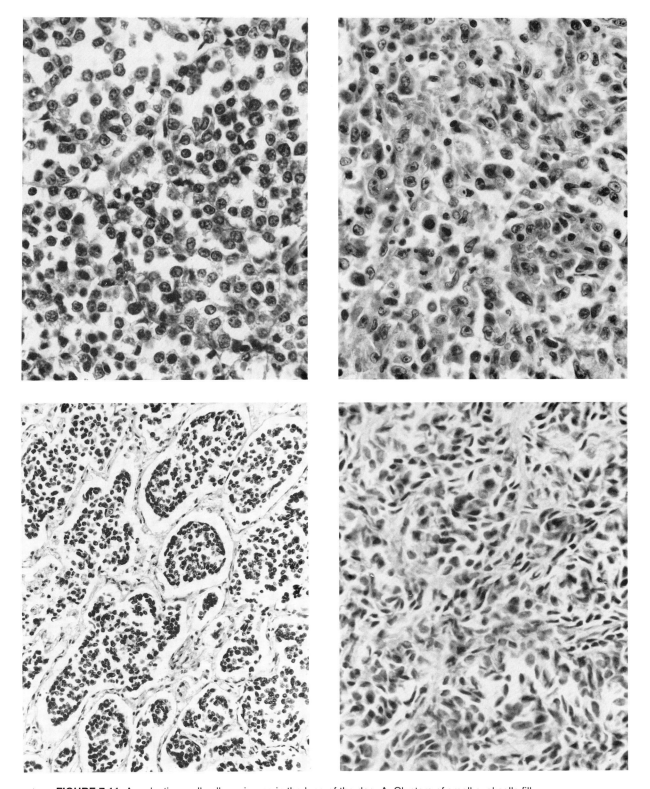

$\begin{array}{c|c} A & B \\ \hline C & D \end{array}$ **FIGURE 7.11.** Anaplastic small cell carcinoma in the lung of the dog. A. Clusters of small oval cells fill alveolar lumens and partly obliterate interalveolar septa. B. Pleomorphic tumor cells with clearly visible cytoplasm. C. Higher magnification of B. Elongated cells ("oat" cell type) filling alveoli. D. Small spindle-shaped cells that occupy the alveolar lumens.

plasm. Some of the cells resemble lymphocytes. The cells are usually densely packed but are sometimes loosely arranged.

The stroma is predominantly delicate and irregular and does not completely separate the cell masses into lobules. Occasionally, coarse strands of stroma are formed, and often cell masses are seen penetrating into this tissue. Inflammatory foci and necrotic areas are also found.

Clinically, anaplastic small cell carcinoma behaves like other lung carcinomas. In all cases in dogs there has been metastasis to the regional lymph nodes; hematogenous metastasis is observed occasionally.

2. *Anaplastic large cell carcinoma.* This rare tumor has been encountered only in the dog. It appears as a differentiated neoplasm with cells in rosettes or as an undifferentiated neoplasm with highly anaplastic cells (figs. 7.12A–C).

In the rosette cell type, the neoplastic cells are larger than those in anaplastic small cell carcinoma, and they often resemble epidermoid cells. The most consistent feature is the presence of cell groups (rosettes) or cells in a palisade arrangement within the alveoli. Occasionally, there is a suggestion of a glandlike pattern. The cells have lighter staining nuclei than those in anaplastic small cell carcinoma, and the cytoplasm is obvious but not abundant.

In the undifferentiated form of anaplastic large cell carcinoma, the cells lack rosette formation and appear in solid sheets that obscure the alveolar architecture. Some of the solid masses of cells contain glandlike clefts. The tumor cells are similar to those in the rosette type, being moderately large and of transitional cell type and having abundant cytoplasm. Stromal fibrosis is usually absent. The neoplastic cells may be found in the lymphatics, but they seldom invade into the stroma. Stromal reaction is minimal or lacking in both types of anaplastic large cell carcinoma.

**Etiology and Transmission.** Exogenous factors that may be associated with lung carcinoma in experimental animals are ionizing radiation, atmospheric pollutants (nickel carbonyl, asbestos, benzopyrene, and other chemicals of the aromatic amine groups), and viruses. By far the most important factor in humans is cigarette smoke.

Auerback *et al.* (1970) trained male beagle dogs to smoke cigarettes through tracheostomas. One group of these experimental dogs smoked nonfiltered cigarettes, another group smoked filtered cigarettes, and a control group smoked no cigarettes. On an equivalent weight basis for humans, each of the dogs smoked approximately 20 to 40 cigarettes per day. The cigarettes contained 34.8 mg of tar and 1.85 mg of nicotine. After 753 days carcinomas were found in the lungs of 24 dogs in the nonfiltered cigarette group, and after 875 days carcinomas appeared in the lungs of 12 additional dogs smoking nonfiltered cigarettes. There were no carcinomas in the group smoking filtered cigarettes or in nonsmoking dogs. The evidence indicated that the lower the tar content, the less harmful the effects of cigarette smoking in the dogs; in other words, the filters removed the carcinogenic products.

Howard (1970) studied 40 dogs that were allowed to inhale $^{239}PuO_2$ particles; 22 of these dogs developed primary lung tumors after 38 to 110 months of exposure. Most neoplasms were located peripherally in the lungs and were of the bronchiolar–alveolar type. There were also five epidermoid carcinomas, three sarcomas, and two primary lymphomas of the lung. Of particular interest in this study were the early changes in the formation of the lung carcinoma. These changes, which occurred in the bronchiolar epithelium, consisted of hyperplasia of the basilar cells of the epithelial layer, cellular atypia, and metaplasia. The longest latent period for neoplastic change was 8 to 9 years. The primary cells undergoing neoplastic change were those of the terminal bronchioles and alveoli.

Three hemangiosarcomas, one fibrosarcoma, and one adenocarcinoma were found in 126 beagles exposed to aerosols of $^{144}Cs$ (Hahn *et al.*, 1973). The tumors developed after 750 to 1,318 days of exposure. The neoplasms usually appeared in the cephalad lobes of the lung, probably because of the higher concentration of the isotope in this region.

**Growth and Metastasis.** Metastasis of the various types of pulmonary neoplasms encountered in animals seems to be similar to that observed in humans. In animals that die from lung carcinoma, metastasis is observed, predominantly in the bronchial lymph nodes, but often metastasis is not found in extrathoracic organs. In cases where the tumor has spread via the bloodstream rather than by lymphatics metastasis is found in extrapulmonary organs.

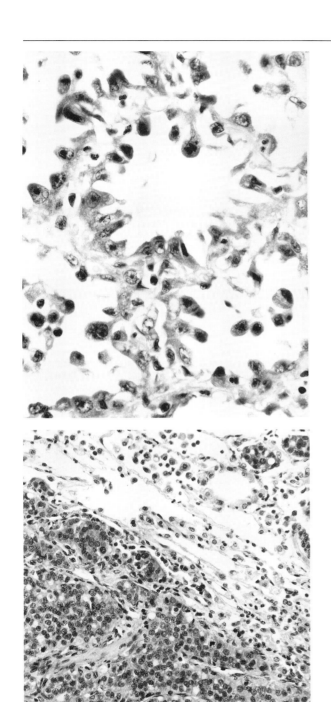

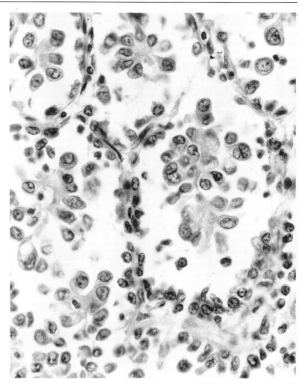

**FIGURE 7.12.** Anaplastic large cell carcinoma. A. Neoplastic cells budding from alveolar walls. B. Neoplastic cells accumulating as rosettes in alveolar lumens. C. More undifferentiated type with cells that lack rosette formation and appear as solid masses filling the alveoli. The solid neoplastic area is adjacent to alveoli only partly filled with tumor cells. (A and B, courtesy of *Vet. Path.*)

Metastasis via the airways, lymphatics, or blood vessels is common within the lungs in most pulmonary carcinomas, and often several lung lobes may show disseminated foci of tumor tissue. Transmigration of neoplastic cells through the airways accounts for many of the so-called multiple lung tumors in dogs, although bronchiolar–alveolar carcinoma probably arises multicentrically. In some instances, spread to the adjacent pleura and pericardium is observed. When comparing the behavior of lung tumors in animals with that in humans, it is important to realize that euthanasia is often carried out in animals before metastasis has had time to develop. It is not possible, therefore, to give any valid statistical data regarding the frequency and localization of metastases in animals.

The reported sites of extrathoracic metastases are the spleen, heart, pericardium, pleura, kidneys, bones, and skeletal muscles. Metastasis to the adrenal glands and brain, which occurs occasionally in humans, is rarely found in animals. The carcinomas also show invasion into the mediastinum, pleura, diaphragm, and pericardium. Almost 100% of epidermoid carcinomas and 90% of anaplastic carcinomas show metastasis (Brodey and Craig, 1965). However, only about 50% of the bronchogenic and bronchiolar–alveolar carcinomas metastasize. The undifferentiated carcinomas of all types metastasize more often than the differentiated ones. The less malignant neoplasms most often spread by direct extension via aerogenous routes and are confined to the pulmonary parenchyma. The more malignant forms spread via the lymphatics and blood vessels.

Among 38 carcinomas in the lungs of cats reported in the literature, two metastasized to the bones (Gustafsson and Wolfe, 1968). One of these carcinomas metastasized from the lung to the ulnar bone by way of the bloodstream, after which metastatic emboli traveled from the bone to the axillary lymph nodes and subsequently reseeded in the lung.

Although rare, lung tumors in cattle usually metastasize to the bronchial or mediastinal lymph nodes, but they also metastasize to other lymph nodes within the thoracic and abdominal cavities and occasionally to peripheral lymph nodes. These carcinomas may also metastasize to the pleura, liver, kidneys, adrenal glands, peritoneum, spinal canal, eyes, and ovaries.

## Carcinoid of the Lung

Carcinoids in the canine lung have been found as large, firm, pale nodules localized in the immediate neighborhood of the main bronchus (Nielsen, 1970; Stunzi, 1971). Metastasis may be present in the bronchial lymph nodes. Carcinoid tumors consist of polygonal cells with broad, slightly granular cytoplasm and round or polygonal nuclei. These cells form cords a few cells wide or large solid masses separated by delicate, well-vascularized stroma. A mosaic and trabecular pattern may be found in the same tumor. In some areas, a whorllike arrangement of the polygonal cells suggests an endocrine tumor. There is usually extensive necrosis. Some of the tumor cells contain small argyrophilic granules in the cytoplasm. The neoplasm resembles the carcinoid of the intestinal tract.

The carcinoid tumors arising in the mucosa of the lungs or alimentary tract form a distinct group with characteristic endocrine function in relationship to their site of origin. In humans, the carcinoids include adrenocorticotropic hormone-secreting bronchial carcinoid, histamine-producing gastric carcinoid, and serotonin-producing ileal and appendiceal carcinoid. On the basis of the morphological and metabolic features of the carcinoid tumors occurring at different sites, it is likely that the tumor is derived from the neuroendocrine cells that embryologically migrate into these sites and mature into the cells with endocrinological function.

## Sarcoma of the Lung

Tumors of connective tissue origin are rare in the lungs of domestic animals, and when present they resemble their counterparts at other sites. In the dog, five probable cases of primary pulmonary osteosarcoma have been reported (Brodey, 1971). Rhabdomyoma and rhabdomyosarcoma, although extremely rare as primary tumors in the lungs of domestic animals, have also been reported. Only three cases of these neoplasms were found in the literature through 1970: one in a lamb (Day, 1922), one in a calf (Siebold, 1946), and more recently, one in the lung of a sheep (O'Donahoo and Seawright, 1971). This latter neoplasm was an invasive, cream-white, rubbery growth, which histologically had irregular bundles of striated muscle fibers that streamed in all directions. It also contained tubular structures lined by ciliated, nonciliated, or mucin-producing epithelial cells. Some of the epithelial structures were surrounded by smooth muscle and by neoplastic skeletal muscle. The authors suspected that this growth was some form of congenital malformation (hamartoma) rather than a true neoplasm. Primary hemangiosarcomas and Schwann cell tumors have occurred rarely in the lungs of dogs.

## Granular Cell Tumor (Myoblastoma) of the Lung

Parker *et al.* (1979) reviewed granular cell tumors in animals and described a case in the lung of a horse (fig. 7.13). This neoplasm has also been called "granular cell myoblastoma," but "myoblastoma" is a misleading term and its use has fallen into disrepute.

Many of these neoplasms in humans have been considered to arise from fibroblastlike precursor cells that share a common origin with Schwann cells or are metaplastic variants of Schwann cells. Some nonneoplastic granular cells develop from smooth muscle, and some granular cell tumors may have a similar origin. The neoplasms tend to occur more frequently at certain anatomical sites in humans, but the distribution gives little indication of the cell of origin. From the few reported cases in domesticated animals, it appears that the lung of the horse and the tongue of the dog are predilection sites of origin for this neoplasm.

Granular cell tumors have been interpreted as neoplasms of myoblastic origin, as a degenerative process, or as a storage disease of muscular, histiocytic, fibroblastic, or neurogenic origin. The currently proposed relationship of granular cell tumors to Schwann cells is supported by the following evidence: the frequent close anatomical relationship of granular cell tumors to peripheral nerves, the presence of substances similar to degradation products of myelin in granular cell tumors, the presence of high concentrations of cerebrosides and gangliosides in granular cell tumors, and the histological similarity between granular cells and Schwann cells near axons undergoing Wallerian degeneration.

Five granular cell tumors have been found in the tongues of dogs, and there is a report of a similar tumor in the cerebrum and meninges of a dog. By contrast, all six previously reported granular cell tumors in horses have arisen in the lungs, usually in close proximity to the major airways. The equine tumors may be associated with hypertrophic osteoarthropathy (Alexander *et al.*, 1965).

Granular cell tumors in domesticated animals have been reported primarily in older animals, with

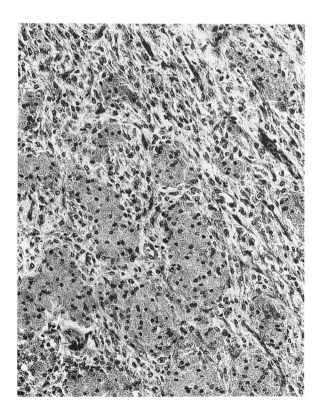

**FIGURE 7.13.** Granular cell tumor (myoblastoma) of the horse. Granular cells are in small clumps or strands and individual granular cells are in a fibrovascular stroma. Granular cells may also be interdigitated between collagen whorls around capillaries. Movat's pentachrome stain. (Courtesy of Dr. G. A. Parker and *J. Comp. Path.*)

no predilection for either sex. Regardless of species or site of origin, all of the tumors have been morphologically and histochemically similar.

## Jaagsiekte or Pulmonary Adenomatosis of Sheep

**General Considerations.** Several sheep diseases are characterized by the development of slowly progressive pneumonia or development of a lung neoplasm. Examples of these are maedi, zwoegerziekte, bouhite, Montana progressive pneumonia, and jaagsiekte. The names maedi, bouhite, zwoegerziekte, and jaagsiekte all have the same connotation, namely dyspnea. Similarities in the pathology and/or symptomatology of some of these diseases have given rise to considerable confusion in the literature as to their exact identity. There seems to be no doubt that certain of these conditions are related. For example, it has been demonstrated that neutralizing antibodies against the causative virus of maedi are present in the serum of sheep suffering from zwoegerziekte and Montana progressive pneumonia, whereas none exist in the serum of sheep suffering from jaagsiekte. The following discussion refers to jaagsiekte, a distinct neoplastic entity.

Jaagsiekte, or pulmonary adenomatosis, as it is also called, is a specific contagious disease of sheep that is characterized by the slow and progressive development of a lung neoplasm. The disease is manifested by a long incubation period, and recoveries from the disease, once the typical signs of the disease are manifested, do not occur. The etiology of jaagsiekte is a type-A or type-D retrovirus. In other words, jaagsiekte is a transmissable neoplasm, just as are feline lymphoma, avian leukosis, myxomatosis in rabbits, bovine papillomatosis, and others. While this disease is known in most overseas countries as jaagsiekte or pulmonary adenomatosis, a more correct appellation would be pulmonary carcinomatosis, since the condition is of neoplastic type that includes metastasis to regional lymph nodes. There is some debate whether the lymph node spread of the tumor cells represents true metastasis or just lymph node "implantation" of cells spreading through lymphatic vessels. Extrathoracic metastases have been seen in cases in Israel.

Any sheep population is vulnerable to jaagsiekte. The disease has now been recognized in many countries, including Iceland, South Africa, India, Peru, Mexico, China, Germany, the Netherlands, Kenya, and Canada. This disease was reported in the United States in 1980 (Cutlip and Young, 1982). Jaagsiekte probably exists in other parts of the world as well. The incidence in different areas varies from 0.2 to 3.6% in sheep, but may be considerably higher in flocks where the infection has been present for several years. The distribution of jaagsiekte is not related to host susceptibility since sheep from regions free of the disease are susceptible when moved to infected areas (Dungal, 1946; Dungal *et al.*, 1938). An outbreak of the disease may result from the introduction of an affected animal into a clean flock, but an interval of 5 to 8 months elapses before appearance of the disease.

The classical example of an epidemic of jaagsiekte is the experience suffered by the farmers of Iceland during the late 1930s when large scale outbreaks occurred. The disease started in 1933 on a farm containing Karakul rams imported from Germany and spread to involve one-third of the sheep in the country (Dungal *et al.*, 1938). Between 1936 and 1938, Iceland had 50 to 80% mortality in some flocks of sheep from jaagsiekte. Because of the climate, the methods of sheep farming in Iceland at that time were conducive to the spread of the disease. In the spring the sheep grazed on pastures close to the farms, and in the summer they were driven into the mountain pastures in the interior of the country where they grazed in common with other flocks. They remained there for 3 to 4 months, and then during autumn, they were driven back to large collecting areas capable of holding as many as 4,000 sheep. There, the sheep were penned together until they were separated into flocks belonging to individual owners and driven to the various farms for the winter. Infection was greatest at this time when the sheep were kept indoors in houses that were poorly ventilated. It is possible that secondary bacterial invasion of the lungs associated with climatic conditions played a role in the rapid course of disease during the winter.

Jaagsiekte must not be confused with maedi, which is also found in many of the same areas, sometimes on the same farm or in the same animal

## Oral Papilloma of the Dog

**Age, Breed, Sex, and Sites.** These tumors mainly affect pups (average age of 1 year), and there is no breed or sex prevalence. Oral papillomas are almost always multiple. They affect the buccal mucosa, tongue, palate, pharynx, and epiglottis. Papillomas of the lip ordinarily grow more slowly than those of the mouth.

**Gross Morphology.** These discrete neoplasms vary from white flattened or smooth nodules a few millimeters in diameter to neoplasms that are gray and pedunculated or cauliflowerlike (fig. 8.2). The experimental neoplasm first appears as a pale, smooth elevation corresponding to the area of scarification. In several weeks the tumor reaches full size and resembles a typical papilloma seen in the skin. With regression the tumor darkens and shrinks; complete regression takes several weeks. Healing occurs without scar formation. Chambers *et al.* (1960) showed that regression is enhanced by injection of "immune" lymphocytes from dogs in which the tumor has regressed.

Watrach *et al.* (1971) studied a natural case of papillomatosis of the oral and pharyngeal cavities in an 18-month-old dog with a squamous cell carcinoma developing in the posterior portion of the right side of the oral cavity. This was the first case of possible malignant transformation of virus-induced oral papilloma in the dog. Such transformation is well recorded in cattle (see Esophagus).

**Histological Features.** The initial change in oral papilloma is a simple hyperplasia of the epithelium. This change increases with a corresponding increase in the cornified layer. The cells of the basal layer remain normal in size, whereas the cells of the outer stratum spinosum enlarge greatly and exhibit intensely stained nuclei. With epithelial proliferation, the surface is thrown into folds that contain connective tissue cores.

Cheville and Olson (1964) described the pathogenesis of experimental canine oral papilloma. In the first stage after experimental infection, there is focal acanthosis (hyperplasia) in the epithelium, that is, a focal exaggeration of the normal process of keratinization. No virus is seen at this stage. In the next stage of papilloma development, the cells are diverted from keratinization to the production of virus. Some of the cells in the acanthotic stratum spinosum are enlarged and have increased cytoplas-

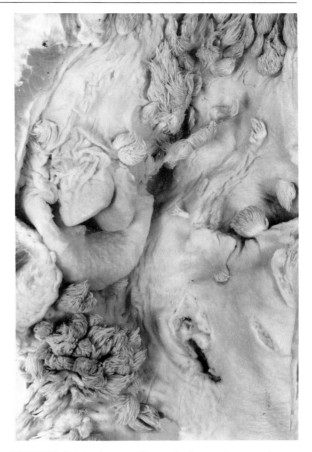

**FIGURE 8.2.** Infectious papillomas in the oropharynx of a young dog.

mic basophilia. At this stage some large cells in the stratum granulosum form intranuclear inclusion material, show loss of nucleoli, and fail to have cytoplasmic differentiation to tonofibrils and keratohyaline granule formation. The cytoplasm may have a swollen vesicular appearance (ballooning degeneration) because of mitochondrial swelling and disorientation of endoplasmic reticulum. This lesion parallels and is probably due to the nuclear change. At this stage the intranuclear body masses are concentrated with viral antigen; DNA-containing virus production is at its maximum.

The virus either stimulates cellular proliferation with formation of papilloma or replicates itself and destroys the cell. Initially the virus replication begins in the stratum germinativum, although virus is not detected there because it is masked in that site just as in the Shope papilloma in the skin of the rabbit or the papilloma in the skin of the cow. Virus particles are first seen in association with the nucleoli in cells of the upper stratum spinosum. Virus soon spreads throughout the nuclei especially in the more superficial cells of the keratogenic zone and most of the normal nuclear material is replaced. Virus particles are demonstrated most easily in the stratum corneum where the cells are undergoing degeneration. Apparently when the neoplastic cells can no longer reproduce themselves, they produce virus.

**Etiology and Transmission.** Oral papillomas in dogs are caused by viruses of the papovavirus group and are considered contagious. The formation of complete virus particles in the superficial part of the papilloma aids transmission. Experimentally, the tumors can be transmitted by scarification with whole cells or cell-free filtrates (De Monbreun and Goodpasture, 1932; M'Fadyean and Hobday, 1898). The incubation period of the experimental disease, 30 to 33 days, may be shorter in malnourished or sickly puppies. The disease lasts 1.5 to 3 months and is followed by spontaneous regression of the tumors. Solid immunity follows experimental or natural infection. The virus can be titered by giving graded doses in the oral mucosa (Konishi *et al.*, 1972).

The virus of oral papilloma exhibits great tissue and host specificity. It multiplies only in the oral or pharyngeal mucosa of the dog with no autotransplantation to extraoral sites. Papillomas fail to develop when the virus is scarified into the skin or vagina of the dog. The virus can be held 64 days at 10°C in 50% glycerol. It withstands 45°C for 60 minutes, but is inactivated by 50°C for 60 minutes (Gründer, 1959).

The prevalence of viral oral papilloma in dogs seems to vary in some districts with time (Borthwick *et al.*, 1982). These authors decribe oral papilloma in older dogs that histologically showed no ballooning degeneration and no inclusion bodies. Also, although it had many cells in mitosis, it did not exhibit cellular atypia. Such "old dog" oral papilloma is rare.

## Squamous Cell Carcinoma of the Gingiva of Dogs and Cats

**Incidence, Age, Breed, and Sex.** In collections of all tumors of the gum, squamous cell carcinoma is often the most common tumor type found in cats and second only to epulides in dogs. It occurs in older age groups: the average age for cats is 10.5 years and for dogs is 8.8 years. No breed predilection is apparent, and the sex predisposition to the male is less marked than for carcinoma in the tonsil of the dog.

**Clinical Considerations and Sites.** The tumor bearers present with halitosis, blood-tinged salivation, and in the late stages, asymmetrical facial swelling and possibly ocular protrusion. Although any site may be involved by these solitary tumors (fig. 8.1), the anterior and posterior upper jaw regions in the dog are most frequently affected (Todoroff and Brodey, 1979).

**Gross Morphology.** Macroscopically, the early lesions are white or pink nodular masses measuring 0.5 to 1 cm in diameter; as they extend they may form fleshy masses around the teeth or form ulcerated plaquelike lesions. Some tumors around the carnasial teeth extend onto the palate making it difficult to decide whether the lesion originated in the gingiva or palate. This neoplasm invades locally, destroys periodontal structures causing loosening of the teeth, and possibly stimulates osteoclasts to erode the bone in front of the advancing tumor. Primary tumors invading the maxilla may extend into the nasal cavity and periorbital tissue. Knecht and Priester (1978) gave a frequency ranking list of a variety of tumors involving the bones in the dog, including 48 squamous cell carcinomas in the maxilla and 54 in the mandible.

**Histological Features.** The tumors are typical squamous cell carcinomas (see chap. 2), but histological grading has not been assessed for these oral tumors. On the basis of radiographs, Todoroff and Brodey (1979) showed that whereas all melanomas and fibrosarcomas are osteolytic, a few squamous cell carcinomas are osteoblastic. Of a clinic population of 20,000 cats and 65,000 dogs, Quigley *et al.* (1972) encountered 4 cats and 1 dog in which the carcinomas in the mandible were unconnected to the overlying epithelium and stimulated fibroblastic disease. No significant difference could be demonstrated related to histological type, mitotic rate, size of nucleoli, depth of pigmentation, lymph vessel invasion, tumor location, volume of tumor, delay between observation and excision, or ablation by scalpel surgery versus cryosurgery.

## Melanocytic Tumors in Other Species

In contrast with the dog, malignant melanotic tumor is rare in the mouth of the cat. In data from 13 universities in the United States and Canada Dorn and Priester (1976) found only one melanoma among 50 cat oropharyngeal tumors, and Cotter (1981), adding data to a literature survey, could find only four melanomas in 169 oropharyngeal neoplasms. Various surveys (e.g., Brodey, 1966) mention that the tumors usually occur on the palate or gum.

Occasionally one encounters melanomas in the horizontal ramus of the mandible of cattle and sheep at the abattoir. Although they may grow sufficiently large to lead to fracture of the ramus, metastasis does not develop. Melanocytes can be demonstrated in the fat and connective tissue around the mandibular nerve of the other ramus, and these may be the source of such tumors. Wiseman *et al.* (1977) reported two cases of large unilateral tumors associated with the vertical ramus of the mandible and surrounding structures of two calves, one a 14-month-old Charolais cross bullock and the other a 9-month-old Ayrshire heifer. In the latter, the tumor had been observed since birth.

Histologically, the neoplasm resembles the human melanotic neuroepidermal tumor of infancy, that is, there are epitheliumlike melanin-containing cells and small lymphocytelike cells set in a fibrous stroma. A tumor at a similar site in a 7-month-old Aberdeen Angus cross steer was shown by Long *et al.* (1981) to have different light and electron microscopic pattern and was considered to be a congenital fibrotic melanoma.

Dorn and Priester (1976) mentioned five melanomas in 29 equine oropharyngeal malignancies but gave no further details.

## Tumors of Soft (Mesenchymal) Tissue

### Fibroma and Fibrosarcoma

**General Considerations.** Transitional forms exist between histologically well-differentiated fibroma durum, fibroma molle, and fibrosarcoma. Even nonencapsulated, invasively growing tumors with many mitotic figures do not often metastasize either to regional lymph nodes or to distant sites, although recurrence following surgery or radiotherapy is common. Most published series of tumors therefore list very few clear-cut benign fibromas in the oropharynx.

**Fibrosarcoma in Dogs.** Fibrosarcoma is common in the dog, but less frequent than melanoma or carcinoma. The mean age (7.6 years) is significantly lower than for the other two types of neoplasms, and the age range (0.5 to 15 years) is wide. Cohen *et al.* (1964) suggested a slight predisposition for males but no breed preference, while Thrall (1981) supports the sex data but notes that 11 of 17 affected dogs were from breeds that weighed more than 50 lb. Dorn and Priester (1976) agreed that there is an increase in relative risk of males developing fibrosarcoma and melanoma but not squamous cell carcinoma. The gum is the commonest site, but the lip, cheek, palate, and tongue may also be involved (fig. 8.1). The tumors are firm with a smooth, sometimes nodular surface that becomes ulcerated but seldom crateriform (cf. carcinoma and melanoma). Using the World Health Organization report (1978) as a basis for staging, Thrall (1981) found that 13 of 17 cases were greater than 4 cm in diameter and that the same number had osseous involvement of mandible, maxilla, or hard palate. Despite this invasion of bone, metastasis even to the ipsilateral mandibular lymph node is rare. For example, Todoroff and Brodey (1979) reported that 5 of 26 tumors metastasized to regional lymph nodes and 6 of 26 to the lung; Thrall (1981) found that 3 of 17 tumors metastasized to regional lymph nodes and 1 of 17 to the lung. Nevertheless, survival time after diagnosis is usually short because the clinical signs of local growth cause the owners to request euthanasia for their pets. Invasion of bone makes surgery unrewarding. Thrall (1981) reported a mean survival time of 6.8 months following orthovoltage radiotherapy (mean time of

3.9 months before local regrowth). Only one of the 17 dogs in this series was alive and free of tumor after 27 months, and this 5-year-old cocker had such a small tumor that the diagnostic biopsy had removed much of it.

**Fibrosarcoma in Cats.** In cats this tumor follows an age and site distribution similar to that of the dog (fig. 8.1). Since melanoma is rare in cats, fibrosarcoma is second in frequency to carcinoma (Brodey, 1970). Local invasive growth and lack of widespread metastasis resemble the pattern in the dog, and the response to therapy is likewise poor, although slightly better than for squamous cell carcinoma. Survival times for cats treated with combined immunotherapy, chemotherapy, and cryosurgery are 382 and 1,205 days for fibrosarcoma of the mandible and hard palate, respectively, compared with 49 and 59 days for carcinoma (Brown *et al.*, 1980). Cats with neoplasms of the skin induced by feline transmissible sarcoma virus (FeSV) may also show lesions on the lips. Such fibrosarcomas are in young cats (usually less than 5 years old) and are usually multicentric rather than solitary (Hardy, 1981). All the virus isolates listed by Hardy have been from subcutaneous tumors. From present evidence it appears that the oral fibrosarcomas are not examples of the relatively rare FeSV-induced multicentric tumor. The report by Kemp *et al.* (1976) of a 3.5 cm tumor arising at the mucocutaneous border of the upper lip of a cat raises an interesting diagnostic problem in this respect. The authors classified the tumor as pseudosarcomatous fasciitis because it had pleomorphic, bizarre, sarcomalike fibroblasts and occasional giant cells, but the tumor was nonmetastasizing. Polyps in the pharynx of cats under 3 years of age should be investigated carefully since their pedicles may originate from the pharyngeal opening of the eustachian tube (Bedford, 1982); they represent a reaction to otitis media.

**Fibrosarcoma in Sheep.** McCrea and Head (1978) reported a high prevalence of tumors in sheep grazing on bracken fern (*Pteris aquilina*) covered moorland in Northeast Yorkshire. The commonest tumor type encountered was a fibrosarcoma; no bladder tumors were found. Most of these fibrous tumors developed in the mandible or maxilla of ewes over 3 years of age, and only on rare occasion did a sheep have more than a single primary tumor of the jaw. The tumors appear to originate around the roots of mandibular or maxillary molar teeth (figs. 8.4A and B). They grew to a very large size, but metastasis was infrequent and only to the regional lymph nodes. Of eight wether lambs fed dried bracken fern continously from 5 months of age onward (McCrea and Head, 1981), one died from acute bracken poisoning after 45 months and the other seven all developed bladder tumors by the time the experiment ended after 62 months. One of these sheep, when examined after 34 months of bracken feeding, showed a moderately sized fibrosarcoma associated with the left molar maxillary teeth and a small fibrous tissue tumor in the fat around the left mandibular nerve. The relationship between these jaw fibrosarcomas and ingestion of bracken fern therefore remains to be elucidated.

## Periodontal Epulis of the Dog

**General Considerations.** The term *epulis* has come down to us from Greek medicine and was used for any localized gingival enlargement. When histological examination was possible, "epulis" could be qualified by adjectives describing the nature of the lesion (e.g., "sarcomatous epulis") or by the origin of the lesion (e.g., "mandibular bone epulis"). All veterinarians know what canine epulides look like, but attempts to formulate an exact definition have exposed our ignorance of the essential nature of the lesion.

**Incidence.** These growths are very common in the dog but rare in other domestic animals (fig. 8.1). Because they can be recognized macroscopically with some degree of accuracy, it is probable that many cases are not submitted for histological examination. Even so, Gorlin *et al.* (1963) reported 253 canine and 1 feline epulides. Langham *et al.* (1965), in a list of 205 canine oral neoplasms, saw 36 fibromatous epuli of periodontal origin and 38 fibrous epuli; the difference between the two was not reported. Bodingbauer (1954) recorded 48 dogs with epuli in 2,307 examined, which is an occurrence of 2.08%. Both sexes are affected and all ages may have lesions, even 1-year-old animals. The average age is between 7 and 8 years. There is no breed prevalence if one considers solitary epuli; multiple epuli, however, occur most often in brachycephalic dogs.

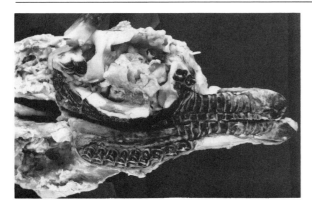

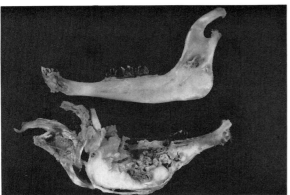

A
—
B

**FIGURE 8.4.** Fibrosarcoma in the jaw of a 5-year-old Swaledale ewe. A. Tumor replacing much of the right maxilla. Note displacement of molar teeth, extension to the hard palate, and the ulcerated necrotic center of the tumor. B. Tumor extending from left mandibular sinus loosens the molar teeth and allows infection to develop.

**Sites and Gross Morphology.** Solitary epuli may be associated with any teeth, but they probably occur most frequently in the molar region, especially around the carnassial teeth, then next in the premolar and canine tooth regions, and least commonly around the incisors. In the series reported by Bodingbauer (1954), 32 of 48 tumors were maxillary and 16 were mandibular. Small masses (0.5 cm in diameter) tend to be sessile and larger ones (1 to 2 cm) may be pedunculate, arising from the periodontal region usually on the labial aspect of the tooth. They are round or elongated and covered by epithelium similar to that of the gum, which may

be smooth or finely nodular. The surface can become ulcerated and infected because of occlusal damage from opposing teeth. The lesions are firm depending on how much bone is present, and this bone may anchor the mass to the jaw bone. In the majority of cases the related tooth is firmly set in its socket and periodontal disease is minimal.

Epuli may start as several discrete lesions, but usually are first seen clinically when they have become confluent and affect both upper and lower jaws. In macroscopic appearance they resemble the solitary epuli, and although they are largest on the labial aspect of the gum, they will progress to surround the teeth and may virtually bury the incisors and premolars (fig. 8.5A). This phenomenon is most common in brachycephalic dogs; thus in the series of epulides reported by Gorlin *et al.* (1963), boxers made up 35% of the cases and Boston terriers 8%. Burstone *et al.* (1952) described four such cases in related boxers under the name "familial gingival hypertrophy." As they pointed out, the boxer breed was relatively new in the United States at that time and could be traced back to relatively few dogs, so that they did not know whether the lesion was peculiar to the boxer breed or to a strain of boxers. Certainly the breed was common in the United Kingdom at the same time and it had about the same frequency of occurrence given by Brodey (1960) for the United States, that is, 30% of boxers over 5 years of age. Gorlin *et al.* (1963) thought that this condition may simulate "idiopathic fibromatosis" of humans, but Burstone *et al.* (1952) mentioned that the tumor in humans lacks bone or epithelium in the stroma.

**Histological Features.** On the basis of a histological section alone, without clinical history, one cannot distinguish between solitary and multiple epuli. The lesion is composed of closely packed, coarse, collagen fibers with moderately numerous spindle or stellate cells and a regular scattering of small blood vessels that, near the epithelial surface, may show a pattern of granulation tissue. Infiltration by plasma cells and lymphocytes is often found unrelated to ulceration of the surface epithelium. The overlying epithelium is not thickened, but extending from it are branching and reuniting cords of epithelium, reminiscent of the exaggerated rete pegs seen in bovine fibropapilloma or some healing skin wounds (fig. 8.5B). The peripheral cells of

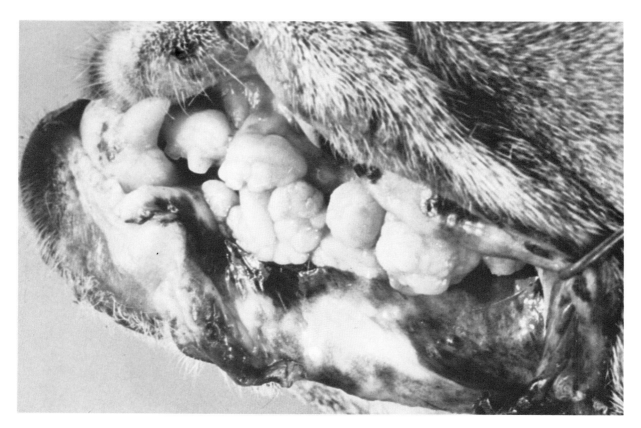

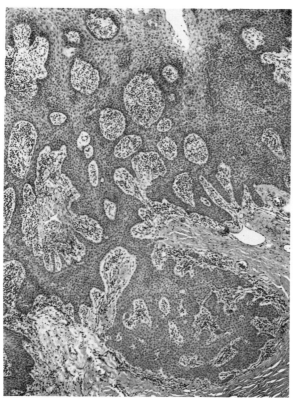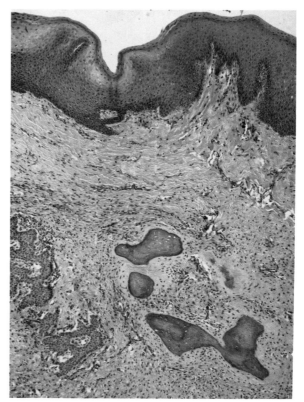

these cords are columnar and in palisade arrangement; the central cells of the larger masses are typical keratinocytes with intercellular bridges, but keratin "pearls" are not found. Occasional cysts lined by stratified squamous epithelium are present in these cords. Mitotic figures are rare in both epithelium and fibrous tissue. In the deeper areas of the lesion, there is osteoid and mature lamellated bone associated with cell-rich bone-forming matrix (figs. 8.5C and 8.6A–D). Sometimes this bone contains fat and marrow tissue between the spicules. Macerated specimens or whole jaw sections show that some bone spicules are exostoses from jaw bone, presumably because of the disturbance of the periosteum, and others are completely separate from the bone and presumably represent metaplasia from fibrous tissue. Occasionally, one can see altered collagen becoming calcified. In addition to this ossification and calcification, a relatively few specimens contain small islands of cementum.

The interpretation of these findings has proved difficult. On the basis of the nature of the epithelium and calcified tissue present in 60% of cases, Gorlin *et al.* (1963) suggested that the tumor had its origin in the periodontal membrane from proliferated cell rests of Malassez (odontogenic epithelial rests). They used the term *fibromatous epulis of periodontal origin* and made two further observations. First, the lesions "may not be a legitimate tumor," and second, epithelial proliferation may be so marked that "erroneous diagnosis of basal cell carcinoma or ameloblastoma were not infrequently made." In another study, Langham *et al.* (1965) listed fibrous epuli and fibromatous epuli of periodontal origin and described an adamantinoma that they considered to be the malignant form of epulis of periodontal origin.

The periodontal epuli are usually hemispherical nodular growths that protrude from the gingiva but grow slowly and may infiltrate the underlying bone but cause little or no bone proliferation. Bodingbauer (1954) divided his 22 histologically examined cases into fibrous epuli (10), telangiectatic epuli (2), bone forming epuli (4), giant cell epuli (2), and predominantly epithelial epuli (4).

The nomenclature recommended by Dubielzig *et al.* (1979*b*) has much to recommend it. They subdivide the group into three categories, namely, fibromatous epulis of periodontal origin, ossifying epulis of periodontal origin, and acanthomatous epulis. This latter growth is the only one that infiltrates into the underlying bone (figs. 8.7A–C), usually the mandible, and is probably equivalent to Langham's adamantinoma. Their conclusion is debatable, namely that periodontal epulides should be classified as dental tumors because they are intimately associated with dental structures and often contain remnants of dental epithelium and dental hard products and because the stroma resembles periodontal membrane. The periodontium comprises the tissues surrounding the tooth, including alveolar bone, periodontal membrane, cementum, and gingival epithelium. It is not surprising that all of these elements are present in proliferative lesions of the region. The term *dental tumor* could be misread as synonymous with *odontogenic tumor,* and epulides are certainly not tooth forming. Whether all these proliferative lesions are neoplastic or not is still undecided.

On the basis of a limited sample of 13 specimens (one of which proved to be a true fibroma), Greenwood and O'Brien (1975) set out the argument in favor of the lesions being localized inflammatory hyperplastic reactions of the gingiva resulting from chronic irritation. All gradations were found from active granulation tissue to relatively avascular masses of fibrous tissue. These authors concluded that the epithelial hyperplasia is not odontogenic, but is rather a reaction of surface epithelium to irritation and infection of a magnitude not likely to be found in the human mouth. They postulate further that collagenase from proliferating gingival epithelium might determine the pattern and extent of new bone formation. This suggestion is not new. Burstone *et al.* (1952) stated that "the bone might be explained as the result of inductive influence of the

**FIGURE 8.5.** Periodontal epuli of the dog. A. Multiple mandibular and maxillary ossifying peripheral epuli in an 11-year-old female boxer. B. Solitary acanthomatous peripheral epulis of mandibular incisor region in a 12-year-old male terrier. C. Solitary ossifying peripheral epulis of maxillary molar region in an 18-year-old female terrier. Note epithelium bottom left and bone trabeculae in center.

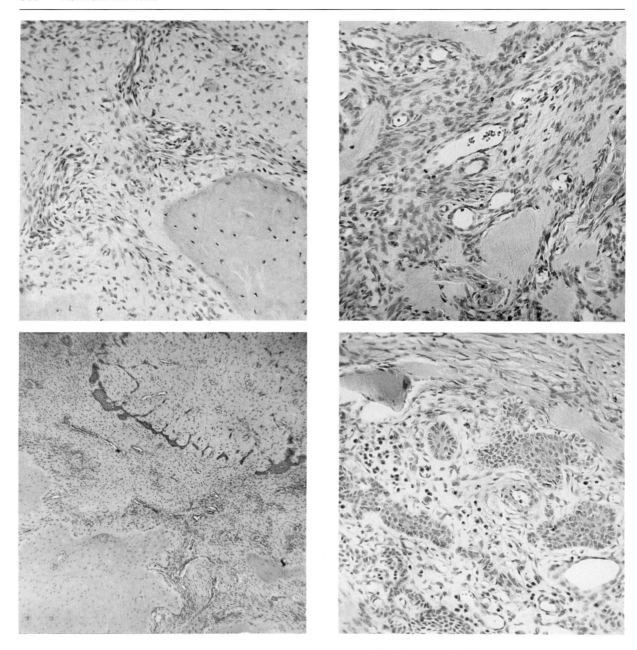

A|B    **FIGURE 8.6.** Epulis in the gingiva of the dog. A. Epulis
C|D    (fibromatous epulis of periodontal origin) showing os-
teoid tissue, epithelial remnants of dental lamina, and fibroblastic stroma. B. Osteoid tissue in an epulis. C. Clumps of
epithelium that are remnants of dental lamina. D. Active fibroblastic tissue around osteoid trabeculae.

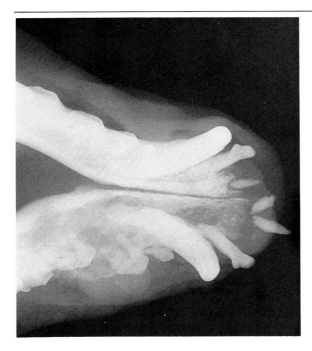

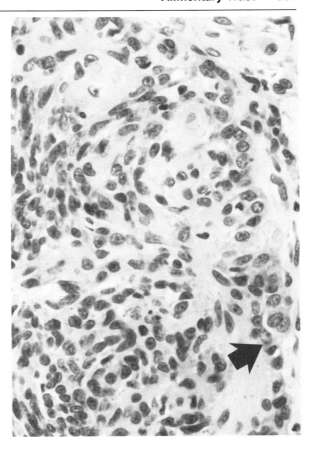

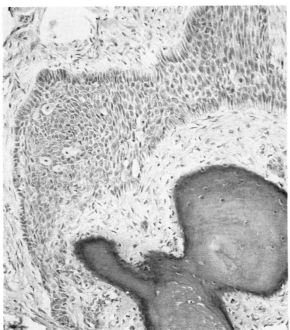

A|B **FIGURE 8.7.** A and B. Acanthomatous epulis in a 10-
C| year-old female Labrador dog. This tumor recurred
twice after surgery. A. Radiograph of the mandible in the dog
illustrating that the neoplasm is infiltrative and osteolytic.
B. Poorly differentiated epithelial mass in the tumor. Observe
on the right (**arrow**) a slight palisading of cuboidal cells at
the periphery of the epithelial mass. C. Tumor in dog. Observe islands of epithelial cells and palisading columnar cells
with basal nuclei at the periphery. Also see the "normal" host
bone spicules adjacent to the invasive cords of epithelium.
This tumor should not be confused with infiltrative squamous
cell carcinoma in the same location.

odontogenic epithelium on the connective tissue." Greenwood and O'Brien (1975), however, have the support of more recent work on collagenolytic activity of inflamed gingival tissue.

**Growth and Metastasis.** Epulides grow slowly and with the exception of acanthomatous epuli, do not invade the underlying bone. Although the growth is progressive, sometimes over a period of years, it is limited and seldom exceeds 2 cm in diameter except in the case of acanthomatous epulides. When the lesion becomes large or multiple, it may trap food, which then decomposes and allows extensive periodontal disease to supervene. Dental calculus is often associated with such lesions. The cases of multiple bilateral epulides in boxers reported by Borthwick *et al.* (1982) surrounded healthy teeth, but in other breeds with the lesion the teeth showed excessive calculus. There is no record of a fibromatous or ossifying epulis undergoing transition to an acanthomatous form. Recurrence following surgical removal is seen in all three forms but especially with the acanthomatous type. New formation must be distinguished from recurrence in early cases of multiple epulis. Metastasis, even to the drainage lymph nodes, is not seen.

Treatment by cryosurgery can produce complete ablation of the tumor. In one of seven cases of epulis subjected to cryosurgery, Werner (1981) reported a recurrence as carcinoma in a 10-year-old male English sheepdog. Thrall *et al.* (1981) stated that 32 patients had an average survival time of 24 months (ranging from 1 to 75 months) after radiotherapy for acanthomatous epulis confirmed by biopsy. In four dogs malignancy developed in 30 to 78 months postirradiation; three tumors were carcinoma and one was osteosarcoma. This phenomenon has three possible explanations: acanthomatous epulides are precancerous lesions, *de novo* neoplasms were induced by radiation, or radiation induced malignant transformation of the lesion. The third alternative could only apply to the carcinoma since no mention is made of metaplasia of the stroma to bone in the biopsy description. In the assessment of these neoplasms, inquiries should be made as to whether the dog has been treated with sodium diphenylhydantoin to control epilepsy because this drug can produce generalized gingival hyperplasia, especially over the incisor teeth (Ross and Baker, 1978).

The biology of the epulides needs careful re-evaluation. First, those lesions that are thought to be inflammatory from clinical and histopathological findings should be classified as inflammatory epuli. The remainder should be subdivided as fibromatous, ossifying, or acanthomatous. Examples of each subgroup should be categorized as solitary or multiple with the location stated and a note made as to whether the lesion is peripheral or invasive.

### Peripheral Giant Cell Granuloma (Giant Cell Epulis)

As the nomenclature implies, these are not giant cell tumors of the jaw bone (osteoclastoma), but apparently arise in the fibrous tissue of the gum. They can therefore be surgically removed, unlike primary bone tumors. This rare tumor, which has been described in cattle, dogs, and cats, presents no problem in histological recognition. It is composed of numerous multinucleate giant cells in a stroma of spindle-shaped connective tissue cells and cavernous blood spaces, sometimes lined by endothelium and sometimes by tumor cells (Head, 1976a). In another case located medial to the right lower canine of a 9-month-old neutered female tabby cat described by Schneck (1975a), there was no recurrence during the 5-month postoperative follow-up.

### Tumors of Muscle Tissue

A large juvenile alveolar rhabdomyosarcoma in a 2-year-old mongrel neutered female apparently centered on the left upper molar teeth region was described by Seibold (1974). This tumor had metastasized widely and was composed of polymorphous cells, but there were "monster multinucleate cells" and binucleate strap- or club-shaped cells with ribbons of cytoplasm suggesting partial muscle differentiation. Seibold describes the way in which mordanting and ripening the phosphotungstic acid hematoxylin stain enabled cross striations to be visualized. Alternatively, electron microscopy can be used to confirm the diagnosis as Peter and Kluge (1970) did in their case that occurred in the mouth of a 2-year-old male German shepherd. In discussing slow-growing rhabdomyosarcoma beneath the epithelium of the laryngeal pharynx of a 6-year-old corgi female, Ladds and Webster (1971) pointed out that since the condition is found in children, it could arise from either mature muscle or immature myoblasts.

## Tumors and Tumorlike Lesions of Blood Vessels

Although cases of tumors of blood vessels are scattered throughout the literature, there are very few detailed case descriptions. Brodey (1966) mentioned three hemangiosarcomas in the oral cavity of the cat, two in the gum, and one in the palate. A recurrent malignant hemangiosarcoma (hemangioendothelioma) in the mandibular incisor gum region of a 7-year-old female Doberman pinscher is mentioned by Borthwick et al. (1982). Dorn and Priester (1976) listed six hemangiosarcomas in 469 canine oral tumors, two in the gingiva, one in the palate, and three in sites not specified.

Sheahan and Donnelly (1981) described two Friesian crossbred heifer calves in which a nodular mass was ablated from the incisor region of the mandible; the masses recurred and were removed again when the calves were 3 and 4 months old, respectively, and no recurrence was found 4 months later. The lesions were composed of vascular channels of varying size with some mitoses in the lining endothelial cells. The authors considered the lesions to be vascular hamartomas, which are nonneoplastic malformations with excessive focal overgrowth of mature cells. The apparent growth in size is due to expansion of the vascular channels and establishment of blood supply to previously dormant areas. Similar lesions have been classified as hemangiomas (Head, 1976a). The ultimate proof of the nature of the lesions would be to see if they continued to grow after the host ceased growing, or if metastasis developed. Even the presence of multiple lesions in a variety of sites can be interpreted as multiple malformations, multiple primary benign tumors, or metastasis of a malignant neoplasm. Thus, Kirkbride et al. (1973) classified the lesions found in an 8-month-old fetus as capillary hemangioma in the tongue and subcutis of the forelimb and as chorioangioma of the placenta. A case that I observed in a 3-week-old calf's skeletal muscle and gums, however, had the histology of a malignant hemangiosarcoma (Head, 1976a).

The problem of assessment of malignancy complicates the evaluation of treatment methods. Crow et al. (1981) recounted the use of electrosurgical resection, chemotherapy, and irradiation to control multiple hemangiomas on the anterolateral edges of the tongue of a 2.5-year-old female Siamese cat. They considered the recrudescences of the lesion not to be new tumor formation, but rather to be growth from the surgical margins; no metastasis was detected 18 months after the first diagnosis. These authors mention that one should look for type-C virus particles in oral hemangiomas because they have been found in a subcutaneous angioma.

Vascular lesions may be composed of lymphatic vessels rather than blood vessels. Such a pedunculate lesion in the roof of the nasopharynx of a 7-year-old German shepherd male was described by Stambaugh et al. (1978). Again the problem of malformation versus true tumor arises.

## Granular Cell Tumor

Gorlin et al. (1959) described a recurrent tumor in an 8-year-old female cat extending from the upper gingiva into the posterior nasal cavity. They tentatively classified this on histological grounds as a malignant granular cell myoblastoma with organoid structure.

In a review of the literature, Giles et al. (1974b) pointed out that granular cell myoblastoma in the dog has a predilection for the tongue and does not recur following removal. They added a fifth case to those in the literature. Histologically, the tumor cells are arranged in small packets of 10 to 20 cells surrounded by reticulum fibers. The nuclei are usually central, and the cytoplasm, which has indistinct margins, is pale, eosinophilic, and faintly granular. The granules are strongly periodic acid–Schiff positive, but unlike mast cell granules they are not metachromatic staining with toluidine blue stain. The granules may be altered myelinlike material since the cells are believed to be of Schwann cell origin.

## Mixed Mesenchymal Sarcoma

Di Bartola et al. (1978) reported an unusual 5 cm mass in the soft palate of a 4.5-year-old male English setter. Histology by light and electron microscopy revealed osteoblastic cells around osteoid, chondrogenic cells in the extracellular matrix, pleomorphic fibroblasts, and unidentified mesenchymal cells. Di Bartola et al. discussed eight canine cases in the literature, and concluded that the term *mixed mesenchymal sarcoma* should be used rather than *soft tissue osteosarcoma*.

## Tumors of Hematopoietic and Related Tissues

Tumors composed of "round" cells need to be stained by the Giemsa method as a first step in their diagnosis. This will separate those to be investigated as mast cell tumors from those to be considered as lymphoid tumors. Division of lymphoid tumors into those derived from the various subsets of T- and B-cells is now becoming possible in veterinary science, but as yet has not been practiced in the oropharyngeal tumors. The site and behavior of 10 lymphoid and 5 mast cell tumors in dogs has been described by Borthwick *et al.* (1982). Gorlin *et al.* (1959) found two canine mastocytomas in the gingiva and one on the hard palate. Werner (1981), reporting on the results of treatment of oral tumors, mentioned three unusual canine gingival tumors: a histiocytoma in a 9-year-old mongrel male with no tumor at 8 months follow-up after surgery; a malignant lymphoreticular tumor in a 14-year-old mongrel female with no tumor 4 months after cryosurgery; and a mastocytoma in a 2-year-old Afghan male with no tumor 8 months after three cryosurgical ablations.

Round cell tumors need more than superficial light microscopic examination to reveal their true identity. The round cells in a 2.5-cm diameter pedunculated tumor described by Ghadially *et al.* (1977) on the gum of the left lower jaw of an 18-year-old terrier cross dog had few of the characteristic features of plasma cells. Further study showed that the tumor cell cytoplasm was pyroninophilic and electron microscopy showed a uniform population of plasma cells apart from rare macrophages. This plasmacytoma had not recurred and there was no evidence of tumor deposits 1 year after surgical removal.

The lymphoid tissue, particularly of the pharynx, may show an exuberant immunological response to chronic inflammation. That such masses are not neoplastic may be suspected on clinical grounds and can be confirmed histologically. One such case with two masses, each measuring 4 × 3 × 2 cm, was reported in a 2-year-old thoroughbred filly by Meagher and Brown (1978).

## Odontogenic Tumors

### General Considerations and Classification

Even in the human subject with regular dental inspection, odontogenic tumors are uncommon. One would not expect to collect a large series of cases on which a classification could be based. An international collaborative effort formed the basis of the World Health Organization classification of human odontogenic tumors (Pindborg *et al.*, 1971). The classification used developed from a system suggested by Pindborg and Clausen that was subsequently modified. Gorlin *et al.* (1963), in an article mainly devoted to human tumors, applied the classification to odontogenic tumors of domestic animals recorded in the literature and to a series of 274 tumors of odontogenic origin collected from 10 major veterinary centers. If one excludes the 255 fibromatous epulides of periodontal origin, only 19 of 1,230 oral tumors were true odontogenic neoplasms.

The classification is based on the inductive effect of one dental tissue on another. This can be broken down into ameloblastic epithelium influencing undifferentiated mesenchyme of the dental papilla, which differentiates into odontoblasts, odontoblasts forming dentine, and dentine having an inductive effect on ameloblasts to form enamel matrix.

It is obvious that understanding of the formation of neoplasms of tooth structures necessitates understanding of the normal embryogenesis of the tooth. As described by Willis (1948), the tooth comes from two embryonic tissues. The enamel cap of the tooth is derived from the dental laminae, which are invaginations of squamous epithelium from the lining of the buccal cavity; all other parts of the tooth, including dentine, cementum, and pulp, come from the embryonic mesenchyme. A better understanding of the genesis of these two embryonic tissues requires an understanding of the structures of the enamel organ (fig. 8.8A). The invaginated epithelium from the dental laminae becomes

found after careful dissection of the area. Tumors of minor salivary glands develop within the various organs of the oropharynx, and their origin is only revealed on histological examination.

## Mixed Tumors

**Definition.** Pleomorphic adenoma, as the name implies, is composed of a mixture of different proportions of epithelium, myoepithelium, hyaline/myxoid/chondroid material, and bone. The epithelium appears as ducts or as squamous cells with intercellular bridges and may show keratinization. The myoepithelium is usually formed by closely packed spindle-shaped cells, but it may be polymorphic. Endochrondral and intramembranous ossification is also seen. Mitoses may be frequent even in benign tumors. Carcinoma in pleomorphic adenoma (malignant mixed tumor) is seen when adenocarcinoma, epidermoid carcinoma, or undifferentiated carcinoma forms in a tumor that is otherwise a typical pleomorphic adenoma.

**Incidence.** This is the commonest human salivary tumor, but it is rare in animals. Wells and Robinson (1975) gave a review of the cases in the literature in the horse, dog, and cow and added their case in a 12-year-old neutered female cat where an extensive 8 cm tumor probably arose from the submandibular salivary gland.

**Age, Breed, Sex, and Sites.** Koestner and Buerger (1965) pointed out that although this neoplasm in humans is common in females, their three cases of salivary mixed tumors in dogs were in males. They comment on the fact that in contrast to the rarity of this salivary tumor, bitches frequently show cartilage in bone from metaplasia of myoepithelium in mammary mixed tumors. My small series of six canine pleomorphic adenomas involved an equal number of male and female dogs. Parotid and submandibular salivary glands are most often the primary sites, but minor glands of the pharynx and tonsil may be affected. This is a tumor of older age groups (7 or more years of age in all species), but an ovine carcinoma in pleomorphic adenoma was in the parotid gland of a 2.5-year-old ram (Head, 1976*a*).

**Growth and Metastasis.** The size of the tumor usually causes the presenting signs. Recurrence may follow removal of even the adenomatous form probably because of residual tumor tissue left *in situ* during what is often an operation in a "difficult site." Tumors of 5 to 10 cm in diameter, however, need several blocks of tissue taken to be sure that enough has been examined histologically to make a proper assessment. Thus, in one canine pleomorphic adenoma reported by Head (1976*a*), only bone spicules, fat, and myxoid tissue were found in the sections examined. The diagnosis of carcinoma in pleomorphic adenoma is usually based on histological features of malignancy rather than on the presence of metastasis. In the case of a parotid tumor reported in a 9-year-old cow (Head, 1976*a*) there was bone in the lymph node metastasis, implying a diagnosis of carcinosarcoma or malignant mixed tumor.

## Monomorphic Adenoma

As the name implies, this tumor exhibits a glandular pattern, but there is little stroma and no myxoid or chondroid areas. The tumor arises from ducts and is well-encapsulated. The cellular pattern is regular, but if there is moderate autolysis, argyrophilic reticulum stains may be needed to reveal the glandular pattern. Two cases have been reported, one in the tongue of a 10-year-old female terrier (Head, 1976*a*) and another in the submandibular gland of a 10-year-old female boxer (Borthwick *et al.*, 1982).

## Mucoepidermoid Tumor

This moderately common tumor in humans is rare in animals. It is easily recognized because, in addition to irregular spaces lined by mucus-secreting columnar epithelium and filled by mucus, there are clumps and strands of squamous epithelium with intercellular bridges, but keratin masses are rare. Sometimes the mucus cysts rupture and provoke a foreign-body inflammatory reaction.

If no mucus-secreting cells can be demonstrated, then the diagnosis must be one of epidermoid carcinoma. There is some doubt as to whether such a salivary epidermoid carcinoma has been reported in animals. Repeated sections of the tumor have revealed either some mucus-secreting epithelium, leading to a diagnosis of mucoepidermoid tumor, or some areas of myoepithelium with chondroid material, leading to a diagnosis of carcinoma in pleomorphic adenoma. Koestner and Buerger (1965) had doubts about their sublingual case in a cat, and Karbe and Schiefer (1967) were similarly hesitant with their case adjacent to the dog's tonsil. Koestner and Buerger described one benign and two malignant mucoepidermoid tumors in dogs, and Karbe and Schiefer described a case in the parotid gland of a 12-year-old male Siamese cat that had metastasis to the lung. Four cases reported by Head (1976*a*) were in old dogs 8 to 14 years of age, three in the parotid gland and one in the submandibular gland. The latter neoplasm metastasized to the drainage lymph nodes, lungs, and liver.

## Acinic Cell Tumor

**Incidence.** This is a rare tumor in humans found only in the parotid gland. In contrast, it is a common tumor in dogs, and because the major salivary glands and most of the minor salivary glands in domestic species are either mixed or serous in type, it can occur at a variety of sites.

**Definition.** It is a tumor of glandular epithelium either in acinic groups or solid sheets; silver stains show the reticulum network and are often helpful in revealing the acinar pattern. The cells are polyhedral with basophilic, sometimes granular cytoplasm, and the nuclei are small. As with the cells of normal serous glands, no mucus can be demonstrated by PAS, Alcian blue, or mucicarmine stains except for small amounts in some of the lumens. The absence of myoepithelial cells and their products differentiates these tumors from pleomorphic adenomas; monomorphic adenomas are distinguished by the fact that they are derived from duct-lining cells and myoepithelial cells or from mucus acini. Sometimes the cells in acinic cell tumors have nonstaining cytoplasm (the so-called clear cell pattern) since stains for mucin are negative.

**Age, Breed, Sex, and Sites.** Koestner and Buerger (1965) reported 11 cases in dogs (5 parotid, 2 submandibular, 2 gum, 1 tongue, and 1 lip) and 1 in the parotid gland of a horse. My collection includes 10 cases in dogs (4 parotid, 3 tongue, 2 gum, and 1 tonsil) and 1 very large mass in the parotid gland of a 15-month-old Angus steer. The mean age for both series in dogs is 9 years (ranging from 3 to 15 years).

**Growth and Metastasis.** The tumor often grows invasively, but metastasis is rare and occurs late in the disease and only to the drainage lymph nodes.

## Adenocarcinoma

**Definition.** Adenocarcinoma may be defined as a malignant glandular tumor forming tubules or solid cords of epithelial cells. Again it must be stressed that several blocks of tissue must be taken for a histological examination to eliminate the diagnosis of mucoepidermoid tumor and of carcinoma in pleomorphic adenoma. Koestner and Buerger (1965) distinguished ductular (papillary) from trabecular adenocarcinoma; in other words, they distinguished tumors that form tubules from tumors that form solid cords. In my experience and that of Karbe and Schiefer (1967), tumors are found exhibiting both histological patterns. As implied above, the tubules sometimes become cystic and the lining shows papillary projections. Mucus secretion may be prominent. The degree of cellular atypia and the number of mitoses often show marked variation within a single tumor.

**Incidence and Sites.** Koestner and Buerger (1965) reported 3 cases in dogs (2 parotid and 1 tongue) and 1 each in the parotid gland of a cat and of a horse. Karbe and Schiefer (1967) reported 4 cases in dogs (2 parotid and 2 submandibular). The author's cases (Head, 1976*a*) were distributed as follows: 1 parotid in a 13-year-old mare; 1 sublingual in an adult cow; 2 parotid, 1 submandibular, and 1 pharyngeal in dogs; and 5 submandibular and 1 pharyngeal in cats. It seems to be the most common salivary gland tumor in the cat, is moderately common in the dog, but is rare in other species. Stackhouse *et al.* (1978) reviewing six surveys of equine tumors representing 1,148 cases found only two equine adenocarcinomas.

**Age.** This is a tumor of older age groups. The mean age for cats is 12 years (8 to 16 years) and for dogs 10 years (3.5 to 13 years).

**Growth and Metastasis.** Growth is often rapid; Borthwick *et al.* (1982) reported regrowth to a 4 cm diameter 3 weeks after cryosurgery. Such rapid growth may be associated with necrosis of the central area of the tumor. Infiltrative growth, especially into lymphatics, leads to local edema and subsequent fibrosis. The swelling produced by the tumor will result in a variety of clinical signs depending on the location of the primary growth. An example of this would be exophthalmos secondary to an adenocarcinoma of the zygomatic salivary gland in an 8-year-old male Labrador (Buyukmihci *et al.*, 1975).

Metastasis to drainage lymph nodes occurs relatively early in the disease. Stackhouse *et al.* (1978) described an interesting adenocarcinoma of the submandibular salivary gland in an 18-year-old Morgan mare. The tumor spread via the deep lymph node chain to form a mass in the anterior thorax, which then led to marked edema of the neck. Biopsy of a superficial lymph node merely showed nonspecific lymphadenitis. About one-third of the reported cases have metastasis in the lungs postmortem. A remarkably widespread series of metastases was recorded by Grevel *et al.* (1978) in an 8-year-old female German pointer. The primary mass was in the sublingual glands and the metastases were in the mandible, humerus, radius, femur, tibia, vertebrae, lungs, heart, kidneys, brain, and multiple lymph nodes.

### Undifferentiated Carcinoma

**Definition.** This tumor is composed of spindle-shaped or round cells that are clearly epithelial and not mesothelial. They are arranged in irregular masses by well-differentiated connective tissue strands, but are not in any of the patterns described in the previous sections. Undifferentiated carcinoma is a definite entity composed of poorly differentiated malignant tumors. This category is not synonymous with "unclassified neoplasms" and is not merely a tumor in which postmortem autolysis has led to a loss of recognizable diagnostic features. In this tumor reticulum fibers tend to surround small groups of individual cells, but the cells do not form into acini, even atypical ones.

**Incidence.** Koestner and Buerger (1965) reported two cases in dogs and Karbe and Schiefer (1967) added another. My collection (Head, 1976*a*) included an additional two tumors in dogs, one in the parotid gland of a 1-year-old sheep, and one each in the parotid glands of two cows (6 and 9 years old, respectively).

In none of the dogs was the parotid gland involved (two submandibular, two pharyngeal, and one sublingual). The mean age was 10 years (range

8 to 13 years). Three carcinomas had metastasized to the drainage lymph nodes and one to the lung and liver.

### Nonepithelial Tumors

Such tumors are rare. Koestner and Buerger (1965) reported an epithelioid or spindle cell pattern in a malignant melanoma in the parotid gland of a dog.

### Allied but Nonneoplastic Conditions

**Ductal Hyperplasia.** An example of this lesion occurred as an incidental finding in routine histology in the parotid gland of a 10-year-old bull (Head, 1976*a*).

**Sialosis.** This bilateral enlargement of salivary glands is due to hypertrophy of serous acinar cells; an example in the parotid gland of a sheep at routine slaughter for meat is mentioned by Head (1976*a*).

**Sialocele (Salivary Mucocele).** Unlike branchial cysts, this fluid-filled cavity seldom has a continuous epithelial lining and it has no neoplastic glandular tissue as in a cystadenoma. It is relatively common in the dog but rare in the cat. Cervical sialoceles are believed to be the result of rupture of the duct of the anterior part of the sublingual gland (Spreull and Head, 1967). In its later stages the inspissated saliva in the lesion becomes organized by granulation tissue. Metaplasia to bone may occur superficially, and the lesion resembles a pleomorphic adenoma.

**Salivary Gland Infarction.** Kelly *et al.* (1979) reported examples of this condition in the submandibular gland of the dog. The extensive ischemic necrosis and regenerative hyperplasia of surviving ductal epithelium might on casual examination be mistaken for an adenocarcinoma with central necrosis.

## Branchioma

**Incidence.** Branchioma, an extremely rare tumor, arises from the vestiges of the branchial apparatus. There is some doubt whether this tumor actually exists in domestic animals. Ball and Auger (1924) reported an osteochondroma at the root of the tongue in a cow to be of branchial origin, and Lucam *et al.* (1944) collected reports on six branchiomas from the literature and added one of their own. Two of these tumors were in horses, and five were in dogs.

**Sites and Structure.** Most of the neoplasms designated as branchiomas were in the head and neck. Histologically, they had the appearance of squamous cell carcinoma. Some of these tumors probably represented metastasis of squamous cell carcinoma from unsuspected sites, such as the tonsil (Cotchin, 1956).

## Nonneoplastic Oropharyngeal Masses

Gorlin *et al.* (1959) described many bacterial granulomatous lesions of the oropharyngeal region, which macroscopically might be confused with neoplasia. Cotter (1981) drew attention to some more obscure infections in this region in cats.

Calcinosis circumscripta is reported in the tongue of dogs occasionally, but histologically it is easily recognized and differentiated from a neoplasm. Macroscopically, the multilocular structure contains chalky, white, friable material and is virtually diagnostic once it has been incised (Douglas and Kelly, 1966).

Madewell *et al.* (1980) described six cases of oral eosinophilic granuloma in Siberian husky dogs under 4 years of age involving lateral and ventral surfaces of the tongue. Thirteen cases of the disease collected over a 10-year period from 1968 by Potter *et al.* (1980) included three cases involving the palate and one case involving both the lingual and palatine regions. They also mentioned an asymptomatic case involving the soft palate of a 1.5-year-old male Samoyed. Light and electron microscopic studies showed well-organized granuloma surrounding foci of degenerate collagen, no causal agents being visualized. Some of the dogs exhibited an absolute eosinophilia on examination of the blood. These lesions are firm, raised, yellowish brown, plaquelike masses that may be ulcerated and covered by a yellowish green exudate; they tend to regress spontaneously, but may then recrudesce. Systemic adrenocorticosteroid therapy is usually successful in treating these lesions. The cause of the condition is not known.

Scott (1975) described in detail the facts relating to 18 cases of the eosinophilic granuloma complex in cats. He divided the lesion into three types: eosinophilic ulcer (mainly involving females, average age 5.7 years), eosinophilic plaque (females, 3.3 years), and linear granuloma (both sexes, 8.4 months). Each of the types can occur on the lip, but only the eosinophilic ulcer in one case was reported in the oral cavity (site not specified). Although sometimes called "rodent ulcer," implying basal cell tumor, there is no possibility of confusing the eosinophilic ulcer on the upper lip with a true tumor, especially if histology is performed. Linear granuloma can be recognized because it is a granuloma around multiple areas of necrobiotic collagen. The eosinophilic plaque may present problems in differentiation from mast cell tumor, but the number of eosinophils always exceeds the number of mast cells in the nonneoplastic disease. Since Scott's (1975) publication, there have been many other reports. Schneck (1975*b*) reported the ulcer in the granuloma in the hard palate where it extended into the nasal passages, and Ochs *et al.* (1978) described nodular granuloma in the dorsoposterior aspect of the tongue of a 2- and an 8-year-old cat.

Many of these lesions respond to cryosurgery (Willemse and Lubberink, 1978).

## TUMORS OF THE ESOPHAGUS AND ESOPHAGEAL REGION OF THE STOMACH

### Tumors Associated with *Spirocerca lupi* in the Dog

**Incidence.** Seibold *et al.* (1955) described tumors of the esophagus in the dog associated with lesions produced by the helminth parasite *Spirocerca lupi*. The relationship has not been proved experimentally (Schwabe, 1955), but it seems highly probable since the incidence of esophageal tumors is generally very low in dogs but significantly high in dogs with these parasites. The percentage of infected dogs that develop tumors is probably quite low. For example, Hanson *et al.* (1957) found only three cases in Cairo, Egypt; Kamara (1964) found only one tumor in 235 infected dogs examined at Freetown, Sierra Leone; Ivoghli (1978) found three fibrosarcomas in 380 dogs with lesions of spirocercosis in Shiraz, Iran; and Chandrasekharon *et al.* (1958) found no neoplasms in 910 dogs with *Spirocerca* infection in Madras, India, but two cases subsequently have been reported there (see Gupta and Singh, 1975). In contrast, Wandera (1976) reported 43 sarcoma cases in 206 infected dogs in Nairobi, Kenya.

*Spirocerca* parasites are widely but unevenly distributed among dogs throughout the world. The frequency of occurrence for dogs in various countries and cities in the world is as follows: Japan, 10%; South Africa, 20%; Indonesia, 40 to 50%; Baghdad, 66%; India, 23 to 42%; Algeria, 70 to 90%; Southern Tunisia and Malawi, 100% in some areas; Mexico, 35%; Sumatra, 40 to 50%; Manila, 45%; Cairo, 46%; and Freetown, Sierra Leone, 57%. Studies with *Spirocerca lupi* from 1951 through 1970 in the southeastern United States have been reviewed by Bailey (1972). Wandera (1976) extended the work of Murray (1968) in Kenya and found 206 dogs with lesions of spirocercosis in 1,607 postmortem examinations between 1964 and 1974 (12.8%). He pointed out that variations in incidence in several East African surveys may be due to the source of the population (e.g., stray rural dogs versus urban dogs).

A significant proportion of larvae taken per orum in the dog probably reach their destination and complete their cycle in the dog, and the difference in rate of infection in different areas is related to exposure to coprophagous (dung) beetles or transport hosts that carry the infection (Bailey, 1963). The infection will not establish in countries without the dung beetle, and when an occasional case appears in such a place, it is usually in a dog brought in from a high incidence country. In a case described by Campbell *et al.* (1964), a female boxer that had lived its first 7 years in Kenya where spirocercosis exists developed a sarcoma in the esophagus 3 years after it had returned to Scotland, a country where no intermediate hosts exist. This animal had been well until 2 weeks before it was destroyed, and the lesions found at necropsy made it probable that this was a *Spirocerca*-associated tumor.

The principal intermediate hosts for the spiurid nematode *Spirocerca lupi* are the coprophagous beetles belonging to the subfamilies Aphodiinae, Coprinae, and Geotrupinae (family Scarabaeidae). The embryonated ova develop to the third stage (infective) larvae or encyst along the tracheal tubes of the beetles. Periods of 4 to 6 weeks are sufficient for the development of spiurid larvae in the susceptible beetle.

Bailey *et al.* (1963) found that six different species of Geotrupes beetles could be infected in the laboratory when exposed to dog feces and cow manure containing eggs. Each species of beetle had its own kind of cyst, and the larvae would emerge actively when the cyst wall was broken. It has been stated that different species of dung beetles probably differ in susceptibility to the spiurids, depending on how well the dung beetle grinds its food (Miller, 1961). If the food is not ground well, as is the case with the Geotrupes (which have less specialized mandibles), the ova are not destroyed. This might account for the higher incidence of infection in dogs with this species of dung beetle.

If the beetle is swallowed by the dog or another suitable host, the larvae continue their development and reach adult stage. If the beetle is swallowed by an intermediate host, the third stage larvae are released from the beetle, reencyst in the mesentery or alimentary canal, and resume their wait for a transport host, which one day may be eaten by an appropriate definitive host. The intermediate (transport) hosts include 9 species of mammals (shrew, hedgehog, genet, Egyptian mongoose, mouse, rabbit, rat, wild ass, and wild boar), 13 species of birds (including the owl, chicken, raven, house sparrow, duck, great gray shrike, and hoopoe), and 7 species of reptiles. Since few beetles are seasonal in their habits, these transport hosts serve as accumulators of larvae and are thus important in the transmission chain (Krahwinkel and McCue, 1967).

The hedgehog is an important transport host in Iraq and China, and the chicken is important in the southern United States, where the practice of feeding viscera of farm-dressed chickens to dogs is probably one of the main factors in the infection (Bailey *et al.*, 1964). The larvae are found mainly in the walls of the esophagus and intestine of the chicken and other birds.

If the transport host or the beetle is eaten by a dog, as is common in scavenger dogs near starvation, the larvae are freed in the stomach and migrate into the stomach wall. From there they pass toward the aorta by way of the walls of the gastric, gastroepiploic, and celiac arteries. When the larvae reach the thoracic part of the aorta, they migrate toward the wall of the lower esophagus by way of the connective tissue between these organs. During their migration, the larvae may form nodular lesions in the adventitia of the aorta. Once the larvae reach the esophagus they become mature in approximately 3 months. The adult parasites are 30 to 80 mm long, approximately 1 mm thick, and bright pink to red in color. In perhaps 0.5 to 5% of infected dogs, adult parasites or larvae can be found at other sites, such as the kidney, urinary bladder, mediastinum, or the wall of the stomach or can be attached to the serosal surfaces of the thoracic or abdominal cavities. Occasionally, involvement of the trachea, bronchi, or lungs results in pneumonia or pulmonary infarction. Irritation of the fascia and periosteum of the vertebrae, especially the posterior thoracic, during migration of the larvae may cause exostosis of the ventral surface of the vertebrae and spondylitis.

**Age, Breed, and Sex.** The age range in dogs with spiurid infection is usually 1 to 7 years. The average age of dogs with esophageal tumors associated with this parasite is 7 years.

Because of the time necessary for migration of the parasite and for development to the adult stage, dogs under 6 months of age are unlikely to have an established lesion (Ribelin and Bailey, 1958). Moreover, the weight of challenge has an influence on the survival of the host. Chhabra's (1973) experiments showed that 3- to 4-week-old puppies given doses of 100 juvenile *Spirocerca lupi* died in 2 weeks as a result of vascular lesions, whereas when adult dogs were dosed with 100 to 200 infective juveniles, a patent infection was produced, the adult worms inducing no clinical signs.

There is no known breed prevalence except that the lesions are seen most often in breed types that are indigenous scavenger dogs, especially in developing countries. Incidence in these countries is much lower in dogs fed adequately by their owners. Sexes of dogs are affected about equally.

Definitive hosts for the parasite other than the dog include seven species of felidae, two species of primates, and five species of canidae.

**Clinical Characteristics and Sites.** Compared with the high incidence of infection, the number with clinical signs is low and most nonmalignant cases go undetected. This may explain the high frequency of tumors in Wandera's (1976) series. Only 39 of his 206 infected dogs had clinical signs of spirocercosis, the majority of the infections being incidental postmortem findings. Of these clinical cases 29 had definite tumors and in 4 others the esophageal nodules were classed as parasarcoma (see Histological Features). Since vomiting was the most common sign (33 cases) and this occurred in dogs with nodules over 4 cm in diameter, it is obvious that a clinically selected postmortem series will favor cases that have undergone neoplastic transformation.

Lesions are found in the esophagus in 15 to 40% of dogs, in the esophagus and aorta in 23 to 86%, and in the aorta in 7 to 30% (Babero *et al.*, 1965; Chandrasekharon *et al.*, 1958; Kamara, 1964; Murray, 1968; Wandera, 1976). Often the aorta alone is involved in dogs less than 1 year of age.

**Gross Morphology**

*Aorta*—Lesions are most common in the thoracic aorta and in the first few centimeters of the abdominal aorta, but they may occur in any area throughout the full length of the aorta (figs. 8.9A and B). *Spirocerca* parasites are found in about 5% of the aortic lesions. The aortic lesion consists of a thickened adventitial mass with central necrosis containing the worms and surrounded by granulation tissue. The intima and media of the aorta are usually greatly thickened, infiltrated with inflammatory cells, and contain much fibroblastic tissue. The lesions in the intima appear as raised plaques that are linear or oval in shape. Irritation and roughening of the aortic endothelium may cause formation of superimposed thrombi. On occasion these thrombi may extend to the bifurcation of the iliac arteries with resultant posterior paralysis. In this connection it must be remembered that the spondylosis of the thoracic vertebrae seen in this disease may also lead to paraplegia.

Almost every aorta has depressed aneurysmal scars, which are evidence of previous parasitic involvement. These scars from previous adventitial invasion do not represent penetrations from the lumen to the adventitia. The scars are 2 to 20 mm in diameter and 1 to 10 mm in depth. They are densely fibrotic and some may have bony plates in their bases.

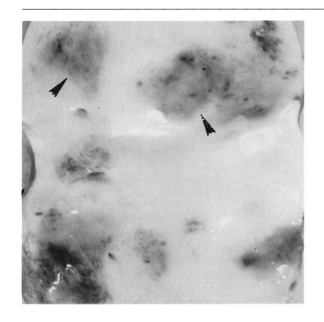
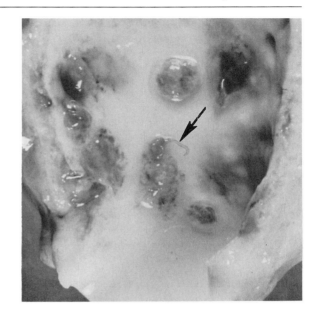
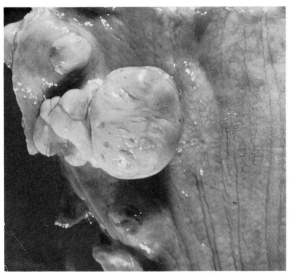
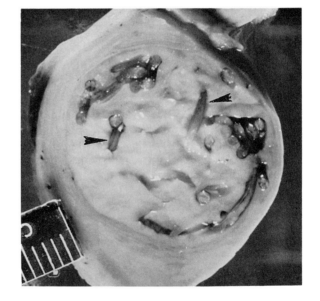

A|B
—
C|D
**FIGURE 8.9.** *Spirocerca lupi* lesions of the dog. A. Hyperemia and hemorrhage (**arrowheads**) under intima of aorta. B. Intimal surface of aorta with part of an immature worm (**arrow**) protruding into the lumen. C. Nonneoplastic pedunculated lesion of the esophagus. D. Cross section of esophageal wall with nonneoplastic mass containing adult worms (**arrowheads**). (Courtesy of Dr. W. S. Bailey and *J. Parasit.*)

The lesions rarely contain calcified and ossified tissue in the media of the aorta, and the ossified tissue may have bone marrow and hematopoietic tissue.

*Esophagus*—The adult worms form a nodule in the esophagus (fig. 8.9C). About 85% of the esophageal nodules are located between the aortic arch and diaphragm, often 2 to 5 cm from the hiatus of the esophagus. The number of esophageal nodules varies from one to eight per animal but usually averages one to two. The worms migrate from the aortic wall at first to an area outside the esophageal wall, where fibrosis may occur, and the lesion may progress into the formation of nodules, often 1 to 5 cm in diameter. The lesion is initially outside the wall, but with increasing size it protrudes into the lumen of the esophagus (fig. 8.9D).

The esophageal lesion often consists of a central cavity containing tightly entwined parasites. Suppuration with fibrotic septa is common in the center of the lesion, and many worms may live in the greenish yellow pus. Each esophageal nodule may contain 1 to 80 worms (usually 6 to 16). The female lays her eggs by extruding herself through a small opening communicating from the cavity of the lesion to the lumen of the esophagus. Purulent fluid and eggs pass through this fistula into the esophagus and are swallowed by the host. Hansen *et al.* (1957) found that only 27 of 43 esophageal lesions had communications into the lumen of the esophagus; thus, only 27 of these dogs had a theoretical chance for egg output into the digestive tract.

The lesions in the esophagus may open into the pleural cavity and cause pleuritis or they may communicate with the aortic lumen and cause bleeding into the esophagus. Also, there may be a communication with the trachea and the development of pneumonia.

The tumors that project into the esophagus are pedunculated, nodular, or fungiform, and they may contain the parasites (fig. 8.10A and B). The shape of the neoplasm depends on the original location of the parasite (Hansen *et al.,* 1957). The tumors measure up to 10 cm in diameter and are fibrous or bony in consistency. The color is generally grayish white. The surface of the tumor is commonly ulcerated.

### Histological Features

*Aorta*—In the early aortic lesions there are tracts

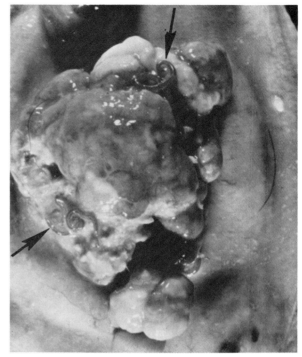

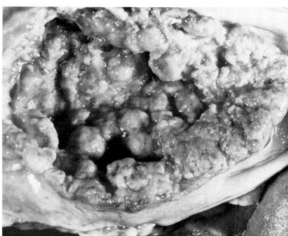

A
―
B

**FIGURE 8.10.** Neoplasms of the esophagus associated with *Spirocerca lupi* infection. A. Pedunculated masses protruding into the lumen; adult worms (**arrows**) embedded in neoplasm. B. Cavitated multinodular sarcoma. (Courtesy of Dr. W. S. Bailey and *J. Parasit.*)

of necrosis resulting from the parasites migrating from the adventitia into the media. This results in severe disruption and destruction of elastic fibers and smooth muscle, followed by fibrosis. A fibrous nodule forms in the outer wall of the aortic adventitia resulting in a loss of elastic fibers and infiltrations of eosinophils, mononuclear cells, plasma cells, and live larvae. Later, the parasites die and become mineralized and surrounded by foreign-body giant cells, and the fibrotic tissue is hyalinized. These are often the only residual changes in the aortic lesion.

The changes in the intima are secondary to the lesion that starts in the adventitia; there is no true atheroma with lipoidal changes present. All intimal plaques appear as collagenous connective tissue, and breaches in the endothelium lead to thrombosis.

With fibrosis and loss of elastic fibers in the wall of the aorta and atrophy of muscle with replacement by collagenous tissue, there may be a pouching of the wall or the formation of a saccular type of aneurysm. Some develop as dissecting types of aneurysms, fill with blood from vessels of the wall, and may rupture to the outside, usually into the thoracic cavity.

*Esophagus*—The pathogenesis of the esophageal lesion has been described (Ribelin and Bailey, 1958). The initial lesion consists of loose, highly vascular, fibroblastic proliferation (fig. 8.11A). Mononuclear cells, numerous neutrophils, worm eggs, and hemorrhages are found in the center of the lesion and to a lesser extent in the fibrous capsule that forms. Plasma cells are especially prominent in the fibrous capsule.

The arteries in the wall of the esophagus may also be affected, showing subendothelial collagenous plaques that almost occlude the lumen. The arteries may also show metaplastic cartilage and bone formation (Murray, 1968).

As the lesion matures, the mononuclear cells and vascular change decrease and the fibroblasts become more numerous. In some lesions there are areas with active fibroblastic tissue and a high mitotic rate (fig. 8.11B). With continued proliferation, the fibroblasts form small neoplastic foci that eventually combine to form a typical fibrosarcoma.

Thus there are cases where the lesion has a distinct compression capsule unlike the established sarcoma case and yet has foci of pleomorphic cells with

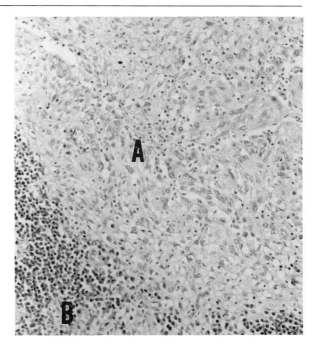

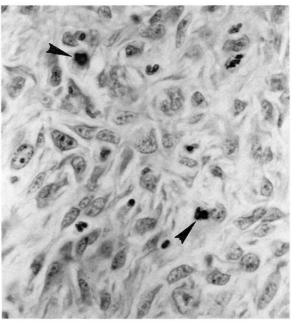

A
B
**FIGURE 8.11.** *Spirocerca lupi* proliferative lesions in the esophagus of the dog. A. Active fibroblastic proliferation (A) surrounded by masses of plasma cells (B). B. Transitional stage between fibroblastic proliferation and sarcoma. Observe mitotic figures (**arrowheads**).

clearly visible mitotic figures. Wandera (1976) has overcome this problem of borderline cases between chronic inflammatory granuloma, fibroma, and fibrosarcoma by using a category termed *parasarcoma*.

Microscopically, the fibrosarcoma appears with closely packed cells, often in sheets or in focal masses. The cells are spindle shaped and have poorly defined, faintly staining cytoplasm, ovoid nuclei, prominent nucleoli, and a large number of mitotic figures. They appear with interwoven collagen bundles. The esophageal mucosal surface is often ulcerated, and there may be secondary infection. Invasion of tumor cells into the blood vessels is sometimes seen.

Some of these tumors display metaplastic transformation of fibroblastic tissue into osteoid, bone, or cartilage. True bone osteoblasts and osteoclasts are sometimes formed. The presence of metaplastic bone and cartilage does not lead to an automatic diagnosis of osteosarcoma, but some reports describe true osteosarcoma formation. Several blocks need to be taken from the nodule as there may be considerable variation in the histological pattern in a single lesion. The sarcomas exhibiting osteoid, bone, and cartilage tend to have an older age distribution. In Wandera's (1976) series, fibrosarcomas had an age range of 1 to 11 years (mean, 5 years), and osteosarcomas, 3 to 15 years (mean, 7.5 years). Moreover, the fibrosarcomas tended to be smaller, only a few being larger than 5 cm in diameter, whereas the osteosarcomas were usually larger than this.

The relationship between *Spirocerca* lesions and neoplasia is based on finding local areas of sarcomatous change within the otherwise chronic inflammatory lesion, some of which contain parasites (Ribelin and Bailey, 1958). When inflammatory changes are no longer recognized, the neoplasm is invariably found in the region where the inflammatory lesions were located. Also, characteristic aortic lesions are found. Epizootiological reports indicate that sarcoma in the esophagus of dogs is confined to countries in which *Spirocerca* infection is reported. The role of spirocercosis in the induction of the neoplasm has not been subject to significant experimental study (Thrasher *et al.*, 1963). Probably, the short time (as little as 4 days) that the parasites remain at the intermediate sites in migration (stomach to aorta) may explain the absence of tumors in these sites. The time that the parasites reside in the esophagus is much longer (several hundred days or more).

Tumors seldom arise in the aortic and vertebral nodules but a few cases have been described (e.g., Wandera, 1976).

During the terminal stage in the esophagus, the parasites mature into adults, copulate, and discharge ova into the lumen of the esophagus. Exuberant proliferation of atypical fibroblasts occurs at this time, especially near the mated adult worms (Thrasher *et al.*, 1963). To date there have been no reports of metabolic or degenerative products or secretions produced during mating and ovulation that might be significant in the inducement of neoplastic change. Bailey (1979) stated his belief that *Spirocerca* is a cocarcinogen with oncogenesis being enhanced by a yet unknown promoting agent(s). He stressed the fact that only a proportion of these neoplasms have worms in them or near them when they are discovered; in his series only 12 out of 50 sarcomas had associated *Spirocerca*. All the other dogs had evidence of previous *Spirocerca* infection, namely spondylosis of the thoracic vertebrae or, more characteristically, scarring of the aorta which persists at least 5 to 8 years after infection. Similar figures are given by Wandera (1976), namely, 13 of 17 fibrosarcoma and 11 of 25 osteosarcoma cases had worms in the tumor mass.

**Growth and Metastasis.** It is of interest that tumors may be recognized in 1-year-old animals. Immature worms may be found in the esophagus of animals as young as 6 months old, but they take 5 months or more to mature. When induced, the sarcoma must be able to grow very rapidly in some cases. Sarcomas may show infiltrative growth both into tissue spaces and blood vessels. Established metastases are observed with varying frequency in 10 to 50% of affected dogs; Wandera (1976) reported that 2 of 17 fibrosarcomas and 12 of 25 osteosarcomas had metastasized. All authors agree that lungs and bronchial lymph nodes are the most common sites for metastasis; myocardium, kidney, liver, spleen, adrenal, and parietal pleura are less commonly affected. Occasionally, the esophageal neoplasms with lung metastasis are associated with hypertrophic osteoarthropathy (Marie's disease). Marie's disease is also seen with esophageal tumors that have not metastasized to the lungs.

## Squamous Cell Carcinoma of the Dog and Cat

**Incidence.** Cotchin (1959) summarized his previous reports to show that carcinoma of the esophagus was common in the cat in the London area, but that sarcoma was rare (22 cases in 151 tumors of the alimentary tract). In the discussion to Cotchin's (1959) paper, I gave the comparable figures for Edinburgh where fewer esophageal tumors had been encountered. This geographical variation in frequency of occurrence was further emphasized by Happé *et al.* (1978) who observed only 2 cases in 494 cats autopsied in Utrecht, the Netherlands, over a 2-year period and by Vernon and Roudebush (1980) who reported a single case and stated that this tumor was rare or nonexistent in U.S. literature. True benign papillomas of the esophagus have not been reported in the cat, although Wilkinson (1970) described multiple papillomatous chronic inflammatory lesions in a 1-year-old cat. These growths decreased in size proceeding cranially from the cardia to the thoracic inlet.

When reviewing the literature, Ridgway and Suter (1979) found that primary tumors in the esophagus of the dog were rare if sarcoma associated with spirocercosis was excluded. They found reports of four squamous cell carcinomas, four undifferentiated carcinomas, one each of scirrhous carcinoma and adenocarcinoma, and five leiomyomas. To this they added eight esophageal tumors observed in 49,229 dogs over an 11-year period; two of these were primary (leiomyoma and squamous cell carcinoma) and six were secondary involvement from other sites (three thyroid, two respiratory tract, and one gastric). There does not seem to be a geographical variation of occurrence in the dog, and most routine diagnostic centers feature only a few examples of esophageal carcinomas in their series. Rarely do the viral or oropharyngeal papillomas of young dogs extend into the esophagus, and when they do, it is in the pharyngeal region.

**Age, Breed, and Sex.** Tumor-bearing cats in all geographical locations are elderly; for example, Cotchin's (1966) series had a mean age of 10.5 years. Castrated males are overrepresented, but there is no breed predisposition. Dogs showed no breed or sex bias, but most were old, ranging from 6 to 11 years of age.

**Sites and Clinical Considerations.** In Cotchin's (1966) series, 24 of the 29 cats had tumors in the middle third of the esophagus at the level of the first two ribs, cranial to the aortic arch. This site probably explains the clinical signs of progressive weight loss, salivation, and regurgitation of food and sometimes fluid a few minutes after intake. A similar site and clinical history are found in most records of other cases in cats and dogs. In addition, where the mucosal surface has become ulcerated, hematemesis may be seen. Ridgway and Suter (1979) stressed the difference between regurgitation and vomiting; only their case of gastric carcinoma with extension into the esophagus showed vomiting.

**Gross Morphology and Histological Features.** The lesion tends to be a single annular thickening completely encircling the tube and extending for a length of up to 8 cm. The neoplasm may not have progressed from plaque to annular lesion by the time of diagnosis. The case described by Krogh (1952) was probably multicentric involving upper and lower thirds of the esophagus. The epithelial surface appears as a white nodularity with some areas of ulceration. This can be detected by endoscopy (McCaw *et al.*, 1980). There are no special histological features, the pattern ranging from a noncornifying to a well-differentiated tumor with keratin pearls. Inflammatory reaction may be extensive because of infection of the ulcerated surface.

**Etiology.** Cotchin (1966) suggested that these tumors in cats were due to ingestion of a carcinogen possibly licked from the fur during self-grooming; the location of the tumor in the esophagus cranial to the aortic arch is due to delayed passage of ingesta. There has been no experimental work concerning this theory, but for other species some interesting ideas have been published. Schoental and Joffe (1974) showed that extracts from cultures of *Fusarium* spp. (fungal contaminants of mouldy cereals) given by stomach tube to rats and mice may be immunosuppressive and can cause hyperplasia of the squamous epithelium of the esophagus and esophageal region of the stomach. This evidence may show that such mycotoxins can be carcinogenic. Many nitrosamine compounds when ingested can induce esophageal papilloma and squamous cell carcinoma in rats. Levinson *et al.* (1979) found that a nitrosamine compound injected intraperitoneally will also produce such multicentric tumors at all levels of the esophagus. Since there were no tumors at the site of injection, the chemical need not act during swallowing but needs enzymatic activation to become carcinogenic, and one site for this may be the esophagus. It has been suggested that in humans the distribution of esophageal carcinoma in parts of the world is the result of mycotoxins and nitrosamines acting as carcinogen and cocarcinogen; moreover, soil deficiencies in different areas are known to make plants more susceptible to fungal attack. Animal protein can also be induced during food processing at certain temperatures in the presence of nitrates to form nitrosamines. The clues may yet lead us to Cotchin's hypothetical carcinogen.

**Growth and Metastasis.** The tumor grows by infiltration of tissue spaces and lymphatic vessels. At its commonest site, direct extension may result in invasion of the wall of the trachea at the entrance to the chest, thus making the case inoperable (e.g., McCaw *et al.*, 1980). Tumors in this region will spread to the caudal cervical, mediastinal, and even bronchial lymph nodes. Distant blood-borne metastasis has been reported in lung, kidney, thyroid, and spleen, but the early onset of clinical signs forestalls extensive metastasis.

## Leiomyoma of the Dog

**Incidence.** These tumors are recorded occasionally in most series published by routine diagnostic laboratories. Brodey and Cohen (1964) reported four cases of gastrointestinal neoplasms in 95 dogs, and Hayden and Nielsen (1973) reported two cases in 39 dogs among 15,215 canine accessions examined over a period of 15 years.

**Age, Breed, and Sex.** The mean age of affected dogs is 12.5 years (ranging from 3 to 18 years) and males are overrepresented. There is no breed predisposition.

**Sites and Clinical Characteristics.** The most common site, unlike that of the carcinoma, is in the distal esophagus often at the cardioesophageal junction. Tumors below 2 cm in diameter are usually asymptomatic incidental findings at autopsy, while larger masses (e.g., 7 cm in diameter) are associated with a history of vomiting soon after eat-ing. The esophagus above the lesion becomes dilated and the wall thickened.

**Gross Morphology and Histological Features.** The tumors are solitary and either partially surround the wall or bulge into the lumen. They grow under the intact mucosa and have a compression capsule. Thus, dilatation up to the area of obstruction of the esophagus can be seen radiographically following a barium meal, but endoscopy merely reveals smooth intact mucosa (cf. carcinoma). In one of Brodey and Cohen's (1964) cases, there was a coexistent small leiomyoma in the pylorus, and in Campbell and Pirie's (1965) case several leiomyomas measuring 1.5 cm in diameter were found in the cardiac region of the stomach. On cut surface they showed a white, glistening, whorled pattern in contrast to the more homogeneous granular cut surface of carcinoma of the stomach. Histologically, the bundles of muscle cells cut in varying directions may show variation in nuclear size, but mitoses and multinucleate giant cells, as seen in leiomyosarcoma of the rectum, are seldom found.

## Papilloma and Squamous Cell Carcinoma in the Upper Alimentary Tract of Cattle

**Incidence.** Statistics from abattoirs suggest that esophageal and forestomach tumors are rare. Brandley and Migaki (1963) found none in 1,000 cattle tumors in the United States, Plummer (1956) found one ruminal carcinoma in 447 cattle tumors in Canada, and Misdorp (1967) found one in 208 bovine tumors in the Netherlands. It must be remembered that recorded frequency depends on the source of the data. Abattoir surveys should only cover reasonably healthy animals, and meat inspectors will detect lesions on the inner linings of viscera of these animals only if they open the organs during the course of inspection. Tumors of the esophagus and rumen that have not yet penetrated the wall will escape detection and those that have penetrated are likely to be extensive and produce clinical signs so that the animal is not consigned to an abattoir and the record of the tumor is lost. Anderson *et al.* (1969) reported one squamous cell carcinoma of the rumen but no esophageal papillomas in 1.3 million cattle examined by U.K.

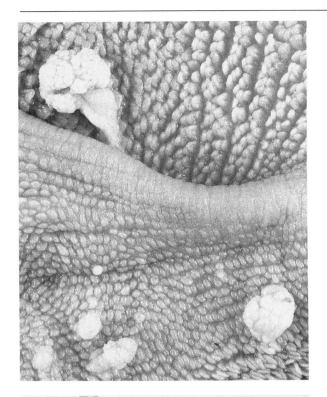

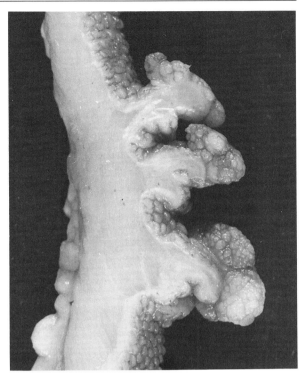

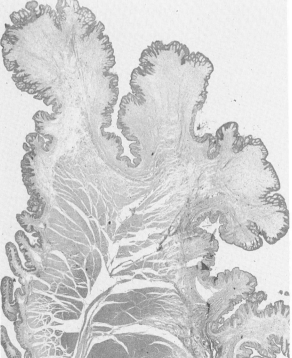

**FIGURE 8.13.** Papilloma in the rumen of sheep. A. Pedunculate and sessile, nodular, and linear papilloma on ruminal pillar. B. Cut surface of rumen fibropapilloma (see millimeter scale at bottom). C. Photograph of rumen pillar showing normal rumen papillae on left and fibropapilloma at the top and right.

ones often pedunculate. On cut surface they show a 1-mm epithelial covering over a white branching stroma (fig. 8.13B). The squamous cell carcinomas we have found in the United Kingdom associated with papilloma of the rumen resemble the larger sessile papillomas macroscopically and are as large as 25 mm in diameter.

**Histological Features.** Although a few of the rumen papillomas are typical squamous papillomas, most are fibropapillomas. They have a normal thickness of covering epithelium from which exaggerated rete pegs extend into a mass of fibrous tissue, which is mainly mature fibrous tissue but shows some areas of more active fibroblasts (fig. 8.13C). The epithelium has few mitotic figures and some cells with large nucleoli. No intranuclear inclusion bodies are found. The cytoplasm of some cells, especially in the keratinized zone, is hydropic, and eosinophilic inclusions may be found in vacuoles. The squamous cell carcinomas arising in these papillomas are well-differentiated and do not penetrate far into the underlying tissues. Georgsson's (1973) case was moderately differentiated without distinctly keratinized pearls.

**Etiology.** Vanselow *et al.* (1982) described multiple cutaneous papilloma on the face and ears of four aged Merino sheep in Australia in which there was progression from virus-induced papilloma to squamous cell carcinoma, possibly under the influence of sunlight. They cite the only other report of papilloma, which was also cutaneous (Gibbs *et al.,* 1975, in England), in which virions of papovavirus type could be demonstrated by electron microscopy. The two affected sheep were 1 and 5 years old, respectively. The papilloma could be transmitted to other sheep but not to cattle. In Edinburgh we have been unable to find virus particles in electron microscopic examination of sections of rumen papilloma, but have found a few papillomalike virions in chemically disrupted ovine rumen papilloma. Immunohistochemical methods have revealed only occasional cells staining for the presence of the ovine alimentary papilloma virus. The virus is found in the cells of the stratum corneum, usually those showing hydropic change. This contrast between the cutaneous ovine papilloma and the ruminal ovine papilloma may mean that there is little mature virus because the cells containing it are shed rapidly. McCrea and Head (1981) found

one small rumen papilloma in one of eight wether lambs fed dried bracken fern for 5 years beginning at 5 months of age. The dried bracken was active since one sheep died of acute bracken poisoning, another developed night blindness, and seven had bladder tumors. This contrasts with the increase in esophageal papillomas reported by Jarrett (1980) in cattle. It should be pointed out, however, that we do not know the number of papillomas present before the bracken feeding started and we did not attempt rumen transmission of the virus in these sheep.

**Growth and Metastasis.** Almost nothing is known of the biology of rumen papilloma in sheep. The tumors seem to be incidental findings when the rumen is examined and we have no record of them producing clinical signs. Likewise, the rumen carcinomas we have encountered have been small, nonmetastasizing tumors recorded either as incidental findings in healthy slaughtered animals or found in animals killed because of the presence of large tumors in other sites. This indicates an interesting species difference in cattle even in geographical areas like the North York moors where the radiomimetic and carcinogenic effects of bracken are well established in sheep.

## Squamous Cell Carcinoma in Monogastric Domestic Animals

**Incidence.** Among monogastric domestic animals, only pigs and horses have a moderately extensive stratified squamous epithelial-lined esophageal region to the stomach. Spontaneous carcinoma of this region is not recorded in the domestic pig, but Plowright *et al.* (1971) reported such tumors in two Kenyan giant forest hogs that grazed the forest clearings where cattle with ruminal carcinoma were herded. Even macroscopic examination without histological follow-up should be sufficient to differentiate common ulceration and inflammatory thickening of this area of the pig's stomach from the rare carcinoma.

Sporadic cases of carcinoma of the esophageal region of the horse stomach have been reported from many parts of the temperate and tropical world. Although they are not particularly common, Tennant *et al.* (1982) found 15 cases in the literature and added 6 of their own. These authors cited Krahnert

(1952) who thought that only 21 of the 50 stomach carcinoma records in the older literature (going back a hundred years) had been carefully studied; 18 of these cases were squamous cell carcinomas of the esophageal region of the stomach and 3 were adenocarcinomas of the glandular region of the stomach. Tennant and co-workers reported that in New York cases had only been observed since 1969 and that the majority of cases described in the literature from the United States and Canada dated from 1970. This may suggest an increasing frequency of occurrence, but we have little baseline population data to verify this. Sundberg *et al.* (1977) used 687 equine necropsies and 635 biopsies examined at Purdue University (Indiana) as the baseline from which they found two squamous cell carcinomas of the stomach and one papilloma of the esophagus.

**Age, Sex, and Breed.** Cotchin (1977) in reviewing the literature gave an age range of 6 to 18 years (mean 12.8 years), whereas Tennant *et al.* (1982) in their collated series of 34 cases gave a range of 6 to 16 years (mean 10.7 years). Tennant and co-workers could not demonstrate a convincing sex distribution (eight females, eight castrated males, and four males), that is, they could not confirm the four to one male to female ratio found by Moore and Kintner (1976). Most authorities agree that no positive breed correlation can be shown. Tennant *et al.* (1982) pointed out that Shetland ponies in the United States are rarely affected by this tumor, but Wester *et al.* (1980) reported that in the Netherlands one of their seven cases was in this breed.

**Clinical Characteristics.** Clinical signs are vague. There is progressive weight loss, intermittent anorexia, and sometimes colic. As the tumor enlarges, signs of obstruction are observable, such as progressive difficulty in feeding and drinking and the occurrence of choking and regurgitation. The latter may result in inhalation pneumonia. Obstruction to the passage of the stomach tube in the late stages may indicate the site of the tumor, and rectal examination may reveal masses near the root of the mesentery. Roberts and Kelly (1979) were able to confirm a carcinoma in the esophagus by fiber optic endoscopic examination. Lesions in the stomach are either not easily reached because of the distance from the nostril to the cardia in a big horse or because the stenosis due to the tumor growth within

the wall of the terminal esophagus prevents the passage of the instrument down to the observably abnormal stomach lining (Keirn *et al.*, 1982). Prior to this method of direct intraluminal observation, exploratory laparotomy was often the only way to establish a diagnosis. If metastasis becomes established on the serous membranes of the abdominal and thoracic cavities, accumulation of fluid may supervene. Exfoliative cytology of such fluid may reveal isolated epithelial cells and cell nests in addition to neutrophils in the ascites fluid (Tennant *et al.*, 1982). Wester *et al.* (1980) illustrated clearly the birefringence of keratinized cells obtained from abdominal fluid smears stained by the Papanicolaou method and examined by polarizing microscopy. The duration between onset of signs and death or euthanasia *in extremis* varies from 3 days to 4 months.

**Sites.** By the time the lesions are recognized they usually cover extensive areas of the esophageal region, which in the horse forms the greater part of the left sac of the stomach. Small growths have also been reported (Damodaran and Sundararaj, 1973), and these lie near the margo plicatus, which is the ridge marking the separation of squamous from glandular lining membrane of the cardiac region. Some tumors apparently arise from areas of squamous metaplasia in the glandular region of the stomach. In this connection it is interesting that a squamous cell carcinoma of the pyloric antrum of a 14-year-old male mixed breed dog was described by Patnaik and Lieberman (1980). Squamous cell carcinoma of the equine esophagus is rare if one excludes the few cases where there has been extension from a primary carcinoma in the stomach. Roberts and Kelly (1979) described such a case at the level of the fifth and sixth cervical vertebrae and gave literature references to another.

**Gross Morphology.** Roberts and Kelly's (1979) case was a 10- to 12-cm-long thickening of the esophageal wall with areas of ulcerations or papilliform and verrucose elevations of the epithelium. Most of the gastric tumors form a large, roughly nodular, cauliflowerlike mass 10 to 30 cm in diameter bulging into the lumen; Moore and Kintner's (1976) case weighed 7 kg. The luminal surface exhibits ulcers 1 to 3 cm in diameter, some areas that are hemorrhagic (red), and other areas that are secondarily infected and necrotic (yellow). The muscular wall becomes infiltrated and thickened as much as 10 cm by the tumor and fibrous reaction. Although there is usually a sharp border to the tumor on the mucosal surface, infiltration in the wall may extend under normal epithelium at the edges.

**Histological Features.** As in many well-differentiated squamous carcinomas, there is a large amount of collagen-rich stroma in this neoplasm, and with the exposed surface likely to become infected, degenerating cells in the centers of the neoplastic cords become liquefied and cystlike structures are formed. At the periphery of the neoplasm the tumor cells may infiltrate into lymphatics and blood vessels where they can be seen some distance beyond the main border of the tumor. Patnaik and Lieberman (1980) described a metaplasia of pyloric gland epithelium to squamous cells in the crypt. They suggested that this metaplasia is likely to be the result of multipotential cells at the base of the crypt glands rather than metaplasia of glandular epithelium or growth of heterotopic squamous cell nests (fig. 8.14).

**Etiology.** Cotchin (1977) summarized the literature that supports the hypothesis that these tumors are directly or indirectly related to damage caused by *Gasterophilus intestinalis* larvae. Damodaran and Sundararaj (1973) report that in India the tumors are related to tumorlike nodules of reaction around *Habronema megastoma*. Tennant *et al.* (1982) do not think that the parasites and tumors are related because the parasites are common and the tumors are rare. However, by analogy with the situation for *Spirocerca lupi* and neoplasms in dogs, such reasoning is suspect. The situation could be multifactorial with an exogenous or endogenous carcinogen such as a nitrosamine acting on the hyperplastic epithelium, as illustrated by Shefstad (1978) adjacent to the parasitic ulcer. Further study of atypical parasitic lesions found in the stomach of routinely slaughtered elderly equines might reveal early tumors and give a lead into this problem. Furthermore, the stomach distant from the established tumor should be examined for metaplasia in the glandular region (fig. 8.14) and for early carcinoma *in situ* formation in the nonglandular region.

**Clinical Laboratory Findings.** Hematological examination often reveals neutrophilia, which may be related to surface ulceration of the tumor, and anemia, which is probably not due to chronic blood

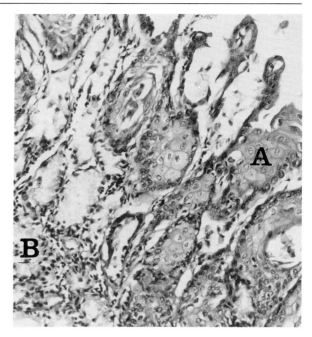

FIGURE 8.14. Squamous cell carcinoma in the stomach of the horse. Superficial mucosa from the fundic region of the stomach showing metaplastic change to squamous epithelial cells (A) from columnar cells (B).

loss. Serum chemistry shows a hypoalbuminemia and/or hyperglobulinemia; thus the albumin to globulin ratio is reduced, an indication of either chronic inflammation or neoplasia. These studies are well covered by Moore and Kintner (1976) and Tennant *et al.* (1982). Menten *et al.* (1978) described an 11-year-old Arabian stallion with lethargy, weight loss, constipation, and anorexia of 3 weeks' duration resulting from a large squamous cell carcinoma of the stomach. The case is of interest because there was marked elevation of serum calcium (18.2 to 19.3 mg/dl). This is an example of pseudohyperparathyroidism; there was no renal failure, the parathyroids were moderately atrophic, and there was no bone reabsorption.

**Growth and Metastasis.** The tumors grow by infiltration of tissue spaces, lymphatic vessels, and small blood vessels. Metastasis to drainage lymph nodes of the stomach and esophagus is common. Infiltrative growth in the stomach leads to direct extension of the carcinoma to contiguous organs and viscera, namely the diaphragm, capsule of the liver, and spleen. Transcelomic deposits may then form on the surface of more distant abdominal structures, and the neoplasm may metastasize from the peritoneum to the pleural surfaces via lymphatic drainage. The latter growths are seldom as advanced as in the abdomen and therefore rarely cause clinical signs. Bloodborne metastasis is found in the liver and less commonly in the lung, kidney, and adrenal gland.

## TUMORS OF THE STOMACH

## Glandular Tumors of the Stomach

**Classification.** Subdivision of glandular tumors of the stomach is difficult; the benign types may be confused with nonneoplastic proliferative lesions. Malignant types often show several histological patterns, and tumors of different histology can have similar macroscopic appearance. The traditional classification for humans as established by Oota and Sobin (1977) is to separate benign adenoma, malignant adenocarcinoma, and carcinoid tumors. Adenomas are flat or polypoid, solitary or multiple, papillary (fingerlike projections of lamina propria covered by atypical epithelium), tubular (branching tubules of epithelium surrounded by lamina propria), or papillotubular (showing both patterns). Adenomas are true tumors so the epithelium is "atypical" in that there is variation in nuclear size and shape and a higher number of mitoses and cell layers. Adenocarcinomas are divided into four types: (1) papillary, (2) tubular, (3) mucinous (where "lakes" of mucus are usually large enough to be seen by the naked eye), and (4) "signet ring" cell, usually as isolated cells in a scirrhous stroma. The signet ring cells have a single droplet of acid mucin or granules of neutral or acid mucin (as in goblet cells). The mucin droplets are located in one part of the cytoplasm, and the nucleus is forced to the periphery of the cell. Each of these types may be subdivided into well, moderately, or poorly differentiated on the basis of the degree of differentiation. Some carcinomas are so poorly organized they are called undifferentiated, that is, they fit into none of these four patterns. Adenocarcinoma is differentiated from adenoma because the papillary and tubular pattern is less defined, there is loss of nuclear

and mucin droplet polarity, mitoses are more frequent, and growth is invasive.

Nevalainen and Jarvi (1977), when describing the ultrastructure of gastric carcinoma, reported that Schmidt as long ago as 1896 noted that some gastric carcinomas were similar to intestinal carcinomas; this observation was expanded later. In human epidemiological and clinical studies, it is now common to use a classification divided into intestinal, diffuse, and indeterminate types of gastric carcinoma. The intestinal type is formed by tubules lined by glandular epithelium that resembles intestinal columnar cells with a brush border and goblet cells. Such tumors have distinct borders, and the adjacent nonneoplastic epithelium may show intestinal type metaplastic change. In the diffuse type of gastric carcinoma, most of the stomach is infiltrated by poorly cohesive rounded cells often of signet ring appearance. Only near the surface are poorly developed tubules found and the tumors do not have a distinct border. The indeterminate type of gastric carcinoma includes those cases where both patterns exist or where the tumor is undifferentiated so that neither pattern can be recognized. In humans intestinal metaplasia is found in some nonneoplastic stomachs and in some gastric adenomas. Some intestinal types of gastric carcinomas apparently arise from normal gastric epithelium (i.e., mucosa not showing intestinal metaplasia). Moreover, it is now becoming clear that intestinal metaplasia is not a single entity (Jass, 1980). Studies of the mucin and enzyme histochemistry show two main types: the "incomplete type," having features of both gastric and small intestinal epithelia, and the "colonic type," having characteristics of the large intestine. Moreover, Nevalailen and Jarvi (1977) on the basis of electron microscopic studies suggested that intestinal type carcinoma cells are similar to intestinal metaplasia, but that diffuse type carcinoma cells resemble the goblet cells of intestinal metaplasia.

Separate from the benign and malignant mucosal tumors described above are the carcinoid tumors. These are derived from basal gastric mucosa, they invade the submucosa early, and therefore seem to be submucosal in origin. Such tumors are composed of uniform cells in sheets or cords. The cells have indistinct borders in light microscopy and may be subdivided on the basis of silver staining into argentaffin carcinoids, which have silver staining cytoplasmic granules that are demonstrated without the use of external reducing agents (Fontana method), and argyrophil carcinoids in which an external reducing agent is needed to reveal the silver staining granules (Bodian method).

Most reports in the veterinary literature have followed some form of the traditional human classification system, but Patnaik *et al.* (1978*a*) used the intestinal and the diffuse systems. These authors have subdivided the intestinal type carcinomas into papillary adenocarcinoma, acinar adenocarcinoma, and solid adenocarcinoma (where only occasional acinar or papillary structures are found). The diffuse type is subdivided into the glandular type (where occasional indistinct glands are formed among the isolated tumor cells) and the undifferentiated type. It is not yet possible, therefore, to say whether this latter system will lead to the delineation of geographical areas of high incidence of gastric tumors of the intestinal type in animals. In the human it has been suggested that intestinal gastric carcinoma may be caused by environmental factors and diffuse type is possibly of genetic origin.

**Incidence.** Lingeman *et al.* (1971) reviewed the recorded cases of gastric tumors and found 61 cases in dogs, 4 in cats, 4 in horses, and 1 each in an ox and a pig. The records for these tumors in oxen, sheep, and pigs are few and sketchy. In the horse, adenocarcinoma is far less common than squamous cell carcinoma of the stomach (e.g., in Krahnert's, 1952, series there are 3 versus 18). Sundberg *et al.* (1977) mentioned 1 papilloma of the horse stomach in a series of 21 tumors from all sites. In the cat, Cotchin (1959) mentioned 4 lymphomas of the stomach, and Brodey (1966) recorded another example, but neither author encountered a gastric carcinoma in their series. Turk *et al.* (1981) found a tubular adenocarcinoma and an undifferentiated carcinoma in a series of gastrointestinal tumors of cats collected between 1967 and 1981. From this group they excluded mast cell tumor and lymphoma.

Among the domestic animals the dog is the most common species to develop spontaneous gastric cancer, but even so it is rare compared with humans. Krook (1956) found 15 cases in the literature going back to 1897 and added four cases from Stockholm. Lingeman *et al.* (1971) brought the total in the literature up to 62 by adding 22 cases, some of which had been previously published from the Registry of Comparative Pathology of the U.S. Armed Forces Institute of Pathology, and included in their analysis 19 cases from London and 2 from Japan. Since then several series of gastric tumors have been published. It is difficult to compare the true incidence in different parts of the world because the baseline varies from tumors collected over a span of years to numbers expressed as percentages of all tumors, of all carcinomas, or of just dog necropsies. Several series agree that gastric carcinomas form about 1% or less of all malignant neoplasms of the dog.

The pattern of gastric tumor types observed in dogs is similar in several parts of the world. Cotchin (1959) listed 1 adenoma, 1 leiomyoma, 4 adenocarcinomas, and 3 sarcomas. Brodey and Cohen (1964) reported 1 adenoma, 10 leiomyomas, 5 adenocarcinomas, 2 fibrosarcomas, 2 leiomyosarcomas, and 3 lymphomas. Over a 15-year period, Hayden and Nielsen (1973) collected 1 adenomatous polyp, 2 leiomyomas, 7 carcinomas, and 1 sarcoma. Sautter and Hanlon (1975), over a 24-year period, saw 2 leiomyomas, 14 carcinomas, 1 leiomyosarcoma, and 3 lymphomas. In 1,961 necropsies performed over 5 years, Gialamas and Schaffraneck (1977) in Vienna recorded only 1 gastric carcinoma, whereas Patnaik *et al.* (1977) in New York found 6 adenomas, 17 leiomyomas, 26 adenocarcinomas, 3 leiomyosarcomas, and 3 lymphomas among 10,270 necropsies. Of these 26 adenocarcinomas, 9 were of the intestinal type and 17 of the diffuse type (Patnaik *et al.*, 1978*a*).

The frequency with which benign glandular neoplasms occur in the stomach of the dog is, from the above data, certainly less than for carcinoma. How many of these are true tumors is problematical. In these series the lesions are found in old dogs in the pyloric region, and they are usually solitary polyps 0.5 to 1 cm in diameter and commonly asymptomatic, occurring as incidental findings at necropsy. Some are probably not true tumors as indicated by Hayden and Nielsen's (1973) nomenclature of adenomatous polyp which had hyperplastic epithelium and occurred in a stomach showing patchy mucosal hyperplastic and atrophic changes. The significance of this differentiation is that true adenoma may be premalignant; thus one of four cases of gastric polyps reported by Murray *et al.* (1972*b*) occurred in a 9.5-year-old miniature poodle that also had a diffuse scirrhous adenocarcinoma and two raised polyps showing focal malignant change. Conroy (1969) described a unique case of a 1- to 1.5-year-old mongrel female with polypoid or sessile growths 2 cm in diameter scattered throughout the stomach; early malignant change was present in some of these "adenomatous polyps."

Carcinoid tumors of the dog's stomach are very rare; one is mentioned by Head (1976*b*).

**Age, Breed, and Sex.** The age for dogs with carcinoma ranges from 3 to 15 years, with the average age from 7.47 (Krook, 1956) to 9.8 (Sautter and Hanlon, 1975) years. Patnaik *et al.* (1977) reported an average age for adenoma in dogs as 9.5 years and for adenocarcinoma, 10 years. The male to female ratio for adenoma was 1:5 and for adenocarcinoma was 17:7. This predisposition to males in carcinoma was demonstrable in several reports but not all, the most marked predisposition being that of Hayden and Nielsen (1973) at 6:1. Such figures may represent a true geographical variation, but need to be compared against the sex distribution of the source population, especially since Patnaik *et al.* (1978*a*) showed a male to female ratio of 7:1 in intestinal type and 2.4:1 in diffuse type from a population of 5,176:4,477 dogs. Most authors could find no breed predisposition, but Else and Head (1980) suggested that in the Edinburgh area, Cairn terriers and West Highland white terriers are overrepresented.

**Clinical Characteristics.** Clinical signs are nonspecific but related to progressive loss of gastric function, particularly due to partial stenosis of the pylorus. Loss of condition with anorexia and intermittent vomiting over a period of 1 to 8 months in an older dog should suggest the possible diagnosis of stomach tumor. Vomiting, often not related to food intake, may consist of mucus or swallowed saliva (foam). It may be stained yellow from bile or contain fresh red blood or brown, granular, partly digested blood. Abdominal pain may be evinced by discomfort on palpation of the anterior abdomen; muscle relaxants may be needed to aid palpation of the tumor mass. Anemia, diarrhea, melena, and hematemesis are not common, but may be seen related to tumor ulceration; if an ulcer bleeds, it is more often a slow leak than a massive hemorrhage. In addition to anemia, hematological examination

can show leukocytosis associated with the ulcer. Dorn *et al.* (1976) found gastroscopy of limited value in confirming the diagnosis in one case, but Sinclair *et al.* (1979) using the same technique were able to demonstrate a large crateriform ulcer associated with the neoplasm. This technique along with biopsy sampling may prove to be of value in the future. The features to be looked for in radiological examination are the absence of the normal changes in the shape of the stomach over several radiographs, filling defects in the pyloric and lesser curvature areas, and delayed emptying with residual barium staining (Murray *et al.*, 1972*b*). Even this diagnostic aid is of limited value; only two of Sautter and Hanlon's (1975) six cases were clearly diagnosed by radiographs. Exploratory laparotomy often establishes a diagnosis, but rapid biopsy examination may be needed to help the surgeon decide between surgical intervention and euthanasia.

**Sites.** The nomenclature of the location of tumors within the stomach varies with different authors, some using surface features as the basis (see Gross Morphology), while others use the various glandular regions of the mucosa. There is general agreement with the finding of Sautter and Hanlon (1975) that although the tumor is usually extensive by the time of diagnosis, most cases are found in the lower two-thirds of the stomach. Involvement of the whole stomach may be seen, but it is rare. The commonest site is the pyloric antrum with extension into the body of the stomach, usually along the lesser curvature. Primary sites in the body of the stomach are the next most common, with the lesser curvature more common than the greater curvature. The cardia is sometimes the center of the tumor, but reports of tumors in the fundus are very rare. Patnaik *et al.* (1978*a*) reports that five of the intestinal type gastric carcinomas were located in the pyloric antrum and that most of the diffuse types involved this area but often extended to other regions. These authors consider that the cells of these intestinal type adenocarcinomas have histological features resembling the gastric glands of the cardiac (three cases) or pyloric (six cases) regions of the stomach.

**Gross Morphology.** The three main patterns of carcinoma given in order of frequency of occurrence are an ulcerated, plaquelike thickening; a diffuse, nonulcerating thickening; and a raised sessile polyp. The tumor is gray-white and firm to fibrous on cut section, clearly with replacement of most of the normal structure of the wall.

Patnaik *et al.* (1978*a*) reported that half of their cases exhibited ulcers equally frequent in intestinal and diffuse types of carcinoma. The ulcer in the plaquelike form may be as large as 5 cm in diameter. The base of the ulcer may be depressed as much as 2 cm below the overhanging margins because the ulcer penetrates through the plaquelike mass bulging into the lumen. The ulcer may extend through the stomach wall so that its floor is only 1 to 2 mm thick and it may even perforate the wall (fig. 8.15A). Omental adhesions to the serosa are common in this region; thus, widespread peritonitis from a perforated ulcerated tumor is rare. Sautter and Hanlon (1975) suggest that the ulceration is due to ischemic necrosis following tumor plugs occluding blood and lymph vessels; this contrasts with the situation in lymphoma and leiomyosarcoma in which blood vessels are occluded by external tumor pressure.

Gastric ulcers may form in carcinoma. Conversely, carcinoma may in theory develop in gastric ulcers. Ulceration of the stomach in dogs has been described but no carcinoma has been recorded in these ulcers. Murray *et al.* (1972*a*) recorded 22 cases of peptic ulceration in dogs, in which 17 were in the duodenum, 3 in the lesser curvature, and 2 in the pyloric antrum of the stomach. Of these 22 cases only 14 presented with clinical signs related to the ulcers. They pointed out that many of these ulcers were related to malignant mast cell tumors or to liver disease. Pancreatic islet cell tumors must be added to these two predisposing factors for ulcers. Zontine *et al.* (1977) illustrated the radiographic diagnosis of duodenal ulceration in dogs and cats and reviewed the literature on the correlation between ulcers and mast cell tumors. They explained that histamine from mast cells stimulates the H-2 receptors, and thus excessive gastric hydrochloric acid secretion occurs.

The mucosal rugae around the ulcer may be thickened or lost. In the diffuse pattern of carcinoma the rugae are also usually obliterated by the thickening of the wall, which is partly due to fibrosis and partly to edema. In both patterns the serosa shows white tumor tissue between the stretched muscle bundles. Delicate threads of plugged vessels

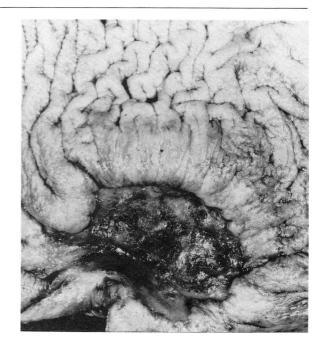

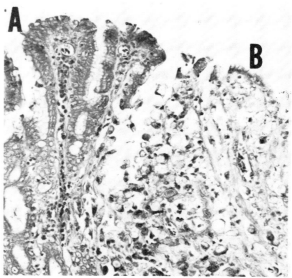

FIGURE 8.15. Carcinoma in the stomach of the dog. A. Mucosal ulcer on lesser curvature distal to cardia of stomach of dog. Microscopic examination of the stomach wall revealed an adenocarcinoma. B. Histological section from margin of this ulcer. Normal mucosa (A) is partially replaced by a diffuse infiltration of undifferentiated carcinoma cells (B). (Courtesy of Dr. C. H. Lingeman and *J. Natl. Cancer Inst.*)

occluded by neoplastic tissue are also seen. Where the diffuse pattern involves most of the stomach, it is sometimes referred to as "leather bottle" or linitis plastica. Diffuse tumors in the pyloric region can obviously become annular and stenosing. Else and Head (1980) pointed out that the unaffected area toward the cardia in such cases becomes dilated giving an hourglass shape to the unopened stomach.

**Histological Features.** The general diagnostic features were discussed in the classification section (above). Lingeman *et al.* (1971) considered that canine gastric carcinoma forms an almost uniform entity that most nearly corresponds to the diffuse human type. They reported that 6 of 17 dogs had intestinal metaplasia of the nonneoplastic gastric mucosa some distance from the carcinoma. Patnaik *et al.* (1978*a*), however, found 9 intestinal type tumors in 26 gastric adenocarcinomas; intestinal metaplasia was found in the gastric epithelium of 6 of the 9 intestinal type carcinomas and 8 of the 17 diffuse types. Not enough attention has been paid in the past to the mucosa of the stomach at sites distant from the primary site of the tumor. Patnaik *et al.* (1978*a*) found epithelial hyperplasia and accentuated mucosal folds in 3 intestinal and 12 diffuse type carcinomas and mucosal atrophy with chronic gastritis in 1 diffuse type carcinoma. Atrophic gastritis can be a precancerous lesion in the human. In some ulcerated plaquelike gastric carcinomas, the ulcer is so large that careful search must be made of the granulation tissue floor of the ulcer and its overhanging edges to find tumor cells. Murray *et al.* (1972*a*) reported that although there was hyperplastic mucus-secreting mucosa surrounding the peptic ulcers, no tumor tissue was found. It is generally agreed that in the dog the ulcer is secondary to the tumor and not the reverse. The junction of gastric carcinoma with surrounding mucosa is sharp in most forms of the tumor (fig. 8.15B), that is, the lesion is solitary without evidence of early satellite malignancies around the main tumor mass.

**Etiology.** There is no definite evidence as to the etiology of gastric neoplasia in dogs. Lingeman *et al.* (1971) pointed out that human stomach carcinoma is thought to be associated with prolonged exposure to unidentified environmental carcinogens, such as polycyclic hydrocarbons formed in the preservation of meat and fish by smoking, or to mycotoxins such as aflatoxin. The relative rarity of

gastric carcinoma in dogs, even in countries where there is a high human incidence of these neoplasms such as Japan and the Soviet Union, suggests that domestic animals are not exposed to these human hazards, are not exposed for a long enough period, or have a species resistance. Certainly, species have a different response to carcinogens; for example, bracken fern extracts given intraperitoneally result in many intestinal type gastric carcinomas in mice after 1 to 2 years but none in rats (C. W. Evans *et al.*, 1982; I. A. Evans *et al.*, 1982). Kurihara *et al.* (1974) produced adenocarcinomas in the stomach of dogs with *N*-ethyl-*N'*-nitro-*N*-nitrosoguanidine.

Hill (1980) explained that nitrate from plants or from farm fertilizers contaminating drinking water supplies could be reduced to nitrite by gut and bladder bacteria; the nitrite could then be absorbed and excreted in body secretions. Similarly, secondary amines produced in the colon by bacteria can be absorbed and excreted. *N*-nitrosamine could then be formed either locally in the stomach (e.g., in patients with pernicious anemia) or as organotropic chemicals formed in the colon but having the stomach as the target organ. Miniature swine fed methylnitrosourea for 4.5 years developed no clinical signs, but all except one had multiple small benign gastric adenomatous polyps with early malignant change; one had a malignant gastric Schwannoma (Stavrou *et al.*, 1976). Shimosato *et al.* (1971) gave four dogs *N*-methyl-*N'*-nitro-*N*-nitrosoguanidine orally in drinking water from 3 months of age for a period of 14 months, and all of the dogs had multiple adenocarcinomas of the stomach when killed at 18 to 34 months of age. These tumors were found at sites throughout the stomach and were papillary, tubular, or signet ring cell type in histological pattern. They showed an intramucosal or superficial pattern of growth and were often microscopic in size and were never more than 1 cm in diameter. These lesions occurred in areas of histologically atrophic but macroscopically normal mucosa. One stomach showed a hemangiosarcoma, and in all four cases there were leiomyosarcomas as large as 9 × 8 × 6 cm in the duodenum or jejunum. No metastasis was found. Kurihara *et al.* (1974) fed four 4-month-old dogs twice daily for 8 months on a pellet diet soaked in *N*-ethyl-*N'*-nitro-*N*-nitrosoguanidine and Tween-60 solution. Endoscopic examination and biopsy revealed tumors in as soon as 176 days, and double contrast radiography revealed tumors in 349 days after feeding. The four dogs died from hematemesis, melena, and vomiting in 277, 395, 546, and 813 days, respectively. The lesions were multiple and ranged from mucosal atrophy with microscopic intramural neoplasms in the earliest death to obvious tumors varying in size from 36 × 24 mm to 55 × 50 mm in the other three dogs. As in the Shimosato *et al.* (1971) series, the tumors were tubular, papillotubular, or signet ring cell carcinomas in histological appearance, but they penetrated into the stomach wall as far as the serosa in two cases. Metastasis was present in the pancreatic and thoracic lymph nodes in the longest survivor. Moreover, with this experimental protocol no sarcomas were produced in the intestines, and the gastric carcinomas were restricted to subcardiac and antrum regions, the presumed sites of longest carcinogen contact.

**Growth and Metastasis.** Murray *et al.* (1972*b*) mentioned a case in which removal of an adenomatous polyp was followed by complete recovery. Surgery on carcinoma cases has been less rewarding because the tumors are well advanced by the time they are diagnosed. Lingeman *et al.* (1971) mentioned a case in a 9-year-old male Irish setter where recurrence in 6 months followed excision of a tumor in the cardiac region. Partial gastrectomy of the pyloric half of the stomach followed by gastroduodenostomy resulted in remission of signs for 2 to 3 months before recurrence necessitated euthanasia of three other dogs (Dorn *et al.*, 1976; Murray *et al.*, 1972*b*; Sinclair *et al.*, 1979).

Very small experimentally induced tumors illustrate the way in which the large spontaneous tumors may have developed. Carcinoma *in situ* is the earliest pattern; the cells show severe atypia but do not invade across the basement membrane of the glands. When the tumor cells invade through the basement membrane into the lamina propria but not through the muscularis mucosa, the tumor is referred to as an intramucosal carcinoma; such a tumor can metastasize via lymphatic and blood vessels. The next stage is extensive lateral spread from the original site both in the lamina propria of the surrounding normal mucosa and through the muscularis mucosa into the underlying superficial submucosa. This superficial spreading carcinoma

growth pattern is not only seen in small early tumors, but also in the large diffuse nonulcerating tumors. The tumor usually invades through the muscle coat within small blood and lymphatic vessels, and these infiltrated structures may become macroscopically visible on the serosa. Such intravascular obstruction can in part be responsible for the marked fibrosis that develops in many tumors, although it is possible that the epithelial cells of such scirrhous carcinomas induce fibroplasia. A few tumors, particularly undifferentiated solid carcinoma, form little stroma and show an intercellular type of invasive growth.

The records of metastasis of gastric carcinoma in the literature vary between series. Sautter and Hanlon (1975) reported 11 of 14 cases with no metastasis despite tumor plugs being present in lymphatics and venules in most animals. In contrast, Patnaik *et al.* (1978*a*) reported 25 of 26 dogs with peritoneal carcinomatosis; 20 of these dogs with local lymph nodes available for examination showed metastasis. The most probable explanation for this variation is that metastasis is a function of the duration of the neoplasm. Lymphatic spread to the gastroduodenal and splenic lymph node groups is the most common distant metastatic site. Bloodborne spread to the liver is next most common. Blood or lymphohematogenous metastasis to the lungs is relatively rare; it should be noted that organs such as the myocardium, kidney, adrenal, and spleen have been involved without visible lung metastasis. Widespread systemic bloodborne metastasis is seldom seen, probably because clinical signs of gastric dysfunction occur relatively early in the disease. Tumor tissue may be visible to the naked eye in the serosa of the stomach and omental adhesions can also be present, but transperitoneal metastasis is rare and ascitic fluid, presumably the result of portal vein congestion, seldom contains tumor cells.

## Nonglandular Tumors of the Stomach

Most authors recording series of stomach tumors in dogs concentrate on carcinomas, but also mention the occurrence of comparable numbers of other types of tumors. Among the latter, smooth muscle tumors are most frequently mentioned, and as Pat-

**Incidence.** Most authors agree that in all species adenoma is less common than adenocarcinoma and that although carcinoma is found occasionally, it is not common except in sheep. Dodd (1960) first reported a high prevalence of adenocarcinoma in the small intestine of sheep in New Zealand where 25 cases were found in 4 years, 17 from animals that had been found dead at a research station. Cordes and Shortridge (1971) extended this study by reporting that adenocarcinoma was the most common tumor type of sheep found in their laboratory, comprising 143 cases in 256 sheep tumors of all types. Only 6 of their cases had been submitted for abattoirs, which is in marked contrast with the series reported by Simpson and Jolly (1974) in New Zealand where all but 5 of 450 cases were obtained from abattoirs. The workers in New Zealand demonstrated a different prevalence in different areas of the country, ranging from 0.2 to 1.6% of ewes slaughtered. McDonald and Leaver (1965) in Australia examined 5 tumor cases in dead or sick sheep from one property where 0.4% of all sheep and 2% of sheep more than 5 years of age had intestinal carcinomas. Ross (1980) in a survey of abattoirs in New South Wales, Australia, recorded a tumor incidence of 0.27% for adult sheep. A similar incidence figure was reported by Head (1967) among ewes slaughtered between 1959 and 1962 at abattoirs in Edinburgh, Scotland. In Iceland, Georgsson and Vigfusson (1973) analyzing data from an abattoir gave an incidence figure of 0.97% of sheep slaughtered at 1 year of age or older. There is a marked difference between these high prevalence countries and countries like South Africa, the United States, and the United Kingdom where only occasional cases have been recorded, as summarized in the report by Pearson and McCaughey (1978). These workers also described 2 cases in ewes in a research flock in Northern Ireland. More recently, Tontis (1982) described 3 cases in Switzerland.

Some of the difference in prevalence of these neoplasms in different countries is due to their misdiagnosis as mesothelioma or chronic peritonitis by meat inspectors (Ross, 1980). This was also pointed out by Head (1967) who examined the earlier records in Edinburgh and found there were cases of peritonitis and peritoneal metastasis from unknown sites, which were probably metastasis from adenocarcinoma of the small intestine. Simpson and Jolly (1974) suggested that the number of cases recorded in sheep has increased since meat inspectors have been trained to recognize the condition. Another possible explanation for altered prevalence rates could be that many of the affected sheep are not examined at necropsy. Head (1967) cited the statement by Brandley and Migaki (1963) to explain the low prevalence of these tumors in the United States where 95% of the sheep slaughtered are lambs since the carcass value of most range ewes does not justify the cost of transportation and slaughter. Despite the problem of obtaining accurate and comparable data, there seems little doubt that there are countries in the world where intestinal adenocarcinoma is very common in sheep.

Incidence figures are difficult to establish, not only because the population at risk cannot always be established but also because the data have been incompletely recorded. Lingeman and Garner (1972) surveyed the literature and added 11 canine and 6 feline cases from the Armed Forces Institute of Pathology files and divided the data into three categories: small intestine, large intestine, and intestine not otherwise specified. The species distribution of adenocarcinoma in these three categories, respectively, was as follows: for the dog, 16, 88, and 11 cases; cat, 45, 13, and 14; cattle, 18, 3, and 15; sheep, 434, 1, and 3; and equine, 1, 5, and 27. Thus, in this and other surveys, the carcinomas in the dog are found mainly in the large intestine; in cats, cattle, and sheep they are mainly in the small intestine; and in the equine there are no specific sites. Intestinal adenocarcinoma was not reported in pigs until Vitovec (1977) recorded 5 cases in the jejunum and 1 in the cecum.

The base population from which these various affected animals are drawn varies. Thus, in dogs Krook (1956) found 9 adenocarcinomas in the intestine in 7,248 necropsies; Schaffer and Schiefer (1968) reported 10 adenocarcinomas in 7,895 postmortems and 4 in 4,261 biopsies (there was one adenoma in their series); and Gialamas and Schaffraneck (1977) found 2 carcinomas in 1,961 necropsies. Turk *et al.* (1981) gave values for cat intestinal adenocarcinoma of 1.2% of 2,494 biopsy and necropsy accessions in contrast to 0.3% of 9,775 accessions for dogs; they note the similarity to the values of Patnaik *et al.* (1976, 1977) of 0.7% of cat necropsies and 0.33% of dog cases. Vitovec

(1977) gave the proportion of intestinal carcinomas in the total cattle tumor count in Czechoslovakia as 1.6%. They also cited Monlux and Monlux (1972), who reported 0.1% incidence in the United States; Damodaran and Parthasarathy (1973), who reported 1.0% incidence in India; and Misdorp (1967), who reported 5.76% incidence in the Netherlands.

Malignant epithelial tumors are not the only neoplasms encountered in the intestine of the dog. In reports by Brodey and Cohen (1964), Hayden and Nielsen (1973), and Head and Else (1981), 27 adenomas were found (10 in the small intestine and 17 in the large intestine); 58 leiomyomas (22 small intestine and 36 large intestine); 16 leiomyosarcomas (10 small intestine and 6 large intestine); and 139 lymphomas (84 small intestine and 55 large intestine). In the same series of cases, 58 adenocarcinomas were reported (23 small intestine and 35 large intestine).

**Age, Breed, and Sex.** In cattle there is no breed predisposition, tumors usually being found in old animals (11 years old and over) at meat inspection in abattoirs. Under dairy and beef production systems, cows are affected, but where draught oxen are used (e.g. in India), bullocks may also be allowed to live to this old age.

In sheep, Dodd's (1960) cases were in 5-year-old or older Romney ewes and Cordes and Shortridge's (1971) series were all in Romney ewes except for one Lincoln ewe and one Romney wether. The sheep were 2 to 11 years old, but mostly between 5 and 7 years old because most sheep are slaughtered at this age. These authors state that sheep are probably not biologically old until they reach 10 to 15 years of age. In Australia, McDonald and Leaver (1965) saw all their cases in wether Merinos, two of which were 5 years old and three of which were 7 years old. It is rare to maintain castrated male sheep beyond fat lamb slaughter age except in "fine wool" producing breeds, so it is unlikely that sex plays any role in the etiology of the tumor.

Georgsson and Vigfusson (1973) found all their cases in the Icelandic sheep breed, the age ranging from 1 to 12 years old (averaging 7.5 years). They report that the usual culling age is 7 years and that if culling were earlier the incidence of observed neoplasms would drop sharply. The cases reported by Pearson and McCaughey (1978) were in 4-year-old and older grayface ewes. The ones reported by McCrea and Head (1978) were in older ewes of the Scots blackface and Swaledale breeds, and those reported by Norval et al. (1981) were in blackface, border Leicester, and half-bred sheep. Most of the cases were in breeds that were dominant in the districts being investigated. Simpson and Jolly (1974) in their survey material compared the prevalence in British breeds (mainly Romneys) as 0.9 to 1.5% with the prevalence in fine wool breeds (Merinos, Merino crosses, and Corriedales) of 0.2 to 0.4%. This observation was confirmed by Ross (1980) who compared fine wool sheep with fine wool cross British breed (border Leicester).

Vitovec's (1977) porcine cases were all in mature or old sows; the exact ages and breeds were not given.

The average age for intestinal carcinoma in dogs is 8 to 9 years (ranging from 4 to 15 years). No sex or breed bias is obvious in most series, but 10 cases reported by Head and Else (1981) were all in males. Canine recto-anal carcinoma has a similar average age range of 8 to 10 years. In Hayden and Nielsen's (1973) series, 2 of 5 recto-anal carcinomas were in German shepherd dogs; 15 of the 34 cases in the literature are in this breed. The male to female ratio in different series is variable. Hayden and Nielsen's (1973) literature survey showed a male to female ratio of 24:9, and in our series the ratio was 5:1. Hayden and Nielsen's own series of tumors, however, had a male to female ratio of 2:3.

Canine colorectal polyps show some interesting age distribution differences from the carcinomas. Although Hayden and Nielsen's (1973) ages for the polyps and carcinomas were similar, the 17 cases of Seiler (1979) had an average age for polyps of 6.7 years (ranging from 1.5 to 12 years). Ours also had a lower mean age for colorectal polyps than for carcinomas. The male:female sex ratios for canine colorectal polyps is as follows: 7:9 (Seiler, 1979), 4:3 (Hayden and Nielsen, 1973), and 2:4 (Head and Else, 1981). No obvious breed predisposition is recorded.

Although these data suggest a difference in age, breed, and sex distribution between benign and malignant tumors at different sites, none of these authors related their data to a base population. Patnaik et al. (1977) used the necropsy population as a baseline and grouped data from all sites. They were able to show that collies and German shepherds were predisposed to all intestinal tumors and to adeno-carcinoma in particular, but no significant pre-disposition to other tumors could be demonstrated. Analysis of the sex distribution by different authors revealed no significant predisposition, but ade-nocarcinomas were more frequent in males and leiomyosarcomas were more frequent in females.

Turk *et al.* (1981) described 42 feline adenocarcinoma cases of their own and added 46 cases from the literature. This series had an average age of 10.6 years (ranging from 2 to 17 years) and a breed pre-disposition to Siamese. Although the literature sug-gested males were affected more often than females by about 3 : 1, the data of Turk and co-workers did not confirm this. This sex bias is not related to the site of tumor as in dogs because rectal carcinoma is rare in cats, none being recorded in Turk *et al.*'s (1981) series and only 2 in the 46 literature cases. Our series confirmed the sex bias for intes-tinal carcinoma (4 male, 7 neutered male, and 2 neutered female) and added a case of rectal carci-noma in a 14-year-old neutered female cat. In view of the rarity of rectal carcinoma, it is interesting that Lingeman and Garner (1972) reclassified as a hyperplastic polyp the 3-cm pedunculated colonic mass removed 7 cm from the anus of a 13-year-old neutered female cat; this lesion had been described as an adenomatous polyp.

**Sites.** Tontis *et al.* (1976) reviewed the literature of cattle intestinal carcinoma; only 17 of the 31 cases had recorded sites, namely, 7 duodenal, 3 je-junal, 3 ileal, 1 ileocecal valve, 2 colonic, and 1 rec-tal. This agrees with Vitovec's (1977) findings of 3 neoplasms in the proximal third of the jejunum, 2 in the middle third jejunum, and 1 in the duo-denum. In contrast, his 6 cases in sows were dis-tributed in the middle or distal third of the jejunum in 5 cases and in the body of the cecum in 1 case.

In sheep most cases occur in the small intestine, mainly jejunal, but a few are reported in the spiral colon, for example, 5 of 450 described by Simpson and Jolly (1974). Most series record none in the duodenum, but Cordes and Shortridge (1971) found 7 of 60 at that site. One of the cases de-scribed by Pearson and McCaughey (1978) had a tumor in the duodenum and another in the middle jejunum.

The site distribution in ruminants is roughly similar to that in cats; for example, Turk *et al.* (1981) found 2 duodenal, 11 jejunal, 6 ileal, and 8 ileocecal tumors at the colic junction and 6 tumors in the colon. As these authors point out, it is some-times difficult to decide whether the tumor should be assigned to ileal or ileocecalcolic sites. All the literature is in agreement that duodenal and rectal tumors are rare, with the most common sites for feline intestinal carcinomas being the ileocecalcolic junction, the ileum, and the jejunum (Patnaik *et al.*, 1981). Patnaik *et al.* (1976) subdivided 20 intestinal adenocarcinomas at each site into four subclasses, namely adenocarcinoma with solid cell groups (car-cinoid), adenocarcinoma with solid acinar cells, pa-pillar adenocarcinoma, and mucinous adenocar-cinoma. The various sites for these subclasses were 2 in the duodenum, 1 in the jejunum, 12 in the ileum, 1 multiple case in the duodenum and je-junum, 1 in the cecocolon, 2 in the colon, and 1 in the rectum. All of these multiple tumors were pa-pillary adenocarcinomas. In contrast, most series of carcinomas in dogs have a similar site distribution to that found by Krook (1956), namely, 1 in the duodenum, 9 in the jejunum, 1 in the ileum, 1 in the colon, and 6 in the rectum. As in the other spe-cies, adenoma is less common than adenocarcinoma so that accurate distribution figures are not avail-able, but the site distribution pattern resembles that of carcinoma given above. More cases of adenoma have been recorded in the rectum of dogs than in any other species. Seiler (1979) stated that colorec-tal polyps, although sometimes found in the colon, are usually in the rectum at or close to the anorectal junction. Patnaik *et al.* (1980*a*) subdivided 31 in-testinal adenocarcinoma cases at each site into five subclasses, namely, acinar, solid, papillary, signet ring cell, and mucinous. The number of carcinomas (all subclasses) and their site distribution were as follows: 7 in the duodenum, 4 in the jejunum, 1 in the ileum, 9 in the colon, and 10 in the rectum.

**Gross Morphology.** Most cases are found be-cause they have produced clinical signs and the lesion is therefore in an advanced state of develop-ment. Early lesions are only encountered in experi-mental situations or in geographical areas where carcinomas are frequent and therefore routine nec-ropsies are likely to reveal asymptomatic tumors (e.g., sheep in Australia or cattle in western Scotland).

Carcinomas are usually solitary in all species. Head and Else (1981), for example, found 2 of 10 carcinomas in the canine small intestine and 1 of 6 in the canine large intestine. All of these were multiple neoplasms. None of 14 carcinomas in the feline intestine were multiple. Jarrett (1980), dealing with high prevalence alimentary carcinomas of cattle in Scotland, found that both benign and malignant intestinal tumors were multiple. These tumors were of several morphologies within the intestine and ranged from multiple (over 50) adenomatous polyps, to sessile plaques of hyperchromatic epithelium, to more markedly proliferative lesions that were especially prevalent in the duodenum and related to the ampula of the bile ducts. In sheep, Simpson and Jolly (1974) found that 6 of 50 consecutive cases had 2 to 4 separate primary tumors and the remainder had single primary tumors in their sheep cases, but pointed out that secondary tumors proximal to the primary tumors could mimic a primary tumor macroscopically. They showed, histologically, that these neoplasms were spreading inward toward the mucosa from the serosa. The colorectal polyps of old dogs are often multiple but seldom exceed 10 in number.

The appearance of carcinoma varies with the extent of its field of origin, its pattern of growth (particularly the method of invasive spread), and the type of tumor, since some tumor cells seem to stimulate the formation of collagenous fibrous stroma. These factors result in tumors that are either intramural or intraluminal and focal or annular as illustrated by Head and Else (1981). Focal intramural benign tumors are seen as nodular leiomyoma; nodular adenoma is rare. Nodular intraluminal benign tumors are the well recognized pedunculate or sessile adenomatous polyps. The other form of focal tumor is plaquelike and intramural. Polypoid adenomas are much more frequent than the plaque form in dogs by a ratio of 6:1.

Malignant focal carcinomas have less defined borders because of their invasive growth pattern, but they can usually be designated as either nodular or plaquelike, the latter often showing a depressed ulcerated mucosal surface. The nodular malignant epithelial tumors tend to grow into the lumen. Thus, a long-standing tumor will eventually come to resemble an intraluminal focal tumor that originated from a polypoid primary tumor in which malignant cells had grown invasively into the submucosa and muscle coats. If the intraluminal mass grows progressively to occlude the lumen, then the intestine above dilates and the muscle coat becomes hypertrophied.

Benign tumors growing in a ring encircling the intestine do not seem to occur. The annular carcinoma may constrict the lumen (annular stenosing) or not alter the lumen diameter (annular fusiform). Most annular stenosing carcinomas are scirrhous in nature possibly because the cells induce fibrosis and they invade along lymphatics, which leads to retention of lymph and fibroplasia. If the tumor is not scirrhous (i.e., medullary carcinoma, lymphoma, or leiomyosarcoma), then infiltration of tumor cells into tissue spaces around the fibers of the muscle coat leads to muscle atrophy. Such tumorous segments of the small intestine tend to balloon outward and may even perforate. The annular stenosing carcinoma in dogs, cats, and sheep is usually 1 to 2 cm long, but in cattle it may be 5 cm long. The mucosal surface is usually smooth, but Vitovec (1977) described his cases in the jejunum of cattle and pigs as having broadly sessile, polypoid, or cauliflowerlike growths into the lumen. The wall at the tumor site is replaced by firm, white, fibrous tissue, but the wall may not be much thickened (only as thick as 0.5 cm). Because of the lymphatic permeation, the white fibrous tumor tissue extends over the mesentery to the drainage lymph nodes. The progressive stenosis results in dilatation of the intestine and often hypertrophy of the muscle coat above the site of the tumor, although Patnaik et al. (1976) mentioned poststenotic dilatation in cats. The annular fusiform carcinoma may be as much as 10 to 15 cm long, and on cut surface the normal structure of the wall is replaced by soft, homogeneous tissue of varying thickness, even as thick as 8 cm in cattle. Sometimes the annular lesion thickens the intestinal wall over a considerable length in an almost parallel-sided fashion. Such lesions may be called diffuse. The adenocarcinomas in dogs and cats are mainly annular stenosing in the small intestine but plaquelike in the rectum.

In canine cases studied by Patnaik et al. (1980a), most solid and mucinous adenocarcinomas were annular, whereas 5 of 13 with an acinar pattern were intraluminal as were all the papillary tumors. Irrespective of the site and whether the tumors were annular or intraluminal, the average length of bowel involved was 2 to 5 cm for acinar carcinoma, 3 to 5 cm for mucinous carcinoma, and 3.5 to 5 cm for solid carcinoma. The papillary adenocarcinoma in the duodenum involved two segments 25 and 95 cm in length and in the colon a segment 10.3 cm in length; thus, it could be called diffuse annular in pattern in contrast to the carcinomas in the rectum which were only 0.5 to 1 cm long. In cats these tumors (Patnaik *et al.*, 1976) were all intramural and mainly stenosing except for a rectal tumor consisting of ulcerated, polypoid, intraluminal growths anterior to the constricted area.

Adenomas may be plaquelike sessile masses or pedunculate polyps with broad or narrow stalks. Whether all carcinomas arise in preexisting adenomas is not known. It is thus important in lesions that are clearly malignant to carefully examine the luminal aspect of the tumor and the adjacent "normal" mucosa for evidence of benign tumor formation. If the hypothetical preexisting adenoma was sessile, then such evidence is difficult or impossible to obtain, but pedunculate lesions may still be present. Simpson and Jolly (1974) have pointed out that polyps may be formed by a late outgrowth of adenocarcinoma; this can be recognized because the muscularis mucosae is carried up into the polyp.

**Histological Features.** There are no special problems in the recognition of most histological patterns of intestinal tumors except the scirrhous form of annular stenosing adenocarcinoma. Such tumors may not be recognized macroscopically because the serosal deposits are much more dramatic than the narrow ring of the primary tumor at the end of the distorted dilated segment of intestine. Histological examination of the serosal deposits will show mainly collagenous fibrous tissue in which the isolated tumor cells may be mistaken for inflammatory cells or the occasional small acini may not be present in the section examined. Sections stained for mucin may help to identify these epithelial tumor cells. Vitovec (1977) suggested that meat inspectors in abattoirs may not recognize the small lesions in the intestine and merely submit the liver or lung metastatic lesions to the histopathologist, who might then suspect a primary bile duct or uterine endometrial carcinoma.

Turk *et al.* (1981) found osseous metaplasia in one-third or less of each of the tubular, mucinous,

and undifferentiated carcinomas they reported in cats; one tubular adenocarcinoma exhibited chondroid metaplasia. Similarly, bone spicules have been reported in scirrhous adenocarcinomas in 3 of 200 tumors in sheep (Simpson and Jolly, 1974). Cotchin (1977) likewise cited references to bony metaplasia in the stroma of adenocarcinomas of the small and large intestines of horses. Patnaik *et al.* (1976), in addition to finding two cases of adenocarcinoma with osseous metaplasia, found another case in the duodenum with squamous metaplasia in some acini.

Recognition of the development of carcinoma *in situ* and other early patterns of tumor growth was discussed above under gastric carcinoma. Benign epithelial tumors must be examined carefully for these stigmata of malignancy. In Seiler's (1979) series, 5 of 17 canine colorectal polyps exhibited cellular atypia of a degree to suggest carcinoma *in situ*. One should be on guard against misinterpreting pseudocarcinomatous invasion associated with twisting of the stalk of polypoid adenoma or with fibrosis interfering with the blood and lymph drainage. Venous congestion may result in hemorrhage into the glands, and if the epithelial lining of the gland desquamates into the lumen, it may mimic a plug in a blood vessel. Hubmann (1982) reported that submucosal radiation fibrosis in the rectum of rats leads to lymph cysts developing and that this allows fragmentation of the muscularis mucosae and thus the appearance of mucosal epithelium in the submucosa. A similar appearance is seen in edematous adenomas and possibly in porcine intestinal adenomatosis.

Patnaik *et al.* (1980a) examined the mucosa adjacent to the primary tumor in the small intestine and observed hyperplasia with branching crypts and an increase in goblet cells; thus there was a resemblance to rectal mucosa. In addition, fused crypt glands with cells resembling tumor cells were observed in the basilar areas of the villi and were interpreted as early tumor formation. Similar but less marked hyperplasia and branching of irregular crypts were seen in the large intestine, but no transition to neoplasia was seen. As Patnaik and co-workers indicate, in such examinations one must take care not to confuse direct extension of the tumor along lacteals and into the villi of adjacent mucosa with true multicentric tumor formation.

It is well recognized that at sites of lymphoid

tissue in the intestine, particularly in the colon, the muscularis mucosae becomes discontinuous and non-neoplastic glands may extend into this lymphoid tissue in postinflammatory reactive states. The observation by Patnaik *et al.* (1980*a*) is therefore of interest in that acinar adenocarcinomas of the colon of dogs, unlike those of the duodenum, are often craterlike and associated with the lymphoid tissue of the region.

Tumors may change their histological pattern as they extend into different tissues. This is clearly shown in adenocarcinoma of the sheep. In the mucosa the tumor is formed by closely packed acini of absorptive cells or mucus-secreting goblet cells. In the latter the acinar lumens are often difficult to see in hematoxylin- and eosin-stained sections. The stroma is minimal, but in the submucosa there is more fibrous tissue. The tumor on the serosa and the peritoneum, however, may have as little as 1% of carcinoma tissue set in collagenous fibrous tissue; the acini here are smaller in size, less mucus is produced, and there are isolated epithelial cells some of which are signet ring cells. The primary mucosal neoplasm is tubular adenocarcinoma in form, thus this is the proper diagnostic term for the whole tumor.

Simpson and Jolly (1974) found that the earliest lesions in sheep were nodules or plaques 0.3 to 0.5 cm in diameter, but that in 20% of established annular stenosing carcinomas, there were one to seven polyps protruding into the lumen. They interpreted these polyps as extensions of tumor growth from the mucosa into the submucosa, which then bulged into the lumen; the overlying mucosa became eroded, leaving a polypoid growth. The muscularis mucosae approaches the lumen surface near the polyp base and the mucosa is lost at this point and over the polyp surface. Cordes and Shortridge (1971) thought that at least some of their tumors arose in polyps.

Electron microscopy indicates that carcinoma in sheep arises from undifferentiated cells of the crypts of Lieberkühn that have undergone neoplastic transformation and then differentiation into absorptive epithelial cells or intestinal goblet cells (Ross and Day, 1979*a;* Simpson and Jolly, 1974). Georgsson and Vigfusson (1973) reached a similar conclusion regarding special differentiation of tumor cells; using light microscopy, they showed a few scattered interchromatin cells in the primary and secondary tumors with Masson–Fontana staining.

**Clinical Considerations.** Carcinomas of the intestine produce their signs by causing progressive, slowly developing obstruction. An animal may be reported to have had signs of obstruction from several days to 9 months or longer on first presentation. By the time the tumor has produced clinical signs, it is usually palpable in the abdomen or per rectum. At first there is evidence of malabsorption with weight loss and vague gastrointestinal tract dysfunction. If the lesion is of a stenosing type in carnivores, vomiting may begin to dominate the clinical picture as the obstruction progresses, depending on the site of the tumor within the intestinal tract. Diarrhea may be seen with some stenosing lesions in the distal tract and with diffuse lesions at any level. Some tumors ulcerate and show hemorrhage; if this is capillary hemorrhage in the upper colon or above, then melena may be suspected because of black feces. If the major vessel is eroded in the lower colorectum or higher in the tract, then fresh red blood will be seen per rectum. Hemorrhage may occur with benign or malignant tumors.

Sudden perforation of the intestine with subsequent peritonitis can be seen either because of a penetrating ulceration of a ballooning fusiform carcinoma or pressure necrosis of tumor on the opposing nonneoplastic wall. Geib and Abrevayn (1965) described such a case in an 8-year-old female mongrel dog in which a 3-cm polypoid tubular adenoma on the mesenteric surface of the duodenum opposed a $1 \times 1.5$ cm ulcer near the openings of the pancreatic and bile ducts. Progressive development of ascites with abdominal swelling may be caused by transcelomic metastasis which can block lymphatic drainage from the abdominal cavity via the diaphragm and flanks. This is common in sheep and is recorded in 3 of 10 dogs and 7 of 13 cats (Head and Else, 1981).

Tumors of the colorectum, as well as giving rise to fresh blood at the anus following defecation, are usually associated with tenesmus, excessive mucus production from the anus, and either diarrhea or constipation (depending on whether defecation is painful and whether the diet results in hard or soft feces). Polypoid tumors near the anorectal junction may prolapse through the anal ring and repeated straining may lead to rectal prolapse. Intestinal tu-

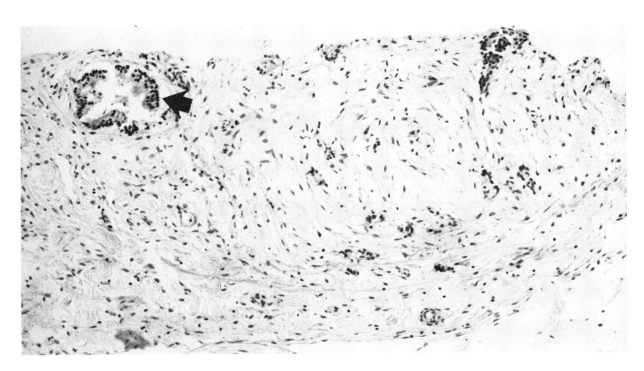

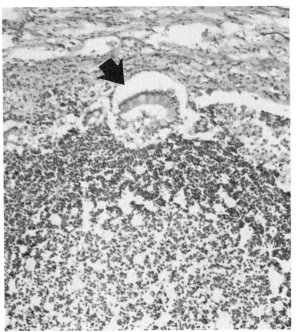

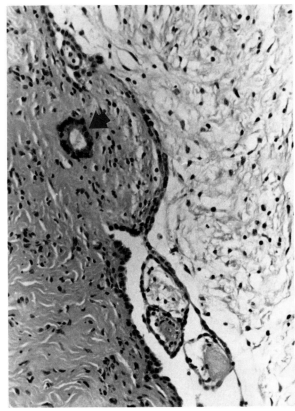

mass (fig. 8.19B). The serosal involvement proximal to the annular tumor is probably the result of retrograde lymphatic flow. Similar coalescing fibrosed plaques on the anteroventral flank peritoneum (fig. 8.19C) and diaphragm may be mistaken at meat inspection for chronic peritonitis. Further transcelomic spread through the diaphragm to the parietal pleura and even to the lung pleura may be seen, and lymphatic spread to the posterior mediastinal lymph node is common (fig. 8.19D). These plaquelike peritoneal and pleural deposits are accompanied by an accumulation of free fluid in which tumor cells, sometimes showing attempts at acinar formation (fig. 8.19E), may be demonstrated in centrifuge deposit. The ascites fluid may measure as much as 4 to 16 liters in advanced cases in sheep, and the pendulous abdomens of these animals simulate pregnancy. Pearson and Cawthorne (1978) recorded two ewes with extension of the tumor from the peritoneum to the ovaries and oviducts. They suggest that instead of the usual gravitational deposition in the anteroventral abdomen, the genitalia become involved with altered position of the gravid uterus when a tumor-bearing ewe becomes pregnant.

Vitovec (1977) mentioned nodular lesions in lymphatics of the mesentery with jejunal carcinomas in cattle and pigs, but he observed no peritoneal metastasis. Despite this, he described three cases in cattle with metastasis to the bronchomediastinal lymph nodes and one to the paraaortic lymph nodes. The lymph nodes in these cattle were yellow on cut surface with areas of necrosis; this contrasts with the white color and the absence of necrosis in sheep lymph nodes with metastasis.

## Tumors of the Diffuse Endocrine System

**General Considerations.** In humans carcinoid tumors are differentiated from carcinoma of the intestinal tract because although they have some of the histological features of epithelial tumors, they would not fit into the classification outlined in the previous section. It came to be realized that these tumors were derived from the enterochromaffin (Kultschitsky) cells of the intestinal mucosa.

Chromaffin cells were thus named because they had cytoplasmic granules that could be visualized after formalin–dichromate fixation because they contained substances with an affinity for chrome salts. Enterochromaffin cells were more easily demonstrated using silver stains. It was then discovered that the granules contained 5-hydroxytryptamine (serotonin or enteramine) and that this amine combined with aldehydes or certain acids to produce compounds with fluorescent and reducing properties. The ability to reduce silver salts to metallic silver (the argentaffin reaction) and the reaction of such reducing substances in Schmorl's ferric ferricyanide technique were more widely used to investigate these cells than the formalin-induced fluorescence. This research showed that some cells had an affinity for silver salts, but did not have reducing substances to effect the argentaffin reaction; metallic silver could, however, be formed if an externally added reducing agent was used. This argyrophil technique revealed granules containing the 5-hydroxytryptamine (5-HT) precursor, 5-hydroxytrytophan. It must be noted that some argyrophil techniques such as that of Grimelius are more successful after Bouin's fluid than after formalin fixation. Another stain that can be used for demonstrating 5-HT is the azo-coupling (alkaline diazonium) technique; this stain has the advantage that gluteraldehyde as well as formaldehyde can be used as a fixative, but there is a disadvantage in that the method seldom gives good results on postmortem material.

Classification of intestinal endocrine cells on the basis of their reaction to argentaffin, argyrophil, and diazonium staining techniques has been superseded by the results of the investigation of these cells using electron microscopy, spectrofluorimetry, and immunocytochemistry. Such studies along with biochemical investigations have revealed that there are many related endocrine cells in the gastrointestinal tract exhibiting neurosecretory granules in their cytoplasm, in addition to those producing 5-HT. This led to the concept of a diffuse endocrine system distributed as scattered cells in the gastrointestinal tract and other endodermally derived organs. It seems probable that each cell type synthesizes and stores a single hormone, with the secretion from these cells being short chain polypeptides and/or biologically active amines. Using pure hormone as antigen to prepare antibody, one can by immunofluorescence or immunoperoxidase techniques identify the cells manufacturing these hormones. Thus, Dawson (1982) identified entero-glucagon, somatostatin, and 5-HT in the stomach cells producing gastrin. In the small intestine, in addition to enterochromaffin cells producing 5-HT, there are cells in which enteroglucagon, secretin, somatostatin, motilin, and gastrin inhibitory polypeptide can be identified. The cells in the gastrointestinal tract and elsewhere with these neurosecretory granules in their cytoplasm have been designated as the amine precursor uptake and decarboxylation (APUD) system. Although this is a convenient name for this group of endocrine cells, it is viewed by some workers with disfavor because not all of these cells can decarboxylate an amine precursor. Such workers prefer to speak of "the diffuse endocrine system."

Although some of the research identifying the cells of the diffuse endocrine system in the gastrointestinal tract was performed in small domestic animals, the application of this work to carcinoids of veterinary interest is in its infancy. It is obvious that a tumor with the histological pattern of a carcinoid should be screened for the presence of granules by more than one technique. Appropriate fixation is the key to success in most methods. Biopsy material is better than postmortem tissue since the former can be fixed more rapidly, thus reducing the loss of active chemicals that tend to diffuse out of the cell. For example, 5-HT is completely lost within 5 to 6 hours of death of the animal, whereas 5-HT precursor remains argyrophilic for as long as the cell structure persists. If a tumor of the diffuse endocrine system is suspected on clinical grounds, then arrangements can be made to carry out a full investigation of the exact tumor type. In most veterinary diagnostic situations, however, a "carcinoid" is only diagnosed on examination of formalin-fixed, paraffin-embedded, hematoxylin- and eosin-stained material. Confirmation should then be attempted both by histochemical stains and by reprocessing the formalin-fixed tissue for electron microscopic studies since some granules may still be detectable. However, subclassification based on size, shape, and structure of the granules cannot be expected from such material. Ideally, small blocks should be fixed and processed for electron microscopy immediately after biopsy or death of the animal as a routine procedure in all gastrointestinal tumor cases.

**Classification.** Willis (1948) preferred the term *argentaffin carcinoma* to carcinoid since this group of tumors is not entirely of benign type; many of the tumors show invasive growth and eventually undergo metastasis. It seems probable that each cell type in the diffuse endocrine system can give rise to a specific tumor. Dawson (1976) suggests that when a single clear function can be attributed to a tumor, one should use the appropriate term. *Gastrinoma,* for example, would be appropriate for a nonargentaffin carcinoid of the duodenum associated with the Zollinger–Ellison syndrome. Records of human tumor sites, histological pattern, ultrastructure, immunolocalization, amine histochemistry, clinicopathological behavior, and biochemical investigation have not been correlated in a sufficient number of cases to allow a detailed classification to be established. Williams *et al.* (1980) divided tumors of the diffuse endocrine system in humans into carcinoid, mucocarcinoid, and mixed carcinoid–adenocarcinoma. Carcinoids are further subdivided into enterochromaffin cell carcinoid (the classic carcinoid, which is strongly argentaffin and argyrophil), G-cell tumor (a carcinoid or gastrinoma that is nonargentaffin and weakly argyrophil), and other carcinoids (those whose relationships to specific cell types in the diffuse endocrine system are not yet clearly established). The mucocarcinoids resemble well-differentiated adenocarcinomas, with differentiation to both mucus-secreting epithelium and to endocrine cells. It must be noted that occasional endocrine cells may be found in many adenocarcinomas, so for a diagnosis of mucocarcinoid the number of granulated cells must exceed some arbitrary level set by the pathologist. The mixed carcinoid–adenocarcinoma differs histologically from the mucocarcinoid in that some areas are carcinoid and others are adenocarcinoma.

**Incidence.** Single cases of these neoplasms have been recorded in the ox, dog, and cat. Only Patnaik *et al.* (1980*a*) have attempted a frequency distribution; they found 4 in 64 dog intestinal tumors from 10,270 necropsies in 1977 and 2 in 22 cat intestinal tumors from 3,145 necropsies in 1976. It would seem that tumors with the classic enterochromaffin cell carcinoid histology are rare in domestic animals; and it is likely that mucocarcinoid and mixed carcinoid–adenocarcinoma exist, but they have rarely been diagnosed.

**Age, Breed, and Sex.** In the dog, tumors have been reported in both sexes (five female, one male), several breeds, and over an age range of 9 to 12 years. The cats with recorded ages were 9 and 13 years of age, respectively, and both were castrated males. Isaksson's (1946) case was in a cow said to be in good health at the time of slaughter.

**Clinical Characteristics.** Williams *et al.* (1980) developed a functional classification for these tumors in addition to devising a morphological classification. Some tumors produce a recognizable clinical syndrome, while in others there is no demonstrable functional disturbance. For several reasons there is not necessarily a correlation between this function and the histological differentiation. The cells may be storing but not releasing hormone, releasing or not storing hormone, or producing only inactive precursors or fragments of hormone. Moreover, some tumors appear to consist of more than one cell type and hence produce more than one hormone. The granule content is therefore not directly related to the functional state. Likewise, the size of the tumor is not proportional to the clinical signs produced; a small active tumor may release the level of hormone needed to produce a clinical syndrome that is only achieved by a relatively inactive tumor when it has increased its bulk by metastasis. The functional disturbance can be due to hypofunction, hyperfunction, or ectopic hormone production. In humans enterochromaffin cell carcinoids release vasoactive amines resulting in the carcinoid syndrome, namely, diarrhea, flushing or cyanosis of the skin, bronchoconstriction, hypertension, pulmonary valvular stenosis, and right heart failure. The other clear-cut clinical state is the Zollinger–Ellison syndrome associated with the G-cell tumor in which there is severe gastric hypersecretion and peptic ulceration. Other less well defined signs such as watery diarrhea are sometimes recorded.

These clinical syndromes have not been reported in animals. Diarrhea and weight loss are common but are also seen in noncarcinoid tumors of the intestine. Likewise, the normocytic, normochromic regenerative anemia reported by Giles *et al.* (1974a) was probably related to an ileal ulcer of the dog in which the carcinoid involved cecum and, to a less extent, ileum. The 5-month history of episodic intestinal hemorrhage reported in the cecal carcinoid

of Sykes and Cooper (1982) may have been related to the partial denudation of the cecal mucosa.

**Sites.** Isaksson (1946) reported a case of multiple tumors in the jejunum of the ox. In the dog, Patnaik *et al.* (1977) had two cases in the duodenum and two in the colon. The case described by Giles *et al.* (1974a) involved the ileocecal junction, that of Patnaik and Lieberman (1981) was in the rectum 4 cm from the anus, and that of Christie and Jabara (1964) was at the anorectal junction. Two of Sykes and Cooper's (1982) cases were removed as pedunculate small (1-cm) nodules protruding from the anus, and the third dog had a 5-cm mass at the cecocolic junction, mainly involving the cecum. Another case reported by Giles *et al.* (1974b) was located in the tongue of the dog. In the cat the ileum was the site for the case of Lahellec and Jancourt (1972) and both cases of Patnaik *et al.* (1976), but Carakostas *et al.* (1979) described thickening of the duodenum and a pancreatic mass $2.5 \times 7$ cm.

**Gross Morphology.** In humans some tumors on cut surface have a yellow to orange color and others are gray but may turn yellow on formalin fixation. This feature has not been reported in animals. The shape of the tumor in the intestine is not diagnostic, ranging from an annular stenosing thickening 3 cm in diameter (Lahellec and Jancourt, 1972), to a nodular mass $3 \times 4$ cm in size with extensions along dilated blood vessels in the serosa of the ileum (Giles *et al.*, 1974a), to a diffuse annular thickening 3.5 to 15 cm long (Patnaik *et al.*, 1980a). In the rectum the tumors appear as nodular, intraluminal, fungating masses measuring 4 to 9.5 cm in greatest width (Christie and Jabara, 1964; Patnaik and Lieberman, 1981). All of these patterns are seen in the other intestinal tumor types.

**Histological Features.** Dawson (1976) summarized the literature to show three basic patterns of these neoplasms in the human. The first pattern involves solid islands of uniform cells with eosinophilic granular cytoplasm and poorly defined cell boundaries. There is palisading of the peripheral rim of cells as in solid basal cell tumors of the skin, but in these cells the nuclei lie toward the center of the island and the granular cytoplasm is peripheral. These peripheral cells often show more distinct granularity with special stains than with the central cells. The fibrous stroma varies in amount, and sometimes the stroma is dominant and the tumor cells form cords or trabeculae up to five cells wide. The second pattern is ribbonlike anastomosing loops one or two cells wide set in a vascular stroma, superficially resembling the Garland form of basal cell carcinoma of the skin. Finally, a third pattern involves irregular masses and broad trabeculae of tumor cells that appear on low power examination to have acini scattered throughout. At high magnification the masses show periodic acid–Schiff (PAS) positive material in the "acini" that might better be called rosettes.

In the latter two patterns, the argyrophil, argentaffin, and diazo positive cells are scattered in an irregular manner through the tumor and are not mainly peripheral in the cell masses as in the first pattern. Undifferentiated anaplastic tumors may be found in which only small areas show one of these three recognizable patterns. Sometimes a single tumor may have a mosaic of lobules each with a different pattern, and (as previously mentioned) the mixed carcinoid–adenocarcinoma tumors have areas of carcinoid in any one of these patterns mixed with areas of adenocarcinoma. If the tumor is well differentiated in the mucocarcinoid, the mucus droplets tend to be above the nucleus near the tubular lumens and the granular differentiated cytoplasm is located below the nucleus toward the periphery of the tubule.

The carcinoids described in animals were mainly of the first pattern (islands of uniform cells), but some with areas of the latter two patterns have been mentioned. Patnaik and Lieberman's (1981) case was of the mixed carcinoid–adenocarcinoma type. Sykes and Cooper (1982) demonstrated amyloid especially around arterioles of the rectoanal carcinoid but not in the cecal tumor. They suggested that this amyloid protein may be from polypeptides of prohormones in the tumor rather than from immunoglobulins. These three tumors were also unusual because some multinucleate cells were present in addition to uniform round cells.

Giles *et al.* (1974a) demonstrated both argyrophil and argentaffin granules; Carakostas *et al.* (1979) and Patnaik and Lieberman (1981) demonstrated positive argyrophil staining with a modified Grimelius stain. Lahellec and Jancourt (1972) used Fontana ammoniacal silver nitrate, and Isaksson's (1946) case was strongly argyrophilic with Foot's silver stain. Although the normal small intestine was positive with the diazonium method, Christie and Jabara (1964) could not show a positive reaction in the tumor. Several of these authors eliminated the possibility of the tumor being of mast cell origin by using toluidine blue, PAS, and Giemsa staining. Carakostas *et al.* (1979) and Giles *et al.* (1974a) used electron microscopy to reveal cytoplasmic granules in the tumor cells. In the three cases described by Sykes and Cooper (1982), all were nonargentaffin, only one was argyrophil with one of the two argyrophil stains used, none showed formaldehyde induced fluorescence, but all showed membrane-bound granules by electron microscopy. The tumor cells did not contain metachromatic granules with appropriate stains, but a few mast cells were scattered through the tumor. Unlike mast cell tumors, no eosinophils were found in these carcinoids. Sykes and Cooper (1982) pointed out that neoplastic mast cells can be differentiated from carcinoid tumor cells by electron microscopy since the membrane bound granules are uniformly large and of various densities in contrast to the pleomorphic, small, uniformly dense carcinoid tumor granules.

**Growth and Metastasis.** Cell morphology in humans cannot be used as a guide to clinical behavior of these tumors since well-differentiated tumors with few mitoses can give rise to metastasis. The site of the primary neoplasm can be a partial guide since carcinoids of the stomach and small intestine are more often invasive than carcinoids of the cecum and colon. The tumors seem to arise deep in the mucosa and invade the submucosa, producing a larger mass here than in the mucosa, which often remains intact over large tumors. Extensive growth, both on a broad front and within the lumens of vessels, occurs into the intestinal muscle coat and serosa. Eventually, invasion of the overlying mucosa may lead to ulceration. Most of the veterinary examples of these neoplasms have moderately numerous mitoses and have metastasized in a manner similar to an adenocarcinoma, except in one respect: the liver when involved shows numerous plugs of tumor cells in portal veins, visible on histological examination but not visible to the naked eye. In the cat metastasis was from ileum to the drainage lymph nodes (Lahellec and Jancourt, 1972) and to the mesentery and omentum (Patnaik *et al.*, 1976) and from the duodenum and pancreas to the pleura and lung (Carakostas *et al.*, 1979). In the dog Giles *et al.*'s (1974*a*) case spread to the liver as did all of Patnaik *et al.*'s (1980*a*) cases, which also showed metastasis to the local lymph nodes, pancreas, and lung. The rectal tumor of Christie and Jabara (1964) showed a 10 × 6.5 cm metastasis to the mesentery of the colon, while that of Patnaik and Lieberman (1981) was remarkable in that metastatic nodules were present in the lung, liver, rib, heart, kidney, and adrenals, as well as the sublumbar, hepatopancreatic, and bronchial lymph nodes. The cells in one of the rectoanal tumors described by Sykes and Cooper (1982) had numerous mitotic figures; the other had few mitotic figures; both were invasive but neither had recurred 2 years after removal. The cecal carcinoid showed emboli in blood vessels, but no metastasis was described.

## Tumors of Soft (Mesenchymal) Tissue

### Tumors of Muscle Tissue

**Classification.** Recognition of smooth muscle tumors of the intestines by light microscopy is not necessarily easy because most trichrome stains give variable results and because the visualization of blunt-ended nuclei versus spindle-shaped fibrous tissue nuclei is not always easy. Also, the mere fact that the tumor lies in the muscle coat is not proof that it is of muscle origin. Furthermore, leiomyoma may mimic neurilemmoma (Schwannoma) by showing nuclear regimentation or palisading (i.e., the arrangement of nuclei into parallel bands). Some connective tissue will be found supporting the tumor. This fibrous tissue may be the dominant cell type in some regions; Christie and Jabara (1964) mentioned mucin associated with such an area of fibroblasts in a leiomyosarcoma of the ileum. Differentiating benign from malignant tumors may even present problems, although diagnosis of leiomyosarcoma is easy if invasive growth and metastasis are present. It is difficult to judge how many mitoses and nuclei are present in relation to cytoplasm in a well-differentiated leiomyosarcoma compared with a leiomyoma. Diagnosis of a highly malignant leiomyosarcoma may call for a detailed search among the pleomorphic cells and mul-

tinucleate giant cells to find an area that betrays its smooth muscle origin.

**Incidence.** Saidu and Chineme (1979) described a leiomyoma 20 cm in diameter in the spiral colon of a 10-year-old white Fulani cow. Along with this study they reviewed the scattered bovine cases in the literature. Most surveys of intestinal tumors in small animals mention a few examples of these tumors, possibly more in dogs than cats. Hayden and Nielsen (1973) found seven leiomyomas in 15,215 canine necropsies. In contrast, Turk *et al.* (1981) reported one leiomyosarcoma in 2,494 feline accessions.

**Age, Breed, and Sex.** In the dog benign and malignant tumors have a similar distribution with no obvious breed or sex predisposition and an age range of 6 to 16 years (mean 10 to 11 years). Similar statements can be made for the far fewer recorded tumors in cats, but the cats were older (12 to 17 years of age).

**Sites.** An interesting variation is present in the larger series of these neoplasms in the literature. All the dog cases of Hayden and Nielsen (1973) were benign; 1 was located in the small intestine, 1 in the cecum, and 5 in the rectoanal region. All 19 dog cases of Patnaik *et al.* (1977) were leiomyosarcomas with a site distribution of 3 in the duodenum, 6 in the jejunum, 1 in the ileum, 4 in the cecum, 3 in the colon, and 2 in the small intestine (specific site not mentioned). The series reported by Head and Else (1981) in 8 dogs had a distribution for leiomyoma of 2 in the ileum, 1 in the cecum, and 1 in the rectum and for leiomyosarcoma, 1 in the duodenum, 1 in the ileum, and 2 in the rectum. No obvious site distribution emerges from the data.

**Gross Morphology.** Small tumors encountered as incidental findings at necropsy clearly arise in the outer muscle coat and not in the muscularis mucosae. In our series (Head and Else, 1981) the intestinal tumors were nodular in pattern except for one that was fusiform, whereas the rectoanal tumors were plaquelike. Tumors range in size from less than 1 cm to 17 cm in diameter; the larger tumors usually cause clinical signs. Hayden and Nielsen (1973) cite reports of two canine leiomyomas in the small intestine, one that weighed 976 g and the other 2 g. All the recorded tumors were solitary.

**Clinical Characteristics.** Eckerlin (1975) described a polypoid leiomyoma in an 8-year-old neutered male Labrador retriever that was found when an intussusception was reduced 20 cm from the ileocolic junction. In a useful survey of the literature he pointed out that most neoplasms cause complete obstruction of the gastrointestinal tract, but intestinal perforation occurs in some before obstruction develops. Most of the cases presented by Hayden and Nielsen (1973) were in the rectoanal region and were associated with tenesmus, restlessness, and unwillingness to sit.

**Growth and Metastasis.** As mentioned above, prediction of growth pattern is difficult. Brodey and Cohen (1964) mentioned resection of a leiomyoma of the intestine and of a leiomyosarcoma of the cecum, neither of which had metastasized 5 months and 7 months later, respectively. Likewise, the leiomyosarcoma described by Christie and Jabara (1964) had extended into the lumen as a mass 9 × 2.5 × 1.5 cm in size and into the mesentery as a mass 7 × 4.5 × 5 cm in size, but the dog was in good health 7 months after resection. These tumors can metastasize, however, as evidenced by the fact that all the leiomyosarcomas of the rectum seen by Head and Else (1981) had metastasized to the iliac lymph nodes by the time of diagnosis and one case showed widespread lymphohematogenous metastasis.

### Other Soft Tissue Tumors

Brodey and Cohen (1964) described two fibrosarcomas, one in the colon of a 5-year-old female Dalmatian, the other in the duodenum of a 7-year-old neutered female collie. Both metastasized following resection. The first metastasized to the liver and spleen in 3 months, and the second metastasized to the liver after 3 years. A colonic fibrosarcoma mentioned by Turk *et al.* (1981) in a 2-year-old female domestic shorthair cat also showed metastasis. As pointed out by Head (1976*b*), some tumors are so undifferentiated that they lack regions with spindle-shaped nuclei set in a fibrillary matrix; Hayden and Nielsen (1973) recorded such an anaplastic sarcoma in the cecum of a 9-year-old spaniel. At the other end of the differentiation scale, Eckerlin *et al.* (1976) described a jejunal mass in a 10-year-old castrated male mongrel dog in which the tumor

cells ranged from fusiform to osteoid and cartilaginous in pattern. This extraskeletal chondroblastic osteosarcoma had metastases in the lymph nodes of the liver and cecum 5 months after removal of the primary mass.

Schwannomas were described in male dogs by Singleton (1956) and Patnaik *et al.* (1977). Singleton's case was 8 years old when the 12.5 × 10 cm tumor was removed from the cecum; the dog was healthy 2 months later. The two duodenal cases described by Patnaik *et al.* (1977) were reported as being massive, solitary, gray-white, multilobate tumors.

A ganglioneuroma, believed to be congenital, was found in the middle jejunum of a 5-week-old male Siamese kitten by Patnaik *et al.* (1978*b*). The tumor thickened the wall to 8 to 10 mm over a segment 6.5 cm long. Histologically, the submucosa and upper two-thirds of the circular muscle coat were replaced by wavy bundles of nerve fibers, Schwann cells, connective tissue, and solitary or groups of large ganglion cells.

When describing the strangulation of the rectum by a pedunculated lipoma in a 15-year-old mare 5 months pregnant, Mason (1978) concluded from a literature survey that this was a well-recognized condition but with few published descriptions. In contrast, tumors of fat cells in other animals are rare in the intestine. Hayden and Nielsen (1973) found a case in the literature of a lipoma of the colon in an aged dog, while Head and Else (1981) recorded an 18-month-old castrated male cat with liposarcoma nodules in ileum, kidney, and mesenteric lymph nodes. Such true tumors of adipose cells must be differentiated from lipomatosis and fibrolipomatosis involving the omentum, mesentery, and retroperitoneum of cattle and less often in dogs.

## Tumors of the Hematopoietic and Related Tissues

### Lymphoid Tumors

**General Considerations.** Lymphomas are covered in general in chapter 6. Lymphocytes may undergo neoplastic transformation at any stage in their life cycle; hence tumors with different functional, anatomical, and cytological patterns are to be expected in the lymphoma family of neoplasms. The intestine has normal lymphoid tissue, therefore it can be the site of primary lymphoma. Dawson *et al.* (1961) determined the clinical criteria needed in humans to establish whether the intestinal lesion is primary lymphoma or an extension from other sites. Head and Else (1981) modified this as follows: (1) the lymphoma must involve the intestine and not just the drainage lymph nodes, (2) the tumor must invade the muscle coat (cf. reactive hyperplasia and inflammatory polyps), and (3) the peripheral lymph nodes must not be involved (to eliminate secondary spread from multicentric lymphoma).

**Incidence.** Because of the confusion between primary alimentary lymphoma and involvement of the intestine in a generalized systemic disease, existing incidence figures are suspect. It is sufficient to say that examples are seen in all species.

**Age, Breed, and Sex.** The tumors in all species are distributed among many breeds and over a wide age range from the very young to the very old; thus Head and Else (1981) give the age range for the dog as 7 months to 16 years and for the cat as 1 year to 18 years. It is obvious then that the mean age will be lower than for epithelial and smooth muscle tumors. Our figures for the dog and cat showed more cases in males than females, whereas all five of the canine cases of Patnaik *et al.* (1977) were in female dogs.

**Clinical Characteristics.** Most affected animals exhibit progressive weight loss and sometimes diarrhea over a variable period ranging from a few weeks to over 1 year. This is associated with the rate at which the tumor growth alters the villous architecture of the intestinal mucosa and the structure of the drainage lymph nodes, thus leading to maladsorption and lymph stasis. The hematological and biochemical changes indicative of this functional disturbance were well described for the horse by Roberts and Pinsent (1975). The timing of vomiting in dogs and cats may indicate the site of the tumor; specifically, 3 to 6 hours after a meal indicates duodenal lymphoma and 16 to 24 hours, ileal lymphoma. Ulceration of the tumor can give rise to hemorrhage detectable as melena or fresh blood depending on the tumor site and the speed of passage of the ingesta. Such cases may develop chronic hemorrhagic anemia. The possibility of related hyperparathyroidism should be considered, although the case of Schonbauer and Kohler (1981) in a 2-year-old stallion with intestinal lymphoma and calcinosis of the heart, lung, and kidney had no evidence of hyperparathyroidism. In cats the co-existence of kidney lesions may lead to the presenting signs originating from renal dysfunction (polydipsia and polyuria) rather than from alimentary dysfunction.

**Sites.** Head and Else (1981) show diagrammatically that the tumors in dogs and cats involve the whole intestinal tract diffusely or only in localized areas. The localized form can be solitary or multiple. The tumors are plaquelike, fusiform, or nodular in shape and intraluminal or intramural in pattern, but intramural fusiform type is most commonly seen. Because the invaded muscle undergoes atrophy leaving rows of lymphocytes supported by parallel bands of delicate reticulum fibers, these fusiform segments of neoplastic gut frequently balloon outward and the thin, mainly tumorous wall may rupture.

**Growth and Metastasis.** Some tumors appear to metastasize as if tumor emboli have spread and established transcelomically to peritoneal surfaces and hematogenously to the liver. Other examples show similar sized lesions in the intestinal tract and kidney, suggesting multicentric origin, whereas others involve lymphoid tissue of the intestine, spleen, and selected lymph nodes as if the circulating tumor lymphocytes were programmed to establish in favored sites. Suspect atypical lymphocytes are sometimes hematologically revealed in the peripheral blood.

**Etiology.** The demonstration of viral etiology of lymphoid tumors in cattle and cats suggests that at least some of the alimentary lymphomas have an infective origin. The variability of biological behavior of the tumor and host suggests that there may be several distinct tumor entities within this group. Recognition of the lymphocyte subsets involved in these intestinal tumors along with detection of the viral genome in the host nucleus may show that a single agent acts on different lymphocytes to produce different disease entities or that more factors than the viral agent are at work.

### Intestinal Mast Cell Tumors

**General Considerations and Incidence.** Similar problems exist with mast cell tumors as with lymphoma. Primary mast cell tumors do occur, and sometimes the lymph nodes draining the alimentary tract are involved in generalized mast cell proliferations. In 1958 I described mesenteric lymph node involvement in systemic mast cell neoplasia in 4 dogs and 2 cats (Head, 1958). Up to that time I had not seen a primary mast cell tumor of the gastrointestinal tract. Patnaik *et al.* (1980*b*) remarked on the sparsity of records in the literature. They described one case in a dog and recorded cases from the literature in the abomasum of a cow and in the intestinal tracts of 24 cats (Alroy *et al.*, 1975). Garner and Lingeman (1970) reviewed the literature of mast cell neoplasms in the domestic cat and found one case described by Nielsen where mast cell neoplasia involved the spleen, liver, lymph nodes, and intestine of a 10-year-old neutered female cat.

**Age, Breed, and Sex.** The dog case reported by Patnaik *et al.* (1980*b*) was a 9-year-old male German shepherd. The 24 cats reported by Alroy *et al.* (1975) had no breed predilection and an average age of 12.3 years; the sex distribution was 12 neutered females, 1 intact female, 9 castrated males, and 2 intact males. Garner and Lingeman (1970) described three cases from the files of the Armed Forces Institute of Pathology in the jejunum and mesenteric lymph node of a 13-year-old male cat; in the mesenteric lymph nodes of the duodenum, liver, and spleen of a 14-year-old cat; and the cecum of a 13-year-old female cat. In the second case, mast cells were present in the peripheral blood smears.

**Site and Gross Morphology.** The dog case reported by Patnaik *et al.* (1980*b*) had an 8-cm ileocecocolic intussusception with a pedunculate intraluminal mass attached to the ileocecal valve. The lesions in the cats studied by Alroy *et al.* (1975) were in the colon in 3 cases and in the intestine at all levels in 21 cases. Regardless of site, the tumors showed a fusiform pattern and intestinal diameters ranging from 1 to more than 7 cm. On opening the gut, cream- to tan-colored tissue replaced the muscle coat centrally, but merged with the normal intestinal layers above and below the segmental thickening. The mucosa was sometimes encroached upon but was not ulcerated.

**Histological Features.** In the dog case the tumor and the adjacent wall and mesentery were replaced by typical mast cells in groups and rows between collagenous stroma. Giemsa staining revealed "typical granules" in the tumor cells.

Garner and Lingeman (1970) pointed out that the cells in their neoplasms were undifferentiated, resembling lymphoreticular cells of lymphoma or plasmacytoma with hematoxylin and eosin staining. In some cells the cytoplasm was well demarcated and in others it was reticular. In Giemsa stained fixed sections, granules were not demonstrable or were only visible in a few cells, whereas in freshly prepared imprints stained with Wright–Giemsa the cells had numerous granules. By contrast, the granules had strongly PAS positive staining in more than 90% of the cells. The implication is that this type of staining reflects immaturity rather than degranulation; this is supported by the fact that blood eosinophils were absent or rare in the sections.

The cat tumors were mainly located in the muscle coat and submucosa, sometimes extending into the lamina propria of the intact mucosa. The tumors of Alroy *et al.* (1975) were composed of polygonal cells in nests separated by delicate collagenous stroma or they had cells in whorls mimicking germinal centers with central polygonal cells surrounded by fusiform cells. With hematoxylin and eosin stain, the cytoplasmic borders were indistinct and the cytoplasm was finely granular and vacuolated, unlike typical mast cells. Also, the nucleus was eccentric, not central as in typical neoplastic mast cells, and mitoses were uncommon. Eosinophils ranged in number from abundant to rare. The characteristic granules were strongly metachromatic in sections stained with acid toluidine blue (pH 2.5). Red granules with aldehyde fuchsin stain were only found in two cases of the six examined. The others showed positive cells scattered among the vacuolated negative cells. In all cases, PAS positive cells were present. Because the polygonal cell masses occurred mainly in the submucosa and muscle, the possibility of carcinoid was considered, but only the enterochromaffin cells in the overlying mucosa had argyrophil, argentaffin, and formalin induced fluorescent granules. Ultrastructurally, the cells had the features of feline cutaneous and visceral mast cell tumor cells, but most had the appearance of degranulated mast cells (i.e., fused and empty "vesicles"). About 5% of the cells had moderately electron dense granulofibrillary material forming the granule, but none had the electron dense or crystalline mast cell granules of neoplastic mast cells of the cat.

Finn and Schwartz (1972) described an annular thickening of the terminal ileum 4 cm long and 2 cm thick in a 12-year-old castrated male shorthair domestic cat. The tumor showed a rupture of the ileal wall opposite a $1.7 \times 1.4 \times 2$ cm contiguous nodular growth on the mesenteric border. The mesenteric nodes, especially the right colic lymph node, had enlarged, active germinal centers, and the Peyer's patches were hyperplastic. No metastases were present. The uniform 8 to 9 $\mu$m diameter cells infiltrated the mesentery, muscle, submucosa, and lamina propria between the glands of the mucosa. The nonlobulated tumor cell nuclei had a dense chromatin pattern, were eccentric, but lacked mitoses, and the cytoplasm contained 8 to 30 large eosinophilic granules shown by hematoxylin and eosin stains. These granules did not stain with Alcian blue, Giemsa, or PAS, but were light brown (rarely black) with phosphotungstic acid hematoxylin stain. With electron microscopy the globules (mean diameter 1.15 to 1.5 $\mu$m) were seen to be membrane bound, electron dense, and homogenous or finely granular, and they occasionally showed dense transverse bands. Finn and Schwartz (1972) suggested that this was a tumor of globule leukocytes; this may add some weight to the suggestion that this is a specific cell type. Both they and Alroy et al. (1975) drew attention to the work of Murray et al. (1968) who presented evidence from rats, cattle, and sheep in Glasgow, Scotland, that in parasitic infections, mast cells tranform into globule leukocytes. There seems little doubt that the Finn and Schwartz tumor has many features in common with both the degranulated mast cell tumors described by Alroy et al. (1975) and the poorly differentiated mast cells of Garner and Lingeman (1970). Perhaps they are different end results of local environmental factors acting on a basic mastocytoma pattern to release the chemicals in the granules in different ways. In any case, this pattern has variations reflecting the lack of differentiation of some tumor cells.

From the above discussion, it is clear that fusiform and nodular tumors of the intestine can be epithelial, endocrine, lymphoid, or mast cell in origin. Touch imprints of the lightly scarified cut surface of such tumors when air-dried and stained with Wright–Giemsa would distinguish lymphoma from mastocytoma and might suggest further investigation of some endocrine tumors. This examination should be made on fresh tumor tissue before it is formalin fixed and lost to more sophisticated diagnostic tests. Biochemical investigation of these tumors might explain why no ulceration of the stomach or duodenum has been reported in association with intestinal mastocytoma, unlike that which occurs with some cutaneous mast cell tumors.

**Growth and Metastasis.** In the dog, Patnaik et al. (1980b) recorded a metastasis 6 cm in diameter in the ileocecal lymph node and tumor masses in the medulla of the mesenteric lymph node; neoplastic mast cells were also present in the bone marrow, liver, and lungs. Alroy et al. (1975) saw metastasis in 16 cases, 14 in the mesenteric lymph nodes, 6 in the liver, 6 in the spleen, 2 in the lung, 1 in the hepatic lymph node, 1 in the cecal lymph node, and 1 in the femoral bone marrow.

## Perianal Tumors

Head (1976) listed a series of tumor types (e.g., melanotic tumors of gray horses), most of which are covered in other chapters in this volume. At this point it is worth noting that in the canine, squamous cell carcinoma, rectal type adenocarcinoma, mucoepidermoid (adenosquamous) carcinoma, lymphoma, and mast cell tumor of the region are usually plaquelike, fixed to the skin, and frequently ulcerated. In contrast, tumors of the apocrine glands and tumors of perianal (hepatoid) glands are usually nodular, and the overlying skin is movable unless ulceration has supervened. McGavin and Fishburn (1975) described an interesting adenoma that grew, despite stilbestrol therapy, from the apocrine glands of the anal skin of a 15-year-old male standard poodle. They cited a case recorded by Diamond and Garner (1972) of a cocker spaniel that had both an apocrine gland adenocarcinoma of the anal sac and a perianal gland adenoma.

Anal sac apocrine gland tumors are described in chapters 2 and 13.

## TUMORLIKE LESIONS

### Lesions that Mimic Epithelial Tumors

Rowland and Rowntree (1972) in Edinburgh, Scotland, described an outbreak of a hemorrhagic bowel syndrome in a herd of pigs involving all ages of animals from 3-week-old piglets to adult sows. Following this outbreak both the survivors and previously unaffected pigs that were 6 to 16 weeks old developed intestinal adenomatosis from which resolution to normal often occurred by the time the pigs were slaughtered for bacon at about 6 to 8 months of age. These authors recorded the previous reports in the literature of similar diseases affecting pigs. From this routine diagnostic observation, a research program developed that showed the presence of microorganisms in the affected cells (Rowland *et al.,* 1973), which were subsequently isolated and named *Campylobacter sputorum* subsp. *mucosalis* (Lawson and Rowland, 1974). These workers went on to suggest that where extensive necrosis occurs in cases of porcine intestinal adenomatosis, excessive granulation tissue is formed in the healing process, hypertrophy of the muscle coat develops, and the lesion resembles regional (terminal) ileitis (Rowland and Lawson, 1975). Workers in the United States, Canada, Sweden, and Australia confirmed this observation, although they altered the terminology for this disease to *porcine proliferative enteritis* for the whole complex and *proliferative hemorrhagic enteropathy* for the lesions exhibiting congestion, hemorrhage, fibrin deposition, and thrombosis of blood vessels. Lomax and Glock (1983) detailed their own and others' attempts to reproduce the disease complex.

Macroscopically, porcine intestinal adenomatosis involves intestine from the ileum to the upper third of the spiral colon including the cecum. Although in some cases the lesions may only be detectable on microscopic examination, in advanced cases the wall of the intestine becomes thickened and the mucosal surface shows deep transverse folds with sessile nodules and even multiple pedunculate 1- to 1.5-cm-diameter polyps, especially in the large intestine.

Transmission experiments using homogenized scrapings of affected intestinal mucosa or cultures of *Campylobacter* given orally result in 10 to 50% of the pigs developing macroscopic lesions and sometimes as many as 75% showing lesions histologically. Although superimposed infections by other pathogens of the intestine, including both bacterial (e.g., *Salmonella* spp. or *Escherichia coli*) and protozoal (e.g., *Balantidium* spp.), may exacerbate the condition, they are not primary etiological factors. The failure to obtain consistent experimental repro-

duction of the disease perhaps points to some other undetected etiological factor.

The earliest lesions observed consist of infiltration by eosinophils and neutrophils, loss of goblet cells, and formation of an exudate containing bacteria in the crypt lumens. The crypts become elongated and branched; their lining epithelium assumes an immature character with the cells showing basophilic cytoplasm, hyperchromatic basal nuclei, and many mitoses; and the cells are sometimes stratified. The lacteals become dilated and macrophages become the dominant infiltrating cell. The immature crypt type epithelium eventually replaces the whole thickness of the mucosa and there is loss of villi. With histochemical techniques the small intestine fails to reveal the common enzymes normally found in mature villous epithelium. In the large intestine goblet cells are absent; these areas, when focal, resemble adenoma. Warthin–Starry silver stained sections reveal curved organisms in the apical cytoplasm of the immature epithelial cells, even in those cells in mitosis, and phagolysosomes in macrophages also contain bacteria. The organisms, which are 1.6 to 2.7 $\mu$m long and 0.2 to 0.3 $\mu$m in diameter, are not seen to be surrounded by host cell membrane on electron microscopic examination, and the parasitized cells have the normal organelles of immature crypt epithelium.

The bacterial organism causing this disease is a normal commensal of the oral cavity. To judge from transmission experiments, the organism administered orally can pass through the stomach lumen unaffected. It enters the cells of the crypt epithelium (for which it seems to have a predilection) via the microvillar free border, and stimulates cell division. In the absence of secondary infection, the fully developed adenomatous proliferation occurs in about 1 month, and then recovery supervenes in about 6 weeks and the intestinal mucosa returns to normal. The role of immune mechanisms in the recovery phase, their possible influence via lymphokines on the proliferation of epithelial cells, and whether or not hypersensitivity reaction plays a role in some forms of the disease have not yet been elucidated. The problems raised by a transient adenomatous hyperplasia and the lack of certainty as to whether the *Campylobacter* is a primary or secondary pathogen make this an important subject in neoplasia of the intestine, even though the lesion is not a true tumor.

The lesions have no premalignant significance since adenocarcinoma in the intestine of pigs is rare. Occasionally, a small number of epithelium-forming gland acini is found in lymphatics in the submucosa of the intestine and even in the cortex of the drainage mesenteric lymph nodes. These are not true metastases, but rather represent extension and release of epithelial fragments along dilated lymphatics. Established lesions have been detected in distant sites, and such displaced acini are uncommon in most series of cases.

Similar lesions associated with intracellular *Campylobacter*-like organisms have been described in the duodenum of guinea pigs by Elwell *et al.* (1981). In their literature survey, they record cases in the ileum of lambs, the ileum of hamsters, and the cecum and proximal colon of blue foxes. To this list of species Duhamel and Wheeldon (1982) added a case in the mid-ileum of a 6-month-old Arabian colt. Vandenberghe and Marsboom (1982) raised the point that all intestinal adenocarcinomas should be examined for *Campylobacter*-like organisms. They described the presence of such bacteria in the cytoplasm of tumor cells in two cases of adenocarcinoma of the colon in Wistar rats. Fox *et al.* (1982) described an outbreak of proliferative colitis in ferrets from which they isolated *Campylobacter fetus* subsp. *jejuni*. They commented that the convoluted, branching, hyperplastic glands in ferrets frequently penetrate into the submucosa, as they do in hamsters but not in pigs.

## Lesions that Mimic Mesenchymal Tumors

The gross appearance of canine granulomatous colitis is thickening and corrugation with bleeding points affecting the descending colon and rectum; advanced cases involve the cecum and colon. The slightly enlarged regional lymph nodes might suggest a lymphoid tumor. Histologically, these changes are due to infiltration of the submucosa and lamina propria by histiocytes that have strongly positive PAS staining cytoplasm. Van der Gaag *et al.* (1978) described a case in a 1-year-old French bulldog, a breed that has the same ancestral origin as the boxer, which is the only breed in which the disease had previously been recorded. In van der Gaag's review of

the literature, credit is given to van Kruiningen and co-workers (1965) who first described the condition in the United States. Since then the disease has been reported in the Netherlands, West Germany, and Australia. The descriptive term *histiocytic ulcerative colitis* is used for the condition. This term was partially adopted by van Kruiningen and Dobbins (1979) when they described a similar lesion in cats that they called *feline histiocytic colitis*. These authors found that bacterial bacilli were present in the macrophages as observed by electron microscopy.

The regional enterocolitis of cocker spaniels described by Strande *et al.* (1954) must not be confused with a tumor because histologically the cellular infiltrate is composed of neutrophils, eosinophils, and macrophages.

Hendrick (1981) pointed out that eosinophilic enteritis in cats shows segmental or diffuse thickenings of the stomach, small intestine, and colon and that the mesenteric lymph nodes, spleen, and liver of these cats may also become involved. Histologically, these lesions of the intestines are not neoplastic, but are composed of mature eosinophils accompanied by some fibrosis. The implication is that there is a spectrum of disease that varies from localized to disseminated eosinophil infiltration and possibly occurs as eosinophilic leukemia.

## MESOTHELIOMA

**General Considerations.** A single layer of flattened mesothelial cells lines the three main celomic cavities, namely, the pleural, pericardial, and peritoneal cavities, the latter extending down the spermatic cord to the surface of the testis. Normal mesothelial cells are difficult to see in paraffin sections because they are cut across their narrowest face, thus one can see the spindle-shaped nucleus but not the cytoplasm. The cytoplasm of these cells can be seen if imprints are taken from the surface or if cell deposits are examined from serous effusions or from fluid washed off serous membranes.

When stimulated, as for example in inflammation, the mesothelial cells increase in thickness and the nuclei become rounded so they may resemble a row of cuboidal cells when seen in section. "Activated" mesothelial cells obtained from rats injected intraperitoneally with crocidolite asbestos were shown by Whitaker *et al.* (1982) to have more glycolytic enzymes and mitochondrial respiration when compared with "resting" mesothelial cells, but to have less reaction product than peritoneal macrophages. Macrophages could be differentiated from activated mesothelial cells because the former contain lipoids but the latter do not. Three forms of mesothelial cells have been described in human serous effusions: recently desquamated small round cells, medium-sized activated cells with large amounts of deeply staining cytoplasm, and large vacuolated cells. In some experimental situations Whitaker *et al.* (1982) showed these vacuoles to contain hyaluronic acid, but it is still uncertain whether this is produced by the mesothelium or is in passage from the subserosal tissue. Electron microscopy shows that activated mesothelial cells have more glycogen than resting cells (PAS reactive in light microscopy), more rough ergastoplasm (thus more ribonucleic acid staining with methyl green-pyronin), and an accentuated development of the Golgi apparatus (thus higher thiamine pyrophosphatase activity).

Harvey and Amlot (1983) showed that cultures of human mesothelial cells, derived from serous effusions, synthesize large amounts of interstitial collagen types I and III, but not basement membrane collagen types IV and V. They discussed the possibility that desquamation changes the pattern of mesothelial cell collagen synthesis from basement membrane type *in vivo* to the interstitial type *in vitro*. In addition, they pointed out that this change could result in the fibrosis that accompanies chronic serous effusions.

It is recognized that distinction between activated or reactive mesothelial cells and neoplastic mesothelium is difficult. Specific marker systems have not yet been devised to separate these two cell types; therefore, differentiation between some types of inflammation of celomic cavities and mesothelioma rests on the interpretation of the histological pattern in, for example, a biopsy sample. Exfoliative cytology even of mesothelioma or secondary transcelomic tumor cases will reveal activated mesothelial cells, some of which may be binucleate, multinucleate, or even exhibit mitosis. In addition to the cuboidal surface mesothelial cell type, primary tumors of the lining of celomic cavities have a spindle cell fibrous component. It is not clear whether tumors can arise from either of these two components of the celomic lining without the other being involved. Willis (1967) holds the view that a purely spindle cell fibrous tumor should be called a fibroma or fibrosarcoma. Until a system has been devised to positively identify these spindle cell elements as intimately related to surface mesothelial cells, this seems a sound course to follow.

There is no doubt that mesotheliomas are rare; thus, Geib *et al.* (1962) cited other workers as having seen one case in 1,000 dogs and three cases in 5,315 dogs. There is also little doubt that some reports in the literature are misdiagnoses of examples of serosal disease secondary to undiscovered primary neoplasms in the neighboring viscera. Willis (1967) considered that many reports of cases in humans are valueless because there were no necropsies or because details were not given to establish the thoroughness of the postmortem examination. Thus, he suggested that the fixed lung should be sectioned with a bacon slicer to eliminate the possibility of metastases from a small undetected primary tumor onto the pleural surfaces. In domestic animals secondary lung tumors are more likely to be the source of such pleural deposits since primary lung tumors are rare. Other sources for pleural metastases are through the chest wall (e.g., from a thoracic mammary carcinoma) or from the anterior mediastinum, either from a secondary tumor in the lymph nodes or from a primary thymic carcinoma. In the abdominal cavity, the ovaries, uterus, alimentary tract, and prostate must be meticulously examined before making a diagnosis of peritoneal mesothelioma. It must also be noted that pleural involvement may develop as a result of spread from the peritoneum via the diaphragm. Spread within subserosal lymphatics suggests a secondary tumor. One must remember that many adenocarcinomas are released into the celomic cavity as isolated cells that deposit with fibrin on the activated mesothelial surface and are then incorporated by the organization of the fibrin into the celomic lining proper. These cells then form recognizable acini and may only then exhibit the property of synthesizing mucin.

In addition to a very careful postmortem examination, including culture for bacteria and fungi, a detailed clinical history should be recorded. As part of the protocol for a diagnosis of mesothelioma one must establish that there was no history of removal of a tumor at a previous date. A history of an earlier acute illness associated with a celomic space should also be viewed with suspicion. For example, spontaneous rupture of the atrium of the heart with fluid in the pericardial sac and an abundance of activated mesothelium can undergo partial resolution to mimic a mesothelioma. The main reaction will be centered on the atrium, and there will be much hemosiderin in the cellular response. Careful search will reveal the site of rupture, said by Stunzi and Ammann-Mann (1973) to be most commonly located between the smooth part of the left atrium and auricle near the site of "jet lesions" from mitral valve mucoid endocardiosis.

**Classification.** Following the scheme adopted for humans by Enzinger *et al.* (1969), one should specify the biological behavior, histological pattern, extent of the lesion, and site for each tumor. Thus, tumors are either benign or malignant mesotheliomas depending on their behavior. Since the tumor arises from mesothelial cells and supporting tissues, it may exhibit a spectrum of histological patterns from predominantly epithelioid to predominantly fibrous. A tumor with both epithelioid and spindle cell patterns of mesodermal cells in more or less equal amounts is called biphasic.

The epithelioid cells can exhibit tubular, papillary, or tubulopapillary growth patterns. Fibroma and fibrosarcoma can be differentiated from predominantly fibrous mesothelioma because they lack the epithelioid component. The extent of the lesion may vary from localized to diffuse, the latter term implying multiple lesions involving extensive areas of the serous cavities. In such diffuse mesothelioma it may be difficult to decide whether one is dealing with a multicentric benign tumor or widespread metastasis of a malignant mesothelioma. The subdivisions often group together so that the two most common groups are benign (predominantly fibrous, localized mesothelioma) and malignant (predominantly epithelioid, diffuse mesothelioma).

**Incidence, Age, Breed, Sex, and Sites.** Mesothelial tumors are rare. Case reports that fulfill the stringent requirements outlined above are so few that incidence figures cannot be given. It is clear that there are two distribution patterns. In cattle and in one sheep case newborn or very young animals are affected, whereas in other species adult or aged animals have been reported with mesothelioma.

Baskerville (1967) extended the summaries of previously published cases noted by Grant (1958) and added his own examples to make a total of 16 mesotheliomas in the bovine. The age ranged from an 8-month-old fetus, to a full-term stillborn calf, to a 4-month-old calf, suggesting that the disease is congenital in nature. The breeds affected were probably those that were locally common. Five were male, five were female, and in six the sex was unrecorded. The peritoneum was affected in 14 cases, with the pelvic region and tunica vaginalis sometimes being the major site, and the peritoneum and pleura were involved in one case and the pleura alone in another. These mesotheliomas were reported from many geographical locations, mainly in Europe. Grant's (1958) cases were discovered during a survey to investigate the incidence of congenital bovine lymphoma in Sweden, and he suggested that some cases may be missed because not all stillborn or aborted calves come to postmortem examination. Some bovine cases have been recorded in older animals. Grant (1958) mentioned one in the mesentery and pleura of a 7-year-old cow, and Ladds and Crane (1976) described one in the scrotum of a mature bull.

There is one case in sheep, reported by Brown and Weaver (1981), in the peritoneal cavity of a 4-month-old Suffolk-cross male lamb, which might be similar to congenital bovine mesothelioma. In contrast, McCullagh *et al.* (1979) described a case in the pleura and anterior mediastinum of a 10-year-old castrated male Saanen goat used for feeding tsetse flies.

Mesothelial tumors in adult horses, dogs, and cats have been found in scattered countries around the world. In horses the peritoneum was involved in the example described by Ricketts and Peace (1976), the pericardium in a case of Carnine *et al.* (1977), and the pleura in animals mentioned by Straub *et al.* (1974) and Kramer *et al.* (1976). The ages of the animals ranged from 6 to 27 years, and three of the four were mares, the fourth being a gelding.

Twenty-seven examples of localized, nonmetastasizing fibrous pleural mesothelioma were reported by Seffner and Fritzsch (1964) as occurring in 654 pigs slaughtered from two large German piggeries.

Thrall and Goldschmidt (1978), in summarizing the site distribution of mesothelioma in several species, showed that the pleura of the dog was affected more often than the pericardial sac and that the peritoneal surfaces were rarely affected. They suggested that there may be a slight bias toward male dogs, but the cases reported by van Ooijen (1978) and Ikede *et al.* (1980) occurred in spayed females. The cases reported in the literature have an age range of 4 to 13 years (mean 7.8 years), and no breed predisposition is apparent.

In cats the peritoneal surfaces were involved in the case described by Raflo and Nuernberger (1978), the pericardium in the case of Tilley *et al.* (1975), and the pleura was the site mentioned by E. J. Andrews (1973) and by Creighton and Wilkins (1975). The cases were in females of Siamese and domestic shorthair breeds ranging in age from 1.5 to 9 years.

**Clinical Characteristics.** Mesothelioma of the pericardial sac may be responsible for clinical signs of congestive heart failure due to the accumulation of fluid in the pericardial sac and subsequent cardiac tamponade if a large enough amount of fluid forms. The volume of fluid needed to produce signs ranges from 3 liters in the horse to 200 ml in the cat. The signs can be relieved by pericardiocentesis, but the fluid reforms (e.g., at a rate of 320 ml every 5 days in the dog). It is not known whether the fluid is produced in excessive amounts by the cells or by the associated vessels, or whether the drainage of normally produced fluid is reduced because of blocked lymphatic drainage.

Likewise, accumulation of fluid in the thoracic cavity associated with pleural mesothelioma can cause dyspnea and alveolar collapse in the cranioventral lung lobes. Intrathoracic lesions are best seen if radiography is performed immediately after thoracocentesis. Fluid volumes to produce signs range from 2 liters in the dog to 60 liters in the horse. The fluid reforms quickly following removal, the rate varying from 1 to 10 liters every 3 days in the dog.

Peritoneal mesothelioma is associated with progressive abdominal distension. In the adult horse there may be up to 30 liters of fluid, and colic has been reported. The congenital form of the tumor in the bovine may cause difficulty in parturition partly because as much as 12 liters of fluid in the abdomen of the fetus may be present and partly because of marked hydrops of the amniotic membranes.

The fluid withdrawn from any of these three sites may show free erythrocytes, usually has low protein content, and does not clot on standing, but often has a moderate number of nucleated cells. These cells may be entirely leukocytes, but often desquamated tumor cells are found, especially in the predominantly epithelioid mesothelioma. The problems of exfoliative cytological diagnosis and the change in the deposit character at different sites and at different times were discussed by van Ooijen (1978). Geib *et al.* (1962) illustrated the use of Papanicolaou stain for smears and cell blocks of the sediment. Since paracentesis will yield a large volume of fluid in these cases, the sample must be processed immediately, first by making a cytospin preparation and then centrifuging the remainder. The pellet from centrifugation can in part be resuspended for smear preparations and processed for light and electron microscopy as detailed by Else (1984).

The differences between activated and malignant mesothelial epithelioid cells have been discussed by Kramer *et al.* (1976). The activated mesothelial cells released into transudates or inflammatory exudates occur singly or in monolayered clumps of four to five cells; the nuclei are central, round to oval, uniform in diameter, occupying as much as one-half of the cell, and having one or more small nucleoli. Binucleate cells are common. The cytoplasm with Romanovsky stain is basophilic, finely vacuolated, may contain phagocytosed cells or particles, and has an indistinct edge. With PAS stain the vacuoles appear as positively reacting glycogen granules since they can be digested with malt diastase. In contrast, neoplastic mesothelial cells occur not only as single cells and clumps of more than five cells, but also in three-dimensional clusters or spheres with solid centers, resembling adenocarcinoma acini. The nuclei vary in size, are often large, and have large eosinophilic nucleoli. The cytoplasm, in addition to the fine glycogen granules, often has large vacuoles that are PAS negative (cf. glycoprotein of adenocarcinoma).

**Gross Morphology.** The tumors are small, discrete nodules 1 to 50 mm in diameter and have either a shaggy surface due to individual fronds being visible or a cauliflowerlike surface due to many complex fissures. The color ranges from gray-white to red or yellow depending on the amount of hemorrhage and its duration with subsequent hemosiderin formation. Where transcelomic spread is a feature, the lesions tend to be larger and may be confluent. Often the parietal serosal surface is more affected than the visceral. The cut surface of the lesions usually shows no evidence of infiltrative growth into the underlying tissue.

**Histological Features.** The most common pattern is of cuboidal epithelioid cells covering papillary projections of a spindle cell fibrovascular core. No basement membrane separating the two cell types could be demonstrated in most light microscopic studies, but Trigo *et al.* (1981) found a continuous basal limiting structure. Although both cuboidal and spindle cells are neoplastic, mitoses are usually rare in both; if present they are mainly seen in the epithelioid cells. Occasionally the epithelioid cells extend into the fibrous core as rosettes or tubules. Some of these cells may exhibit vacuoles that may contain refractile material. Ricketts and Peace (1976) pointed out that this material is of unknown nature and is nonreactive with PAS, Alcian blue, mucicarmine, and oil red O stains. Ciliated epithelioid cells can be demonstrated in light microscopy, as in one of Misdorp's (1965) calf cases and the dog pericardial mesothelioma of Ikede *et al.* (1980). Trigo *et al.* (1981) in an electron microscopic study recorded well-developed microvilli, desmosomes, numerous mitochondria, and abundant rough endoplasmic reticulum.

The branching treelike central core is composed of argyrophilic and collagenous fibers. It exhibits a variable, usually weak metachromasia with Alcian blue, methyl violet, or toluidine blue stain at pH 4.5. This is probably hyaluronic acid because there is no metachromatic staining after digestion with testicular hyaluronidase. As Breeze and Lander (1975) pointed out, such material would dissolve to some extent in aqueous fixatives. This variation in ground substance has been reported in other species in addition to the ox and dog; thus McCullagh *et al.* (1979) described the stroma of their goat case as "myxomatous," and E. J. Andrews (1973) stated that in the cat case the stroma macroscopically slightly resembled soft cartilage. In the lamb Brown and Weaver (1981) noted that islands of cartilage developed in the larger masses of spindle-shaped cells. Dubielzig (1977) introduced the term *sclerosing mesothelioma* for tumors composed of thick fibrous serosal masses containing isolated large anaplastic cells. In addition to the cartilaginous metaplasia there are reports of the loose connective tissue forming osteoid and mineralized bone, which must be differentiated from dystrophic calcification associated with necrosis. Sometimes multinucleated giant cells are scattered throughout the tumor. This, along with the macroscopic appearance of the lesions resembling "grape lesions" of tuberculous serositis, prompted Grant (1958) and Misdorp (1965) to stress that a search for acid-fast organisms should be made in congenital calf lesions.

**Etiology.** There is considerable epidemiological evidence linking asbestos inhalation with human disease. The subject has been little studied in domestic animals. Asbestos is the name given to a group of fibrous minerals similar in appearance, but having a variety of complex chemical compositions. Different forms of asbestos have different degrees of carcinogenicity. Thus, chrysolite (white asbestos) with curly fibers 0.5 to 3 in. long penetrates less far down the bronchial tree and has a British Standard atmospheric contamination acceptance of 1 fiber/ml as opposed to 0.5 fiber/ml for the straight fibers of amosite (brown asbestos) and 0.2 fiber/ml for the short, straight, brittle fibers of crocidolite (blue asbestos). Four types of disease in humans are associated with asbestos inhalation: pleural plaques of fibrous tissue, which calcify in 20 years; progressive pulmonary fibrosis and epithelialization of an interstitial pneumonia; rarely, mesothelioma occurring 20 to 40 years after exposure; and lung cancer, which is dose related, occurring 10 to 15 years after exposure, and for which cigarette smoking acts synergistically.

The visualization of asbestos can be done by light microscopy, but only large fibers are detected and these more easily when coated by iron-containing protein. These ferruginous bodies are best detected in sections stained by Perls' method, since hematoxylin may mask fine positive fibers. Alternatively, the tissue may be digested in potassium hydroxide and the deposit examined by phase contrast. Electron microscopy will detect smaller fibers, and if tissue is ashed the resistant fibers in a large volume of tissue can be monitored using the transmission or scanning electron microscope.

Pulmonary macrophages with phagocytosed dust particles exhibit "pleural drift," that is, they move through alveolar walls toward the pleura. In doing so they may penetrate bronchioles and be transported by the mucociliary staircase, or they may

Hayden, D. W., and Nielsen, S. W. (1973) Canine Alimentary Neoplasia. *Zbl. Vet. Med.* 20A, 1–22.

Head, K. W. (1958) Cutaneous Mast-Cell Tumours in the Dog, Cat and Ox. *Brit. J. Dermatol.* 70, 389–408.

———. (1967) Breed and Geographical Variations in the Occurrence of Tumours in Domesticated Mammals. In: Shivas, A. A., ed., *Racial and Geographical Factors in Tumour Incidence*. Pfizer Med. Monograph. No. 2. Edinburgh University Press (Edinburgh), 251–275.

———. (1976a) International Histological Classification of Tumours of Domesticated Animals. XI. Tumours of the Upper Alimentary Tract. *Bull. Wld. Hlth, Org.* 53, 145–166.

———. (1976b) International Histological Classification of Tumours of Domestic Animals. XII. Tumours of the Lower Alimentary Tract. *Bull. Wld. Hlth. Org.* 53, 167–186.

Head, K. W., and Else, R. W. (1981) Neoplasia and Allied Conditions of the Canine and Feline Intestine. *Vet. Ann.* 21, 190–208.

Hendrick, M. (1981) A Spectrum of Hypereosinophilic Syndromes Exemplified by Six Cats with Eosinophilic Enteritis. *Vet. Path.* 18, 188–200.

Henson, W. R. (1939) Carcinoma of the Tongue in a Horse. *J. Amer. Vet. Med. Assoc.* 94, 124.

Hill, M. J. (1980) Bacterial Metabolism and Human Carcinogenesis. *Brit. Med. Bull.* 36, 89–94.

Hill, M. J., Morson, B. C., and Busey, H. J. R. (1978) Aetiology of Adenoma–Carcinoma Sequence in Large Bowel. *Lancet* 1, 245–247.

Holt, P. F. (1981) Transport of Inhaled Dust to Extrapulmonary Sites. *J. Path.* 133, 123–129.

Hubmann, F.-H. (1982) Proctitis Cystica Profunda and Radiation Fibrosis in the Rectum of the Female Wistar Rat after X-Irradiation. *J. Path.* 138, 193–204.

Ikede, B. O., Zubaidy, A., and Gill, C. W. (1980) Pericardial Mesothelioma with Cardiac Tamponade in a Dog. *Vet. Path.* 17, 496–500.

Isaksson, A. (1946) Multiple karcinoider i tunntarmen hos Notkreatur. *Skand. Vet. Tidskr.* 36, 86–92.

Ivoghli, B. (1978) Esophageal Sarcomas Associated with Canine Spirocercosis. *Vet. Med.* 73, 47–49.

Jackson, C. (1936) The Incidence and Pathology of Tumours of Domesticated Animals in South Africa: A Study of the Onderstepoort Collection of Neoplasms with Special Reference to the Histopathology. *Onderstepoort J. Vet. Sci. and Anim. Indust.* 6, 1–460.

Jarrett, W. F. H. (1980) Bracken Fern and Papilloma Virus in Bovine Alimentary Cancer. *Brit. Med. Bull.* 36, 79–81.

Jass, J. R. (1980) Role of Intestinal Metaplasia in the Histogenesis of Gastric Carcinoma. *J. Clin. Path.* 33, 801–810.

Kamara, J. A. (1964) The Incidence of Canine Spirocercosis in the Freetown Area of Sierra Leone. *Bull. Epiz. Dis. Afr.* 12, 465–468.

Karbe, E., and Schiefer, B. (1967) Primary Salivary Gland Tumours in Carnivores. *Can. Vet. J.* 8, 212–215.

Keirn, D. P., White, K. K., King, J. M., and Tennant, B. C. (1982) Endoscopic Diagnosis of Squamous Cell Carcinoma of the Equine Stomach. *J. Amer. Vet. Med. Assoc.* 180, 940–942.

Kelly, D. F., Lucke, V. M., Denny, H. R., and Lane, J. G. (1979) Histology of Salivary Gland Infarction in the Dog. *Vet. Path.* 16, 438–443.

Kemp, W. B., Abbey, L. M., and Taylor, L. A. (1976) Pseudo-Sarcomatous Fasciitis of the Upper Lip of a Cat. *Vet. Med. Small Anim. Clin.* 71, 923–925.

Kipnis, R. M. (1978) Focal Cystic Gastropathy in a Dog. *J. Amer. Vet. Med. Assoc.* 173, 182–184.

Kirkbride, C. A., Bicknell, E. J., and Robl, M. G. (1973) Hemangiomas of a Bovine Fetus with a Chorioangioma of the Placenta. *Vet. Path.* 10, 238–240.

Knecht, C. D., and Priester, W. A. (1978) Musculoskeletal Tumours in Dogs. *J. Amer. Vet. Med. Assoc.* 172, 72–74.

Koestner, A., and Buerger, L. (1965) Primary Neoplasms of the Salivary Glands in Animals Compared to Similar Tumours in Man. *Path. Vet.* 2, 201–226.

Konishi, S., Tokita, H., and Ogata, H. (1972) Studies on Canine Oral Papillomatosis. I. Transmission and Characterization of the Virus. *Jp. J. Vet. Sci.* 34, 263–268.

Krahnert, R. (1952) Zum Magenkrebs des Pferdes. *Mh. Vet. Med.* 7, 399–404.

Krahwinkel, D. J., Jr., and McCue, J. F. (1967) Wild Birds as Transport Hosts of *Spirocerca lupi* in the Southeastern United States. *J. Parasit.* 53, 650–651.

Kramer, J. W., Nickels, F. A., and Bell, T. (1976) Cytology of Diffuse Mesothelioma in the Thorax of a Horse. *Equine Vet. J.* 8, 81–83.

Krogh, G. (1952) Ett fall av kronisk esofagit och primart esofaguskarcinom hos hund. *Nord. Vet. Med.* 4, 893–900.

Krook, L. (1956) On Gastrointestinal Carcinoma in the Dog. *Acta Path. Microbiol. Scand.* 38, 47–57.

Kurihara, M., Shirakabe, H., Murakami, T., Yasui, A., Izumi, T., Sumida, M., and Igarashi, A. (1974) A New Method for Producing Adenocarcinomas in the Stomach of Dogs with N-Ethyl-N-Nitro-N-Nitrosoguanidine. *Gann* 65, 163–177.

Ladds, P. W., and Crane, C. K. (1976) Scrotal Mesothelioma in a Bull. *Aust. Vet. J.* 52, 534–535.

Ladds, P. W., and Webster, D. R. (1971) Pharyngeal Rhabdomyosarcoma in a Dog. *Vet. Path.* 8, 256–259.

Lahellec, M., and Jancourt, A. (1972) Étude clinique et histologique d'une tumeur carcinoide du grêle chez un chat. *Bull. Acad. Vét. Fr.* 45, 363–365.

Langham, R. F., Keahey, K. K., Mostosky, U. V., and Schirmer, R. G. (1965) Oral Adamantinomas in the Dog. *J. Amer. Vet. Med. Assoc.* 146, 474–480.

Langham, R. F., Mostosky, U. V., and Schirmer, R. G. (1969) Ameloblastic Odontoma in the Dog. *Amer. J. Vet. Res.* 30, 1873–1876.

———. (1977) X-Ray Therapy of Selected Odontogenic Neoplasms in the Dog. *J. Amer. Vet. Med. Assoc.* 170, 820–822.

Lawson, G. H., and Rowland, A. C. (1974) Intestinal

Adenomatosis in the Pig: A Bacteriological Study. *Res. Vet. Sci.* 17, 331–336.

Levinson, D. A., Hopwood, D., Morgan, R. G. H., Coghill, E., Milne, G. A., and Wormsley, K. G. (1979) Oesophageal Neoplasia in Male Wistar Rats due to Parenteral Di-(2-Hydroxyprophyl)-Nitrosamine. *J. Path.* 129, 31–36.

Lingeman, C. H., and Garner, F. M. (1972) Comparative Study of Intestinal Adenocarcinomas of Animals and Man. *J. Natl. Cancer Inst.* 48, 325–346.

Lingeman, C. H., Garner, F. M., and Taylor, D. O. N. (1971) Spontaneous Gastric Adenocarcinoma of Dogs: A Review. *J. Natl. Cancer Inst.* 47, 137–153.

Lomax, L. G., and Glock, R. D. (1982) Naturally Occurring Porcine Proliferative Enteritis: Pathologic and Bacteriologic Findings. *Amer. J. Vet. Res.* 43, 1608–1614.

Long, G. G., Leathers, C. W., Parish, S. M., and Breeze, R. G. (1981) Fibrotic Melanoma in a Calf. *Vet. Path.* 18, 402–404.

Lownie, J. F., Altini, M., Austin, J. C., and Le Roux, P. L. (1981) Verrucous Carcinoma Presenting in the Maxilla of a Dog. *J. Amer. Anim. Hosp. Assoc.* 17, 315–319.

Lucam, F., Tisseur, H., and Simintzis, G. (1944) Les Branchiomes. *Rev. Méd. Vét.* 95, 97–105.

MacVean, D. W., Monlux, A. W., Anderson, P. S., Silberg, S. C., and Roszel, J. F. (1978) Frequency of Canine and Feline Tumours in a Defined Population. *Vet. Path.* 15, 700–715.

Madewell, B. R., Stannard, A. A., Pulley, L. T., and Nelson, V. G. (1980) Oral Eosinophilic Granuloma in Siberian Husky Dogs. *J. Amer. Vet. Med. Assoc.* 177, 701–703.

Mason, B. J. E. (1974) Temporal Teratomata in the Horse. *Vet. Rec.* 95, 226–228.

Mason, T. A. (1978) Strangulation of the Rectum of a Horse by the Pedicle of a Mesenteric Lipoma. *Equine Vet. J.* 10, 269.

McCaw, D., Pratt, M., and Walshaw, R. (1980) Squamous Cell Carcinoma of the Oesophagus in a Dog. *J. Amer. Anim. Hosp. Assoc.* 16, 561–563.

McCrea, C. T., and Head, K. W. (1978) Sheep Tumours in North East Yorkshire. I. Prevalence on Seven Moorland Farms. *Brit. Vet. J.* 134, 454–461.

———. (1981) II. Experimental Production of Tumours. *Brit. Vet. J.* 137, 21–30.

McCullagh, K. G., Mews, A. R., and Pinsent, P. J. R. (1979) Diffuse Pleural Mesothelioma in a Goat. *Vet. Path.* 16, 119–121.

McDonald, J. W., and Leaver, D. D. (1965) Adenocarcinoma of the Small Intestine of Merino Sheep. *Aust. Vet. J.* 41, 269–271.

McGavin, M. D., and Fishburn, F. (1975) Perianal Adenoma of Apocrine Origin in a Dog. *J. Amer. Vet. Med. Assoc.* 166, 388–389.

Meagher, D. M., and Brown, M. P. (1978) Lymphoid Masses in the Pharynx of a Thoroughbred Filly. *Vet. Med. Small Anim. Clin.* 73, 171–174.

M'Fadyean, J. (1890) The Occurrence of Tumours in the Domesticated Animals. *J. Comp. Path. Therap.* 3, 41–42, 147–149.

M'Fadyean, J., and Hobday, F. (1898) Note on the Experimental Transmission of Warts in the Dog. *J. Comp. Path.* 11, 341–344.

Miller, A. (1961) The Mouth Parts and Digestive Tract of Adult Dung Beetles (Coleoptera-Scarabaeidae) with Reference to the Ingestion of Helminth Eggs. *J. Parasit.* 47, 735–742.

Misdorp, W. (1965) Tumors in Newborn Animals. *Path. Vet.* 2, 328–343.

———. (1967) Tumours in Large Domestic Animals in The Netherlands. *J. Comp. Path. Therap.* 77, 211–216.

Mohanty, J., Ojha, S. J., Mitra, A. K., and Rao, A. T. (1971) A Case of Adamantinoma in a Heifer. *Indian Vet. J.* 48, 99–101.

Moore, J. N., and Kintner, L. D. (1976) Recurrent Esophageal Obstruction Due to Squamous Cell Carcinoma in a Horse. *Cornell Vet.* 66, 590–597.

Murray, M. (1968) Incidence and Pathology of *Spirocerca lupi* in Kenya. *J. Comp. Path.* 78, 401–405.

Murray, M., Miller, H. R. P., and Jarrett, W. F. H. (1968) The Globule Leukocyte and its Derivation from the Subepithelial Mast Cell. *Lab. Invest.* 19, 222–234.

Murray, M., Robinson, P. B., McKeating, F. J., Baker, G. J., and Lauder, I. M. (1972*a*) Peptic Ulceration in the Dog: A Clinico-Pathological Study. *Vet. Rec.* 91, 441–447.

———. (1972*b*) Primary Gastric Neoplasia in the Dog: A Clinico-Pathological Study. *Vet. Rec.* 91, 474–479.

Nevalainen, T. J., and Jarvi, O. H. (1977) Ultrastructure of Intestinal and Diffuse Type Gastric Carcinoma. *J. Path.* 122, 129–136.

Norval, M., Head, K. W., Else, R. W., Hart, H., and Neill, W. A. (1981) Growth in Culture of Adenocarcinoma Cells from the Small Intestine of Sheep. *Brit. J. Exp. Path.* 62, 270–282.

Ochs, D. L., Irving, G. H., and Casey, H. W. (1978) Eosinophilic Granuloma in the Cat: Two Cases Involving the Tongue. *Vet. Med. Small Anim. Clin.* 73, 1275–1277.

Oota, K., and Sobin, L. H. (1977) Histological Typing of Gastric and Oesophageal Tumours. In: *International Histological Classification of Tumours,* No. 18. World Health Organization (Geneva).

Palminteri, A. (1966) The Surgical Management of Polyps of the Rectum and Colon of the Dog. *J. Amer. Vet. Med. Assoc.* 148, 771–777.

Pamukcu, A. M., Erturk, E., Yalciner, S., Milli, U., and Bryan, G. T. (1978) Carcinogenic and Mutagenic Activities of Milk from Cows Fed Bracken Fern (*Pteridium aquilinum*). *Cancer Res.* 38, 1556–1560.

Pamukcu, A. M., Göksoy, S. K., and Price, J. M. (1967) Urinary Bladder Neoplasms Induced by Feeding Bracken Fern (*Pteris aquilina*) to Cows. *Cancer Res.* 27, 917–924.

Patnaik, A. K., and Lieberman, P. H. (1980) Gastric Squamous Cell Carcinoma in a Dog. *Vet. Path.* 17, 250–253.

———. (1981) Canine Goblet-Cell Carcinoid. *Vet. Path.* 18, 410–413.

Patnaik, A. K., Hurvitz, A. I., and Johnson, G. F. (1977) Canine Gastrointestinal Neoplasms. *Vet. Path.* 14, 547–555.

———. (1978*a*) Canine Gastric Adenocarcinomas. *Vet. Path.* 15, 600–607.

———. (1980*a*) Canine Intestinal Adenocarcinoma and Carcinoid. *Vet. Path.* 17, 149–163.

Patnaik, A. K., Johnson, G. F., Greene, R. W., Hayes, A. A., and MacEwen, E. G. (1981) Surgical Resection of Intestinal Adenocarcinoma in a Cat, with Survival of 28 Months. *J. Amer. Vet. Med. Assoc.* 178, 479–481.

Patnaik, A. K., Lieberman, P. H., and Johnson, G. H. (1978*b*) Intestinal Ganglioneuroma in a Kitten—A Case Report and Review of Literature. *J. Small Anim. Pract.* 19, 735–742.

Patnaik, A. K., Liu, S-K., and Johnson, G. F. (1976) Feline Intestinal Adenocarcinoma. A Clinicopathologic Study of 22 Cases. *Vet. Path.* 13, 1–10.

Patnaik, A. K., Twedt, D. C., and Marretta, A. M. (1980*b*) Intestinal Mast Cell Tumour in a Dog. *J. Small Anim. Pract.* 21, 207–212.

Pearson, G. R., and Cawthorne, R. J. G. (1978) Intestinal Adenocarcinoma in a Ewe. *Vet. Rec.* 103, 409, 477.

Pearson, G. R., and McCaughey, W. J. (1978) Two Cases of Intestinal Adenocarcinoma in Aged Ewes. *N.Z. Vet. J.* 26, 123–124, 129.

Pearson, H. (1979) Pyloric Stenosis in the Dog. *Vet. Rec.* 105, 393–394.

Peter, C. P., and Kluge, J. P. (1970) An Ultra Structural Study of a Canine Rhabdomyosarcoma. *Cancer* 26, 1280–1288.

Pindborg, J. J., Kramer, I. R. H., and Torloni, H. (1971) Histologic Typing of Odontogenic Tumours, Jaw Cysts, and Allied Lesions. In: *International Histological Classification of Tumours,* No. 5. World Health Organization (Geneva).

Pirie, H. M. (1973) Unusual Occurrence of Squamous Carcinoma of the Upper Alimentary Tract in Cattle in Britain. *Res. Vet. Sci.* 15, 135–138.

Plowright, W., Linsell, C. A., and Peers, F. G. (1971) A Focus on Rumenal Cancer in Kenyan Cattle. *Brit. J. Cancer* 25, 72–80.

Plummer, P. J. G. (1956) A Survey of Six Hundred and Thirty-Six Tumours from Domesticated Animals. *Can. J. Comp. Med.* 20, 239–251.

Potter, K. A., Tucker, R. D., and Carpenter, J. L. (1980) Oral Eosinophilic Granuloma of Siberian Huskies. *J. Amer. Anim. Hosp. Assoc.* 16, 595–600.

Quigley, P. J., Leedale, A., and Dawson, I. M. P. (1972) Carcinoma of Mandible of Cat and Dog Simulating Osteosarcoma. *J. Comp. Path.* 82, 15–18.

Raflo, C. P., and Nuernberger, S. P. (1978) Abdominal Mesothelioma in a Cat. *Vet. Path.* 15, 781–783.

Ragland, W. L., and Gorham, J. R. (1967) Tonsillar Carcinoma in Rural Dogs. *Nature* 214, 925–926.

Rao, A. T., Nayak, B. C., and Choudary, C. (1972) A Case of Adamantinoma in a Newly Born Jersey Crossbred Male Calf. *Indian J. Anim. Sci.* 42, 353–354.

Ribelin, W. E., and Bailey, W. S. (1958) Esophageal Sarcomas Associated with *Spirocerca lupi* Infection in the Dog. *Cancer* 11, 1242–1246.

Ricketts, S. W., and Peace, C. K. (1976) A Case of Peritoneal Mesothelioma in a Thoroughbred Mare. *Equine Vet. J.* 8, 78–80.

Ridgway, R. L., and Suter, P. F. (1979) Clinical and Radiographic Signs in Primary and Metastatic Esophageal Neoplasms of the Dog. *J. Amer. Vet. Med. Assoc.* 174, 700–704.

Roberts, M. C., and Kelly, W. R. (1979) Squamous Cell Carcinoma of the Lower Cervical Oesophagus in a Pony. *Equine Vet J.* 11, 199–201.

Roberts, M. C., and Pinsent, P. J. N. (1975) Malabsorption in the Horse Associated with Alimentary Lymphosarcoma. *Equine Vet. J.* 7, 166–172.

Roberts, M. C., Groenendyk, S., and Kelly, W. R. (1978) Ameloblastic Odontoma in a Foal. *Equine Vet. J.* 10, 91–93.

Ross, A. D. (1980) Small Intestinal Carcinoma in Sheep. *Aust. Vet. J.* 56, 25–28.

Ross, A. D., and Baker, R. (1978) Gingival Hyperplasia Induced by Sodium Diphenylhydantoin in the Dog: A Case Report. *Vet. Med. Small Anim. Clin.* 73, 585–587.

Ross, A. D., and Day, W. A. (1979*a*) Some Ultrastructural Changes Associated with Sheep Intestinal Carcinoma. *N.Z. Med. J.* 90, 516.

———. (1979*b*) Intestinal Polyps in a Lamb. *N.Z. Vet. J.* 27, 172–173.

Rowland, A. C., and Lawson, G. H. K. (1975) Porcine Intestinal Adenomatosis: A Possible Relationship with Necrotic Enteritis, Regional Ileitis and Proliferative Haemorrhagic Enteropathy. *Vet. Rec.* 97, 178–180.

Rowland, A. C., and Rowntree, P. G. M. (1972) A Hemorrhagic Bowel Syndrome Associated with Intestinal Adenomatosis in the Pig. *Vet. Rec.* 91, 235–241.

Rowland, A. C., Lawson, G. H. K., and Maxwell, A. (1973) Intestinal Adenomatosis in the Pig: Occurrence of a Bacterium in Affected Cells. *Nature* 243, 417.

Saidu, S. N. A., and Chineme, C. N. (1979) Intestinal Leiomyoma in a Cow. *Vet. Rec.* 104, 388–389.

Sautter, J. H., and Hanlon, G. F. (1975) Gastric Neoplasms in the Dog: A Report of 20 Cases. *J. Amer. Vet. Med. Assoc.* 166, 691–696.

Schaffer, E., and Schiefer, B. (1968) Incidence and Types of Canine Rectal Carcinomas. *J. Small Anim. Pract.* 9, 491–496.

Schneck, G. W. (1975*a*) A Case of Giant Cell Epulis (Osteoclastoma) in a Cat. *Vet. Rec.* 97, 181–182.

———. (1975*b*) Eosinophiles Granulom bei einer Katze. *Dtsch. Teirärztl. Wschr.* 83, 162–163.

Schoental, R., and Joffe, A. Z. (1974) Lesions Induced in Rodents by Extracts from Cultures of *Fusarium poae* and *F. sporotrichioides. J. Path.* 112, 37–42.

Schonbauer, M., and Kohler, H. (1981) Calcinosis in Horse Jointly Occurring with Lymphatic Leucosis of the Small Intestine and the Mesenteric Lymph Nodes. *Zbl. Vet. Med.* 28A, 742–749.

Schutte, K. H. (1968) Esophageal Tumours in Sheep:

Some Ecological Observations. *J. Natl. Cancer Inst.* 41, 821–824.

Schwabe, C. W. (1955) Helminth Parasites and Neoplasia. *Amer. J. Vet. Res.* 16, 485–488.

Scott, D. W. (1975) Observations on the Eosinophilic Granuloma Complex in Cats. *J. Amer. Anim. Hosp. Assoc.* 11, 261–270.

Seffner, W., and Fritzsch, R. (1964) Uber gehäuftes Auftreten von Pleuramesotheliomen bei Schweinen. *Arch. Exp. Vet. Med.* 18, 1395–1405.

Seibold, H. R. (1974) Juvenile Alveolar Rhabdomyosarcoma in a Dog. *Vet. Path.* 11, 558–560.

Seibold, H. R., Bailey, W. S., Hoerlein, B. F., Jordan, E. M., and Schwabe, C. W. (1955) Observations on the Possible Relation of Malignant Esophageal Tumours and *Spirocerca lupi* Lesions in the Dog. *Amer. J. Vet. Res.* 16, 5–14.

Seiler, R. J. (1979) Colorectal Polyps of the Dog: A Clinicopathologic Study of 17 Cases. *J. Amer. Vet. Med. Assoc.* 174, 72–75.

Sheahan, B. J., and Donnelly, W. J. C. (1981) Vascular Hamartomas in the Gingiva of Two Calves. *Vet. Path.* 18, 562–564.

Shefstad, D. K. (1978) Scanning Electron Microscopy of Gasterophilus Intestinalis Lesions of the Equine Stomach. *J. Amer. Vet. Med. Assoc.* 172, 310–313.

Shimosato, Y., Tanaka, N., Kogure, K., Fujimura, S., Kawachi, T., and Sugimura, T. (1971) Histopathology of Tumours of Canine Alimentary Tract Produced by N-Methyl-N'-Nitro-N-nitrosoguanidine, with Particular Reference to Gastric Carcinomas. *J. Natl. Cancer Inst.* 47, 1053–1070.

Silverberg, S. G. (1971) Carcinoma Arising in Adenomatous Polyps of the Rectum in a Dog. *Dis. Colon Rectum* 14, 191–194.

Simpson, B. H., and Jolly, R. D. (1974) Carcinoma of the Small Intestine in Sheep. *J. Path.* 112, 83–92.

Simu, G., Ivascu, I., and Simu, G. (1975) A Bovine Ameloblastic Tumour with Peculiar Stromal Pattern Suggesting a Predentinic Ameloblastoma. *Zbl. Vet. Med.* 11A, 791–796.

Sinclair, C. J., Jones, B. R., and Verkerk, G. (1979) Gastric Carcinoma in a Bitch. *N.Z. Vet. J.* 27, 16–18.

Singleton, W. B. (1956) An Unusual Neoplasia in a Dog (a Probable Neurilemoma of the Caecum). *Vet. Rec.* 68, 1046–1047.

Spreull, J. S. A., and Head, K. W. (1967) Cervical Salivary Cysts in the Dog. *J. Small Anim. Pract.* 8, 17–35.

Stackhouse, L. L., Moore, J. J., and Hylton, W. E. (1978) Salivary Gland Adenocarcinoma in a Mare. *J. Amer. Vet. Med. Assoc.* 172, 271–273.

Stambaugh, J. E., Harvey, C. E., and Goldschmidt, M. H. (1978) Lymphangioma in Four Dogs. *J. Amer. Vet. Med. Assoc.* 173, 759–761.

Stavrou, D., Dahme, E., and Kalich, J. (1976) Induction of Tumours of the Stomach in Miniature Swine by the Administration of Methylnitrosourea. *Res. Exp. Med.* 169, 33–43.

Strafuss, A. C., and Bozarth, A. J. (1973) Liposarcoma in Dogs. *J. Amer. Anim. Hosp. Assoc.* 9, 183–187.

Strande, A., Sommers, S. C., and Petrak, M. (1954) Regional Enterocolitis in Cocker Spaniel Dogs. *Arch. Path.* 57, 357–362.

Straub, R., von Tscharner, C., Pauli, B., Lazary, S., and Schatzmann, U. (1974) Pleuramesotheliom bei einem Pferd. *Schweiz. Arch. Tierheilk.* 116, 207–211.

Stünzi, H., and Ammann-Mann, M. (1973) Nicht-traumatische Rupturen des Herzvorhofs beim Hund. *Zbl. Vet. Med.* 20, 409–418.

Stünzi, H., and Rusterholz, P. (1958) Zür Klinik und pathologischen Anatomie des Tonsilenkarzinomas beim Hund. *Schweiz. Arch. Tierheilk.* 100, 271–277.

Summers, P. M., Wells, K. E., and Adkins, K. F. (1979) Ossifying Ameloblastoma in a Horse. *Aust. Vet. J.* 55, 498–500.

Sundberg, J. P., Burnstein, T., Page, E. H., Kirkham, W. W., and Robinson, F. R. (1977) Neoplasms of Equidae. *J. Amer. Vet. Med. Assoc.* 170, 150–152.

Sykes, G. P., and Cooper, B. J. (1982) Canine Intestinal Carcinoids. *Vet. Path.* 19, 120–131.

Tennant, B., Keirn, D. R., White, K. K., Bentinck-Smith, J., and King, J. M. (1982) Six Cases of Squamous Cell Carcinoma of the Stomach of the Horse. *Equine Vet. J.* 14, 238–243.

Thackray, A. C., and Sobin, L. H. (1972) Histological Typing of Salivary Gland Tumours. In: *International Histological Classification of Tumours*, No. 7. World Health Organization (Geneva).

Thorsen, J., Cooper, J. E., and Warwick, G. P. (1974) Esophageal Papillomata in Cattle in Kenya. *Trop. Anim. Hlth. Prod.* 6, 95–98.

Thrall, D. E. (1981) Orthovoltage Radiotherapy of Oral Fibrosarcomas in Dogs. *J. Amer. Vet. Med. Assoc.* 179, 159–162.

Thrall, D. E., and Goldschmidt, M. H. (1978) Mesothelioma in the Dog: Six Case Reports. *J. Amer. Vet. Radiol. Soc.* 19, 107–115.

Thrall, D. E., Goldschmidt, M. H., and Biery, D. N. (1981) Malignant Tumour Formation at the Site of Previously Irradiated Acanthomatous Epulides in Four Dogs. *J. Amer. Vet. Med. Assoc.* 178, 127–132.

Thrasher, J. P., Ichinose, H., and Pitot, H. G. (1963) Osteogenic Sarcoma of the Canine Esophagus Associated with *Spirocerca lupi* Infection. *Amer. J. Vet. Res.* 24, 808–818.

Tilley, L. P., Owens, J. M., Wilkins, R. J., and Patnaik, A. K. (1975) Pericardial Mesothelioma with Effusion in a Cat. *J. Amer. Anim. Hosp. Assoc.* 11, 60–65.

Todoroff, R. I., and Brodey, R. S. (1979) Oral and Pharyngeal Neoplasia in the Dog: A Retrospective Study of 361 Cases. *J. Amer. Vet. Med. Assoc.* 175, 567–571.

Tomlinson, M. J., McKeever, P. J., and Nordine, R. A. (1982) Colonic Adenocarcinoma with Cutaneous Metastasis in a Dog. *J. Amer. Vet. Med. Assoc.* 180, 1344–1345.

Tontis, A. (1982) Signet-Ring Cell Carcinoma in the

Small Intestine of Sheep. *Schweiz. Arch. Tierheilk.* 124, 359–362.

Tontis, A., and Luginbuhl, H. (1976) Plattenepithelkarzinom am Zahnfleisch eines Rindes. *Schweiz. Arch. Tierheilk.* 118, 535–537.

Tontis, A., Schatzmann, H., and Luginbuhl, H. (1976) Colloid Carcinoma in the Jejunum of a Cow. Surgery, Pathology and Course. *Schweiz. Arch. Tierheilk.* 118, 535–537, 543–545.

Trigo, F. J., Morrison, W. B., and Breeze, R. G. (1981) An Ultrastructural Study of Canine Mesothelioma. *J. Comp. Path.* 91, 531–537.

Turk, J. R., and Leathers, C. W. (1981) Light and Electron Microscope Study of the Large Pale Cell in a Canine Malignant Melanoma. *Vet. Path.* 18, 829–832.

Turk, M. A. M., Gallina, A. M., and Russell, T. S. (1981) Non-Hematopoietic Gastrointestinal Neoplasia in Cats: A Retrospective Study of 44 Cases. *Vet. Path.* 18, 614–620.

Turner, C. B. (1974) An Oral Papilloma in a Young Calf. *Vet. Rec.* 95, 367–369.

Vandenberghe, J., and Marsboom, R. (1982) Campylobacter-like Bacteria in Adenocarcinoma of the Colon in Two Wistar Rats. *Vet. Rec.* 111, 416–417.

van der Gaag, I., Happé, R. P., and Wolvekamp, W. (1976) A Boxer Dog with Chronic Hypertrophic Gastritis Resembling Menetrier's Disease in Man. *Vet. Path.* 13, 172–185.

van der Gaag, I., Van Toorenburg, J., Voorhout, G., Happé, R. P., and Aalfs, R. H. G. (1978) Histiocytic Ulcerative Colitis in a French Bulldog. *J. Small Anim. Pract.* 19, 283–290.

van Kruiningen, H. J. (1977), Giant Hypertrophic Gastritis of Basenji Dogs. *Vet. Path.* 14, 19–28.

van Kruiningen, H. J., and Dobbins, W. O. (1979) Feline Histiocytic Colitis. A Case Report with Electron Microscopy. *Vet. Path.* 16, 215–222.

van Kruiningen, H. J., Montali, R. J., Strandberg, J. D., and Kirk, R. W. (1965). A Granulomatous Colitis of Dogs with Histologic Resemblance to Whipple's Disease. *Path. Vet.* 2, 521–544.

van Ooijen, P. G. (1978) Exfoliative Cytology in the Diagnosis of a Diffuse Mesothelioma in the Dog. *T. Diergeneesk.* 103, 1116–1120.

Vanselow, B. A., Spradbrow, P. B., and Jackson, A. R. B. (1982) Papilloma Viruses, Papillomas and Squamous Cell Carcinomas in Sheep. *Vet. Rec.* 110, 561–562.

Vernon, F. F., and Roudebush, P. (1980) Primary Esophageal Carcinoma in a Cat. *J. Amer. Anim. Hosp. Assoc.* 16, 547–550.

Vitovec, J. (1977) Carcinomas of the Intestine in Cattle and Pigs. *Zbl. Vet. Med.* 24A, 413–421.

Wagner, J. C., Berry, G., and Pody, F. D. (1980) Carcinogenesis and Mineral Fibres. *Brit. Med. Bull.* 36, 53–56.

Wandera, J. G. (1976) Further Observations on Canine Spirocercosis in Kenya. *Vet. Rec.* 99, 348–351.

Watrach, A. M., Small, E., and Case, M. T. (1971) Ca-

nine Papilloma: Progression of Oral Papilloma to Carcinoma. *J. Natl. Cancer Inst.* 45, 915–920.

Weiss, E., and Frese, K. (1974) International Histological Classification of Tumours of Domestic Animals. VII. Tumours of the Skin. *Bull. Wld. Hlth. Org.* 50, 79–100.

Weller, R. E., and Hornof, W. J. (1979) Gastric Malignant Lymphoma in Two Cats. *Mod. Vet. Pract.* 60, 701–704.

Wells, G. A. H., and Robinson, M. (1975) Mixed Tumour of Salivary Gland Showing Histological Evidence of Malignancy in a Cat. *J. Comp. Path.* 85, 77–85.

Werner, R. E., Jr. (1981) Canine Oral Neoplasia: A Review of 19 Cases. *J. Amer. Anim. Hosp. Assoc.* 17, 67–70.

Wester, P. W., Franken, P., and Hani, H. I. (1980) Squamous Cell Carcinoma of the Equine Stomach. A Report of 7 Cases. *Vet. Q.* 2, 95–103.

Whitaker, D., Papadimitriou, M., and Walters, M. N.-I. (1982) The Mesothelium: A Cytochemical Study of "Activated" Mesothelial Cells. *J. Path.* 136, 169–179.

Wilkinson, G. T. (1970) Chronic Papillomatous Oesophagitis in a Young Cat. *Vet. Rec.* 87, 355–356.

Willemse, A., and Lubberink, A. A. M. E. (1978) Cryosurgery of Eosinophilic Ulcers in Cats. *T. Diergeneesk.* 103, 1052–1056.

Williams, E. D., Siebenmann, R. E., and Sobin, L. H. (1980) Histological Typing of Endocrine Tumours. In: *International Histological Classification of Tumours,* No. 23. World Health Organization (Geneva).

Willis, R. A. (1948) *Pathology of Tumours.* Butterworth & Co. (London).

———. (1967) *Pathology of Tumours.* 4th ed. Butterworth & Co. (London).

Wiseman, A., Breeze, R. G., and Pirie, H. M. (1977) Melanotic Neuro-Ectodermal Tumour of Infancy (Melanotic Progonoma) in Two Calves. *Vet. Rec.* 101, 264–266.

Withers, F. W. (1938) Squamous-Celled Carcinoma of the Tonsils in the Dog. *J. Path. Bact.* 49, 429–432.

World Health Organization. (1978) Consultation on the Biological Behaviour and Therapy of Tumours of Domestic Animals. VPH/CMO/78.15 (Geneva).

Young, P. L. (1978) Squamous Cell Carcinoma of the Tongue of the Cat. *Aust. Vet. J.* 54, 133–134.

Zontine, W. J., Meierhenry, F., and Hicks, R. F. (1977) Perforated Duodenal Ulcer Associated with Mastocytoma in a Dog. A Case Report. *J. Amer. Vet. Radiol. Soc.* 18, 162–165.

## 9

*James A. Popp*
# Tumors of the Liver, Gall Bladder, and Pancreas

## TUMORS OF THE LIVER

### Hepatocellular Carcinoma

**Incidence.** Hepatocellular carcinoma has been identified in numerous species, including dogs (MacVean *et al.*, 1978; Mulligan, 1949*b;* Patnaik *et al.*, 1980, 1981*a;* Rooney, 1959; Strombeck, 1978; Trigo *et al.*, 1982), cats (Patnaik *et al.*, 1975), cows (Monlux *et al.*, 1956; Kithier *et al.*, 1974), sheep (Anderson and Sandison, 1967; Monlux *et al.*, 1956), pigs (Anderson and Sandison, 1967; Ramachandran *et al.*, 1970), fowl (Campbell, 1949, 1969; Omata *et al.*, 1983; Wadsworth *et al.*, 1978), woodchucks (Snyder *et al.*, 1982), and trout (Sinnhuber *et al.*, 1977). The precise incidence in the various species and a comparison of incidence among species are not available because the incidence data reported in the literature are based on a selected population such as that from a single, small geographical area. In addition, the literature does not always distinguish hepatocellular carcinoma from hepatocellular adenoma. However, information from abattoirs in the United Kingdom indicates that hepatocellular and biliary neoplasms are 4 times more common in cattle than sheep and nearly 18 times more common in cattle than pigs (Anderson and Sandison, 1967). These authors also reported that hepatic and biliary neoplasms account for 10%, 31%, and 4% of all neoplasms in cattle, sheep, and pigs, respectively. Several reports of large series of these carcinomas in dogs (Mulligan, 1949*b;*Patnaik *et al.*, 1980, 1981*a, b;* Rooney, 1959) suggest that

dogs may have a high incidence compared with other domestic species, although such reports may simply reflect a disproportionate interest in neoplasms of dogs. The incidence of the carcinoma in dogs has been reported as 1.6 per 100,000 dogs (MacVean *et al.*, 1978). An incidence of less than 1% of all neoplasms of dogs was reported by Bastianello (1983).

Hepatocellular carcinoma has been reported to be both more common (Mulligan, 1949*b;* Patnaik *et al.*, 1980) and less common (Bastianello, 1983; Rooney, 1959) than cholangiocarcinoma in dogs. On the basis of a very small number of cases, hepatocellular carcinoma in cats appears to be more common than cholangiocarcinoma (Patnaik *et al.*, 1975).

The age distribution of animals with this neoplasm is apparently variable from species to species. The average age of affected dogs is 10 to 11 years, although the neoplasm has been reported in animals as young as 4 years of age (Patnaik *et al.*, 1980; Rooney, 1959). In contrast to dogs, in which hepatocellular carcinoma is found in older animals, this neoplasm has been reported in sheep less than 1 year of age (Anderson and Sandison, 1967; Monlux *et al.*, 1956) and in pigs less than 6 months of age (Anderson and Sandison, 1967). Since this information is derived from abattoir data, the complete age distribution of pigs, sheep, and cattle with the carcinoma is not known. In dogs, the neoplasm is more frequent in males than in females (Patnaik *et al.*, 1981*a*). No breed predilection has been identified for this neoplasm in dogs (Patnaik *et al.*, 1980) or any other species of domestic animals. Both species and strain differences in the incidence of hepatic neoplasms have been well documented in laboratory rodents.

**Clinical Characteristics.** Dogs with hepatocellular carcinoma may have nonspecific clinical signs including anorexia, vomiting, ascites, lethargy, and weakness (Mulligan, 1949b; Patnaik et al., 1980; Strombeck, 1978; Trigo et al., 1982). Less frequently, affected dogs have jaundice, weight loss, and diarrhea. Hepatomegaly is a common feature with this neoplasm. Abdominal enlargement and a palpable abdominal mass are more readily detected with hepatocellular carcinoma than with cholangiocarcinoma (Trigo et al., 1982). Seizures may sometimes be due to hepatoencephalopathy (Patnaik et al., 1980; Strombeck, 1978).

Abnormalities in clinical laboratory parameters are common in dogs with hepatocellular carcinoma (Patnaik et al., 1980; Strombeck, 1978; Trigo et al., 1982). Most affected animals have elevations in serum concentrations of alkaline B-phosphatase, asparate amino transferase, and alanine amino transferase. Total bilirubin and serum lactic dehydrogenase are elevated in a few affected animals. Hypoglycemia is occasionally found. The clinical pathology alterations are simply indicative of hepatic disease and do not aid in differentiating this carcinoma from other primary hepatic neoplasms, including cholangiocarcinoma.

Hematological changes are seen in slightly over half of the dogs reported to have this carcinoma (Patnaik et al., 1980). Red blood cell counts are decreased, and total white blood cell counts are elevated when alterations are noted.

Inadequate information is available on the clinical signs associated with this carcinoma in species other than dogs.

**Gross Morphology.** Hepatocellular carcinomas vary from small, round, discrete lesions several centimeters in diameter to large diffuse masses that may be greater than 10 cm in diameter (Monlux et al., 1956; Mulligan, 1949b; Patnaik et al., 1981a; Rooney, 1959). The larger lesions usually have an irregular to multinodular surface and an irregular shape; they are never umbilicated. Smaller lesions are more likely to be spherical or oval in shape, similar to benign neoplasms of hepatocellular origin. The carcinoma frequently protrudes above the surface of the liver. The edge of the lesion is usually grossly identifiable, even when the lesion is large and of irregular size and shape. Adhesions may be observed between the neoplasm and the diaphram or other adjacent structures (Trigo et al., 1982).

The color and consistency are extremely variable between tumors as well as within a single tumor (Patnaik et al., 1981a; Rooney, 1959; Trigo et al., 1982). The smaller growths usually resemble normal liver. The larger growths have a mottled appearance with some areas resembling normal liver, while other areas are light tan to gray in color. In some instances, the entire neoplasm will be light tan to light yellow because of lipid infiltration of the neoplastic hepatocytes. In the larger neoplasms, dark red areas are due to hemorrhage secondary to necrosis. Nonhemorrhagic necrotic areas are light gray to white in color and are most frequently found toward the center of the neoplasm. The carcinoma is usually soft and friable; this feature aids in distinguishing the tumor from cholangiocarcinoma, which has a firm consistency. Because of the friable nature of this carcinoma, rupture of the surface results in hemoperitoneum or blood clots on the capsular surface of the neoplasm.

Hepatocellular carcinoma is found in any lobe of the dog liver, although it is most common in the left lateral lobe (Patnaik et al., 1980). The reason for this preferential location is unknown. Neoplasms may be found in more than one liver lobe due to multiple primary lesions or to intrahepatic metastasis of a single neoplasm.

**Histological Features.** The histological appearance of the neoplasm varies depending on either the degree of differentiation of the individual hepatocytes or the histological arrangement of the cells (Patnaik et al., 1981a; Ponomarkov and Mackey, 1976; Trigo et al., 1982). This wide spectrum of histological appearance has led to a proposed classification system for the carcinoma (Patnaik et al., 1981a). In the more differentiated neoplasms, the histological arrangement and cytology bear a close resemblance to normal liver (fig. 9.1). The neoplastic cells form thin cords, but they may appear as thickened trabeculae. It is not unusual to find a cord of neoplastic hepatocytes that is 5 to 10 cells thick and occasionally as much as 20 cells thick. Necrosis may be found in the center of the wide trabeculae.

Although the trabecular pattern is probably the most common histological form of the tumor in domestic animals, numerous other patterns have been recognized (Rooney, 1959). The neoplastic cells can form pseudoglandular structures or solid sheets with no apparent pattern. In other cases, the neoplasm has widely dilated sinusoids that separate trabeculae of tumor cells, or irregular clusters of cells. In a minority of neoplasms, thin strands of connective tissue separate clusters of neoplastic cells. These histological patterns are not mutually exclusive; several different patterns may be identified within a single neoplasm. Cystic spaces can be found in the various histological types of the neoplasm, but are most common in the neoplasm having a pseudoglandular pattern.

The cytology is also variable in hepatocellular carcinoma (Patnaik *et al.*, 1981*a;* Ponomarkov and Mackey, 1976; Rooney, 1959; Trigo *et al.,* 1982). The cells of the well-differentiated carcinoma strongly resemble normal hepatocytes, with central, round nuclei and usually moderately eosinophilic cytoplasm (fig. 9.1). The cytoplasm, however, may be pale staining or even vacuolated if filled with glycogen or lipid. Bile pigment is occasionally found in the neoplastic hepatocytes (Rooney, 1959). At the other end of the spectrum, the undifferentiated neoplasm has very pleomorphic cells that are not readily recognized as hepatocytic in origin (fig. 9.2). The nuclei of these cells are variable in both size and shape; it is not unusual for the nuclei to vary in diameter by threefold. The cytoplasm of the cells is generally basophilic and greatly reduced in volume, resulting in an obviously increased nuclear to cytoplasmic ratio. The neoplastic cell often lacks the square shape of the sectioned normal hepatocyte. The cells may assume a round shape or rarely a

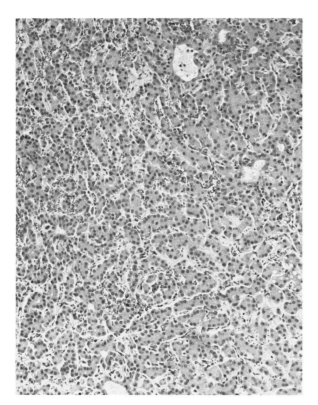

**FIGURE 9.1.** Hepatocellular carcinoma of the dog having a trabecular pattern. Note the well-differentiated hepatocytes forming abnormally thickened and irregular cords. (Courtesy of Dr. A. K. Patnaik and *Vet. Path.*)

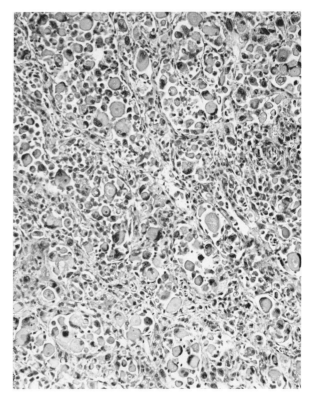

**FIGURE 9.2.** Hepatocellular carcinoma of the dog composed of anaplastic cells. (Courtesy of Dr. A. K. Patnaik and *Vet. Path.*)

spindle shape. Nucleoli tend to be enlarged in most cells irrespective of the general state of differentiation. Individual giant cells are sometimes found in the undifferentiated neoplasms. Mitotic figures occur more often in the carcinoma than in the corresponding benign neoplasm, but they are relatively rare in differentiated carcinoma.

Some rare carcinomas have the histological and cytological characteristics of both hepatocellular carcinoma and cholangiocarcinoma (Campbell, 1949; Patnaik *et al.*, 1981*a*). In some cases, these carcinomas appear to have arisen as single masses, but in others they arise as independent neoplasms that have merged through mutual invasion. In either case, such tumors with clear hepatocellular and bile ductular components are best designated as "hepatocholangiocarcinoma," although they are also referred to as "combined hepatocellular and cholangiocarcinoma."

Special techniques have been used to characterize spontaneously occurring hepatocellular carcinoma in animals. Ultrastructural studies of the tumor from pigs (Ito *et al.*, 1972) have not been helpful in diagnosing this lesion. α-Fetoprotein was found in the serum of two out of four cases of spontaneous hepatocellular carcinoma in cows (Kithier *et al.*, 1974). These results in cattle parallel those in humans and laboratory rodents in which α-fetoprotein is found in the serum of some but not all individuals with the neoplasm.

The nonneoplastic liver tissue is usually histologically normal in animals with hepatocellular carcinoma. In contrast to humans, cirrhosis is rarely found in the livers of dogs (Patnaik *et al.*, 1981*a*) or cows (Monlux *et al.*, 1956) with this carcinoma. Cirrhosis and chronic inflammation are associated with the carcinoma in ducks (Omata *et al.*, 1983) and woodchucks (Snyder *et al.*, 1982), both of which also have hepatitis virus in the neoplasm. Cirrhosis is also associated with chemically induced hepatocellular carcinoma in pigs (Graw and Berg, 1977; Shalkop and Armbrecht, 1974).

A diagnosis of this carcinoma is based on first finding histological evidence that the growth is of hepatocytic origin. While hepatocytic characteristics are easy to recognize in the more differentiated neoplasms, this distinction is often difficult in the less well-differentiated tumors. Fortunately, most neoplasms will have at least some areas with hepa-

tocellular characteristics. The distinction between well-differentiated hepatocellular carcinoma and hepatocellular adenoma is also difficult (Ponomarkov and Mackey, 1976). When tumor cell invasion is lacking, the diagnosis is based on the degree of cytological alteration.

Difficulty may also arise in distinguishing hepatocellular carcinoma with a pseudoglandular pattern from cholangiocarcinoma. In this case, a distinction can be made by examining the cytological characteristics as well as the general histological pattern. In addition, the cholangiocarcinoma usually has an extensive collagenous stroma. Hepatocellular carcinoma must also be distinguished from primary hepatic carcinoid. This is done on the basis of histological appearance and the use of silver impregnation stains that demonstrate secretory granules in carcinoid cells (Patnaik *et al.*, 1981*c*; Ponomarkov and Mackey, 1976).

Metastatic neoplasms from other organs are easily distinguished from primary hepatocellular carcinoma with the exception of metastatic endocrine neoplasms. The multiplicity of metastatic sites in endocrine carcinoma is helpful in differential diagnosis.

**Growth and Metastasis.** Hepatocellular carcinoma progressively invades the adjacent hepatic tissue. Invasion tends to occur by clusters of neoplastic cells and rarely as individual neoplastic cells; it does not occur uniformly around the periphery of the neoplasm, but may occur only in a few areas. This feature necessitates examining multiple sections of questionably malignant tumors. Invasion of blood vessels and lymphatics occurs, but is rarely obvious within a single lesion; thus it should not be considered a necessary requirement for diagnosis of malignancy in the neoplasm. Vascular invasion is more common than lymphatic invasion.

Metastasis occurs most commonly in the lung and hepatic lymph nodes (Patnaik *et al.*, 1981*a*; Ponomarkov and Mackey, 1976). While the local lymph nodes may contain metastatic neoplastic cells, they are rarely massively enlarged. Metastatic sites in the lung are usually numerous and relatively small. The earliest metastatic foci are located in the capillaries of the alveolar wall indicating a hematogenous spread. The carcinoma is also known to occasionally metastasize to the heart, spleen, kidney, intestine, brain, and ovary via the vascular system

(Campbell, 1949, 1969; Patnaik *et al.*, 1981*a*; Rooney, 1959). The neoplasm also spreads by direct extension to the omentum and peritoneum (Rooney, 1959; Shalkop and Armbrecht, 1974; Trigo *et al.*, 1982). This occurs when neoplastic cells from a friable neoplasm are dispersed within the peritoneal cavity after rupture of the primary tumor. The anaplastic and pleomorphic neoplasms tend to metastasize more often than the more differentiated neoplasms (Patnaik *et al.*, 1981*a*). The metastatic rate for hepatocellular carcinomas in dogs is 61% (Patnaik *et al.*, 1981*a*).

Metastasis generally occurs late in the course of neoplastic development. In general, the primary neoplasm is large while the metastases are small. Therefore, the resulting debilitation of the affected animal is usually due to the primary neoplasm and not to the metastasis.

**Etiology.** The etiology of the spontaneously occurring carcinoma in domestic animals is generally unknown. However, studies on the etiology of the human tumor and information from experimental studies in both laboratory and domestic animals would suggest either a viral or chemical etiology. A viral etiology has been proposed for humans (Blumberg and London, 1981), woodchucks (Snyder *et al.*, 1982), and ducks (Omata *et al.*, 1983). In each case, there is a correlation between the presence of a hepatitis virus and the carcinoma.

Extensive information is available concerning a chemical etiology for this neoplasm. Several chemicals experimentally cause the carcinoma in common domestic animals (Allison *et al.*, 1950; Graw and Berg, 1977; Hirao *et al.*, 1974; Shalkop and Armbrecht, 1974; Stula *et al.*, 1978) and in trout (Sinnhuber *et al.*, 1977). While some of these chemicals probably do not pose a threat to domestic animals because of the lack of naturally occurring exposure, aflatoxin and nitrosamines are common in the environment and are potential causes of the carcinoma in domestic animals. Exposure, albeit to low doses, can occur through the ingestion of feeds contaminated with these chemicals. These carcinogens are potent as shown by the fact that pigs can develop hepatocellular carcinoma after being fed diets containing aflatoxin at a concentration of 1 ppm (Shalkop and Armbrecht, 1974) or given diethylnitrosamine at a daily dose of 0.4 mg/kg body weight (Graw and Berg, 1977). Dogs given diethylnitrosamine in drinking water at the rate of 50, 100, or 500 ppm develop a variety of hepatic neoplasms including hepatocellular carcinomas (Hirao *et al.*, 1974).

## Hepatocellular Adenoma

**Incidence.** Hepatocellular adenoma has been reported in dogs (Allison *et al.*, 1950; Dagle *et al.*, 1984; Trigo *et al.*, 1982), cattle (Anderson and Sandison, 1967), sheep (Anderson and Sandison, 1967; Monlux *et al.*, 1956), pigs (Anderson and Sandison, 1967; Graw and Berg, 1977; Shalkop and Armbrecht, 1974), and fowl (Wadsworth *et al.*, 1978). The distinction between benign and malignant neoplasms of hepatocytic origin has not been made in all of these reports. While this neoplasm is found in a wide range of species, it is relatively uncommon as a spontaneous neoplasm in domestic animals. The lack of reported benign lesions of hepatocellular origin in two surveys (Bastianello, 1983; MacVean *et al.*, 1978) and the low incidence of benign versus malignant neoplasms in an additional survey (Trigo *et al.*, 1982) indicate that hepatocellular adenoma is less common than hepatocellular carcinoma in dogs. Information on sex and breed incidence of the adenoma is unavailable because of the limited number of reports and the frequent lack of distinction between benign and malignant neoplasms. Although the adenoma is generally found in older animals, it has also been reported in young lambs and pigs (Anderson and Sandison, 1967).

**Clinical Characteristics.** Because of the relatively small size and lack of spread of adenoma, it is usually not clinically apparent. Most single lesions are recognized as incidental findings at necropsy. When the neoplasm is found in conjunction with severe or chronic liver disease, the clinical course is dictated by the related liver disease and not by the neoplasm.

**Gross Morphology.** The adenoma may be single or multiple. When multiple, it is usually associated with chronic liver disease, which may result in chronic fibrosis and nodular hyperplasia. Whether single or multiple, the adenoma is an obvious proliferative growth that may either protrude above the surface of the liver or compress the surrounding liver if located deep. The tumor is usually not encapsulated. It ranges in size from a few millimeters to several centimeters in diameter. The color of an individual lesion is consistent throughout, but may vary from the dark red color of normal liver to light tan or white. The lighter color of some lesions is due to the intracellular accumulation of lipid. Hepatocellular adenoma is rarely hemorrhagic. Most benign hepatocellular tumors have a normal liver consistency, although the lipid-filled lesions may be soft and friable like any other lipid-containing hepatic tissue. Fibrosis is not found in the adenoma, thus it never has a firm consistency. The tumor is generally spherical in shape since it grows by simple expansion in all directions.

The gross morphology of the adenoma is similar in all animals including domestic animals and laboratory rodents and in humans, although it is well established that animals exhibit different hepatic reactions to varius toxic agents.

**Histological Features.** Hepatocellular adenoma is characterized by a uniform histological appearance throughout the lesion, although the appearance of one mass may be slightly different from another in the same liver. In all cases, the adenoma is clearly demarcated from the surrounding liver, although it is not encapsulated. In a few adenomas a pseudocapsule may be formed by aggregation of normal hepatic connective tissue framework as the lesion expands and adjacent hepatocytes become necrotic from compression. Normal hepatocytes at the edge of the tumor are frequently atrophic and may have a variety of nonspecific degenerative changes. Also, the normal lobular architecture of the adjacent liver tissue is disrupted by the compression.

Within the adenoma, cords of hepatocytes are irregular or inapparent due to collapse of sinusoidal spaces. When cords of neoplastic hepatocytes are seen, they will usually be perpendicular to the edge of the neoplasm where they tend to accentuate the border. In contrast to the single-cell thickness of the cords of hepatocytes in the normal liver, the cords in the adenoma are often 2 to 3 cells thick (Ponomarkov and Mackey, 1976). Massively thickened cords 5 to 10 cells thick as in malignant neoplasms, however, are not present in benign tumors.

Cytological characteristics of the benign neoplastic cells clearly indicate a hepatocellular origin, although the morphology does not completely resemble normal liver. Typically, the cells are near normal in size and contain a moderate amount of eosinophilic cytoplasm and a central nucleus. The cytoplasm may be slightly more basophilic or vacuolated than that in normal hepatocytes. When vacuolated, the cytoplasm usually contains an excess of lipid or glycogen (Anderson and Sandison, 1967; Ponomarkov and Mackey, 1976). Special stains to determine the composition of the cytoplasmic material do not help in establishing a diagnosis. The nuclei are slightly hyperchromatic and variable in size. The nucleoli, when observed, are enlarged and reflect the enhanced metabolic activity of the proliferating cell population. Mitotic figures are seen but are not numerous.

Because of the differentiated state of the benign hepatocellular neoplastic cells, it is easy to distinguish them from cells of other benign neoplasms of the liver. The major differential diagnostic problem is distinguishing hepatocellular adenoma from hepatocellular carcinoma and from nodular hyperplasia. The lack of local and vascular invasion aids the distinction between adenoma and carcinoma, although invasion is not always a readily seen feature of carcinoma. Therefore, the distinction is frequently based on other histological characteristics. A general arrangement of cells, including the lack of massively thickened cords, supports a diagnosis of adenoma. Also, a relative homogeneity of cell and nuclear size and a uniform cell shape are strong indicators of the benign tumor.

A greater differential diagnostic problem arises when hepatocellular adenoma must be differentiated from nodular hyperplasia of the liver (Patnaik et al., 1980). Unfortunately, no well-established criteria have been devised to distinguish these two lesions in domestic animals. Much of the pathology literature uses the terms *hepatocellular adenoma* and *nodular hyperplasia* interchangeably. Cytological factors are probably best used to distinguish these two lesions. In general, hyperplastic nodules are expected to have cytological characteristics similar to normal liver, while hepatocellular adenomas have slightly altered cytological characteristics. A lesion should be diagnosed as a hyperplastic nodule if it is expansile causing compression of adjacent tissue but retaining a normal lobular architecture. By comparison, a hepatocellular adenoma does not retain a normal lobular architecture, although it may contain trapped remnants of portal triads. Some workers consider hyperplastic nodules to be multiple and hepatocytic adenomas to be generally single (Ponomarkov and Mackey, 1976).

Hepatocellular adenoma must also be distinguished from hepatoblastoma. With the exception of sheep (Cotchin, 1975; Manktelow, 1965), however, hepatoblastoma has not been described in domestic animals. Adequate information is not available to determine if the lesion in sheep is comparable to hepatoblastoma found in humans and laboratory animals or if it should be considered as hepatocellular adenoma.

**Growth and Metastasis.** The adenoma grows by direct expansion resulting in compression of adjacent tissues including normal liver or biliary passages. Compression of major biliary passages could conceivably result in icterus, although this effect has not been reported. As a benign lesion, the adenoma neither invades locally nor metastasizes.

**Etiology.** The etiology of adenoma is unknown, although a wide range of synthesized and natural chemicals are known to cause liver neoplasms in many species of domestic animals. The contamination of animal feeds containing nitrosamines and aflatoxin, known hepatocarcinogenic agents, suggests a possible chemical etiology through the diet. (See also under Hepatocellular Carcinoma.)

## Nodular Hyperplasia

**Incidence.** Despite the fact that nodular hyperplasia is a common spontaneous lesion, a limited number of references are available in the literature concerning the various pathological characteristics of the lesion. Nodular hyperplasia of the liver has been observed in several domestic species, but appears to be most common in dogs (Bergman, 1985; Fabry *et al.*, 1982; Mulligan, 1949*a*) and pigs (Hayashi *et al.*, 1983). The lesion reportedly occurs in 15 to 60% of old dogs, but is rarely found in younger animals. The incidence of pigs is reported at 4 per 100,000 animals, but it should be noted that this value is based on a young slaughter-aged population.

**Clinical Characteristics.** No clinical signs have been described in association with nodular hyperplasia of the liver. The lack of reported clinical findings probably reflects that most lesions are too small to cause clinical problems. The lesion is therefore first recognized as an incidental finding at necropsy or in the abattoir.

**Gross Morphology.** The literature presents a very confusing picture concerning the pathological characteristics of hyperplastic nodules because not all authors have carefully distinguished hyperplastic lesions from benign neoplastic lesions of hepatocytic origin. It is clear that hyperplastic lesions cannot be distinguished from benign neoplastic lesions based on gross observation alone. However, hyperplastic lesions appear grossly as variably sized masses that usually protrude slightly above the capsular surface. Their most striking characteristic is a light or dark color that makes them clearly distinguishable from the surrounding normal liver (fig. 9.3). Hyperplastic lesions are generally spherical in shape. As with neoplastic lesions, hyperplastic nodules do not have a grossly observable capsule. They may be found as an individual nodule or as a nodular change throughout the liver, which is usually associated with extensive hepatic fibrosis.

**Histological Features.** The hyperplastic nodule is poorly defined histologically in the literature for all species of domestic animals. Based on published descriptions, it is clear that lesions described as hepatocellular adenomas by some authors are referred to as hyperplastic nodules by others. The term *hyperplastic nodule* should be reserved for those proliferative lesions that clearly have an increased number of cells, yet retain the normal liver lobular architecture (Mulligan, 1949*b*). By this definition, hyperplastic nodules of the liver retain a relatively normal arrangement of central veins and portal triads. Adjacent liver tissue may be compressed by the proliferative lesion, which is never encapsulated. The nodules do not have an increase in fibrous connective tissue even when fibrosis is present in the surrounding liver. The cords of hepatocytes within the hyperplastic nodule are either one or two cells thick. The hepatocytes are normal in size or enlarged due to various cytoplasmic alterations. Accumulations of either lipid or glycogen are the most frequent changes observed. Nuclei are normal in size and shape, but nucleoli are sometimes enlarged, as a reflection of enhanced metabolic activity in proliferating hepatocytes. Hypertrophied cells have been identified in livers containing hyperplastic nodules (Bergman, 1985).

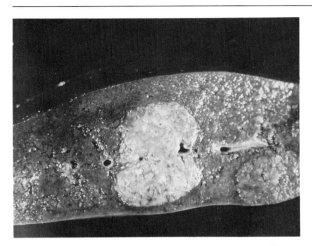

**FIGURE 9.3.** Nodular hyperplasia in the liver of a dog. Two lesions are noted on cross section of the liver and are distinguished from the surrounding liver because of their pale color. (Courtesy of Dr. D. J. Meuten.)

Problems in differential diagnosis are restricted to distinguishing hyperplastic nodule from hepatocellular adenoma. Although no uniform agreement exists, the retention of normal lobular architecture is the best available criterion for distinguishing these two lesions. Additional information is needed on the reversibility of the lesions after removal of the inciting agents before a better histological basis can be established to distinguish hyperplastic from benign neoplastic lesions.

**Etiology.** The etiology of spontaneously occurring hyperplastic nodules is unknown. However, it should be remembered that nodular hyperplasia and hepatocytic neoplasia can be experimentally induced by chemicals in a wide range of animals including domestic species. Specifically, nitrosamines and aflatoxin should be considered as potential causes of nodular hyperplasia since these chemicals are frequently found in animal feeds, although the concentrations are generally low.

## Cholangiocarcinoma

**Incidence.** Cholangiocarcinoma (bile duct carcinoma) has been reported in dogs (Bastianello,

1983; MacVean *et al.*, 1978; Patnaik *et al.*, 1980, 1981*b;* Rooney, 1959; Strafuss, 1976; Trigo *et al.*, 1982), cats (Hou, 1964; Patnaik *et al.*, 1975), sheep (Anderson and Sandison, 1967; Monlux *et al.*, 1956), cattle (Anderson and Sandison, 1967; Monlux *et al.*, 1956; Strafuss *et al.*, 1973), and horses (Rehmtulla, 1974). As with hepatocellular carcinoma, adequate information is not available to compare the incidence among the various species. The incidence of cholangiocarcinoma is reported as 1.6 per 100,000 in dogs (MacVean *et al.*, 1978).

Although cholangiocarcinoma should not be considered a rare neoplasm, it occurs less frequently than most types of neoplasms in domestic species. In dogs it accounts for less than 1% of all neoplasms (MacVean *et al.*, 1978; Strafuss, 1976). When compared with other primary hepatic neoplasms, cholangiocarcinoma in dogs is reported to be either more common (Bastianello, 1983; Rooney, 1959) or less common (Mulligan, 1949*b;* Patnaik *et al.*, 1980) than hepatocellular carcinoma. Neoplasms are much more common in the intrahepatic bile ducts of dogs than in the extrahepatic bile ducts and gall bladder (Hayes *et al.*, 1983; Patnaik *et al.*, 1980).

Cholangiocarcinoma tends to occur in older animals, but limited information is available in many species. In dogs 65% of the cases are found in animals more than 10 years of age (Patnaik *et al.*, 1980). The age distribution in dogs is different than in meat producing animals. Hepatocellular carcinoma is found in cattle less than 3 years of age, in sheep less than 1 year, and in pigs less than 6 months, while cholangiocarcinoma is not found in the same groups (Anderson and Sandison, 1967). Precise information on the age of animals with cholangiocarcinoma, however, is not known since it is based on abattoir data. When all bile duct carcinomas are considered, males and sexually intact females have the same relative risk; spayed females have a 1.5 times greater risk than intact females (Hayes *et al.*, 1983). No breed predilection has been found for this neoplasm in dogs (Hayes *et al.*, 1983; Patnaik *et al.*, 1981*b*).

**Clinical Characteristics.** Available information on clinical signs in animals with this carcinoma is limited to dogs. The signs tend to be nonspecific, and the dogs frequently have anorexia, lethargy, ascites, vomiting, weight loss, and dyspnea (Patnaik *et al.*, 1981*b*; Trigo *et al.*, 1982). Clinical evidence of icterus is found in only 13% of cases.

Available clinical pathology demonstrates that dogs with cholangiocarcinoma often have leukocytosis and elevated serum alkaline phosphatase (Patnaik *et al.*, 1980, 1981*b*). It is surprising that the total bilirubin and serum aspartate amino transferase are not elevated (Patnaik *et al.*, 1980). It should be noted, however, that clinical pathology information on affected animals is limited to a few cases.

**Gross Morphology.** Cholangiocarcinoma lesions can be either large and diffuse or small and nodular (Patnaik *et al.*, 1981*b*; Trigo *et al.*, 1982). The large tumor can be greater than 10 cm in diameter and extend from the lobe of origin to adjacent lobes. It is usually lobulated. The small nodular tumor is frequently 1 cm in diameter. Irrespective of size, the border between the neoplasm and adjacent liver tissue is relatively distinct but often irregular. The neoplasm can extend above the surface of the liver, and it may have a central depression (fig. 9.4). Small tumors can be completely embedded in the liver and are not visible from the capsular surface.

The carcinoma is usually gray-white in color, but may also be light brown (Patnaik *et al.*, 1981*b*; Trigo *et al.*, 1982). The light color is primarily due to the extensive connective tissue stroma, which also accounts for the typically firm consistency. The tumor is frequently solid but may also be cystic. Cystic spaces are variable in distribution, even within a single neoplasm, and usually contain a light yellow gelatinous material. Necrotic spaces are sometimes found and tend to be near the center of the tumor and are filled with blood-tinged fluid.

This neoplasm is found in any lobe of the liver of dogs (Patnaik *et al.*, 1980). The available literature offers insufficient information to determine if any particular lobe is preferentially affected. It is not uncommon to find cholangiocarcinomas in more than one lobe of the liver in an affected animal, but it is often difficult to determine if the multiple sites represent multiple primary neoplasms or intrahepatic metastases from a single neoplasm.

**Histological Features.** The carcinomas are histologically similar in all species. Many of these tumors are composed of small glandlike structures or packets of neoplastic cells embedded in an obvious connective tissue stroma that may have fibrosis

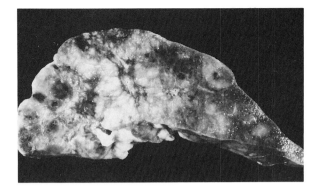

**FIGURE 9.4.** Cholangiocarcinoma of the dog. The lesion is large, protruding above the surface of the liver, is irregular in color, and has several depressions on the capsular surface. (Courtesy of Dr. D. J. Meuten.)

(Anderson and Sandison, 1967; Ponomarkov and Mackey, 1976; Trigo *et al.*, 1982). The glandular structures are usually irregular in size and shape. The stroma may be composed of immature collagenous connective tissue and lacks inflammatory cell infiltrate unless necrosis is present.

A second histological type of cholangiocarcinoma is characterized by dilated cystic spaces lined by neoplastic bile duct epithelial cells (Patnaik *et al.*, 1981*b*). This variation has been called a *bile duct cystadenocarcinoma* to indicate the cystic characteristic of the tumor. This subclassification of the neoplasm probably has limited prognostic value since the cystic form has the same rate of metastasis as other forms of the neoplasm (Patnaik *et al.*, 1981*b*). The lumen of the glandular structures and cystic spaces contain mucin that appears as an eosinophilic secretion on routine histological stains but stains positively for mucin by the Alcian blue or periodic acid–Schiff (PAS) techniques (Trigo *et al.*, 1982). Bile pigment is usually not observed within the neoplasm.

The cytology of the individual cells reflects the degree of differentiation of the neoplasm (Ponomarkov and Mackey, 1976). The cells are usually moderately differentiated and are cuboidal or columnar in shape with variable amounts of light basophilic cytoplasm. The cytoplasm is light eosinophilic or clear in some cases. In the more anaplastic growths the cells are pleomorphic. The nuclei are round to oval and uniform in size and shape, and they may be hyperchromatic with the chromatin uniformly

**Histological Features.** The most striking histological feature of cystic hyperplasia of the gall bladder is the presence of variably sized cysts containing large amounts of mucus. Each cyst is lined by a continuous single layer of epithelium (Kovatch *et al.*, 1965). Fronds of hyperplastic epithelium protrude between the cysts and project into the lumen of the gall bladder. Individual epithelial cells may appear in different forms: normal columnar, hypertrophic, reduced in size to a cuboidal shape, or (rarely) squamous type. The cells and mucous material in the cysts usually stain with the PAS technique. Mitotic figures are rarely observed. Smaller cysts appear to develop from ducts or the mucin-secreting glands normally found in the gall bladder mucosa. The surface epithelium over the areas of cystic hyperplasia is usually reduced to a cuboidal cell type. The diffuse nature of the lesion and lack of histological evidence of neoplasia make cystic hyperplasia of the gall bladder easily recognizable.

**Etiology.** The cause of gall bladder cystic hyperplasia is not known for sure, but there is some evidence to suggest a hormonal basis. In the ewe, cystic hyperplasia of the gall bladder is associated with pregnancy, suggesting that hormonal factors, perhaps continued progesterone stimulation, are the underlying cause of the lesion (Fell *et al.*, 1983). This contention is supported by a case report where cystic hyperplasia was found in a dog given progestational compounds (Mawdesley-Thomas and Noel, 1967). Cystic hyperplasia of the gall bladder in dogs is not the result of inflammation since inflammatory cells are not observed in the lesion (Kovatch *et al.*, 1965).

## TUMORS AND HYPERPLASIA OF THE EXOCRINE PANCREAS

### Carcinoma of the Exocrine Pancreas

**Incidence.** Carcinoma of the exocrine pancreas has been reported in dogs (Bastianello, 1983; Mulligan, 1963; Priester, 1974), cats (Banner *et al.*, 1979; Priester, 1974), horses (Priester, 1974; Rowlatt, 1967; Sundberg *et al.*, 1982), and cattle (Rowlatt, 1967; Priester, 1974), but was not detected in pigs or sheep in a large survey of domestic animals (Priester, 1974). Carcinoma of the exocrine pancreas is slightly more common than carcinoma of pancreatic islet cell origin (Anderson and Johnson, 1967; Bastianello, 1983; Priester, 1974; Rowlatt, 1967). Tumors of the pancreatic islets are discussed in chapter 13.

Most pancreatic carcinomas are found in older dogs, although the neoplasm has also been observed in dogs as young as 3 years of age (Anderson and Johnson, 1967; Priester, 1974). Likewise, a high proportion of pancreatic carcinomas occurs in aged cats (Priester, 1974). Since the number of cases reported in the literature is small, an association with age cannot be made in other species. The Airedale terrier appears to have a higher risk for pancreatic carcinoma than other breeds, but this information is based on a small number of cases. This breed is known to have a high predisposition for all types of cancer. Available information indicates that the boxer breed has the second highest risk for pancreatic cancer. No sex differences are found in animals with this carcinoma (Priester, 1974).

The overall incidence of pancreatic carcinoma is comparable in dogs and humans, but the sex distribution is different (Priester, 1974). In humans pancreatic carcinoma is found predominantly in males, but no such sex difference has been observed in dogs. The incidence of this neoplasm is increasing in humans; comparable information is not available for domestic animals.

**Clinical Characteristics.** The most common signs of carcinoma of the exocrine pancreas are abdominal pain, vomiting, weight loss, depression, and a palpable abdominal mass (Anderson and Johnson, 1967; Rowlatt, 1967). Since pancreatic carcinomas often cause obstruction of the common bile duct, typical clinical signs may be confounded by signs of secondary liver involvement, such as icterus and biliary cirrhosis. Ascites is associated with extensive peritoneal implantation of the neoplasm or with compression of the portal vein or its major branches. Rarely, the first clinical signs arise as a result of distant metastasis.

Limited clinical pathological information is available on animals having pancreatic carcinoma (Anderson and Johnson, 1967). Absolute neutrophilia occurs in most dogs, but it is usually the result of hemoconcentration and dehydration. A moderate left shift in the white blood cell count is observed in a few cases.

**Gross Morphology.** Most carcinomas of the exocrine pancreas are found in the middle portion rather than the duodenal or splenic portions of the pancreas (Anderson and Johnson, 1967; Rowlatt, 1967) (fig. 9.10). The tumor forms a single discrete mass in the pancreas or occurs as multiple masses throughout the entire pancreas. When individual nodules are found, they usually measure several centimeters in diameter. They are gray-white or pale yellow in color and usually have a firm consistency. The center of the tumor may be necrotic.

Mineralization is sometimes found with or without apparent necrosis. Fat necrosis is frequently observed in the adipose tissue adjacent to the affected pancreas.

**Histological Features.** The histological features of pancreatic carcinoma are extremely variable between neoplasms as well as within a single neoplasm (Anderson and Johnson, 1967; Kircher and Neilsen, 1976). The neoplastic cells form tubular structures (fig. 9.11), acini (fig. 9.12), or solid sheets of undifferentiated cells (fig. 9.13), thus providing fea-

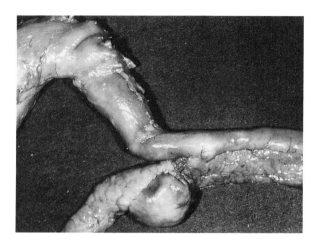

**FIGURE 9.10.** Carcinoma in the exocrine pancreas of a cat. A single nodular lesion is found near the middle of the pancreas. (Courtesy of Dr. L. T. Pulley.)

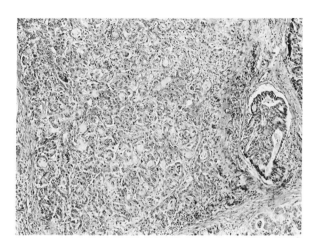

**FIGURE 9.12.** Carcinoma of the exocrine pancreas in a dog. The neoplastic cells form acinar structures. (Courtesy of Dr. R. C. Cattley and Auburn University, Alabama.)

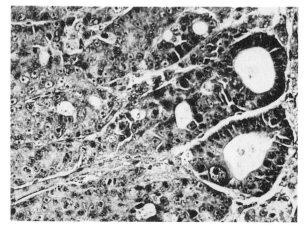

**FIGURE 9.11.** Carcinoma in the exocrine pancreas of a dog. Note the tubule formation by the neoplastic cells. (Courtesy of Dr. J. Alroy and *Amer. J. Path.*)

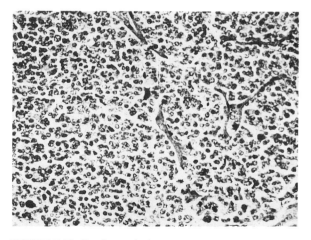

**FIGURE 9.13.** Carcinoma in the exocrine pancreas of a dog. The undifferentiated neoplastic cells form solid sheets of cells. (Courtesy of Dr. J. Alroy and *Amer. J. Path.*)

tures for a subclassification of the neoplasm (Kircher and Nielsen, 1976). Tubular structures are lined by either cuboidal or columnar cells. The histological pattern and the degree of differentiation often vary within a single neoplasm.

The individual carcinoma cell usually has pale eosinophilic cytoplasm that occasionally contains bright eosinophilic zymogen granules. Columnar cells sometimes have clear vacuoles in the apical cytoplasm. The nuclei are round, small to medium in size, and contain modest amounts of chromatin. Only in the most undifferentiated neoplasms are the nuclei variable in size and shape. The nuclear to cytoplasmic ratio can be extremely variable. While the nuclei are relatively uniform in size in most neoplasms, the cytoplasm can vary widely depending on the cell structure and the degree of differentiation. Columnar cells are generally well-differentiated with extensive cytoplasm in the apical end of the cell; the basal part of the cell has a moderately sized nucleus. Cuboidal cells lack the polarity of columnar cells and contain much less cytoplasm. As expected, undifferentiated carcinomas have a high nuclear to cytoplasmic ratio because of the small amounts of cytoplasm in the neoplastic cells. The nucleoli are generally small. Mitotic figures are rarely seen in the well-differentiated neoplasm that forms tubular or acinar structures, but they are relatively common in the undifferentiated neoplasm that forms solid sheets of cells.

The stroma of the neoplasm is variable. In the well-differentiated neoplasm the stroma consists of a delicate network surrounding the small tubules and acini of neoplastic cells. In other tumors, especially the poorly differentiated ones, the stroma is densely fibrotic (fig. 9.14). More extensive stroma is found in the neoplasm composed of large tubules. Hemorrhage and necrosis are common in the carcinoma containing densely fibrotic (scirrhous) stroma. A fibrous capsule is never complete.

Carcinoma of the exocrine pancreas must be distinguished from carcinoma of the pancreatic islet cells and metastases from stomach and intestinal neoplasms. The tendency of the exocrine-derived neoplasm to form tubular or glandular structures distinguishes it from islet cell neoplasm. However, it may be difficult to distinguish the cell of origin in the undifferentiated pancreatic exocrine carcinoma. The neoplasm is distinguished from invading tumors of the gastrointestinal tract on the basis of

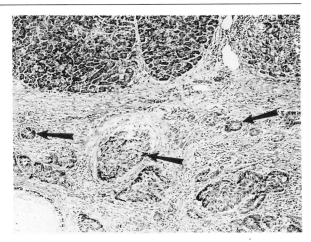

**FIGURE 9.14.** Carcinoma in the exocrine pancreas of a dog. The packets of neoplastic cells (**arrows**) are surrounded by scirrhous stroma. (Courtesy of Dr. R. C. Cattley and Auburn University, Alabama.)

gross appearance and cytological characteristics.

The exact histological origin of exocrine pancreatic carcinoma of domestic animals has never been clarified. The two obvious sites of origin are the acinar and ductular epithelial cells. The tubular arrangement of many neoplasms suggests a ductular origin, but this has been discounted on the basis of electron microscopic evaluation of cases in the dog and cat in which demonstration of zymogen granules was cited as evidence for an acinar cell origin of the neoplasm (Banner *et al.*, 1978, 1979).

**Growth and Metastasis.** Pancreatic carcinoma is a relatively aggressive neoplasm that invades locally and metastasizes to distant sites. Local invasion may result in obstruction of the common bile duct with corresponding effects on the clinical signs. Histologically, invasion is found in the adjacent pancreatic tissue, blood vessels, and lymphatics. Neoplastic cells are found in the perineurium as they extend along the perineurial lymphatics. Pancreatic carcinoma most frequently metastasizes to the liver, lungs, peritoneal surfaces, and local lymph nodes, but it has also been found in the spleen, diaphragm, and kidney (Anderson and Johnson, 1967; Rowlatt, 1967). The carcinoma usually metastasizes before clinical signs are seen (Kircher and Nielsen, 1976).

**Etiology.** The cause of pancreatic acinar carcinoma is unknown for all species of domestic animals. In humans it has been hypothesized that carcinogen-containing bile refluxes from the common bile duct into the pancreatic duct where the two ducts meet as they enter the intestine. While this hypothesis has some validity, it cannot account for all of the pancreatic neoplasms in domestic animals since the common bile duct does not enter the intestine in conjunction with the pancreatic duct in all species (Priester, 1974).

## Adenoma of the Exocrine Pancreas

**Incidence.** Adenoma of the exocrine pancreas is an extremely rare neoplasm. Few cases have been reported in the literature and true incidence data are unavailable. On the basis of reported cases (Rowlatt, 1967), adenoma of the pancreas appears to be most common in cattle and dogs. It must be stressed that a literature review does not provide incidence data for a single species or comparative incidence data between species. Also, proliferative lesions of the exocrine pancreas are not always distinguishable from proliferative lesions of the endocrine pancreas. In addition, there are no clear morphological criteria to distinguish benign tumors from hyperplastic lesions; thus published reports of adenomas probably include hyperplastic lesions of the exocrine pancreas. Despite the lack of solid incidence data for adenoma, this tumor is undoubtedly less common than carcinoma of the exocrine pancreas.

**Clinical Characteristics.** Since adenoma of the exocrine pancreas is usually a small tumor, no clinical signs are observed. The neoplasm is found incidentally at necropsy or when tissues are examined histologically.

**Gross Morphology.** Adenoma of the exocrine pancreas usually measures only a few millimeters in diameter. It protrudes above the surface of the pancreas but is usually inapparent because of a slight difference in color compared with the surrounding tissue (fig. 9.15). Some tumors contain small cysts.

**Histological Features.** The adenoma usually compresses the surrounding pancreatic tissue and has a thin fibrous capsule. It has a tubular or acinar pattern (Kircher and Nielsen, 1976). Tumors with a tubular pattern have cystic spaces lined by cuboidal or columnar epithelial cells that may form papillary projections into the lumens of cysts. A thin col-

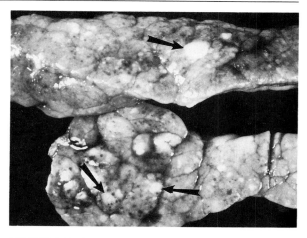

**FIGURE 9.15.** Adenoma in the exocrine pancreas of a dog. The proliferative lesion is causing compression of adjacent pancreatic tissue. (Courtesy of Dr. L. T. Pulley.)

lagenous connective tissue stroma is found throughout the growth. The morphology suggests that the neoplasm arises from ducts, although detailed studies on the pathogenesis are lacking.

The acinar pattern in this neoplasm is rare, and when present the lesion is often diagnosed as a hyperplastic nodule. The acinar formations consist of cells that have a relatively normal acinar epithelial appearance. The cytoplasm is red and granular in hematoxylin- and eosin-stained sections and rarely contains zymogen granules.

In both histological patterns the nuclei are round and vesicular. Mitotic figures are rarely observed.

Adenoma of exocrine pancreatic tissue must be distinguished from hyperplastic nodules and malignant exocrine neoplasm. This distinction must be made on the general histological characteristics since no well-defined criteria have been described. Since the adenoma has a well-differentiated appearance, it cannot be confused with neoplasms that originate in other organs such as the stomach or intestine.

**Growth and Metastasis.** As a benign tumor, the adenoma grows and compresses the adjacent tissue but does not metastasize. The pathogenesis of adenoma and carcinoma has not been well studied in domestic animals. It is uncertain whether the adenoma is an end-stage tumor or one that can progress to carcinoma. The apparent rarity of adenoma compared with carcinoma suggests that carcinoma arises *de novo* rather than from adenoma.

## Nodular Hyperplasia of the Exocrine Pancreas

**Incidence.** Since nodular hyperplasia has little clinical significance, this lesion has been rarely reported in the literature. Nevertheless, nodular hyperplasia is a common lesion of the exocrine pancreas particularly in older dogs, cats, and cattle. Although detailed data are lacking, nodular hyperplasia is certainly more common in older than in younger animals.

**Clinical Characteristics.** No clinical effects of nodular hyperplasia of the exocrine pancreas are known. The lesion is usually an incidental finding at necropsy.

**Gross Morphology.** Nodular hyperplasia is occasionally seen as a solitary lesion, but it is more commonly multiple. The individual lesion is small, rarely measuring over several millimeters in diameter. When located on the surface of the pancreas, it appears as multiple, small, white lesions against the light pink to light tan normal pancreatic tissue. Hyperplastic nodules rarely protrude above the surface of the pancreas.

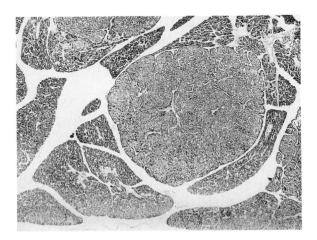

**FIGURE 9.16.** Nodular hyperplasia in the exocrine pancreas of a dog. Multiple small pale nodules are noted on the surface of the pancreas (**arrows**). (Courtesy of Dr. D. J. Meuten.)

**Histological Features.** Hyperplastic nodules are not encapsulated and do not compress the adjacent tissue (Kircher and Nielsen, 1976) (fig. 9.16). In the common acinar type lesion, the cells tend to form normal appearing lobules. Nodular hyperplasia is easily recognized histologically because of abnormal staining and the size of the acinar cells. The cytoplasm is usually very eosinophilic and sometimes has a clear vacuolated appearance. The individual cells are either larger or smaller than the normal cells in adjacent lobules. Rarely, a hyperplastic lesion is found within a dilated pancreatic duct. In such a lesion, the duct is lined by hyperplastic epithelium that often forms folds within the lumen.

**Growth and Metastasis.** All histological characteristics suggest that this proliferative change is hyperplastic, but it is not known if it has the potential to progress to neoplasia.

## REFERENCES

Allison, J. B., Wase, A. W., Leathem, J. H., and Wainio, W. W. (1950) Some Effects of 2-Acetylaminofluorene on the Dog. *Cancer Res.* 10, 266–271.

Anderson, L. J., and Sandison, A. T. (1967) Tumors of the Liver in Cattle, Sheep and Pigs. *Cancer* 21, 289–301.

Anderson, N. V., and Johnson, K. H. (1967) Pancreatic Carcinoma in the Dog. *J. Amer. Vet. Med. Assoc.* 150, 286–295.

Anderson, W. A., Monlux, A. W., and Davis, C. L. (1958) Epithelial Tumors of the Bovine Gall Bladder—A Report of Eighteen Cases. *Amer. J. Vet. Res.* 19, 58–65.

Banner, B. F., Alroy, J., Pauli, B. U., and Carpenter, J. L. (1978) An Ultrastructural Study of Acinic Cell Carcinomas of the Canine Pancreas. *Amer. J. Path.* 93, 165–182.

Banner, B. F., Alroy, J., and Kipnis, R. M. (1979) Acinar Cell Carcinoma of the Pancreas in a Cat. *Vet. Path.* 16, 543–547.

Bastianello, S. S. (1983) A Survey on Neoplasia in Domestic Species over a 40-Year Period from 1935 to 1974 in the Republic of South Africa. VI. Tumors Occurring in Dogs. *Onderstepoort J. Vet. Res.* 50, 199–220.

Benjamin, S. A., Hahn, F. F., Chiffelle, T. L., Boecker, B. B., Hobbs, C. H., Jones, R. K., McClellan, R. O., and Snipes, M. B., (1975) Occurrence of Hemangiosarcomas in Beagles with Internally Deposited Radionuclides. *Cancer Res.* 35, 1745–1755.

Bergman, J. R. (1985) Nodular Hyperplasia in the Liver of the Dog: An Association with Changes in the Ito Cell Population. *Vet. Path.* 22, 427–438.

Blumberg, B. S., and London, W. T. (1981) Hepatitis B Virus and the Prevention of Primary Hepatocellular Carcinoma. *N. Eng. J. Med.* 304, 782–784.

Campbell, J. G. (1949) Spontaneous Hepatocellular and Cholangiocellular Carcinoma in the Duck. An Experimental Study. *Br. J. Cancer* 3, 198–210.

———. (1969) Tumours of Epithelial Tissue. In: *Tumours of the Fowl.* W. Heinemann (London), 131–148.

Cotchin, E. (1975) Spontaneous Tumours in Young Animals. *Proc. Roy. Soc. Med.* 68, 653–655.

Dagle, G. E., Bristline, R. W., Lebel, J. L., and Watters, R. L. (1984) Plutonium-Induced Wounds in Beagles. *Hlth. Physics* 47, 73–84.

Erturk, E., Atassi, S. A., Yoshida, O., Cohen, S. M., Price, J. M., and Bryan, G. T. (1970) Comparative Urinary and Gallbladder Carcinogenicity of N-[4-(5-Nitro-2-Furyl)-2-Thiazolyl] Formamide and N-[4-(5-Nitro-2-Furyl)-2-Thiazolyl] Acetamide in the Dog. *J. Natl. Cancer Inst.* 45, 535–542.

Fabry, A., Benjamin, S. A., and Angleton, G. M. (1982) Nodular Hyperplasia of the Liver in the Beagle Dog. *Vet. Path.* 19, 109–119.

Fell, B. F., Robinson, J. J., and Watson, M. (1983) Cystic Hyperplasia of the Gall Bladder in Breeding Ewes. *J. Comp. Path.* 93, 171–178.

Fraumeni, J. F., Jr., and Kantor, A. F. (1982) Biliary Tract. In: Schottenfeld, D., and Fraumeni, J. F., Jr., eds., *Cancer Epidemiology and Prevention.* W. B. Saunders (Philadelphia), 683–691.

Gourley, I. M., Popp, J. A., and Park, R. D. (1971) Myelolipomas of the Liver in a Domestic Cat. *J. Amer. Vet. Med. Assoc.* 158, 2053–2057.

Graw, J. J., and Berg, H. (1977) Hepatocarcinogenetic Effect of DENA in Pigs. *Z. Krebsforch.* 89, 137–143.

Hayashi, M. A., Tsuda, H., and Ito, N. (1983) Histopathological Classification of Spontaneous Hyperplastic Liver Nodules in Slaughtered Swine. *J. Comp. Path.* 93, 603–612.

Hayes, H. M., Jr., Morin, M. M., and Rubenstein, D. A. (1983) Canine Biliary Carcinoma: Epidemiological Comparisons with Man. *J. Comp. Path.* 93, 99–107.

Hirao, K., Matsumura, K., Imagawa, A., Enomoto, Y., Hosogi, Y., Kani, T., Fujikawa, K., and Ito, N. (1974) Primary Neoplasms in Dog Liver Induced by Diethylnitrosamine. *Cancer Res.* 34, 1870–1882.

Hou, P. C. (1964) Primary Carcinoma of Bile Duct of the Liver of the Cat (*Felis catus*) Infested with *Clonorchis sinensis. J. Path. Bact.* 87, 239–244.

———. (1965) Hepatic Clonorchiasis and Carcinoma of the Bile Duct in a Dog. *J. Path. Bact.* 89, 365–367.

Ikede, B. O., and Downey, R. S. (1972) Multiple Hepatic Myelolipomas in a Cat. *Can. Vet. J.* 13, 160–163.

Ito, T., Miura, S., Ohshima, K., and Numakunai, S. (1972) Fine Structure of Hepatocellular Carcinoma in Swine. *Jap. J. Vet. Sci.* 34, 33–37.

Jeraj, K., Yano, B., Osborne, C. A., Wallace, L. J., and Stevens, J. B. (1981) Primary Hepatic Osteosarcoma in a Dog. *J. Amer. Vet. Med. Assoc.* 179, 1000–1003.

Kircher, C. H., and Nielsen, S. W. (1976) Tumors of the Pancreas. *Bull. Wld. Hlth. Org.* 53, 195–202.

Kithier, K., Al-Sarraf, M., Belamaric, J., Radl, J., Valenta, Z., Zizkovsky, V., and Masopust, J. (1974) Alpha-Fetoprotein in Bovine Hepatocellular Carcinoma. *J. Comp. Path.* 84, 133–141.

Kovatch, R. M., Hildebrandt, P. K., and Marcus, L. C. (1965) Cystic Mucinous Hypertrophy of the Mucosa of the Gall Bladder in the Dog. *Path. Vet.* 2, 574–584.

Ladds, P. W. (1983) Vascular Hamartomas of the Liver of Cattle. *Vet. Path.* 20, 764–767.

Lombard, L. S., Fortna, H. M., Garner, F. M., and Brynjolfsson, G. (1968) Myelolipomas of the Liver in Captive Wild Felidae. *Path. Vet.* 5, 127–134.

MacVean, D. W., Monlux, A. W., Anderson, P. S., Jr., Silberg, S. L., and Roszel, J. F. (1978) Frequency of Canine and Feline Tumors in a Defined Population. *Vet. Path.* 15, 700–715.

Manktelow, B. W. (1965) Hepatoblastomas in Sheep. *J. Path. Bact.* 89, 711–714.

Mawdesley-Thomas, L. E., and Noel, P. R. B. (1967) Cystic Hyperplasia of the Gall Bladder in the Beagle, Associated with the Administration of Progestational Compounds. *Vet. Rec.* 80, 658–659.

Monlux, A. W., Anderson, W. A., and Davis, C. L. (1956) A Survey of Tumors Occurring in Cattle, Sheep, and Swine. *Amer. J. Vet. Res.* 17, 646–677.

Montali, R. J., Hoopes, P. J., and Bush, M. (1981) Extrahepatic Biliary Carcinomas in Asiatic Bears. *J. Natl. Cancer Inst.* 66, 603–608.

Mulligan, R. M. (1949a) *Neoplasms of the Dog.* Williams and Wilkins (Baltimore), 111.

———. (1949b) Primary Liver-Cell Carcinoma (Hepatoma) in the Dog. *Cancer Res.* 9, 76–81.

———. (1963) Comparative Pathology of Human and Canine Cancer. *Ann. N.Y. Acad. Sci.* 108, 642–690.

Omata, M., Uchiumi, K., Ito, Y., Yokosuka, O., Mori, J., Terao, K., Wei-Fa, Y., O'Connell, A. P., London, W. T., and Okuda, K. (1983) Duck Hepatitis B Virus and Liver Diseases. *Gastroenterol.* 85, 260–267.

Patnaik, A. K., Hurvitz, A. I., and Lieberman, P. H. (1980) Canine Hepatic Neoplasms: A Clinicopathologic Study. *Vet. Path.* 17, 553–564.

Patnaik, A. K., Hurvitz, A. I., Lieberman, P. H., and Johnson, G. F. (1981a) Canine Hepatocellular Carcinoma. *Vet. Path.* 18, 427–438.

———. (1981b) Canine Bile Duct Carcinoma. *Vet. Path.* 18, 439–444.

Patnaik, A. K., Lieberman, P. H., Hurvitz, A. I., and Johnson, G. F. (1981c) Canine Hepatic Carcinoids. *Vet. Path.* 18, 445–453.

Patnaik, A. K., Liu, S.-K., Hurvitz, A. I., and McClelland, A. J. (1975) Nonhematopoietic Neoplasms in Cats. *J. Natl. Cancer Inst.* 54, 855–860.

Ponomarkov, V., and Mackey, L. J. (1976) XIII. Tumours of the Liver and Biliary System. *Bull. Wld. Hlth. Org.* 53, 187–194.

Priester, W. A. (1974) Data from Eleven United States

and Canadian Colleges of Veterinary Medicine on Pancreatic Carcinoma in Domestic Animals. *Cancer Res.* 34, 1372–1375.

———. (1976) Brief Communication: Hepatic Angiosarcomas in Dogs: An Excessive Frequency as Compared with Man. *J. Natl. Cancer Inst.* 57, 451–454.

Ramachandran, K. M., Rajan, A., Mony, G., and Maryamma, K. I. (1970) Hepatocellular Carcinoma in a Pig. *Ind. Vet. J.* 47, 304–306.

Rehmtulla, A. J. (1974) Occurrence of Carcinoma of the Bile Ducts: A Brief Review. *Can. Vet. J.* 15, 289–292.

Rooney, J. R. (1959) Liver Carcinoma in the Dog. *Acta Path. Microbiol. Scand.* 45, 321–330.

Rowlatt, U. (1967) Spontaneous Epithelial Tumours of the Pancreas of Mammals. *Br. J. Cancer* 21, 82–107.

Shalkop, W. T., and Armbrecht, B. H. (1974) Carcinogenic Response of Brood Sows Fed Aflatoxin for 28 to 30 Months. *Amer. J. Vet. Res.* 35, 623–627.

Sinnhuber, R. O., Hendricks, J. D., Wales, J. H., and Putnam, G. B. (1977) Neoplasms in Rainbow Trout, A Sensitive Animal Model for Environmental Carcinogenesis. *Ann. N.Y. Acad. Sci.* 298, 389–408.

Snyder, R. L., Tyler, G., and Summers, J. (1982) Chronic Hepatitis and Hepatocellular Carcinoma Associated with Woodchuck Hepatitis Virus. *Amer. J. Path.* 107, 422–425.

Sternberg, S. S., Popper, H., Oser, B. L., and Oser, M. (1966) Gallbladder and Bile Duct Adenocarcinomas in Dogs after Long Term Feeding of Aramite. *Cancer* 13, 780–789.

Strafuss, A. C. (1976) Bile Duct Carcinoma in Dogs. *J. Amer. Vet. Med. Assoc.* 169, 429.

Strafuss, A. C., Vestweber, J. G. E., Njoku, C. O., and Ivoghli, B. (1973) Bile Duct Carcinoma in Cattle: Three Case Reports. *Amer. J. Vet. Res.* 34, 1203–1205.

Strombeck, D. R. (1978) Clinicopathologic Features of Primary and Metastatic Neoplastic Disease of the Liver in Dogs. *J. Amer. Vet. Med. Assoc.* 173, 267–269.

Stula, E. F., Barnes, J. R., Sherman, H., Reinhardt, C. F., and Zapp, J. A., Jr. (1978) Liver and Urinary Bladder Tumors in Dogs from 3,3′-Dichlorobenzidine. *J. Environ. Path. Tox.* 1, 475–490.

Sundberg, J. P., Reilly, M. J., Wyand, D. S., and Fichandler, P. D. (1982) Pancreatic Adenocarcinoma in a Coyote–Dog Cross. *J. Wild. Dis.* 18, 513–515.

Trigo, F. J., Thompson, H., Breeze, R. G., and Nash, A. S. (1982) The Pathology of Liver Tumours in the Dog. *J. Comp. Path.* 92, 21–39.

Wadsworth, P. F., Majeed, S. K., Brancker, W. M., and Jones, D. M. (1978) Some Hepatic Neoplasms in Non-Domesticated Birds. *Avian Path.* 7, 551–555.

Waller, T., and Rubarth, S. (1967) Haemangioendothelioma in Domestic Animals. *Acta Vet. Scand.* 8, 234–261.

Watt, D. A. (1970) A Hepatocholangioma in a Sheep. *Austral. Vet. J.* 46, 552.

# 10

*Svend W. Nielsen and Jack E. Moulton*

# Tumors of the Urinary System

## TUMORS OF THE KIDNEY

Renal tumors are rare in animals and comprise the following types (in order of decreasing frequency): renal cell carcinoma, most frequently seen in dogs and cattle; embryonal nephroma, most frequently seen in pigs, chickens, and puppies; and renal adenoma, occasionally seen in horses and cattle. Renal lymphoma is frequent in cats, cattle, and chickens. Mesenchymal tumors of the renal stroma, fibroma, leiomyoma, lipoma, hemangioma, and their corresponding malignant counterparts are extremely rare in domestic animals. Renal pelvic transitional cell (urothelial) tumors, squamous cell carcinomas, and adenocarcinomas are rare but have been seen, mostly in dogs and cats.

## Adenoma

**Incidence.** In domestic animals benign tumors derived from renal tubular epithelium are rare and occur less often than their malignant counterparts. Renal adenomas are usually found incidentally at necropsy or slaughter in older animals. These tumors occur in all domestic species, but have been reported most often in the horse and ox. There are no valid statistics on age, breed, or sex prevalence of this neoplasm.

**Gross Morphology.** Adenomas are usually solitary, small, well-circumscribed, grayish white or yellow masses in the cortex of the kidney. In the horse and ox, adenomas may be quite large and the cut surfaces may have discolored areas due to necrosis and hemorrhage. Multiple and bilateral adenomas occur rarely. In humans renal adenomas are often found coincidentally in scarred contracted kidneys, but a similar association does not occur in domestic animals.

**Histological Features.** Microscopically, the tumors form tubular or papillary structures or sheets of epithelial cells. Mixtures of each are usually present. The tumor cells are cuboidal or columnar. In the former, the cytoplasm is scanty and basophilic or eosinophilic, and in the latter, it is pale or clear. Mitotic figures are uncommon.

In the absence of metastasis or invasion through the capsule, the distinction between renal adenoma and renal carcinoma (and hence predictable behavior) is quite arbitrary. Many pathologists classify human well-differentiated renal epithelial tumors less than 2 cm in diameter as adenomas, whereas larger ones are called carcinomas.

Small, well-differentiated carcinomas may metastasize, but tumors with a similar histological appearance may become massive to the extent that they displace adjacent organs, but without metastasis. For accurate evaluation, several blocks of tissue should be examined. A tumor that is circumscribed in one area may not be so in another.

# Carcinoma

**General Considerations.** There are many names for carcinoma of the kidney—hypernephroma, Grawitz's tumor, malignant nephroma, and clear cell carcinoma, which arises from the tubular epithelium of the kidney. The so-called clear cell type is rare in domestic animals but fairly common in humans. Since the cells of the clear cell carcinoma resemble those of the zona fasciculata of the adrenal gland, this neoplasm was once believed to arise from embryonal rests of adrenal tissue in the kidney and was called hypernephroma. This theory has been discarded. The clear cells in this tumor are known to be cells with fatty metamorphosis or hydropic degeneration and have no relationship to adrenal tissue. Rarely there is ectopic adrenal tissue in the kidney, but this has never been known to be the origin of neoplasia in domestic animals. Carcinoma of the kidney is a pure epithelial tumor arising from tubular epithelium rather than from embryonal nephrogenic tissue.

**Incidence.** Renal carcinomas are not common in any of the domestic species. They are most frequently encountered in the dog and ox and have been reported in the cat, horse, sheep, pig, and cottontail rabbit (Baskin and DePaoli, 1977; Carlton and Dietz, 1977; Flir, 1952; Hashek *et al.*, 1981; Sundberg and Nielsen, 1980). The incidence of renal carcinoma is 1.5 per 100,000 for dogs and 0.7 per 100,000 for cats (Lucke and Kelly, 1976; Nielsen, 1976).

**Age, Breed, and Sex.** Carcinoma usually occurs in older animals. Although the tumor has been reported in a 3-year-old dog, the average age in this species is 8 years. There is no known breed predisposition.

Male dogs are overrepresented in some reports. This male preponderance was evident at the University of California where the authors found 15 canine renal tumors (14 carcinomas and 1 adenoma), 12 of which were from males and 3 from females. The incidence in male dogs is 2.1 per 100,000 and the incidence in the bitch is 0.9 per 100,000. There is no sex predisposition in cats. In cattle these tumors have usually been reported from biased abattoir surveys where aged females are more frequently encountered. Information concerning sex predisposition in other species is not available.

**Clinical Characteristics.** Reports concerning clinical signs associated with renal carcinomas are limited mainly to the dog. Presenting signs are usually vague and nonspecific for renal disease, including listlessness, anorexia, vomiting, and weight loss. The more specific triad of hematuria, a palpable mass in the sublumbar region, and sublumbar pain are usually recognized late in the course, often after the tumor has metastasized. Coughing, reflecting metastasis to the lung, rear leg paresis representing metastasis to vertebrae, and vomiting following neoplastic obstruction of the bowel have been presenting signs in dogs with renal carcinomas. Laboratory tests may indicate anemia, hematuria, and occasionally uremia, the latter appearing only in dogs with coexisting nephritis. Polycythemia associated with the elaboration of erythropoietin by these tumors is observed occasionally in humans (Harrison and Mahoney, 1971). A similar association of polycythemia and renal carcinoma has been referred to by Osborne *et al.* (1972). Tumor cells may be present in the urine sediment. Radiological examination often reveals abnormalities of size or contour of the affected kidney, and excretory urography will usually demonstrate a space-occupying lesion. The tumor can be confirmed by needle biopsy; however, in the absence of metastasis, use of biopsy should be weighed against the possibility of facilitating metastasis or extension of the neoplasm via the needle tract. A laparotomy anticipating nephrectomy would probably be more appropriate.

**Sites.** The tumors are generally unilateral, but some with metastasis to the opposite kidney (Lacroix, 1942) give the false impression of bilateral origin. Incidence favors neither kidney. The tumor customarily originates in the cortex of the kidney and often develops in one pole.

**Gross Morphology.** Most carcinomas of the kidney are roughly spherical and become quite large (Flir, 1952; Schlegel, 1927). One in an ox weighed approximately 40 kg. The larger tumors replace the kidney partly or completely (figs. 10.1A and B). Some carcinomas are well-demarcated from adjacent renal tissue and are difficult to distinguish from adenomas at gross autopsy. The smaller tumors can be embedded within the cortex and are invisible. Some carcinomas extend into the peri-

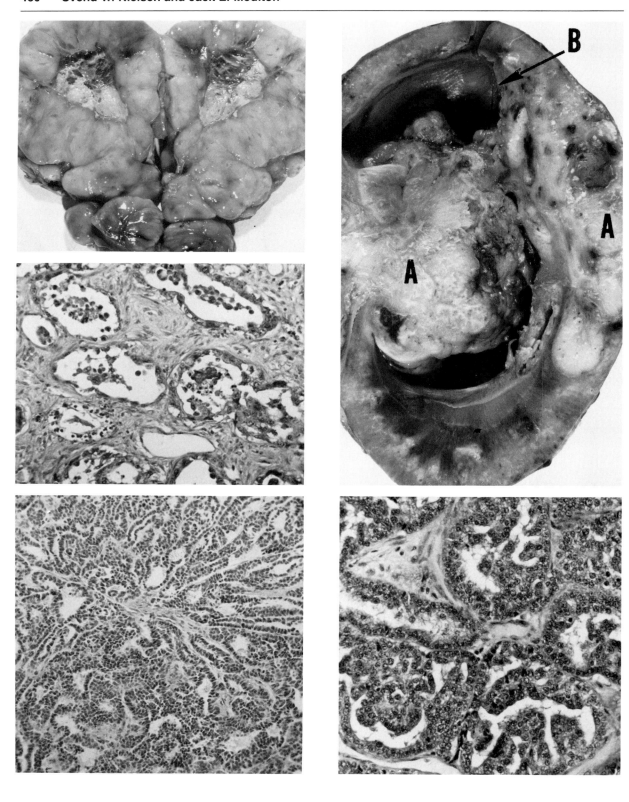

nephric tissues and form adhesions to neighboring structures (Wright, 1936). The renal pelvis and ureter may be involved (Borchmann, 1941). The tumor invades the renal artery or vein, vena cava, and aorta (Monlux *et al.,* 1956; Nielsen and Archibald, 1955), an observation the surgeon should be mindful of when contemplating nephrectomy. The tumors are usually multinodular and soft or hard and fibrous. They are also papillary and cystic (Anderes, 1948; Haigler, 1943). The color is white, gray, or yellow with red or yellow foci. As with neoplastic involvement of any organ, determining whether a renal tumor is primary or a metastasis from some other site depends on a thorough examination during surgical exploration or at necropsy. Adrenal carcinoma, for instance, may spread to the kidney via their shared vasculature and is mistaken clinically for primary renal tumor because the major mass of neoplastic tissue is in the kidney.

**Histological Features.** The tumors are classified according to their predominant pattern and cell type, but there is no indication that the biological behavior differs from one morphological type to another. The most common type in domestic animals is the papillary tubular adenocarcinoma. A second type is clear cell adenocarcinoma, which is rare in animals but is seen in cattle; this type is the most common form in humans (Nielsen *et al.,* 1976; Valade, 1935). The microscopic appearance often varies considerably from area to area within the same tumor, with tubular, acinar, solid, or filiform papillary formations (figs. 10.1C–E). The usual neoplastic cell is cuboidal, columnar, or polygonal and has a dark staining nucleus that is commonly located at one end of the cell. Mitotic figures are common. Some of the more undifferentiated tumors exhibit cells that are small, round, and hyperchromatic. In most tumors the cells display slightly acidophilic cytoplasm. Clear cell tumors consist primarily of large cells with clear cytoplasm containing lipid and glycogen. Some tumor cells have squamous metaplasia. The stroma is scanty or abundant and densely fibrous. The tumors are well vascularized and often exhibit hemorrhage and necrosis.

Predicting the behavior of these tumors on the basis of their histological appearance is sometimes difficult. Although the usual criteria for malignancy apply (anaplasia and invasion of adjacent tissue and vessels), some tumors consisting of well-differentiated tubular or papillary structures, not unlike adenomas, may also metastasize.

**Etiology and Transmission.** A causative agent for spontaneous renal carcinoma has not been demonstrated in domestic mammals or humans. Hormones may play a modulating role, as suggested by the higher incidence of this tumor in male dogs. Renal adenocarcinomas in humans and in Syrian hamsters may have a similar hormonal dependence. In the leopard frog, chicken, and gray squirrel, a causal relationship exists between renal tubular tumors and viruses. The Lucké adenocarcinoma of leopard frogs is caused by a herpes virus, which produces large intranuclear inclusion bodies in tumor cells (Lucké, 1952). The tumor has a distinct regional distribution occurring in northern New England, the province of Quebec, Minnesota, and Wisconsin and is present in as many as 9% of leopard frogs. In domestic chickens injected with certain strains of the avian leukosis oncornavirus, a few renal tubular adenomas occurred in addition to the much more common nephroblastoma and the lymphoid, myeloid, erythroid, endothelial, and fibrous tumors (Guillon and Chouroulinkov, 1964). The poxvirus of the eastern gray squirrel, in addition to the common cutaneous fibroma, is occasionally associated with renal tubular adenoma, bronchiolar–alveolar adenoma, and salivary adenoma. The tumorous epithelium contains large cytoplasmic poxvirus inclusions (O'Connor *et al.,* 1980).

Tubular renal adenocarcinoma has been observed in feral rats from a city garbage dump (Kilham *et al.,* 1962). The adenocarcinoma was believed to have been caused by inhalation of fumes containing

**FIGURE 10.1.** Carcinoma in the kidney of the dog. A. Almost complete replacement of the kidney by carcinoma. B. Neoplastic tissue in the cortex and medulla (A) and renal obstruction with dilatation of the renal pelvis (B). C. Neoplastic tubules lined by cuboidal cells. D. Papillary form of renal carcinoma. E. Irregular tubular formation with small papillary ingrowths of neoplastic cells.

lead from burning refuse. Experimentally, long-term administration of lead salts (phosphates and acetates) to rats and mice produced tubular hyperplasia, adenoma, and adenocarcinoma (Van Esch *et al.*, 1962).

**Growth and Metastasis.** The neoplasm is faster growing than embryonal nephroma and more prone to metastasis. Metastasis has usually occurred by the time the tumor is diagnosed. Renal adenocarcinomas in both humans and animals have a propensity for invasion of the renal vein and ascend up the posterior vena cava with early and frequent formation of pulmonary metastasis. The secondary growths may be widespread; renal and other lymph nodes, lung, liver, adrenals, and vertebrae are the most common sites (Kast, 1957; Stunzi, 1953). Secondary growths also occur in the opposite kidney, pancreas, spleen, heart, peritoneum, skeletal muscle, and other bones. In dogs a usual site for metastasis of this tumor is the skin. When such sites occur, the tumor can easily be mistaken for primary apocrine sweat gland adenocarcinoma; this diagnostic error can cause serious consequences for the clinician (Nielsen, 1976). In contrast to the high rate of metastasis in humans and dogs, a low rate is seen in nonhuman primates. In a study of 43 monkeys (mostly *Macaca mulatta*) with renal tubular carcinoma, only 2 showed metastasis (Jones and Casey, 1981). It is noteworthy that a renal carcinoma in a dog was found to be functioning and produced an abnormal erythropoietin, causing polycythemia (Peterson and Zanjani, 1981).

## Embryonal Nephroma

**General Considerations.** Embryonal nephroma has many names because of its morphological variations and the different concepts of its histogenesis. It also has been called renal or embryonal adenosarcoma, nephroblastoma, and Wilm's tumor. In 1907, Day called attention to tumors that he called embryonal adenosarcomas in the kidneys of slaughtered swine inspected in the abattoir. Since then, embryonal nephromas in domestic animals have been described a number of times. Feldman (1930, 1932, 1933) gave the first detailed description of the tumor in animals in a series of papers and in his monograph on animal neoplasms. Sullivan and

Anderson (1959) briefly reviewed the literature in their report dealing with the tumor in swine, as did Migaki *et al.* in 1971. The tumor is common in chickens (Guillon *et al.*, 1963).

Several reports described the tumor in dogs; these were reviewed by Baskin and DePaoli (1977). The tumor is not uncommon in young calves (Sandison and Anderson, 1968), and a few reports are available for cats (Cotchin, 1959; Potkay and Garman, 1969). The tumor is rare in sheep (Pamakcu, 1956) and horses (Lombard, 1959).

While some controversy still surrounds the histogenesis of this tumor, most workers believe it develops from the metanephric blastema. Electron microscopic studies support this concept. According to Willis (1948), the neoplasm arises from the metanephros or its primordium. The neoplasm is composed of multipotent and undifferentiated vestigial renal tissue that retains its primitive characteristics. The nephrogenic origin of this neoplasm is suggested by the tubules and glomerulus-like structures formed by the neoplastic cells. The tumor may be likened in some respects to an embryonic kidney persisting in a primitive form and never developing to a functional stage.

Besides epithelial tissue, some embryonal nephromas form smooth and skeletal muscle, cartilage, bone, and fat. These tissues are probably products of aberrant differentiation of the same primitive renal blastema that forms the epithelium.

**Incidence.** Embryonal nephromas are rare in all domestic species except the pig and chicken, in which they are common. The results of abattoir surveys in which large numbers of animals have been examined suggest that the incidence of embryonal nephroma in swine varies considerably from one geographic region to another. Embryonal nephroma is the most common tumor of swine in the United States where the estimated incidence is 20 per 100,000, with a much higher incidence in some localities (Brandley and Migaki, 1963). Anderson *et al.* (1969) reported 13 nephroblastomas in a survey of 3.7 million swine slaughtered in the United Kingdom, which is an incidence of 0.35 per 100,000. In an early survey, Jackson (1936) described 10 examples of embryonal nephroma in domestic animals in South Africa, but specifically observed that no cases occurred in swine. At the time of this survey the tumor was being observed with regularity in the United States and, to a lesser extent, in Europe.

**Age, Breed, and Sex.** Since these neoplasms arise in fetal (Roberto and Damiano, 1981) or early postnatal animals, the age group affected is younger than that affected with almost any other tumor. In swine 77% of these tumors are present by the age of 1 year, and 92% are in animals less than 2 years of age (Davis *et al.*, 1933; Sandison and Anderson, 1968; Sullivan and Anderson, 1959); however, the neoplasms are usually not recognized until market age (1 to 2 years of age). Usually the tumors are found in other domestic animals less than 1 year old also. The neoplasms infrequently occur in adults. The age incidence in dogs is similar to that in swine. The tumor has been reported in bovine fetuses (Kirkbride and Bicknell, 1972; Misdorp, 1967) and in a 3-week-old calf (Walker, 1943). Information regarding the breeds of affected swine with embryonal nephroma is not available in the literature, although this information could have a bearing on the regional variation of reported cases. There is no information on breed predilection in other domestic species.

Sullivan and Anderson (1959) recorded a male to female ratio of 2 : 1 in swine, but no sex predisposition was found in the smaller number of cases from the United Kingdom reported by Sandison and Anderson (1968). In six case reports of embryonal nephroma in the dog, four were in males and two were in females. We have observed embryonal nephromas in five dogs and all were males.

**Clinical Characteristics.** Embryonal nephroma often goes unnoticed and is usually observed as a coincidental finding in slaughtered swine in the abattoir.

Often no sign of renal impairment appears in swine since the uninvolved kidney undergoes hypertrophy and takes over the function of the other. In dogs and cats abdominal distention due to a large palpable sublumbar mass is the usual sign. In addition, reduced appetite and weight loss may occur. Gross or microscopic hematuria may be present. Hypoglycemia, which returned to normal following removal of an embryonal nephroma, was reported by Coleman *et al.* (1970). Mowder (1940) found a dog with an embryonal nephroma that ruptured, leading to hemoperitoneum and death.

**Sites.** The neoplasms are usually unilateral. A few are extrarenal, located in the sublumbar region.

The tumors usually occupy one pole of the kidney and are solitary but may be multiple or bilateral. The nephromas usually originate in the renal cortex. The tumor usually extends above the surface of the kidney and when large is often adherent to the omentum. Inward expansion of the tumor may extend to the medulla and renal pelvis. The remaining part of the involved kidney is often compressed into a thin shell at the periphery of the tumor.

**Gross Morphology.** The nephromas are firm, pale, spherical masses having nodular or lobulated external and cut surfaces. A distinct fibrous capsule usually surrounds and transects the tumor, delineating it from adjacent parenchyma and resulting in its lobular appearance. Sullivan and Anderson (1959) recorded considerable variation in the sizes of embryonal nephromas in swine, with tumors measuring 3 mm to 60 cm in diameter and some weighing over 30 kg. Most neoplasms in swine measure 2.0 × 3.5 cm to 17 × 30 cm. In the dog and cat the tumors are often large and displace other abdominal organs by the time they are recognized clinically.

Embryonal nephroma is firm but may contain soft areas of necrosis. The tumor is grayish white on cross section. Areas of muscle, bone, and cartilage are found in some of the neoplasms, particularly in the pig (Jackson, 1936) and chicken (Helmboldt and Jortner, 1966). Focal red or yellow discoloration associated, respectively, with necrosis and hemorrhage is often seen in cut surfaces. Cysts may also be recognized during gross examination of the tumor.

**Histological Features.** While the histological features of embryonal nephroma vary considerably, they are unique for this neoplasm. Regardless of whether the tumor consists predominantly of epithelial or mesenchymal elements, it is embryonic in its microscopic appearance. Typically, the tumor simulates embryonic renal tissue in varying degrees of disarray.

Epithelium predominates in the tumors in swine and connective tissue predominates in the tumors in ruminants (Sullivan and Anderson, 1959). These neoplasms can be pure epithelial tissue and have connective tissue present only as stroma or may consist of equal parts of both epithelial and connective tissue. The epithelial elements vary from well-differentiated tubules to lobular masses of undiffer-

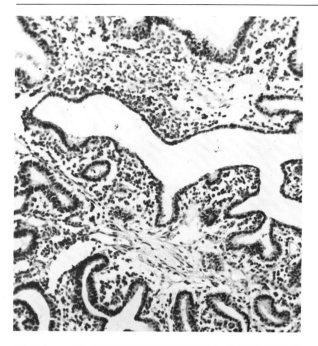

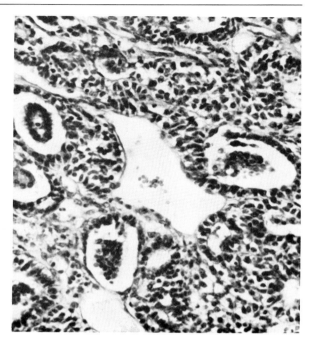

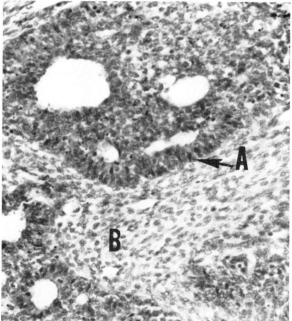

**FIGURE 10.2.** Embryonal nephroma. A. Tumor in a pig showing irregular tubular structure and abundant stroma. B. Nephroma in a dog with tuftlike invaginations of epithelial cells that resemble embryonic glomeruli. C. Tumor in a dog with epithelial masses of neoplastic cells (A) separated by highly cellular sarcomalike stroma (B).

entiated cells. The epithelial cells are also present in solid, branching cords and in nests. Structures resembling developing tubules (fig. 10.2A) surrounded by and blending imperceptibly with masses of undifferentiated cells are often present. The more differentiated tubules consist of single layers of cuboidal or columnar cells resting on basal lamina. Basal lamina are not present around the immature or formative tubular structures. Occasionally, epithelial structures form cysts or contain mucus-secreting cells or form nests of squamous epithelium. The cysts are lined by epithelium, which may exhibit squamous metaplasia with desquamation of keratin into the cystic cavities (Monlux et al., 1956). Some epithelial cells in these neoplasms exhibit marked mitotic activity. Primitive, dark staining, flattened epithelial cells form glomerulus-like invaginations (fig. 10.2B) as though attempting to form visceral and parietal layers of glomerular epithelium. Usually no capillaries are present in these structures; the epithelial cells practically fill the cavities.

The mesenchymal component of the tumor may consist of a sparsely cellular connective tissue stroma. The predominant neoplastic component of the tumor may consist of sarcomatous tissue forming lobular masses and sheets of polygonal cells dispersed in random fashion or it may consist of spindle cells forming whorls and herringbone patterns (fig. 10.2C). While differentiation of the sarcomatous element of the tumor can develop along several different cell lines, fibrosarcoma with collagen production is the most common form of differentiation. In some cases smooth or striated muscle fibers are found and, infrequently, bone or cartilage. When the latter two components are prominent, they probably represent a metaplastic change.

**Etiology and Transmission.** In the chicken, embryonal nephromas have been experimentally produced by the oncornavirus of the avian leukosis complex as an etiological agent (Guillon and Chouroulinkov, 1964). No such agent has been demonstrated in the tumors of other species.

**Growth and Metastasis.** The large and sometimes massive size attained by these tumors in young animals attests to their capability for rapid growth. Although the tumors may be large or multiple within a kidney, metastasis infrequently occurs in swine. The large size indicates infrequent metastasis (Feldman, 1928); if metastasis occurred, the host would be killed before the tumor had time to grow so large. This does not appear, however, to be the case in dogs; out of 11 cases metastasis was present in 8. In cats, although the number of reported cases is small, metastasis has been described. The same is true in other domestic species. It appears that recognizing embryonal nephroma in a live animal other than swine warrants corrective action as appropriate for any such malignancy in the host. Either epithelial or connective tissue components of the tumor are involved in metastasis; in some cases both parts metastasize (Feldman, 1933). Mitotic activity and cellular anaplasia are not correlated with a tendency to metastasize. Metastatic secondaries are found in the sublumbar, renal, mesenteric, and bronchial lymph nodes (Drew et al., 1972). Metastatic cells are also found in the lungs, liver, peritoneum, or opposite kidney (Savage and Isa, 1954). Nodular implantations can be seen in the peritoneum, omentum, and mesentery (Medway and Nielsen, 1954).

## TUMORS OF THE RENAL PELVIS AND URETERS

Tumors in the renal pelvis and ureters are extremely rare, but have been described in the cat and dog (Bloom, 1954; Nielsen, 1964). The same histological types occur here as in the urinary bladder, with the transitional cell (urothelial) papilloma or carcinoma being the most important. Small cauliflowerlike lesions without invasion are papillomas, whereas large ones with invasion are carcinomas. Large lesions may result in obstruction and subsequent hydronephrosis. Squamous cell carcinoma and adenocarcinoma are extremely rare in both animals and humans.

## TUMORS OF THE URINARY BLADDER AND URETHRA

### Transitional Cell (Urothelial) Papilloma

In cattle papillomas account for approximately 17% of primary tumors of the bladder and in dogs, 14% (Pamukcu, 1974). The incidence is not known in other domestic species. This neoplasm usually

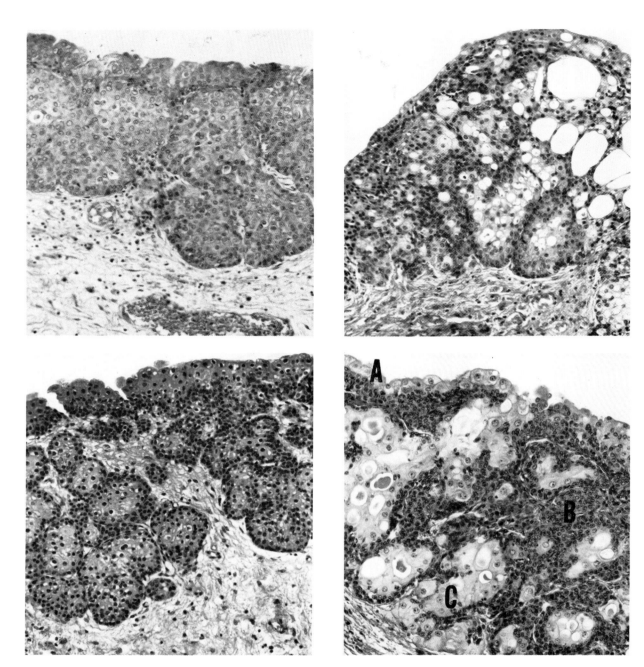

A|B
C|D

**FIGURE 10.3.** Neoplasia of the urinary bladder of dogs, experimentally induced with 2-naphthylamine. A. Preneoplastic epithelial hyperplasia showing thickened epithelial layers (approximately 10 instead of 4 or 5 cells thick). In general, cells retain polarity and are similar to normal transitional cells. Papilloma would probably follow this change. B. Early papilloma showing outward projection of transitional cells and considerable squamous metaplasia. Tumor has not yet become organized into separate papillae with connective tissue stalks. C. Nodular thickening com-posed of transitional cells in early papillomatous change. Next growth would be outward, or growth might continue as downward penetration forming invasive transitional cell carcinoma. D. Squamous metaplasia within nodular thickening of transitional cells. Single layer of less affected transitional cells (A) is at surface. Small, dark cells (B) are undifferenti-ated transitional cells; large, vacuolated ones (C) are squamous cells. The neoplasm may grow outward as papilloma or downward as invasive carcinoma. (Courtesy of *J. Natl. Cancer Inst.*)

nary bladder through the urine, as in experimental urinary bladder tumors of dogs. The tumors are usually confined to the mucous membrane, but when malignant they may invade the muscular wall of the bladder. Tumors of the pelvis, kidney, and ureters may also occur along with enzootic hematuria, but they are not common. If they do occur, they are of the same type as those found in the bladder. Some cows with bladder tumors also develop carcinoma of the pharynx and esophagus (Dobereiner *et al.*, 1967).

**Gross Morphology.** The gross appearance of these neoplasms is generally similar to that described for bladder tumors in this chapter. The tumors appear polypoid, may be single growths or occur in aggregations, and are often pedunculated or sessile (Goto *et al.*, 1954). Some contain mucin cysts.

**Histological Features.** Many types of urinary tumors, both mesenchymal and epithelial, are seen in cattle with enzootic hematuria. Papilloma, adenoma, adenocarcinoma, urothelial carcinoma, squamous cell carcinoma, fibroma, hemangioma, and hemangiosarcoma occur (figs. 10.7A and B).

Histological changes affect the bladder before or at the same time as the neoplasms; these were summarized by Datta (1953*b*). They consist of focal hyperemia, edema, petechial hemorrhages, and occasional ulcers. The mucosal and submucosal blood vessels are dilated and may become ruptured with hemorrhage resulting. Edema sometimes separates the mucosal layer from the submucosal layer. Endarteritis obliterans and detachment of vascular endothelium are also observed.

**Etiology and Transmission.** The etiology of naturally occurring urinary bladder tumors in cattle is not known, but numerous factors have been suggested to be of causal significance. These include dietetic deficiencies, ingestion of poisonous plants, deficiency of lime or excess molybdenum in the soil, and infectious agents (bacterial, mycotic, or protozoal). The geographical distribution and endemic nature of this disease parallel the importance of these factors in industrial cancers of the bladder in humans (Bryan *et al.*, 1963). However, contrary to industrial cancers of the human bladder, for which at least three aromatic amines have been implicated as causative factors, the etiology of naturally occurring bovine urinary bladder tumors remains obscure.

A number of experimental investigations have suggested that bracken fern is implicated in the etiology of enzootic hematuria and bladder neoplasms in cattle. Rosenberger and Heeschen (1960) produced hematuria, but not tumors, in 5 cows fed bracken fern for 15 months. Pamukcu (1963) produced the syndrome in cattle fed the fern for 46 to 365 days. One cow developed a papilloma of the urinary bladder after 360 days. In another experiment, Pamukcu *et al.* (1967) harvested bracken fern from an enzootic area in Turkey and fed it to 18 cattle. Of this group, 10 developed bladder tumors, 3 of which were carcinomas. The cattle that had neoplasms were fed low levels of fern for an average period of 550 days. Price and Pamukcu (1968) also produced bladder tumors in cattle fed the fern for 510 to 1,920 days. Transitional cell carcinoma, hemangioma, and papilloma predominated. All animals had hematuria for months or years before developing neoplasms.

Bracken fern has also been found to be carcinogenic when fed to rats; neoplasms occur in the urinary bladder and intestine (Evans and Mason, 1965; Pamukcu and Price, 1969; Pamukcu *et al.*, 1970).

No viral agent has been consistently recovered from the naturally occurring bovine bladder tumors. The agent of bovine cutaneous papillomatosis, however, has been found capable of producing fibromalike lesions when injected into the submucosa of the urinary bladder of cattle (Brobst and Olson, 1965; Olson *et al.*, 1959, 1962). Pamukcu (1963) produced fibropapillomas in the skin of calves with inoculation of different bladder tumor materials.

## REFERENCES

Anderes, R. L. (1948) Nephroma with Pulmonary Metastasis. *N. Amer. Vet.* 29, 654.

Anderson, A. C. (1963) Carcinoma of the Bladder in a Beagle. *J. Amer. Vet. Med. Assoc.* 143, 30–33.

Anderson, L. J., Sandison, A. T., and Jarrett, W. F. H. (1969) A British Abattoir Survey of Tumors in Cattle, Sheep, and Pigs. *Vet. Rec.* 84, 547–551.

Bankier, J. C. (1943) Enzootic Bovine Haematuria (Redwater of Cattle) in British Columbia. *Canad. J. Comp. Med.* 7, 101–106, 146–151, 178–181.

Baskin, G. B., and DePaoli, A. (1977) Primary Renal Neoplasms of the Dog. *Vet. Path.* 14, 591–605.

Bloom, F. (1954) *Pathology of the Dog and Cat: The Genitourinary System, with Clinical Considerations.* American Veterinary Publications (Evanston, Illinois).

Bonser, G. M. (1943) Epithelial Tumours of the Bladder in Dogs Induced by Pure B-Naphthylamine. *J. Path. Bact.* 55, 1–3.

Bonser, G. M., Clayson, D. B., and Jull, J. W. (1951) An Experimental Inquiry into the Cause of Industrial Bladder Cancer. *Lancet* 261, 286–288.

Borchmann, H. M. (1941) Adenocarcinoma in the Kidney. *Cornell Vet.* 31, 78–80.

Brandley, P. J., and Migaki, G. (1963) Types of Tumours Found by Federal Meat Inspectors in an Eight-Year Survey. *Ann. N.Y. Acad. Sci.* 108, 872–879.

Brobst, D. F., and Olson, C. (1965) Histopathology of Urinary Bladder Tumors Induced by Bovine Cutaneous Papilloma Agent. *Cancer Res.* 25, 12–19.

Bryan, G. T., Brown, R. R., and Price, J. M. (1963) Studies on the Etiology of Bovine Bladder Cancer. *Ann. N.Y. Acad. Sci.* 108, 924–937.

Bull, L. B., Dickenson, C. G., and Dann, A. T. (1932) *Enzootic Haematuria (Haematuria Vesicalis) of Cattle in South Australia.* Council of Science and Industrial Research Australia. Pamphlet 33, 24–27.

Carlton, W. W., and Dietz, J. M. (1977) Two Renal Tumors in Cottontail Rabbits (*Sylvilagus floridanus*). *Vet. Path.* 14, 29–35.

Coleman, G. L., Gralla, E. J., Kirsch, A. K., and Stebbins, R. B. (1970) Canine Embryonal Nephroma: A Case Report. *Amer. J. Vet. Res.* 31, 1315–1320.

Conzelman, G. M., Jr., and Moulton, J. E. (1972) Dose-Response Relationships of the Bladder Tumorigen 2-Naphthylamine: A Study in Beagle Dogs. *J. Natl. Cancer Inst.* 49, 193–205.

Cotchin, E. (1959) Some Tumours in Dogs and Cats of Comparative Veterinary and Human Interest. *Vet. Rec.* 71, 1040–1054.

Datta, S. (1952) Chronic Bovine Haematuria. I. History of the Disease. *Indian Vet. J.* 29, 187–209.

———. (1953a) Chronic Bovine Haematuria. *Indian Vet. J.* 30, 1–33.

———. (1953b) Chronic Bovine Haematuria. V. The Lesions. *Indian Vet. J.* 30, 96–119.

Davis, C. L., Leeper, R. B., and Shelton, J. E. (1933) Neoplasms Encountered in Federally Inspected Establishments in Denver, Colorado. *J. Amer. Vet. Med. Assoc.* 83, 229–237.

Day, L. E. (1907) *Embryonal Adenosarcoma of the Kidney of Swine.* 24th Annual Report of the Bureau of Animal Industry (Washington, D.C.), 247.

Dobereiner, J., Tokarnia, C. H., and Canella, C. F. C. (1967) Ocorrencia da hematuria enzootica e de carcinomas epidermoide no trato digestivo superior em bovinos no Brasil. *Pesquisa Agropec. Bras.* 2, 489–504.

Drew, R. A., Done, S. J., and Robins, G. M. (1972) Canine Embryonal Nephroma: A Case Report, *J. Small Anim. Pract.* 13, 27–39.

Druckrey, H. (1967) Quantitative Aspects in Chemical Carcinogenesis. In: Truhaut, T., ed., *Potential Carcinogenic Hazards from Drugs.* UICC Monograph Series, Vol. 7. Springer-Verlag (New York), 60–78.

Evans, I. A., and Mason, J. (1965) Carcinogenic Activity of Bracken. *Nature* 208, 913–914.

Feldman, W. N. (1928) A Study of the Histopathology of the So-Called Adenosarcoma of Swine. *Amer. J. Path.* 4, 125–138.

———. (1930) Extranephric Embryonal Nephroma in a Hog. *J. Cancer Res.* 14, 116–119.

———. (1932) *Neoplasms of Domesticated Animals.* W. B. Saunders (Philadelphia), 410.

———. (1933) Embryonal Nephroma in a Sheep. *Amer. J. Cancer* 17, 743–747.

Flir, K. (1952) Die primaren Nierengeschwulste der Haussäugetiere. *Wiss. Z. Humboldt-Univ.* 2, 93–119.

Geib, L. W., Bellhorn, R. W., and Whitehead, J. E. (1967) Transitional Cell Carcinoma of the Urinary Bladder in a Dog with Unusual Clinical Signs. *Anim. Hosp.* 3, 22–27.

Goto, J., Kato, S., and Hoshikawa, N. (1954) Pathological and Morphological Study on the Hematurial Cystic Tumor in Formosan Cattle. *Jap. J. Vet. Sci.* 16, 209–218.

Guillon, J. C., and Chouroulinkov, I. (1964) Les Tumeurs Rénales chez le Poulet. *Econ. Med. Anim.* 4, 238–247.

Guillon, J. C., Chouroulinkov, I., and Renault, L. (1963) Les Tumeurs Rénales Spontanées des Gallinaces. *Bull. Cancer.* 50, 593–620.

Hadwen, S. (1917) Bovine Haematuria. *J. Amer. Vet. Med. Assoc.* 51, 822–830.

Haigler, S. W. (1943) Adenocarcinoma of the Kidney in a Dog. *J. Amer. Vet. Med. Assoc.* 102, 469–471.

Harrison, J. H., and Mahoney, E. M. (1971) Tumors of the Kidney. In: Strauss, M. B., and Welt, L. G., eds., *Diseases of the Kidney.* 2d ed. Little, Brown and Co. (Boston), 1319–1348.

Harrold, M. W., Edwards, C. N., and Garvey, F. K. (1964) Treatment of Bladder Tumors by Direct Instillation of 5-Fluorouracil: Experimental Observations in Dogs. *Invest. Urol.* 2, 47–51.

Hashek, W. M., King, J. M., and Tennant, B. C. (1981) Primary Renal Cell Carcinoma in Two Horses. *J. Amer. Vet. Med. Assoc.* 179, 992–994.

Hayes, H. M., Jr., Hoover, R., and Tarone, R. E. (1981) Bladder Cancer in Pet Dogs: A Sentinel for Environmental Cancer? *Amer. J. Epid.* 114, 229–233.

Helmboldt, C. F., and Jortner, B. S. (1966) Histologic Features of the Avian Embryonal Nephroma. *Avian Dis.* 10, 452–462.

Hueper, W. C. (1969) *Occupational and Environmental Cancers of the Urinary System.* Yale University Press (New Haven, Conn.), 191–228.

Hueper, W. C., Wiley, F. H., and Wolfe, H. D. (1938) Experimental Production of Bladder Tumors in Dogs by Administration of Betanaphthylamine. *J. Ind. Hyg. Toxicol.* 20, 46–84.

Hurov, L., Ellet, E. W., and O'Hara, P. J. (1966) Bilateral Hydronephrosis Resulting from a Transitional Epithelial Carcinoma in a Dog. *J. Amer. Vet. Med. Assoc.* 149, 412–417.

Huynen, E. (1912) Hydronephrosis Caused by Vesicular Cancer in a Dog. *Am. Vet. Rev.* 41, 610–611.

Jabara, A. G. (1968) Three Cases of Primary Malignant

Neoplasms Growing in the Canine Urinary System. *J. Comp. Path.* 78, 335–339.

Jackson, C. (1936) The Incidence and Pathology of Tumours of Domesticated Animals in South Africa: A Study of the Onderstepoort Collection of Neoplasms with Special Reference to their Histopathology. *Onderstepoort J. Vet. Sci. Anim. Indust.* 6, 1–460.

Jewett, H. J. (1954) Tumors of the Bladder. In: Campbell, M. F., ed., *Urology.* Vol. II. W. B. Saunders (Philadelphia).

Jonas, A. M., and Wyand, D. S. (1963) Primary Adenocarcinoma of the Canine Urinary Bladder. *J. Amer. Vet. Med. Assoc.* 146, 1059–1065.

Jones, S. R., and Casey, H. W. (1981) Primary Renal Tumors in Nonhuman Primates. *Vet. Path.* 18, 89–104.

Kast, A. (1956) Die Epithelgeschwulste der ableitenden Harnwege bei den Haussäugetieren. *Mh. Vet. Med.* 11, 483–490.

———. (1957) Das Nierenkarzinom des Hundes. *Mh. Vet. Med.* 12, 154–156.

Kilham, L., Low, R. J., Conti, S. F., and Dallenbach, F. D. (1962) Intranuclear Inclusions and Neoplasms in the Kidney of Wild Rats. *J. Natl. Cancer Inst.* 29, 863–885.

Kirkbride, C. A., and Bicknell, E. J. (1972) Nephroblastoma in a Bovine Fetus. *Vet. Path.* 9, 96–98.

Lacroix, J. V. (1942) Adenocarcinoma of Kidney. *N. Amer. Vet.* 23, 667.

Lombard, C. (1959) La Prédisposition aux Tumeurs Rénales Spontanées dans le Monde Animal. *Bull. Cancer* (Paris), 46, 460–464.

Lucké, B. (1952) Kidney Carcinoma in the Leopard Frog: A Virus Tumor. *Ann. N.Y. Acad. Sci.* 54, 1093–1109.

Lucke, V. M., and Kelly, D. F. (1976) Renal Carcinoma in the Dog. *Vet. Path.* 13, 264–276.

Marshall, V. F., Green, J. L., and Harris, J. J. (1956) Hormonal Influences on the Experimental Production of Bladder Tumors in Dogs. *Cancer,* 9, 622–625.

Martincinc, M. (1955) Haematuria vesicalis cancerogenes bovis. *Vet. Sarajevo,* 4, 525–612.

McDonald, D. F., and Lund, R. R. (1954) The Role of the Urine in Vesical Neoplasm: I. Experimental Confirmation of the Urogenous Theory of Pathogenesis. *J. Urol.* 71, 560–570.

Medway, W., and Nielsen, S. W. (1954) Canine Renal Disorders. II. Embryonal Nephroma in a Puppy. *N. Amer. Vet.* 35, 920–923.

Migaki, G., Nelson, L. W., and Todd, G. C. (1971) Prevalence of Embryonal Nephroma in Slaughtered Swine. *J. Amer. Vet. Med. Assoc.* 159, 441–442.

Misdorp, W. (1967) Tumors in Large Domestic Animals in the Netherlands. *J. Comp. Path.* 77, 211–216.

Monlux, A. W., Anderson, W. A., and Davis, C. L. (1956) A Survey of Tumors Occurring in Cattle, Sheep and Swine. *Amer. J. Vet. Res.* 17, 646–677.

Morris, H. P., and Eyestone, W. H. (1953) Tumors of the Liver and Urinary Bladder of the Dog after Ingestion of 2-acetylamino-fluorene. *J. Natl. Cancer Inst.* 13, 1139–1165.

Mostofi, F. K. (1962) Pathology of Cancer of the Bladder. *Acta Ohio Intern. Contra Cancrum* 18, 611–615.

Mowder, W. H. (1940) An Embryonal Adenosarcoma of the Kidney. *Vet. Med.* 35, 659.

Mugera, G. M., Nderito, P., and Sorheim, A. O. (1969) The Pathology of Urinary Bladder Tumours in Kenya Zebu Cattle. *J. Comp. Path.* 79, 251–254.

Mulligan, R. M. (1963) Comparative Pathology of Human and Canine Cancer. *Ann. N.Y. Acad. Sci.* 108, 642–690.

Nelson, A. A., and Woodard, G. (1953) Tumors of the Urinary Bladder, Gall Bladder, and Liver in Dogs Fed O-Aminoazotoluene or p-Dimethylaminoazobenzene. *J. Natl. Cancer Inst.* 13, 1497–1509.

Nielsen, S. W. (1964) *Neoplastic Disease in Feline Medicine and Surgery.* Catcott, E. J., ed. American Veterinary Publications (Santa Barbara), 156–176.

———. (1976) *CRC Handbook of Laboratory Animal Science.* Vol. 3. Melby, E. C., and Altman, N. H., eds. Chemical Rubber Company (Cleveland).

Nielsen, S. W., and Archibald, J. (1955) Canine Renal Disorders. III. Renal Carcinoma in Three Dogs. *N. Amer. Vet.* 36, 36–40.

Nielsen, S. W., Mackey, L. J., and Misdorp, W. (1976) Tumours of the Kidney. *Bull. Wld. Hlth. Org.* 53, 237–240.

O'Connor, D. J., Diters, R. W., and Nielsen, S. W. (1980) Poxvirus and Multiple Tumors in an Eastern Gray Squirrel. *J. Amer. Vet. Med. Assoc.* 177, 792–795.

Olson, C., Luedke, A. J., and Brobst, D. F. (1962) Induced Immunity of Skin, Vagina and Urinary Bladder to Bovine Papillomatosis. *Cancer Res.* 22, 463–468.

Olson, C., Pamukcu, A. M., Brobst, D. F., Kowalczyk, T., Satter, E. J., and Price, J. M. (1959) A Urinary Bladder Tumor Induced by a Bovine Cutaneous Papilloma Agent. *Cancer Res.* 19, 779–782.

Osborne, C. A., Low, D. G., and Finco, D. R. (1972) *Canine and Feline Urology.* W. B. Saunders (Philadelphia), 358–359.

Osborne, C. A., Low, D. G., Perman, V., and Barnes, D. M. (1968) Neoplasms of the Canine and Feline Urinary Bladders: Incidence, Etiologic Factors, Occurrence, and Pathologic Features. *Amer. J. Vet. Res.* 29, 2041–2055.

Pamukcu, A. M. (1955) Investigation on the Pathology of Enzootic Bovine Hematuria in Turkey. *Zbl. Vet. Med.* 2, 409–429.

———. (1956) An Annotation on the Occurrence of Tumours in Sheep. *Brit. Vet. J.* 112, 499–506.

———. (1957) Tumors of the Urinary Bladder in Cattle and Water Buffalo Affected with Enzootic Bovine Hematuria. *Zbl. Vet. Med.* 4, 185–197.

———. (1963) Epidemiologic Studies on Urinary Bladder Tumors in Turkish Cattle. *Ann. N.Y. Acad. Sci.* 108, 938–947.

———. (1974) Tumors of the Urinary Bladder. *Bull. Wld. Hlth. Org.* 50, 43–52.

Pamukcu, A. M., and Price, J. M. (1969) Induction of Intestinal and Urinary Bladder Cancer in Rats by

Feeding Bracken Fern (*Pteris aquilina*). *J. Natl. Cancer Inst.* 43, 275–281.

Pamukcu, A. M., Goksoy, S. K., and Price, J. M. (1967) Urinary Bladder Neoplasms Induced by Feeding Bracken Fern (*Pteris aquilina*) to Cows. *Cancer Res.* 27, 917–924.

Pamukcu, A. M., Yalciner, S., Price, J. M., and Bryan, G. T. (1970) Effects of the Coadministration of Thiamine on the Incidence of Urinary Bladder Carcinomas in Rats Fed Bracken Fern. *Cancer Res.* 30, 2671–2674.

Peterson, M. E., and Zanjani, E. D. (1981) Inappropriate Erythropoietin Production from a Renal Carcinoma in a Dog with Polycythemia. *J. Amer. Vet. Med. Assoc.* 179, 995–996.

Potkay, S., and Garman, R. (1969) Nephroblastoma in a Cat: The Effects of Nephrectomy and Occlusion of the Caudal Vena Cava. *J. Small Anim. Pract.* 10, 345–349.

Price, J. M., and Pamukcu, A. M. (1968) The Induction of Neoplasms of the Urinary Bladder of the Cow and the Small Intestine of the Rat by Feeding Bracken Fern (*Pteris aquilina*). *Cancer Res.* 28, 2247–2251.

Rehn, L. (1895) Blasengeschwulste bei Fuchs-Arbeitern. *Arch. Klin. Chir.* 50, 588–600.

Roberto, F., and Damiano, S. (1981) Nephroblastoma in an Ovine Foetus. *Zbl. Vet. Med.* 28A, 504–507.

Rosenberger, C., and Heeschen, W. (1960) Adleriarn (*Pteris aquilina*) die Crsache der sog. Stallrotes der Rindern (Haematuria vesicalis bovis chronica). *Dtsch. Tierärztl. Wschr.* 67, 201–208.

Ryan, C. P., and Holshuh, H. J. (1981) Urethral Adenocarcinoma in a Dog. *Vet. Med.* 76, 1315–1317.

Sandison, A. T., and Anderson, L. J. (1968) Tumors of the Kidney in Cattle, Sheep, and Pigs. *Cancer* 21, 727–742.

Savage, A., and Isa, J. M. (1954) Embryonal Nephroma with Metastasis in a Dog. *J. Amer. Vet. Med. Assoc.* 124, 185–186.

Schade, R. O. K., and Swinney, J. (1968) Precancerous Changes in Bladder Epithelium. *Lancet* 2, 943–946.

Schlegel, M. (1927) Riesenhaftes Cystocarcinoma papilliferum der Niere beim Rind. *Arch. Wiss. Prokt. Tierheilk.* 56, 285–287.

Scott, W. W., and Boyd, H. L. (1953) A Study of the Carcinogenic Effect of Beta-Naphthylamine on the Normal and Substituted Isolated Sigmoid Loop Bladder of Dogs. *J. Urol.* 70, 914–925.

Stalker, L. K., and Schlotthauer, C. F. (1936) Carcinoma of the Urethra of a Female Dog. *Amer. J. Cancer* 28, 591–594.

Stunzi, H. (1953) Carcinoma renale beim Hund. *Schweiz. Arch. Tierheilk.* 9, 238–257.

Sullivan, D. J., and Anderson, W. A. (1959) Embryonal Nephroma in Swine. *Amer. J. Vet. Res.* 20, 324–332.

Sundberg, J. P., and Nielsen, S. W. (1980) *Bovine Medicine and Surgery.* Vol. 1. Amstutz, H. E., ed. American Veterinary Publications (Santa Barbara, California), 605–647.

Valade, P. (1935) Néphrome à cellules claires (hypernéphrome) du chien. *Rec. Méd. Vét.* 111, 577–582.

Valade, P., and Pataud, P. (1939) Cancer du basinet du cheval. *Rec. Méd. Vét.* 115, 226–232.

Van Esch, G., Van Genderen, H. J., and Vink, H. H. (1962) The Induction of Renal Tumours by Feeding of Basic Lead Acetate to Rats. *Brit. J. Cancer.* 16, 289–297.

Walker, R. (1943) Embryonal Nephroma in a Calf. *J. Amer. Vet. Med. Assoc.* 102, 7–10.

Walpole, A. L., Williams, M. H. C., and Roberts, D. C. (1954) Tumours of the Urinary Bladder in Dogs after Ingestion of 4-aminodiphenyl. *Brit. J. Ind. Med.* 11, 105–109.

Willis, R. A. (1948) *Pathology of Tumours.* Butterworth & Co. (London).

Wright, J. G. (1936) Primary Carcinoma of the Kidney in the Dog: Operation of Nephrectomy. *Vet. J.* 92, 261–262.

Yoshikawa, T., and Oyamada, T. (1975) Histopathology of Papillary Tumors in the Bovine Urinary Bladder. *Jap. J. Vet. Sci.* 37, 277–287.

A few canine Sertoli cell tumors exhibit formation of intracellular and extracellular fibrillar bodies that tinctorially and ultrastructurally suggest secretion of basement membrane material by the neoplastic Sertoli cells (Hauser and Wild, 1978).

The fine structure of cells in canine Sertoli cell tumors shows that they have no intercellular junctions or crystals as do normal Sertoli cells. The tumor cells differ from seminoma and Leydig tumor cells by their elongated shape, orientation, intracytoplasmic filaments, lipids, mitochondrial cristae, and abundance of other organelles (Von Bomhard *et al.*, 1978).

*The intratubular form*—Most Sertoli cell tumors display well-formed tubules separated by connective tissue septa (figs. 11.1C and D). The tumor cells are multilayered in the tubules and are generally arranged with their long axes perpendicular to the basement membrane. The cells in the center of the tubule may become detached. The palisaded tumor cells are long and fusiform, with thin cytoplasmic prolongations and indistinct cell borders. The nuclei are small, hypochromatic, elongated, round or oval, and stain lightly basophilic. The cytoplasm is vacuolated, and lipochrome pigment granules in the tumor cells are frequent. In some areas intratubular neoplastic cells spill out of the tubules into the stroma, forming solid infiltrating cords or broad sheets.

*The diffuse form*—Malignant tumors are usually of the diffuse type, being more infiltrative with less tendency to remain in the tubules. The tumor cells may invade the tunica albuginea, rete testis, epididymis, and even scrotal skin. Local lymphatics and veins are frequently invaded. The cells are more irregular in size and shape and are round, polyhedral, or ovoid rather than spindled or fusiform. The cells in the malignant tumors have less tendency to palisade and possess larger, more hyperchromatic nuclei. The cytoplasm exhibits a fine vacuolation or none at all. Mitotic figures are uncommon even in the most malignant tumors of the diffuse type and are extremely rare in the benign intratubular type. Some tumor cells line up in multiple layers and form cystic cavities containing homogeneous acidophilic fluid.

A few anaplastic Sertoli cell tumors have areas resembling those of seminoma. There is often no clear demarcation between seminomalike areas and the rest of the tumor. It is not clear whether this represents atypical differentiation or dedifferentiation of Sertoli cells or whether it is a true mixed or collision tumor of Sertoli and seminoma cells (Cotchin, 1960*b;* Nielsen and Lein, 1974; Scully and Coffin, 1952). The histogenesis of this intermediate cell type between Sertoli cell and seminoma cell is difficult to explain with our current knowledge of gonadal embryology.

**Growth and Metastasis.** Metastasis occurs in 10 to 14% of Sertoli cell tumors. Since the probability is low that a malignant tumor will develop in the opposite testicle, bilateral orchidectomy, as often practiced, is not required (Dow, 1962). Metastatic lesions can be found in the sublumbar, internal iliac, inguinal, mesenteric, and periaortic lymph nodes and in the liver, lungs, kidneys, spleen, adrenals, and pancreas. The metastatic cells resemble the cells of the primary tumor except that they generally form fewer tubules. The metastatic cells are as capable of producing hormones as are the primary tumor cells.

It is important that clinicians recognize that an initial gradual disappearance of the feminizing signs and lesions of a Sertoli cell tumor occurs after removal of the involved testis, but may be followed by reappearance of feminization 4 to 8 months later. This usually indicates the presence of internal metastases that have reached sufficient size and estrogen production to cause refeminization (Coffin *et al.*, 1952).

## Interstitial (Leydig) Cell Tumor

**General Considerations.** The interstitial (Leydig) cells of the testis pass through all stages of cellular activity from quiescence to physiological hyperplasia to neoplasia. It is difficult to distinguish between nodular hyperplasia and adenoma of the interstitial cells. Criteria that suggest hyperplasia rather than neoplasia include multiple origin, bilateral involvement, small size, and senility in the host. An arbitrary way is to classify grossly viable nodules more than 2 mm in diameter as tumors and small microscopic proliferations as nodular hyperplasias.

**Incidence.** This neoplasm is very common in the dog, infrequent in the bull, and very rare in the cat, stallion, boar, and ram (Ball and Douville, 1926; Smith, 1954). McEntee (1958) reported interstitial cell tumors in 12 bulls. All of the tumors were yellowish brown, soft, and bulging and measured a few millimeters to over 6 cm in diameter. They were often multiple and bilateral.

**Age, Breed, and Sex.** Dogs with interstitial cell tumors are usually 8 years old or more; the average age is 11 years. Incidence increases with age, but the tumor has been found in dogs as young as 4 years of age. There is no breed prevalence.

**Clinical Characteristics.** The interstitial cells of the normal animal secrete male hormones and are responsible for the secondary sex characteristics of the male. Tumors of these cells, however, have no hormonal effect on either the opposite testicle or other organs and tissues, and libido is not increased (Huggins and Pazos, 1945). Clinical changes have been reported (Lipowitz *et al.*, 1973), such as prostatic disease, perianal gland tumors, alopecia, and perineal hernia, but these changes are common in old dogs with or without interstitial cell tumors.

**Sites.** Interstitial cell adenomas may be either solitary or multiple in the same or opposite testis. About half are bilateral, and an equal number are multiple in the same testicle. An enlarged testicle is found in 16% of cases, but other clinical signs are uncommon. Some interstitial cell adenomas are found in cryptorchid testicles, but the association is rare compared with the other testicular tumors.

**Gross Morphology.** In dogs about 60% of the tumors measure less than 1 cm in diameter, about 30% are 2 to 3 cm in diameter, and some occupy the major part of the testicle. The tumors are usually round, discrete, and encapsulated. They are much softer than the other testicular tumors and frequently bulge on cut section. Their color is yellow-orange or brown, sometimes with red mottling, and some are cystic.

**Histological Features.** The tumor cells are arranged in three main patterns: (1) solid diffuse type, (2) pseudoadenomatous, and (3) cystic–vascular (angiomatoid). The solid diffuse type is arranged either diffusely in large sheets of uniform cells or as cords separated by thin, delicate septa. The tumor cells may be arranged in a palisade fashion around blood vessels, with the cell nuclei situated away from the vessel wall forming a rosettelike structure. The pseudoadenomatous type has lobules of 20 to 30 cells surrounding empty spaces that are not lined by endothelium but may contain acidophilic-staining

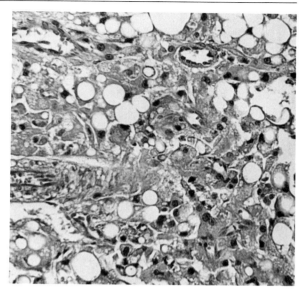

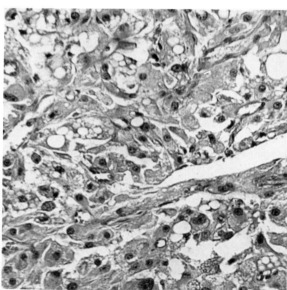

A
B
**FIGURE 11.2.** Interstitial cell adenoma in the testis of the dog. A. Tumor cells with lipid vacuoles. B. Diffuse arrangement of tumor cells.

either glandular or solid masses of cells, similar to an anaplastic seminoma. There may be areas of acinar, tubular, or papillary formations. A 7-year-old standardbred horse with a papillary adenocarcinoma pattern and serum α-ketoproteins was recently reported (Valentine and Weinstock, 1986).

## Gonadoblastoma

This is an extremely rare tumor of the testis consisting of a mixture of germ cells, immature interstitial lutein cells, and Sertoli granulosa cells. The latter may form Call–Exner bodies. A 15-year-old Shetland sheepdog has been reported with this interesting tumor (Turk *et al.*, 1981).

## Teratoma of Gonads

**Definition.** A teratoma is a tumor composed of multiple tissues foreign to the part in which they arise. As a true tumor, and unlike congenital malformation or hamartoma, teratoma displays progressive autonomous growth. A teratoma contains multiple tissues from different germ layers, such as epithelium, brain, bone, and cartilage. A mixed tumor such as that of the canine mammary gland also contains multiple tissues, but it is not a teratoma since the epithelium and connective tissue parts are normal components of the mammary gland and the bone and cartilage originate from metaplasia of myoepithelial cells. Embryonal nephroma also contains multiple tissues, but it is not a teratoma; it is an aberrant differentiation of embryonic tissues of the kidney.

**Classification.** It is artificial to subdivide teratomas into solid or cystic types, according to the number of germ layers present, or into types composed of mature and immature tissues. Solid ones may be cystic, and cystic ones may have solid parts. The number of germ layers seen usually indicates only how thoroughly the tumor has been examined.

The most common teratomas of the human gonads have been referred to as ovarian dermoids or dermoid cysts because they consist primarily of cysts lined by squamous epithelium and contain hair, keratin, or sebaceous material. They represent true teratomas and consist of two or three germ layers. The term *dermoid* should not be used in referring to this neoplasm, since it is also applied to nonneoplastic congenital and acquired lesions of the skin and cornea. The dermoid cyst in the skin is a congenital or traumatically derived cyst of epidermis and adjacent adnexal structures capable of forming hair, sebum, and sweat. The dermoids that grow on the cornea are congenital malformations of heterotopic skin containing adnexal glands and hair. They are found on the corneas of dogs, cattle, and other domestic animals.

Since all degrees of maturity are found in tissues of teratomas, subdivision into embryonic or adult types is not warranted. The type of tissue observed often depends on which part of the tumor is sectioned.

**Histogenesis.** The teratoma, because of its unusual recapitulation of two or more embryonic layers, has given rise to a variety of theories as to its origin. Evidence now supports development from parthenogenetic germ cells. However, some of the evidence is contradictory, and it is not clear whether all teratomas that arise in the gonads develop by the same mechanism.

Teratomas have been produced experimentally in roosters by injecting zinc or copper salts into the testes (Bagg, 1937; Falin, 1940; Michalowsky, 1926). The tumors grow rapidly and contain skin, feathers, respiratory and alimentary tract epithelium, nervous tissue, cartilage, bone, and muscle. There is a seasonal difference in the growth of these teratomas; injections made during the first 3 months of the year produce the greatest number. During that season spermatogenesis is most active in the rooster. Inoculation of pituitary gonadotrophic hormone prolongs spermatogenesis and extends the period when these tumors can be produced.

Teratoma has been transplanted experimentally from one chicken to another (Baker, 1931). Tissues from a spontaneous ovarian teratoma, implanted intramuscularly and intraperitoneally, produced a teratoma similar to the primary tumor. The transplanted tumor secreted ovarian hormone because of the theca cells present.

**Incidence.** Testicular teratoma has been reported most commonly in the horse. It is extremely rare in the dog, cat, ox, and pig. Conway and McCann (1966) reviewed three reports of teratoma in the testicles of horses but found that none of these cases was a teratoma according to the criteria of Willis (1947). They described one case of their own

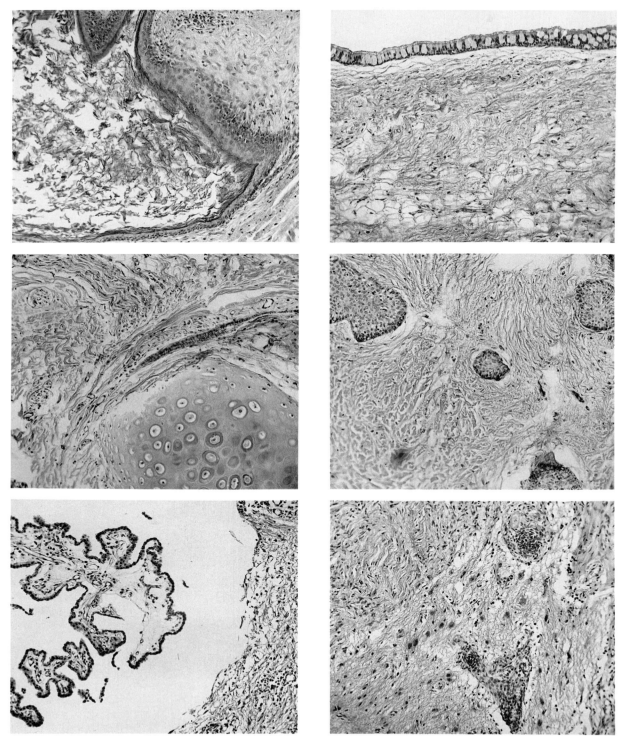

A B  
C D  
E F  

**FIGURE 11.6.** Teratoma in the ovary of a bitch. A. Cyst lined by stratified squamous epithelium with keratosis. This suggests epidermis. B. Ciliated columnar epithelium showing mucin production. This resembles respiratory epithelium. C. Large plate of hyaline cartilage. D. Clumps of squamous epithelium. E. Cyst containing papillary structure covered by cuboidal epithelium, suggestive of tela choroidea. F. Nerve fibers adjacent to central nervous gray matter.

in a draft horse where the tumor had cartilage, skin with hair, epithelial ducts, dentigerous cyst formation, mammary tissue, and nerves.

**Age, Breed, and Sex.** The age for teratoma in the horse ranges from 1 to 5 years, averaging 2 years. Dogs are affected at 1 year or older; most dogs are 8 years old or more. Other animals are usually adults when affected, although the tumors have been reported in several young calves. A majority of the tumors in horses have been in males, whereas those in dogs and cats have usually been in females. All but one of the 35 teratomas in horses reported were in the testes. A few were bilateral and some were multiple in the same testis. At least one-fourth of the teratomas in horses have been found in cryptorchid testicles (Crew, 1922; Shaw and Roth, 1986).

Teratoma in the dog usually involves the ovary. A teratoma was reported in the abdominal cavity of a calf (Hjärre, 1924). The single case of teratoma in the pig was ovarian.

**Gross Morphology.** Teratomas are usually round, ovoid, or of irregular shape. They may or may not be encapsulated. The majority have solid areas and cysts containing semisolid greasy material, hair, and teeth. The solid parts of teratomas are usually grayish white, often with yellow, fatty areas. Some teratomas have grossly visible nodules of cartilage and spicules of bone.

**Histological Features.** A great variety of mature embryonic tissues are present (figs. 11.6A–F). Cysts are lined by squamous epithelium, simple or stratified columnar or cuboidal epithelium, ciliated columnar epithelium, or ependymal cells. Many teratomas contain areas of nervous tissue with neuroglia, neurons, and ganglion cells. Fluid-filled clefts may be lined with secreting choroid plexus epithelium. Myelinated or nonmyelinated nerves, smooth or skeletal muscle, teeth, and sebaceous and sweat glands are all encountered. Cartilage and bone, fat, blood vessels, lymphoid tissue, and many forms of glandular tissue are observed. Teratomas may contain almost any form of tissue normally found in the adult animal.

The arrangement of the various tissues in a teratoma is not always haphazard and disorderly. Some associations of tissues resemble those of normal organs. Cavities lined by respiratory epithelium are often associated with cartilage, and cavities lined by intestinal epithelium are commonly surrounded by smooth muscle. Some nervous tissue is enclosed by meningeal type tissue and by bone and cartilage. The teeth have an orderly arrangement of enamel and dentin and are set in bony sockets. Schwann cells may surround nerves or ganglion cells.

**Growth and Metastasis.** Teratomas in animals, in contrast to those in humans, are almost always benign. The practice of early castration of horses results in detection and removal of many of the teratomas before they have had a chance to become malignant (Willis, 1948).

## Other Tumors

Other tumors of the testis are extremely rare in domestic animals and include mesothelioma, fibroma, and hemangioma with their malignant counterparts. The mesothelioma is either a papillary tumor, as seen in the laboratory rat, or a glandular tumor, as it appears in humans. In the rat it originates on the serosal covering of the testis or epididymis and is characterized by rows of hyperchromatic cells placed on papillary projections of delicate stroma.

Fibrous and vascular tumors of the testis are similar to their counterparts elsewhere in the body.

## TUMORS OF THE PROSTATE

### Canine Prostatic Hyperplasia

**Incidence.** Hyperplasia of the prostate is very common in old dogs. The condition is seldom seen in dogs younger than 4 years of age. The incidence increases with advancing years. There is no clear histological distinction between a normal gland and early stages of hyperplasia.

Prostatic hyperplasia is associated with androgen secretion by the testicle and may be present in dogs with normal, atrophic, or cryptorchid testicles, but it does not develop in castrated dogs. Castration causes involution of both normal and hyperplastic prostate glands, and prostatic secretion ceases within 3 months of castration. The epithelium becomes flattened, the acini have small lumens, and the stroma is relatively increased (Huggins and Clark, 1940). Estrogen, endogenously derived from a Sertoli cell tumor or exogenously, either accidentally in

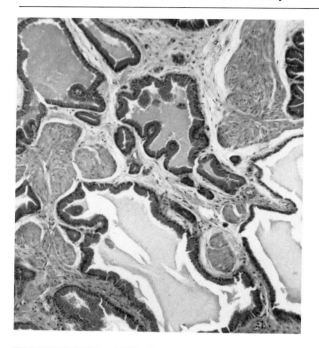

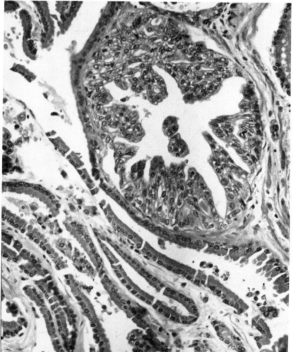

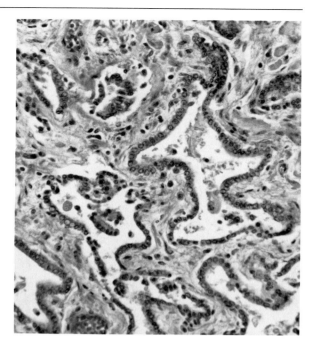 FIGURE 11.7. A. Hyperplasia of prostate gland in a dog. Dilated acini are lined by columnar cells often located on fronds of connective tissue. Acinar lumens contain glandular secretory fluid. B. Early carcinoma change in dog prostate. Irregular acini are lined by cuboidal cells. Another part of this neoplasm had diffuse infiltration of carcinoma cells. C. Focus of early neoplasia in dog prostate.

feed or by injection as a therapeutic measure, may slow the growth of a hyperplastic gland, but it may also cause squamous metaplasia of the epithelium.

Prostatic enlargement in the dog, unlike that in humans, does not cause urethral obstruction, but may result in rectal obstruction with constipation.

**Gross Morphology.** The hyperplastic gland is uniformly enlarged. The outer surface is smooth or nodular and both lobes are involved, although one may be more involved than the other. The normal bilobed appearance of the gland is sometimes masked by the enlargement. On cross section multiple cysts as much as 3 cm in diameter are distributed throughout the gland but particularly in the cortex, and they often contain clear or cloudy secretory fluid.

**Histological Features.** The normal prostate of

**Etiology and Transmission.** This neoplasm is caused by the bovine papilloma virus and is transmitted naturally during copulation, which accounts for the high incidence in some herds of breeding stock. An experimental subcutaneous injection of papilloma virus obtained from a skin papilloma or a genital fibropapilloma of a cow induces fibroblastic proliferation in the connective tissue with minimal proliferation of epithelium. Since cutaneous papillomas are common in cattle, there is ample opportunity for the mucosa of the penis, vulva, or vagina to become infected with papilloma virus (Monlux and Monlux, 1972).

**Growth and Metastasis.** This is a benign lesion that frequently will regress and disappear in a few months. If surgical removal is attempted, neoplasms often recur, especially in bulls less than 15 months old (Formston, 1953). Recurrence occurs because of regrowth of infected fibroblasts or because the normal tissue is exposed to virus during surgery. Surgical prognosis is better in older animals. Tumor infiltration into neighboring tissue is not uncommon, with adhesions forming between the penis and sheath.

## Transmissible Genital Papilloma (Condyloma) of the Pig

Parish (1961, 1962) reported papillomalike growths on the prepuce of mature pigs and was able to transmit the tumor via cell-free extracts injected into the genital mucosa of pigs. Naturally occurring and experimentally induced neoplasms grew for a time and then regressed. Parish demonstrated the presence of papilloma virus antigen by gel diffusion at the stage of maximum growth of the tumor. The nature of the antibody response that resulted in regression was not determined, although cell-mediated immunity was suspected. After regression, pigs were immune to subsequent challenges of virus.

These tumors were circular and round and projected about 1 cm from the mucosal surface, and their maximum diameter was 3 cm. Some were pedunculated, and others were filiform with secondary papillary formation.

Histologically, the growths studied by Parish were characterized as being similar to condyloma acuminatum of humans, with excessive and rapid thickening of the stratum spinosum and marked prolongation of the rete pegs. Mitotic figures were frequent in the basilar layers of the growth. The lesions resembled papillomas, with extensive and uneven acanthosis covered by a thin layer of keratinized cells. Both basilar and suprabasilar layers continued to have actively dividing cells. There was little proliferation of underlying connective tissue.

## Squamous Cell Papilloma and Carcinoma of the Penis in the Horse

**Incidence.** These are fairly common neoplasms in the horse and the most important ones of the genitalia (Kast, 1957). They mainly affect adult or aged horses, show no breed predilection, and occur with equal frequency in stallions and castrated males. Smegma of the penis is suggested as an etiological factor. Plaut and Kohn-Speyer (1947) tested the carcinogenic properties of equine smegma on the skin of mice and found that within 36 to 423 days some mice developed papillomas, squamous cell carcinomas, and fibrosarcomas at the sites of application. No tumors were found in control mice. The results were the same whether whole smegma or a nonsaponifiable fraction was used. Nothing has yet been proved about the effect of smegma on the horse.

**Sites and Structure.** These tumors occur principally on the glans penis but are found also on other areas of the penis, such as the inner lining of the prepuce. The neoplasms are sessile, of cauliflower or mulberry shape, and variable in size. Histologically, they show the same structure as squamous cell tumors in any other mucosal or skin site. The neoplasms commonly recur after surgery, and some exhibit metastasis to the regional lymph nodes and lungs. It may be difficult to distinguish penile papillomas from carcinomas because transitional forms are common. Carcinomas have atypical cells, mitoses, loss of cellular polarity, and show invasion at the base with lymphatic invasion. Metastasis is rare but may be found in deep or superficial inguinal lymph nodes.

## Transmissible Venereal Tumor of the Dog

**Classification.** The exact cell of origin of the transmissible venereal tumor of the dog is not definitely known. At various times it has been described as a tumor of lymphocytes (De Monbreun and Goodpasture, 1934), histiocytes (Mulligan, 1949), reticular cells (Kaalund-Jørgensen and Thomsen, 1937), and mature end cells of the reticuloendothelial series (Bloom *et al.*, 1951). It has been called an infectious or venereal granuloma, "Sticker" tumor, transmissible sarcoma, lymphosarcoma, and contagious venereal tumor (Jackson, 1936, 1944; Nanta *et al.*, 1949; Novak and Craig, 1927; Wade, 1908).

**Incidence.** This tumor was first described in 1820 and transplanted from dog to dog in 1876 by Novinsky. The neoplasm is seen where dogs are intensively bred and there are infected studs or breeding bitches, where dogs are in close contact, or where many dogs exist as strays or wild dogs with unrestrained sexual activity, as in congested cities of developing countries. It is enzootic in Puerto Rico and in the Bahamas, where it is the most common tumor of dogs. The tumor is unknown in Sweden, Denmark, and the United Kingdom. It is reported from other parts of Europe and from Ireland, South America, Japan, China, Java, Kenya and other African countries, and Indonesia. The incidence varies in the United States (Karlson and Mann, 1952); it was high in New York City and Philadelphia during the first part of this century, but later decreased.

**Age, Breed, and Sex.** Venereal tumors of the dog are most common during the years of greatest sexual activity. There is no heritable breed prevalence. When first introduced into the United States, this neoplasm was confined to the English bulldog, in which it was common in the United Kingdom at that time (Dunstan, 1904; Glass, 1923). By 1933, however, the tumor had spread first to the Boston terrier and then to other breeds in the United States, and now any breed may be affected (Gleason, 1947). When certain breeds experience a higher incidence, it is usually because they are being intensively bred, and much-used studs or breeding bitches are spreading the tumor. This accounts for a high incidence in greyhounds in Ireland. The female is more suscep-

tible than the male; the tumor is never found in the virgin female.

**Sites.** Venereal tumor is solitary or multiple and is almost always on the external genitalia, but may occur in oral, nasal, and conjunctival mucosa and in the skin. In the male dog the tumor is usually on the more caudal part of the penis (fig. 11.10A) from the crura to bulbis glandis or the area of the glans penis and is found occasionally on the prepuce. In the female dog the neoplasm is usually found in the posterior part of the vagina, often at the junction of the vestibule and vagina (fig. 11.10B). It sometimes surrounds the urethral orifice, and if it is near the entrance to the vagina, it protrudes from the vulva.

There have been a number of reports of venereal tumors in extragenital sites of the skin (Ajello, 1949; Feldman, 1929; Lacroix and Riser, 1947; Mulligan, 1949). Higgins (1966) suggested that many of the skin sites where the tumors are found represent lesions caused by biting and scratching, common in stray dogs (fig. 11.10C), which predisposes the skin to tumor implantation. He observed scars in the skin above subcutaneous tumors, suggestive of previous wounds. Skin tumors were found on the back, flank, neck, head, and limbs of dogs. They were as much as 6 cm in diameter, often ulcerated, and bled. Some were found in and around the eyes or even in the buccal cavity. The ones in the eyes grew into the orbit and caused blindness. Histologically, the metastatic neoplasms were identical to the primary growths with sheets of uniform polyhedral cells with prominent nuclei, frequent mitotic figures, and variable eosinophilic cytoplasm. It is likely that some of the nongenital tumors reported have been confused with (1) histiocytoma, the most common neoplasm of the skin in the young dog, (2) cutaneous lymphoma, or (3) poorly differentiated mastocytoma, a tumor that also has the skin of the external genitalia as a preferred site. The venereal tumor is definitely not associated with the aortic body cells, as once suggested by Jackson (1936).

**Gross Morphology.** This neoplasm may be cauliflowerlike, pendunculated, nodular, papillary, or multilobulated. It ranges from a small nodule 5 mm in diameter to a large mass measuring more than 10 cm. The neoplasm is firm though friable, and the superficial part is commonly ulcerated and inflamed. Some neoplasms are as large as 10 to 15 cm in di-

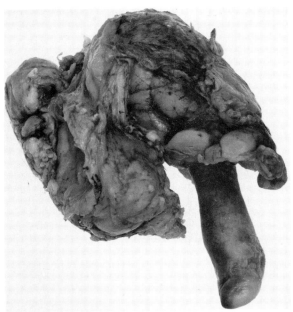

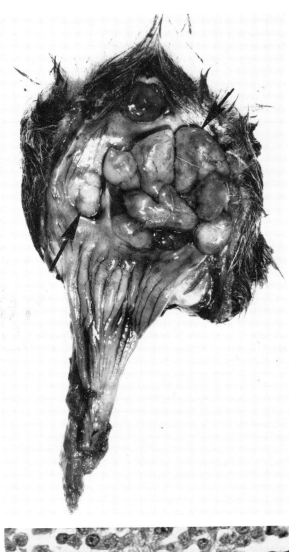

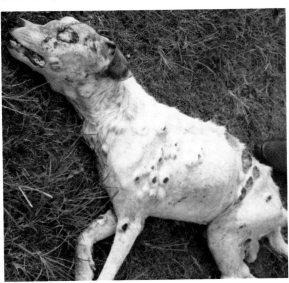

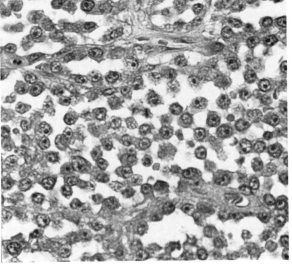

A | B
C | D

**FIGURE 11.10.** Transmissible venereal tumor of the dog. A. Lateral view of the penis of a dog showing a large tumor involving caudal parts of the penis. The dorsoventral measurement of this tumor is 10 × 12 cm. Approximately 6 cm of the normal penis is visible. B. Multiple polypoid growths (**arrows**) in the vagina of a bitch. C. Mongrel stray dog with advanced tumor involvement of the skin and subcutaneous, periorbital, and buccal tissues. Many of the lesions are ulcerated and hemorrhagic. D. Microscopic features showing uniform size tumor cells that resemble immature lymphocytic cells but are not of lymphocytic origin. (A, courtesy of Dr. J. M. Howell and *Vet. Rec.*; C and D, courtesy of Dr. D. A. Higgins and *Vet. Rec.*)

ameter and, if on the glans penis, may protrude from the preputial opening.

**Histological Features.** The cells are in compact masses or sheets and sometimes grow in rows, cords, or loose in a delicate stroma (fig. 11.10D). The stroma is variable but usually minimal, similar in amount to that seen in histiocytoma and lymphoma. The cells are round, ovoid, or polyhedral in shape. They have large, round, hyperchromatic nuclei, distinctly marginal chromatin, and large central nucleoli. They have a moderate amount of faintly eosinophilic cytoplasm, and the outline of the individual cell may be indistinct. Many mitotic figures are found; sometimes six to eight are seen per high power field.

As the tumor mass increases in size, the cells become tightly packed and irregularly ovoid, and fibroblastlike cells appear, possibly indicative of a transformation of the tumor cells (Kennedy et al., 1977). Many lymphocytes, few plasma cells, and occasional macrophages are scattered throughout the tumor.

The number and type of infiltrating inflammatory cells depend on whether the venereal tumor is in a progressive, steady, or regressive state (Chandler and Yang, 1981). Reticular fibers may invest small groups of tumor cells in some areas; there is no evidence that the tumor cells produce these fibers. The neoplastic cells sometimes show extensive necrosis, and tumors often have an ulcerated surface with hemorrhage and secondary infection.

**Electron Microscopy.** Using electron microscopy the tumor cells are seen to have no specific ultrastructural features. The cytoplasm is abundant with many free ribosomes, granular endoplasmic reticulum, and large mitochondria. The Golgi apparatus is of moderate proportion, and there are cytoplasmic projections that interdigitate with neighboring cells (Drommer and Schultz, 1969; Yang et al., 1973). The ultrastructural characteristics are those of a lymphoreticular tumor.

Virus particles are inconsistently seen (Kennedy et al., 1977; Murray et al., 1969; Yang et al., 1976b).

**Karyotypic Appearance.** Highly significant and constant karyotypic differences exist between normal dog cells and cells of the tumor. The normal chromosome count for the dog is 78, and all but 2

are acrocentric chromosomes. In transmissible venereal tumor there are usually 58 to 59 chromosomes, with 13 to 17 metacentric and 42 acrocentric. This is a constant variation in karyotype, found worldwide (Barski and Cornefert-Jensen, 1966; Makino, 1963; Murray et al., 1969; Weber et al., 1965).

When this neoplasm is grown in cell culture, the cell population changes from a mixture of tumor cells and a few fibroblasts to a culture of pure fibroblasts; the tumor cells die out more rapidly than they can divide, and fibroblasts take over (Ajello, 1956; Bloom et al., 1951; Yang et al., 1973).

**Etiology and Transmission.** This is one of the few tumors of animals that is transmitted to the genitals by coitus. Transfer is from either the female or male. The violent exertions associated with coitus in the dog render both sexes prone to genital injury and susceptible to transplantation of the tumor cells (Feldman, 1929). In one case an infected male dog transmitted the tumor to 11 of 12 susceptible females in mating (Smith and Washbourn, 1898). The tumor is also transmitted when a susceptible dog licks the genitals of an affected dog and then his own or those of another susceptible dog (Bloom, 1954).

Experimentally, this tumor has been passed through 40 generations of dogs during a period of 17 years (Karlson and Mann, 1952). Of 564 dogs involved, 68% developed the tumor. During this passage there were no changes in histology or the ability of the tumor to become established.

Transmission of venereal tumor occurs only by transplantation of viable tumor cells and not by a virus that may transform the cells in a susceptible host (Cohen, 1974; De Monbreun and Goodpasture, 1934; Stubbs and Furth, 1934). The tumor cannot be produced with cells that have been frozen, heated, treated with glycerin, or desiccated, and cell-free filtrates will not induce tumor formation.

The neoplasm will develop following subcutaneous, intraperitoneal, or subarachnoid injections of viable tumor cells (Sticker, 1904; Thiéry, 1954). Injection or scarification of the skin or mucosa of the genital organs also results in tumor transmission, but placing the cells on the intact mucosa is unsuccessful (Stubbs and Furth, 1934). Upon inoculation of viable cells in suspension from laboratory passaged tumor, the tumor developed in over 88% of the recipient adult dogs and in 100% of neonatal pups (Yang and Jones, 1973). The latent period for these tumors was remarkably consistent (approximately 16 days).

The origin of the tumor is not known, but based on the following findings, the stemline linear hypothesis seems reasonable: (1) transmission is by transplantation with intact viable tumor cells, (2) new tumors develop only by multiplication of transplanted cells as seen in labeled thymidine studies, and (3) karyotypic appearance is uniform worldwide. The first clone of tumor cells may have originated by a mutation in lymphohistiocytic cells by a virus, chemical, or radiation. This clone of tumor cells was disseminated by dogs through coital allogenic transplantation. There are still many questions regarding how this tumor can overcome the histocompatibility barriers present.

Since the tumor cells are foreign to the host and not rejected immediately, as would be expected in a homograft reaction, they are passed from animal to animal like a parasite. They are maintained by the animal until immune mechanisms cause regression of the tumor or until the growth or secondary complications kill the host. There is some analogy to human choriocarcinoma, where its nonself cell overcomes normal histocompatibility barriers. The venereal tumor can be transplanted into closely related canids, such as coyotes, wolves, jackals, and the red fox. There are two additional species with unique properties on which transplantation has been achieved; the *nude* mouse and the hamster cheek pouch.

**Growth and Metastasis.** Growth of the tumor is rapid at first and slow later, indicative of immune inhibition of growth (Cohen and Steel, 1972). Cohen (1973) carried out a study to elucidate the role played by the immune response in determining the course of tumor growth. Tumors in dogs given whole-body X-irradiation showed malignant behavior; tumors in nonirradiated animals showed more benign and variable behavior.

Metastasis is uncommon. It occurs in a few dogs, probably less than 5% of reported cases (Karlson and Mann, 1952; Oduye *et al.*, 1973). The superficial inguinal lymph nodes are usually involved in the male and the superficial inguinal and external il-

iac nodes in the female. Metastases are also seen in the kidney, liver, spleen, eye, brain, pituitary, skin and subcutis, mesenteric lymph nodes, and peritoneum (Adams and Slaughter, 1970; Howell *et al.*, 1969; Manning and Martin, 1970; McLeod and Lewis, 1972; Novak and Craig, 1927; Rust, 1949). Most metastatic growths, particularly in the skin, occur from trauma and mechanical implantation of tumor cells from the genital areas. Metastasis also occurs by implantation to the internal genital tract of the female, specifically, the cervix, uterus, and Fallopian tubes.

**Immunity and Regression.** Subcutaneous inoculation of tumor cells produces a tumor 3 to 6 mm in diameter in 2 to 3 weeks (Bloom *et al.*, 1951). Size is maximum in 5 to 7 weeks, and spontaneous regression follows. The lesion almost completely disappears within 6 months of implantation (Karlson and Mann, 1952). The high incidence of regression under natural conditions indicates that caution must be used in interpreting the effects of therapeutic agents.

Histologically, the regressive neoplasm demonstrates a decrease in number of tumor cells and their eventual disappearance. Regression is associated with edema, hemorrhage, and infiltration of neutrophils, lymphocytes, and plasma cells (Yang *et al.*, 1976*a*). Fibrosis may develop in the terminal stages of regression.

Dogs with regressing venereal tumors are usually immune to subsequent implantations unless large numbers of cells are used (Beebe and Ewing, 1906; De Monbreun and Goodpasture, 1934). Regression of tumors can be brought about also by injecting whole blood or serum from recovered dogs (Crile and Beebe, 1908; Powers, 1966). Newborn puppies from "immune" dams (mothers with antibodies to the tumor) show a longer latent period for tumor development, and neoplasms in these puppies are smaller and show more rapid regression (Prier and Brodey, 1963). Regression is due to the formation of IgG in the sera of dogs after a period (40 days) of tumor growth (Cohen, 1972). An increasing amount of antibody forms during the course of tumor growth. The antibody can be demonstrated on the cell surface membrane by the direct immunofluorescence method (Epstein and Bennett, 1974).

Peripheral lymphocytes of dogs with regressing tumors have been shown to be cytotoxic to tumor cells, whereas lymphocytes from normal dogs or from dogs with progressive venereal tumors were not (Chandler and Yang, 1981; Cohen, 1980).

The peripheral blood leukocyte adherence inhibition (LAI) test is an excellent *in vitro* indicator of tumor-specific cellular immunity. In this test nonadherence of leukocytes is associated with active phagocytosis. Dogs with regressing tumors have much higher LAI activity than normal dogs or dogs with progressing tumors (Harding and Yang, 1981*a,b*).

A venereal tumor-associated soluble antigen has recently been identified and characterized physiochemically (Palker and Yang, 1981). This antigen may block or modify the host defense mechanism to the tumor.

## TUMORS OF THE OVARY

Tumors of the ovary fall into three broad categories: (1) "surface epithelial" tumors, originating from the modified celomic mesothelial cell covering of the ovary; (2) sex cord–gonadostromal tumors; and (3) germ cell tumors. The tumors will be described and classified in a manner similar to the WHO classification (Nielsen *et al.*, 1976).

### Surface Epithelial Tumors

The "surface epithelial" tumors constitute a group of tumors common in female dogs and humans but uncommon in the mare, cat, and cow. The average age of affected dogs is about 9 years, and there is no breed predisposition. The canine tumors may be associated with such secondary changes as cystic endometrial hyperplasia, metritis, or vaginal hemorrhage. There are four main histological patterns: papillary adenoma, papillary adenocarcinoma, cystadenoma, and cystadenocarcinoma. Transitional forms and poorly differentiated tumors occur frequently.

**Sites and Gross Morphology.** The neoplasms are either unilateral or bilateral and are characteristically papillary or cystic with frequent focal solid areas (figs. 11.11A and B). The size is variable, usu-

ally 7 to 10 cm in diameter. Some exhibit extensions through the ovarian capsule. The cysts often contain brown or clear watery fluid. Detached epithelial fronds or cyst fluid containing tumor cells frequently escape from primary carcinoma and produce neoplastic implantations in the abdominal cavity that may result in ascites. The malignant tumors in the bitch show a more solid appearance than benign tumors.

**Histological Features.** The papillary tumors probably arise from ovarian surface epithelium or from underlying epithelial nests in the ovarian cortex, whereas the cystic tumors may also develop from either surface epithelium or from the rete ovarii. Both adenoma and carcinoma exhibit multibranched papillae that arise multicentrically with single or multiple layers of columnar or cuboidal epithelial cells covering delicate connective tissue stalks (fig. 11.11C). The epithelial cells are usually well-oriented and have round or ovoid nuclei and large nucleoli. It is often difficult to distinguish between papillary adenoma and papillary adenocarcinoma. The following differential features are used: (1) size of the tumor; (2) mitotic activity; (3) invasion into ovarian stroma; (4) extension into the mesovarian, ovarian bursa, or peritoneum; and (5) implantation metastasis.

Cystadenoma and cystadenocarcinoma have lumen formations that range in size from small, evenly sized glands mimicking the rete ovarii to larger, thin-walled cysts measuring as much as 1 cm in diameter. The lining is cuboidal or flattened epithelium. The cyst lumen commonly contains a homogeneous acidophilic material that represents secretion of the tumor cells. The malignant form is distinguished from the benign form by the size of the tumor, cellular atypia, and the infiltrative growth characteristics of the tumor cells. Carcinomas grow faster and become larger than adenomas and usually infiltrate into the mesovarial connective tissues of surrounding ovarian stroma.

Papillary tumors and cystadenocarcinomas of the ovary in domestic animals metastasize most often by implantation into the peritoneal cavity, and rarely by way of the lymph or blood.

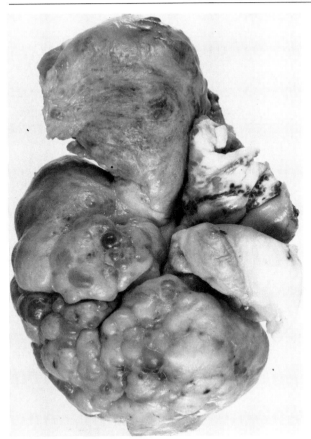

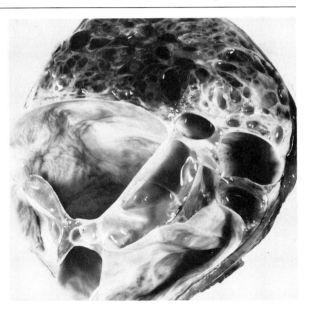

A|B
C| **FIGURE 11.11.** Papillary cystadenoma and cystadeno-carcinoma of the ovary. A. Surface view of adenocarcinoma of left ovary in a bitch. B. Multiple cystic structure of adenoma in a cow. C. Cystadenoma with multibranched papillae in a dog. (B, courtesy of Dr. E. Cotchin and *Res. Vet. Sci.*)

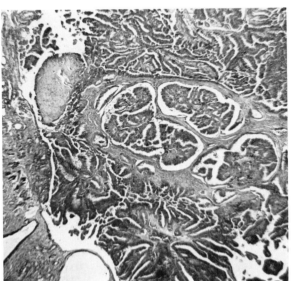

## Sex Cord–Gonadostromal Tumors

Sex cord–gonadostromal tumors of the ovary are (in order of decreasing frequency) granulosa cell tumor, thecoma, and luteoma. Lack of agreement on clinical behavior and histology makes strict subdivision of these tumors difficult. Distinguishing these neoplasms on the basis of the hormone secreted is not possible because relatively few hormone analyses have been made and because androgenic activity in an ovarian tumor may be the result of disturbed chemistry in a primary estrogen-producing neoplasm.

These tumors are derived from, or mimic in growth, constituents of the sex cords and gonadal stroma and are differentiated from other ovarian neoplasms such as surface epithelial tumors, teratomas, and dysgerminomas by their capacity to form hormonally active steroids. However, the proportion of neoplasms derived from one stromal element or another differs considerably among species.

**Incidence and Clinical Features.** The literature on sex cord–gonadostromal tumors of the ovary in various domestic species was reviewed by Norris *et al.* (1968, 1969*a,b*, 1970) and Tontis *et al.* (1982). These tumors are fairly common in the bitch, mare, and cow and less common in the sow and ewe; there is no breed predilection in any species. The neoplasms may be found at a slightly younger age than are most neoplasms in the bitch. The tumors are found in the mare at 7 to 16 years of age (average 9 years). They usually occur in older animals, although they are sometimes found in animals less than 4 years of age.

## Granulosa Cell Tumor

This is the most common of the sex cord–gonadostromal tumors in all species of animals and is usually a unilateral tumor. In the bitch it varies from 4 to 16 cm in diameter and is smooth to coarsely nodular. The growth has solid and cystic areas and often contains hemorrhages. It is firm and grayish white to yellow. Signs of hyperestrinism, such as pyometra, cystic endometrial hyperplasia, prolonged estrus, and enlarged nipples and vulva are found in association with approximately half of these tumors in dogs (Cotchin, 1961; Norris *et al.,* 1970). In the cat prolonged estrus and loss of hair with thinning of the hair coat have been observed.

In the cow and mare most of the tumors are large, ranging from 10 to 23 cm in diameter, lobulated, and ovoid or spherical. They may be soft or firm and are usually encapsulated and limited to the ovary (Cordes, 1969). Occasionally, malignant tumors grow beyond the limits of the ovary. The color is yellowish gray, sometimes with red stippling. The tumor has both solid and cystic areas (fig. 11.12A). The cysts contain clear, reddish brown or yellow watery fluid. Focal necrosis and hemorrhage are common. Cows with granulosa cell tumors have shown signs of nymphomania and relaxation of the pelvic ligaments. Less commonly, masculine behavior patterns have been observed. Lactation may occur in virgin heifers with granulosa cell tumors, and some cows have endometrial hyperplasia.

Mares with sex cord–gonadostromal tumors have three main behavioral patterns: (1) anestrus, (2) continuous or intermittent estrus, and (3) stallion-like behavior. Most granulosa cell tumors in the mare are associated with significant increases of testosterone levels in the blood. Aggressive male behavior is confined to those mares whose testosterone levels are above 100 pg/ml of plasma. The fluid present in the cysts of equine granulosa cell tumors may have high concentrations of testosterone, reaching 75,000 pg/ml (Stickle *et al.,* 1975). Human granulosa cell tumors of the Sertoli cell type with virilizing effects are called *arrhenoblastomas,* and those without chemical evidence of masculinization are named *androblastomas.* Norris *et al.* (1969*b*) claimed that the Sertoli cell tumor of the ovary is not the same as the arrhenoblastoma seen in human females because of the absence of Leydig cells and lack of immature mesenchymal structures in the Sertoli cell neoplasm.

Mares with virilizing testosterone levels from granulosa cell tumors will often resist handling, rectal palpation, and perineal examination (Bosu *et al.,* 1982). Increased estrogen levels are less clearly related to behavioral patterns. Some mares exhibiting persistent sexual receptivity have slightly increased plasma levels of estrogen. The uninvolved ovary is invariably small and inactive. This is a useful diagnostic feature allowing differentiation of mares bearing these tumors from mares with other types of ovarian tumors or nonneoplastic causes of ovarian enlargement, such as ovarian cysts and hematomas (Hughes *et al.,* 1980; Meagher *et al.,* 1977).

**Histological Features.** The classification of these tumors depends on the predominance of cell types and histological patterns, as several types often coexist in the same tumor. Granulosa cell tumors, which are the most frequent, are also the most variable in histological appearance. They may be of three types. The first type is well-differentiated and has a uniform population of small cells closely mimicking the cells of the Graafian follicle, occasionally with groupings of cells surrounding pink proteinaceous or clear fluid, forming the so-called Call–Exner bodies. The latter are common in humans and are most frequently seen in benign tumors of the cat, cow, and dog. The second type has long strands or islands surrounded by septa of connective tissues, with areas that resemble the Sertoli cell tumor of the testis. In this subtype of granulosa cell

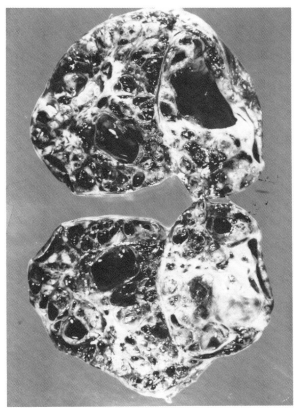

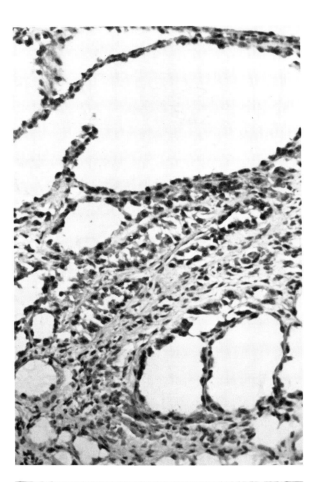

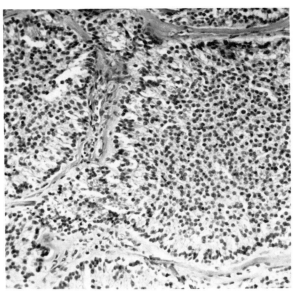

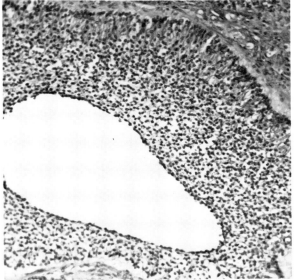

A|B
C|D

**FIGURE 11.12.** Granulosa cell tumor in the ovary of a mare. A. Sectioned tumor showing multicystic character. B. Acinar structure lined by single layers of cells. C. Solid and cystic clusters of cells with peripheral rim of cells in palisade arrangement. D. Folliclelike structure with space in center.

tumor, the tumor cells are clear with indistinct cell borders, often lipid filled, tall, triangular, and placed on a basement membrane. The nuclei are small, hypochromatic, and lack mitoses. The third type consists of ovoid, poorly delineated granulosa cells arranged in a diffuse sarcomatous pattern. Luteinization may occur in some granulosa cell tumors. The frequency of histological subtypes varies between species and necessitates a separate description for each species.

In the bitch the granulosa cell tumor has cells similar to those of the developing follicles with occasional Call–Exner bodies. The tumor cells are round in outline and have small, dark staining nuclei that are more hyperchromatic and variable in size than in the normal follicle. Mitotic figures are common. A few cells have light staining or foamy cytoplasm, but usually the cells have darkly eosinophilic-staining cytoplasm. Myxoid change may appear in the intercellular matrix; a spindle cell pattern is occasionally observed. A Sertoli cell pattern is not unusual, and it is composed of tubular columns, cords, or clusters of epithelial cells separated by delicate connective tissue septa. The cells are elongated and frequently have pointed ends. Characteristically, they have clear or foamy cytoplasm and uniform small nuclei. Mitotic figures, cellular pleomorphism, and anaplasia are minimal.

In the mare most granuloma cell tumors are cystic, and the gross appearance may be that of a multilobulated cyst. The neoplasms have prominent microcysts with follicles and tubules lined by double layers of cells with basally oriented nuclei. There is a prominent supporting stroma of spindle cells. Leydig-like cells are commonly seen among the theca cells and beneath the nests of granulosa cells. These cells appear to be most abundant in those cases in which masculine behavior is most pronounced. Other granulosa cell neoplasms may have abundant light staining cells resembling testicular Sertoli cells (Mills *et al.*, 1977).

In the cow the granulosa cell tumor may have a microfollicular pattern with follicles of variable size lined by cells resembling the follicular epithelium of the normal Graafian follicle. These cells are one to three or more layers deep (fig. 11.12B). When stratified, the basilar layer of cells is usually well-oriented (fig. 11.12C). The lumens of many of the folliclelike structures contain a homogeneous or granular acidophiliclike staining material. The cells lining the follicular structures sometimes project into the lumen, suggesting a cumulus oophorus, or show multiple papillary infoldings simulating papillary cystadenocarcinoma. In some, the entire lumen of the follicle is filled with tumor cells, whereas in others the follicles are cystic and lined by flattened cells (fig. 11.12D). The tumor cells less commonly form solid masses, small rosettes resembling Call–Exner bodies, or a pattern suggesting embryonic follicles.

The neoplastic cells are round or ovoid and resemble normal follicular cells, but they are more variable in size and have more hyperchromatic nuclei. The cytoplasm is often vacuolated, and the nuclei are round or ovoid and hyperchromatic. There are a moderate number of mitotic figures, but often several may be seen in a high power field. In some tumors it is possible to see columnar and vacuolated cells that resemble luteal cells or testicular Sertoli cells. The Sertoli cell types have fewer cysts and less hemorrhage and necrosis. The growth is tubular, with connective tissue septa separating columns or cords of tumor cells. The tumor cell cytoplasm is frequently vacuolated and amphophilic in staining. Cytoplasm shows positive PAS and lipid staining reactions. The tumor cells may be elongated, often with pointed ends; rarely, spindle cells are present. The nuclei are uniformly small and slightly vesicular with inapparent nucleoli. Mitotic figures are uncommon. Small foci of a granulosa cell pattern may be found.

The origin of the Sertoli cells in this neoplasm is still in doubt. It may be from the rete ovarii, granulosa cell nests, or from male-directed cells in the ovary. The latter is the most likely origin since the testis and ovary are from the same anlage and, early in gestation, appear morphologically identical. Thus, the testis and ovary contain cells that retain the potential to form tumors resembling developmental stages of the other.

In the cat, granulosa cell tumors are composed of small cells containing eccentrically located hyperchromatic nuclei that have microfollicular arrangement with Call–Exner bodies, and tumor cells are radially arranged around eosinophilic material. Mitotic figures and cellular atypia are prominent.

**Growth and Metastasis.** The behavior of granulosa cells varies with species. In general, more me-

mors of the Testis. I. Water and Electrolyte Content of Testicular Tumors and of Normal, Cryptorchid, and Estrogenized Testis. *Cancer Res.* 4, 447–452.

Huggins, C., and Moulder, P. V. (1945) Estrogen Production by Sertoli Cell Tumors of the Testis. *Cancer Res.* 5, 510–514.

Huggins, C., and Pazos, R. (1945) Studies on Tumors of the Testis. II. The Morphology of Testicular Tumors of Dogs. *Amer. J. Path.* 21, 299–310.

Hughes, J. P., Kennedy, P. C., and Stabenfeldt, G. H. (1980) Pathology of the Ovary and Ovarian Disorders in the Mare. *Int. Cong. An. Repro. AI (Madrid)* 9, 203–222.

Innes, J. R. M. (1942) Neoplastic Diseases of the Testis in Animals. *J. Path. Bact.* 54, 485–498.

Jackson, C. (1936) The Incidence and Pathology of Tumours of Domesticated Animals in South Africa: A Study of the Onderstepoort Collection of Neoplasms with Special Reference to the Histopathology. *Onderstepoort J. Vet. Sci. Anim. Indust.* 6, 1–460.

———. (1944) The Cytology of the Contagious (Venereal) Tumour of the Dog. *Onderstepoort J. Vet. Sci. Anim. Indust.* 20, 97–118.

Jensen, R., and Flint, J. C. (1963) Intratubular Seminomas in Testes of Sheep. *J. Comp. Path.* 73, 146–149.

Joest, E. (1929) *Spezielle Pathologische Anatomie der Haustiere.* R. Schoetz (Berlin).

Jones, T. C., and Friedman, N. B. (1950) Pathologic and Clinical Features of Canine Testicular Tumors. *Bull. Int. Assoc. Med. Mus.* 31, 36–53.

Kaalund-Jørgensen, O., and Thomsen, A. S. (1937) Det Overførbare Veneriske Sarkom hos Hunde. *Maanedsskr. Dyrlaeger* 48, 561–578.

Karlson, A. G., and Kelly, M. D. (1941) Choriohemangioma of the Bovine Allantois-Chorion. *J. Amer. Vet. Med. Assoc.* 99, 133–134.

Karlson, A. G., and Mann, F. C. (1952) The Transmissible Venereal Tumor of Dogs: Observations on Forty Generations of Experimental Transfers. *Ann. N.Y. Acad. Sci.* 54, 1197–1213.

Kast, V. A. (1957) Die Präputialkarzinome bei den Haussäugern. *Mh. Vet. Med.* 12, 212–216.

Kennedy, J. R., Yang, T. J., and Allen, P. L. (1977) Canine Transmissible Venereal Sarcoma: Electron Microscopic Changes with Time after Transplantation. *Brit. J. Cancer.* 36, 375–385.

King, N. W. (1973) *Comparative Pathology of the Uterus.* In: International Academy of Pathology, Monograph No. 14. Williams & Wilkins (Baltimore), 489–557.

Knudsen, O., and Schantz, B. (1963) Seminoma in the Stallion: A Clinical, Cytological and Pathologicoanatomical Investigation. *Cornell Vet.* 53, 395–403.

Lacroix, J. V., and Riser, W. H. (1947) Transmissible Lymphosarcoma of the Dog. *N. Amer. Vet.* 28, 451–453.

Ladds, P. W., and Saunders, P. J. (1976) Sertoli Cell Tumours in the Bull. *J. Comp. Path.* 86, 503–508.

László, F. (1936) Endometriose und Verwandte Veränderungen. *Dtsch. Tierärztl. Wschr.* 44, 706–708.

Leav, I., and Ling, G. V. (1968) Adenocarcinoma of the Canine Prostate. *Cancer* 22, 1329–1345.

Leav, I., Cavazos, L. F., and Ofner, P. (1974) Fine Structure and $C_{19}$-Steroid Metabolism of Spontaneous Adenocarcinoma of the Canine Prostate. *J. Natl. Cancer Inst.* 52, 789–804.

Letulle, M., and Petit, G. (1928) L'endométriome utérin chez la chienne. *Bull. Assoc. Franç. Étude Cancer* 17, 12–18.

Lipowitz, A. J., Schwartz, A., Wilson, G. P., and Ebert, J. W. (1973) Testicular Neoplasms and Concomitant Clinical Changes in the Dog. *J. Amer. Vet. Med. Assoc.* 163, 1364–1368.

Makino, S. (1963) Some Epidemiologic Aspects of Venereal Tumors of Dogs as Revealed by Chromosome and DNA Studies. *Ann. N.Y. Acad. Sci.* 108, 1106–1122.

Manning, P. J., and Martin, P. D. (1970) Metastasis of Canine Transmissible Venereal Tumor to the Adenohypophysis. *Path. Vet.* 7, 148–152.

Mawdesley-Thomas, L. E., and Sortwell, R. J. (1968) Proliferative Lesions of the Canine Uterus Associated with High Dose Oestrogen Administration. *Vet. Rec.* 82, 468–469.

McEntee, K. (1950) Fibropapillomas of the External Genitalia of Cattle. *Cornell Vet.* 40, 304–312.

———. (1958) Pathological Conditions in Old Bulls with Impaired Fertility. *J. Amer. Vet. Med. Assoc.* 132, 328–331.

McEntee, K., and Nielsen, S. W. (1976) Tumours of the Female Genital Tract. *Bull. Wld. Hlth. Org.* 53, 217–226.

McLeod, C. G., and Lewis, J. E. (1972) Transmissible Venereal Tumor with Metastases in Three Dogs. *J. Amer. Vet. Med. Assoc.* 161, 199–200.

Meagher, D. M., Wheat, J. D., Hughes, J. P., Stabenfeldt, G. H., and Harris, B. A. (1977) Granulosa Cell Tumors in Mares—A Review of 78 Cases. *Proc. Amer. Assoc. Equine Pract. Conv.* 23, 133–143.

Meier, H. (1956) Carcinoma of the Uterus in the Cat: Two Cases. *Cornell Vet.* 46, 188–200.

Michalowsky, I. (1926) Die experimentelle Erzeugung einer teratoiden Urisbildung der Hoden beim Hahn. *Zbl. Allg. Path. Path. Anat.* 38, 585–587.

Migaki, G., Carey, A. M., Turnquest, R. U., and Garner, F. M. (1970) Pathology of Bovine Uterine Adenocarcinoma. *J. Amer. Vet. Med. Assoc.* 157, 1577–1584.

Mills, J. H. L., Fretz, P. B., Clark, E. G., and Ganjam, V. K. (1977) Arrhenoblastoma in a Mare. *J. Amer. Vet. Med. Assoc.* 171, 754–757.

Monlux, A. W., Anderson, W. A., Davis, C. L., and Monlux, W. S. (1956) Adenocarcinoma of the Uterus of the Cow: Differentiation of Its Pulmonary Metastasis from Primary Lung Tumors. *Amer. J. Vet. Res.* 17, 45–73.

Monlux, W. S., and Monlux, A. W. (1972) *Atlas of Meat Inspection Pathology. Agriculture Handbook No. 367.* U.S. Department of Agriculture. (Washington, D.C.), 6–8.

Morgan, R. V. (1982) Blood Dyscrasias Associated with Testicular Tumors in the Dog. *J. Amer. Anim. Hosp. Assoc.* 18, 970–975.

Mulligan, R. M. (1944) Feminization in Male Dogs: A Syndrome Associated with Carcinoma of the Testis and Mimicked by the Administration of Estrogens. *Amer. J. Path.* 20, 865–876.

———. (1949) *Neoplasms of the Dog.* Williams and Wilkins (Baltimore).

Murray, M., James, H., and Martin, W. B. (1969) A Study of the Cytology and Karyotype of the Canine Transmissible Venereal Tumour. *Res. Vet. Sci.* 10, 565–568.

Nanta, Bazex, Bru, Lasserre, Puget, Bonneau, and Lacour. (1949) Les tumeurs vénériennes du chien et de la chienne dans la région Toulouseaine. *Rev. Méd. Vét.* 99, 529–531.

Nielsen, S. W. (1964) *Neoplastic Diseases in Feline Medicine and Surgery.* Catcott, E. J., ed. American Veterinary Publications (Santa Barbara), 156–176.

Nielsen, S. W., and Lein, D. H. (1974) Tumours of the Testis. *Bull. Wld. Hlth. Org.* 50, 71–78.

Nielsen, S. W., Misdorp, W., and McEntee, K. (1976) Tumours of the Ovary. *Bull. Wld. Hlth. Org.* 53, 203–215.

Norris, H. J., Taylor, H. B., and Garner, F. M. (1968) Equine Ovarian Granulosa Tumors. *Vet. Rec.* 82, 419–420.

Norris, H. J., Garner, F. M., and Taylor, H. B. (1969a) Pathology of Feline Ovarian Neoplasms. *J. Path.* 97, 138–143.

Norris, H. J., Taylor, H. B., and Garner, F. M. (1969b) Comparative Pathology of Ovarian Neoplasms. II. Gonadal Stromal Tumors of Bovine Species. *Path. Vet.* 6, 45–58.

Norris, H. J., Garner, F. M., and Taylor, H. B. (1970) Comparative Pathology of Ovarian Neoplasms. IV. Gonadal Stromal Tumors of Canine Species. *J. Comp. Path.* 80, 399–405.

Novak, E., and Craig, R. G. (1927) Infectious Sarcoma ("Venereal Granuloma") of the Vagina in Dogs. *Arch. Path.* 3, 193–202.

Oduye, O. O., Ikede, B. O., Esuruoso, G. O., and Akpokodje, J. U. (1973) Metastatic Transmissible Venereal Tumour in Dogs. *J. Small Anim. Pract.* 14, 625–637.

O'Rourke, M. D., and Geib, L. W. (1970) Endometrial Adenocarcinoma in a Cat. *Cornell Vet.* 60, 598–604.

O'Shea, J. D. (1963) Studies on the Canine Prostate Gland. II. Prostatic Neoplasms. *J. Comp. Path.* 73, 244–252.

Palker, T. J., and Yang, T. J. (1981) Identification and Physicochemical Characterization of a Tumor-Associated Antigen from Canine Transmissible Venereal Sarcoma. *J. Natl. Cancer Inst.* 66, 779–787.

Parish, W. E. (1961) A Transmissible Genital Papilloma of the Pig Resembling Condyloma Acuminatum of Man. *J. Path. Bact.* 81, 331–345.

———. (1962) An Immunological Study of the Transmissible Genital Papilloma of the Pig. *J. Path. Bact.* 83, 429–442.

Pierrepoint, C. G., Galley, J. M., Griffiths, K., and Grant, J. K. (1967) Steroid Metabolism of a Sertoli Cell Tumour of the Testis of a Dog with Feminization and Alopecia and of the Normal Canine Testis. *J. Endocr.* 38, 61–70.

Plaut, A., and Kohn-Speyer, A. C. (1947) The Carcinogenic Action of Smegma. *Science* 105, 391–392.

Powers, R. D. (1966) Serum Factors Associated with the Regression of Canine Transmissible Venereal Sarcoma. *Amer. J. Path.* 48, 7a.

Preiser, H. (1964) Endometrial Adenocarcinoma in a Cat. *Path. Vet.* 1, 485–490.

Prier, J. E., and Brodey, R. S. (1963) Canine Neoplasia: A Prototype for Human Cancer Study. *Bull. Wld. Hlth. Org.* 29, 331–344.

Rewell, R. E. (1947) Tubular Adenoma of the Testis and Oestrogenic Activity. *J. Path. Bact.* 59, 321–324.

Riser, W. H. (1942) Chorioepithelioma of the Bitch. *J. Amer. Vet. Med. Assoc.* 100, 65–66.

Rust, J. H. (1949) Transmissible Lymphosarcoma in the Dog. *J. Amer. Vet. Med. Assoc.* 114, 10–14.

Schlotthauer, C. F. (1939) Primary Neoplasms of the Genito-Urinary System of Dogs: A Report of Ten Cases. *J. Amer. Vet. Med. Assoc.* 95, 181–186.

Schlotthauer, C. F., McDonald, J. R., and Bollman, J. L. (1938) Testicular Tumors in Dogs. *J. Urol.* 40, 539–550.

Scully, R. E., and Coffin, D. L. (1952) Canine Testicular Tumors: With Special Reference to Their Histogenesis, Comparative Morphology and Endocrinology. *Cancer* 5, 592–605.

Shaw, D. P., and Roth, J. E. (1986) Testicular Teratocarcinoma in a Horse. *Vet. Path.* 23, 327–328.

Shortridge, E. H., and Cordes, D. O. (1969) Seminomas in Sheep. *J. Comp. Path.* 79, 229–232.

Siegel, E. T., Forchielli, E., Dorfman, R. I., Brodey, R. S., and Prier, J. E. (1967) An Estrogen Study in the Feminized Dog with Testicular Neoplasia. *Endocr.* 80, 272–277.

Siller, W. G. (1956) A Seroli Cell Tumour Causing Feminization in a Brown Leghorn Capon. *J. Endocr.* 14, 197–203.

Smith, G. G., and Washbourn, J. W. (1898) Infective Venereal Tumours in Dogs. *J. Comp. Path.* 11, 41–51.

Smith, H. A. (1954) Interstitial Cell Tumor of the Equine Testis. *J. Amer. Vet. Med. Assoc.* 124, 356–359.

Sticker, A. (1904) Transplantables Lymphosarkom des Hundes. *Z. Krebsforsch.* 1, 413–444.

Stickle, R. L., Erb, R. E., Fessler, J. F., and Runnels, L. J. (1975) Equine Granulosa Cell Tumors. *J. Amer. Vet. Med. Assoc.* 167, 148–151.

Stubbs, E. L., and Furth, J. (1934) Experimental Studies on Venereal Sarcoma of the Dog. *Amer. J. Path.* 10, 275–286.

Sundberg, J. P., and Nielsen, S. W. (1980) *Bovine Medi-*

*cine and Surgery.* Vol. I. Catcott, E. J., ed. American Veterinary Publications (Santa Barbara), 615–647.

Taylor, P. A. (1973) Case Report: Prostatic Adenocarcinoma in a Dog and a Summary of Ten Cases. *Can. Vet. J.* 14, 162–166.

Teilum, G. (1976) *Special Tumors of Ovary and Testis, Comparative Pathology and Histological Identification.* 2d ed. Munksgaard (Copenhagen).

Terlecki, S., and Watson, W. A. (1967) Adenocarcinoma of the Uterus of a Ewe. *Vet. Rec.* 80, 516–518.

Thiéry, G. (1954) Culture *in vivo* du sarcome de Sticker dans le liquide cephalo-rachidien. *Rec. Méd. Vét.* 130, 232–233.

Tontis, A., König, H., and Luginbühl, H. (1982) Granulosa and Theca Cell Tumours in the Bovine. *Schweiz. Arch. Tierheilk.* 124, 233–243.

Turk, J. R., Turk, M. A. M., and Gallina, A. M. (1981) A Canine Testicular Tumor Resembling Gonadoblastoma. *Vet. Path.* 18, 201–207.

Valentine, B. A., and Weinstock, D. (1986) Metastatic Testicular Embryonal Carcinoma in a Horse. *Vet. Path.* 23, 92–96.

Von Bomhard, D., Pukkavesa, C., and Haenichen, T. (1978) The Ultrastructure of Testicular Tumours in the Dog. Parts I, II, and III. *J. Comp. Path.* 88, 49–73.

Wade, H. (1908) An Experimental Investigation of Infective Sarcoma of the Dog, with a Consideration of its Relationship to Cancer. *J. Path. Bact.* 12, 384–425.

Watt, D. A. (1971) Seminoma in a Sheep. *Australian Vet. J.* 47, 405–406.

Weber, W. T., Nowell, P. C., and Hare, W. C. D. (1965) Chromosome Studies of a Transplanted and a Primary Canine Venereal Sarcoma. *J. Natl. Cancer Inst.* 35, 537–541.

Weiss, E. (1962) Das Prostatakarzinom des Hundes. *Munch. Tierärztl. Wschr.* 75, 145–150.

Williams, W. L., Gardner, W. U., and DeVita, J. (1946) Local Inhibition of Hair Growth in Dogs by Percutaneous Application of Estrone. *Endocr.* 38, 368–375.

Willis, R. A. (1947) Teratomas and Mixed Tumours in Animals and Their Bearings on Human Pathology. *Proc. R. Soc. Med.* 40, 635–636.

———. (1948) *Pathology of Tumours.* Butterworth & Co. (London).

Wilmes, H. (1937) Zum Vorkommen der Adenomyosis Uteri bei Haustieren. *Dtsch. Tierärztl. Wschr.* 45, 385–387.

Wolke, R. E. (1963) Vaginal Leiomyoma as a Cause of Chronic Constipation in the Cat. *J. Amer. Vet. Med. Assoc.* 143, 1103–1105.

Yang, T. J., and Jones, J. B. (1973) Canine Transmissible Venereal Sarcoma: Transplantation Studies in Neonatal and Adult Dogs. *J. Natl. Cancer Inst.* 51, 1915–1918.

Yang, T. J., Kennedy, J. R., and Andrews, R. B. (1976b) Rosette Formation of Human Erythrocytes of Canine Transmissible Venereal Sarcoma Cells. *Amer. J. Path.* 83, 359–366.

Yang, T. J., Roberts, R. S., and Jones, J. B. (1976a) Quantitative Study of Lymphoreticular Infiltration into Canine Transmissible Venereal Sarcoma. *Virchows Arch. B Cell Path.* 20, 197–204.

Yang, T. J., Wang, N. S., and Jones, J. B. (1973) A Study of the Cytology and Cell Culture of the Canine Transmissible Venereal Sarcoma. *Experientia* 29, 1133–1134.

**12**

*Jack E. Moulton*
# Tumors of the Mammary Gland

## MAMMARY TUMORS OF THE DOG

**Incidence, Age, and Breed.** Mammary tumors rank second (behind skin tumors) as the most common neoplasms in dogs of both sexes; they are by far the most common tumors in the bitch.

General reviews of mammary tumors in dogs have been presented by Cotchin (1956), Misdorp *et al.* (1971, 1972, 1973), Moulton *et al.* (1970), Mulligan (1944), Priester (1979), and Taylor *et al.* (1976). According to Bloom (1954) they represent 25 to 30% of all tumors of the bitch. Figures vary considerably on the percentage of mammary tumors among all tumors of dogs. This was reported as 10% by Dobberstein and Matthias (1942), 12% by Kronberger (1961), 13% by Dorn *et al.* (1968), 14% by Überreiter (1960) and Poppensiek (1961), 18% by Cotchin (1954), 41% by Da Silva *et al.* (1947), and 44% by Sticker (1902).

About 65% of mammary tumors in dogs are benign mixed tumors, and 25% are carcinomas (Dahme and Weiss, 1958; Mulligan, 1949; Nieberle, 1933); the rest are hyperplasias, adenomas, malignant mixed tumors, and myoepitheliomas. These figures vary considerably because of different methods of classifying the tumors, especially the separation of mixed tumor from carcinoma.

Prier and Brodey (1963) compared mammary tumors in dogs and humans and found that behavior and histological origin were similar but that frequency of types differed.

Canine mammary tumors have been reported in all parts of the world; there is no indication of any geographical difference in frequency.

The age distribution of mammary tumors closely follows the age distribution of most tumors in dogs. Mammary tumors are rare in dogs less than 2 years old, but incidence begins to increase sharply at 6 to 7 years of age, which is the onset of the "cancer age." Males, which rarely get these tumors, are almost 1 year older than females at the onset of tumors. A plot of the age distribution of mammary tumors is a bell-shaped curve. Age specific rates of incidence that correct for the smaller population of older dogs indicate a much higher risk of mammary cancer in old than in young females (Dorn *et al.,* 1968). Benign mixed tumor begins to appear 1 to 2 years earlier than does carcinoma.

The onset of mammary tumors in dogs compares with the onset of mammary carcinomas in women. The risk of developing these tumors increases markedly beginning at about 6 years of age in the dog and at 40 years in women. These ages correlate well in the age conversion table of Lebeau (1953), in which a dog at 2 years is equivalent to a human at 24 years and each year after 2 years in the dog equals 4 years in humans. A correction must be made for different breeds of dogs. For example, the giant breeds of dogs are "old" at 5 to 8 years, when the smaller breeds are only "middle aged."

Mammary neoplasms occur at an earlier age in X-irradiated dogs than in control dogs (Andersen and Rosenblatt, 1969; Moulton *et al.,* 1970, 1986).

The total incidence of tumors is the same, but the age specific incidence differs in the control and irradiated dogs. This difference is due to the shortening effect of irradiation on lifespan.

When total numbers of each breed in an area are considered, there is an indication of breed prevalence of mammary tumors. The greatest frequency of these tumors is found in sporting breeds (pointers, retrievers, English setters, and spaniels), poodles, Boston terriers, and dachshunds. Some of the differences in breed incidence are striking. For example, in a study near Tulsa, Oklahoma, MacVean et al. (1978) found an incidence of 3.6% in the pointer, 1.1% in the poodle and Boston terrier, and 0.35% in cross-bred dogs. The incidence was higher in intact (nonovariectomized) than in neutered bitches except for the pointer. The higher prevalence in the dachshund was found both in Germany (Dahme and Weiss, 1958; Sandersleben, 1958) and the United States (Frye et al., 1967; Moulton et al., 1970).

**Endocrine Influences.** Mammary tumors occur almost exclusively in female dogs, with only occasional occurrence in males. A literature survey reveals only 22 recorded cases of mammary tumors in male dogs since 1895. Many of these tumors were associated with hormonal abnormalities in the dog, such as estrogen-secreting Sertoli cell tumor of the testis.

The stage of development of the mammary gland during the estrous cycle probably has some influence on the occurrence of mammary neoplasms in females, although the exact nature of this influence is not known (see review by Hamilton, 1975).

The mammary gland of the normal female dog is controlled by the hormonal climate, which regulates the initial development of the gland at sexual maturation (about 10 to 14 months of age) and the gland's cyclic development during the estrous cycle and pregnancy. The duration of the stages of the estrous cycle is as follows (Sekhri and Faulkin, 1970): proestrus, about 9 days; estrus, 9 days; and metestrus, 70 to 80 days. Ovulation is spontaneous at estrus. During metestrus the mammary gland undergoes its fullest development and then begins to regress. Development of the gland after ovulation and consequent corpus luteum formation are similar in both bred and unbred dogs. Biopsy of the gland at metestrus reveals duct and alveolar proliferation that continues until the 6th week after estrus. At the time of maximum lobular development during metestrus, the individual cuboidal alveolar cells form fat droplets and microvesicles indicative of lactation. A small amount of secretion is seen within each alveolar lumen. If the animal has not been bred, involution begins at this time. Involution is characterized by shrinking of the lobules, proliferation of the connective tissue surrounding each lobule, and degeneration of the epithelial cells. The mammary gland during the resting stage has poor lobular development; alveolar buds and ducts are present but alveoli are absent.

Mammary gland development is even more extensive during pregnancy. Proliferation of the lobular ductules can be observed within 3 days after conception. The lumen of each ductule is compressed and lined by epithelium varying in thickness from one to three cells. Ductular proliferation continues until about 4 weeks after conception, at which time alveolar formation begins. Lobulation of the gland is quite distinct by the 42nd day of gestation, and the alveoli develop lumens. The alveolar cell cytoplasm has evidence of secretory activity, with vesicles of protein secretion and lipid formation.

Upon parturition and full lactation, the mammary epithelium undergoes even more extensive development and the lumen of each alveolus becomes distended with secretion and lined by flattened epithelium. This distension will vary with the frequency of nursing and the amount of milk removed. During lactation the epithelial cells contain hypertrophied Golgi apparatuses and increased numbers of mitochondria and ribosomes. The endoplasmic reticulum is highly organized and glycogen granules are absent. In the surface toward the lumen the epithelial cells show microvilli and emptying secretion vesicles.

Different parts of the normal active gland are not always in synchrony and their histology varies from one area to another. In some areas the alveoli are filled with secretion (milk) and their lumens are wide and their walls dilated and thin; in others the lumen is narrow and the epithelium is thickened. The cells are cylindrical, conical, or flattened. In the small excretory ducts the epithelium is cubical or even low cylindrical. Regression after nursing, with return to resting state, is never complete because alveoli never disappear completely. Involution in old age leaves the mammary lobule with only a few scattered ducts, but no alveoli. At this stage the epithelium may be the seat of neoplastic change. In old age the interlobular connective tissue becomes less cellular, as though the intercellular fibrillar tissue were melting down into a homogeneous mass.

Separating the litter from the dam initiates regression of the mammary glands. Although variations exist between lobules, the most prominent early changes associated with regression are alveolar collapse and disorganization of the cells. The lumens of the ducts and alveoli contain granular and foamy secretion as well as portions of cells. Many of the epithelial cells have pyknotic nuclei and the stroma appears edematous. These changes occur within 2 weeks of weaning, although the secretory epithelium does not atrophy completely until 1 month after lactation has ceased. During this time there is gradual elimination of the necrotic parenchyma and an increase in the stroma surrounding the ducts. After the initial pregnancy, the mammary parenchyma never completely atrophies to ducts only, for remnants of the lobular alveoli remain.

The benign mammary mixed tumors are said to enlarge and become soft during proestrus, estrus, and early metestrus and then become small and firm during late metestrus and anestrus (Bloom, 1954; De Vitta, 1939). It is not clear, however, whether these changes occur in the mammary neoplasm or in the tissue surrounding the neoplasm that is not directly involved in the tumor, but is undergoing normal cyclical hyperplastic change.

Strong evidence (Dorn *et al.*, 1968; Mulligan, 1945) supports the hypothesis that ovariectomy has a sparing effect on tumor formation, especially when performed prior to the first estrous cycle. Frye *et al.* (1967) reported that the risk of mammary tumors was four times greater in intact females than in neutered females. Schneider *et al.* (1969) showed that the chance of developing mammary tumors was 1 in 100 in bitches neutered before their first estrous cycle, 1 in 12 in bitches neutered after one estrous cycle, and 1 in 4 in bitches neutered after two estrous cycles. This sparing effect occurred only if the bitches were neutered before 2 years 6 months of age (stage of maturity when development of the mammary gland ceases), paralleling that of women neutered (artificial menopause) at 26 years of age.

The effect of ovariectomy on the course of established neoplasms is uncertain. Meier (1962) reported that ovariectomy results in temporary regression of existing mammary tumors, but Jabara (1960a) claimed that ovariectomy only relieves hyperplastic changes surrounding the neoplasm and has no effect on an established neoplasm of the mammary gland. In premenopausal women ovariectomy will sometimes cause regression of the breast tumor, although the regression is often temporary.

Dozza and Coluzzi (1963) found increased urinary estrogen in bitches with mammary neoplasms. Mulligan (1947) observed enlargement of the mammary glands in bitches injected with estrogenic compounds, whereas Gardner (1941) found only the nipples enlarged.

Many investigators (Andersen, 1965; Beckman, 1945; Bloom, 1954; De Vitta, 1939; Riser, 1947) have reported that mammary tumors are associated with endocrinic disorders such as irregular estrous cycle, ovarian follicular cysts, persistent corpora lutea, hyperplastic endometrium, pseudopregnancy, pyometra, and the unnatural sexual life of household pets. Brodey *et al.* (1966) had an opposing view. In a study of 57 bitches with mammary tumors and 244 normal bitches, they found no significant differences between the two groups in regularity of the estrous cycle, pseudopregnancy, or pregnancy. This observation was confirmed by Schneider *et al.* (1969).

The relationship between mammary neoplasia and exaggerated pseudopregnancy is controversial. Pseudopregnancy is a normal part of the canine estrous cycle, but in some bitches it gives rise to pronounced clinical signs such as excessive milk secretion and behavioral changes. Bitches with pseudopregnancy may have unusually high progestogen levels in their serum. During normal metestrus, progestogens cause alveolar growth in the mammary gland and milk secretion, along with myoepithelial cell proliferation.

Some workers (De Vitta, 1939; Else and Hannant, 1979; Mulligan, 1963; Überreiter, 1960) found an association between pseudopregnancy and hyperplastic nodules or neoplasia in the mammary gland. Others (Brodey *et al.*, 1966; Fidler and Brodey, 1967; Schneider *et al.*, 1969) found no such relationship. Obviously, the hormonal milieu of the canine is not fully understood.

Many features of mammary neoplasms are common to women and dogs, including age of onset, morphological appearance, frequent metastasis, and the general course of the neoplastic diasease. The presence of estrogen receptors on the tumor cells is also similar in women and dogs (D'Arville and Pierrepoint, 1979; Hamilton *et al.*, 1977). Whether estrogen receptors in dogs indicate hormone dependency as they do in women is as yet unknown. Hamilton *et al.* (1977) found estrogen receptors in 52% of canine mammary carcinomas, a figure lower than that for human mammary tumors but higher than for cats. Thus far, no correlation has been found between the histological type of neoplasm in bitches and the presence or absence of epithelial cell estrogen receptors. Estrogen receptors are seen in both benign mixed tumors and carcinomas of the canine mammary gland; their occurrence in benign tumors is half that of malignant tumors (Evans and Pierrepoint, 1975).

The presence of estrogen receptors in some of these tumors might indicate that the bitch will benefit from hormonal therapy, but to date insufficient data have been collected to allow meaningful conclusions.

Briggs (1980) and Kwapien *et al.* (1980) reported on the long-term effects of treating dogs with human contraceptive steroids (progestogens, estrogens, or progestogen–estrogen combinations) and found a few hyperplastic nodules in the mammary glands of treated dogs but no malignant neoplasms. Using short-term treatment (8 weeks) with progestogens, El Etreby and Wrobel (1978) observed lobuloalveolar development of the mammary gland, similar to that of the last few months of pregnancy.

Data are scant that compare the incidence of mammary tumors in virgin bitches with that in bitches that have had litters. Bloom (1954) reported fewer tumors in bitches that had one or more litters.

**Etiology.** There is little evidence that mammary tumors in dogs are associated with virus. Although type-A intracysternal oncornavirus particles are occasionally observed within the neoplastic cells by electron microscopy, there is no experimental evidence that they cause the tumors.

**Sites.** Both benign and malignant mammary tumors occur with increasing frequency from the most cephalad to most caudal mammary glands. (The bitch has five sets of mammary glands; the cranial and caudal thoracic glands, the cranial and caudal abdominal glands, and the inguinal glands. For convenience here, these are numbered 1 to 5, cranial to caudal.) The two most caudal glands are the sites of almost 60% of mammary tumors. The reason for more tumors in the caudal glands is unknown. Mulligan (1947) suggested that the increasing frequency might be associated with the greater proliferative change in the larger, more caudal glands in response to estrogen. More significant, Cameron and Faulkin (1971) and Warner (1976) found more hyperplastic nodules in the caudal mammary glands, suggesting that since these nodules were preneoplastic, they accounted for the greater number of tumors in the caudal glands. Recent observations have shown that carcinomas do not necessarily follow the same frequency pattern in the different glands as do hyperplastic nodules and benign tumors (Moulton *et al.*, 1986). Fewer carcinomas appear in the first (most cephalad) pair of mammary glands, but their frequency is not significantly different in the remaining glands (2 to 5).

Mammary glands of some aged bitches contain dozens of nodules ranging in diameter from a few millimeters to 10 mm (fig. 12.1). The frequency of these nodules increases with age, starting with a very few at 2 to 3 years of age and progressing to several hundred at 12 years of age or older. Cameron and Faulkin (1971), who carefully examined the mammary glands from eight beagle bitches ranging in age from 7 years 7.2 months to 8 years 6 months, found 742 atypical mammary nodules, of which 78% were alveolar hyperplasia, 14% were neoplasms, and 8% were inflammatory lesions. Separate neoplasms from the same individual encompassed a wide range of morphological types.

Bloom (1954) reported that multiple involvement with tumors occurred 50% of the time. Mulligan (1944) found a 20% occurrence of two mixed tumors in the same or different glands, a 5 to 10% occurrence of mixed tumor plus coexisting carcinoma in the same or another gland, and independent carcinomas in separate mammary glands rarely. Primary malignant tumors often occupy more than a single gland, through direct extension or metastasis.

**Classification.** The methods of classifying canine mammary tumors vary considerably. There is fairly good agreement on including categories such as adenoma, carcinoma, and benign and malignant

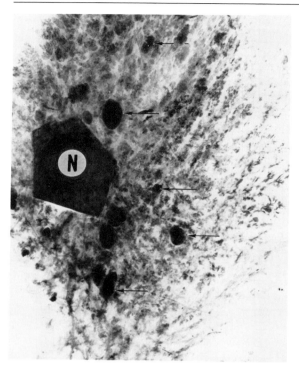

**FIGURE 12.1.** Entire (unsectioned) axillary mammary gland of an aged bitch. The fat has been removed and the specimen stained with hematoxylin and cleared. The pentagonal dark mass is skin left on the surface of the mammary gland (the skin was removed from the rest of the gland); the white circular area (N) in the center is the site of the nipple. A total of 19 densities were observed, 5 marked with arrows, representing hyperplastic nodules and benign tumors. (Courtesy of Dr. L. J. Faulkin.)

mixed tumors. Variation is considerable, however, in the use of other categories: adenoma is confused with hyperplasia or misdiagnosed as carcinoma; fibroadenoma has been listed as a separate tumor or included among the mixed tumors; myoepithelioma has now come into common use as a diagnostic term (Cotchin 1958; Moulton *et al.,* 1970; Mulligan, 1949).

The classification used here is perhaps outdated, but it is a simple one that avoids detailed subdivision (table 12.1). It is based on the most prominent histological feature in the tumor. The general categories for benign mammary tumors are adenoma, mixed tumor, and benign myoepithelioma. Nodu-

lar hyperplasia is included for comparative purposes. The categories for malignant tumors are carcinoma, malignant mixed tumor, and malignant myoepithelioma. The rare Paget's disease of the nipple in the bitch and fibroepithelial hyperplasia in the cat are also included.

Not included in this chapter are tumors of the skin of the mammary gland. Examples are papilloma (including papilloma of the teat skin), adnexal tumors, lipoma, hemangioma, fibroma, and fibrosarcoma. These neoplasms are indistinguishable from their counterparts in the skin and subcutis (see chap. 2).

## Hyperplasia

Hyperplasia (unilobular or multilobular) of the mammary gland of the bitch usually involves multiple lobules and forms a distinct nodular mass in the mammary gland. Hyperplastic nodules are present in one or more mammary glands in the same bitch, and may arise at the same time or as much as 1 year apart. The distinction between lobular hyperplasia and lobular adenoma may be difficult. In general, lobular hyperplasia is similar to

### TABLE 12.1. Classification of Mammary Growths in the Dog

Benign
  Multilobular hyperplasia
  Adenoma, lobular and papillary
  Mixed tumor
  Benign myoepithelioma

Malignant
  Carcinoma (infiltrating and noninfiltrating)
    Lobular carcinoma, noninfiltrating and infiltrating, solid (origin in mammary lobules from alveoli or ductules)
    Papillary carcinoma, includes papillary cystic type (origin in intra- or interlobular ducts)
    Squamous carcinoma (squamous metaplasia of tumor cells)
    Scirrhous (fibrosing) carcinoma (alveolar or duct origin, diffusely infiltrating)
  Malignant mixed tumor (carcinomatous and/or chondrosarcomatous or osteosarcomatous)
  Malignant myoepithelioma
  Paget's carcinoma of nipple

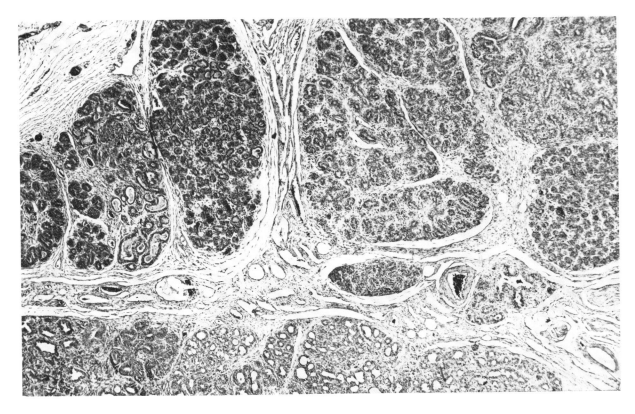

A
─
B

**FIGURE 12.2** Multilobular hyperplasia of the canine mammary gland. A. Hyperplastic nodule showing multiple lobules in different stages of hyperplasia. B. Lobule in resting state with central alveolar ductule and lacking alveolar development.

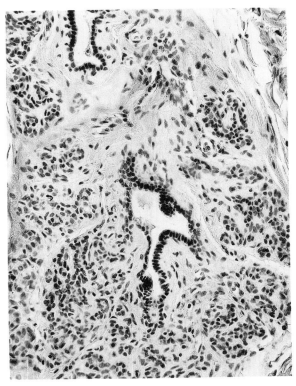

physiological hyperplasia during pregnancy or lactation, but it usually has more atypical histology than the normal change. One encounters 3 different patterns: (1) lobules with uniform alveolar cell proliferation, such as in physiological hyperplasia (fig. 12.2A); (2) alveolar cells containing vesicles and alveolar lumens filled with acidophilic, vacuolated secretory material; and (3) lobules in the resting state (fig. 12.2B). In the first two changes, the mammary lobules become greatly enlarged, and the interlobular stroma forms a thin trabecular framework.

## Adenoma

**Classification.** In the classification of mammary neoplasms prepared by Hampe and Misdorp (1974) for the World Health Organization (WHO), the benign tumors are divided into adenoma, duct papilloma, fibroadenoma of pericanalicular and intracanalicular types (noncellular and cellular), and benign mixed tumor. Adenoma in the pure state is less common than hyperplastic nodule or mixed tumor. In the pure state, it appears as lobular adenoma arising from the alveoli, or as a papillary adenoma arising from multiple sites within the intralobular or interlobular duct system. All gradations exist between lobular adenoma and lobular carcinoma and between papillary adenoma and papillary carcinoma (Moulton *et al.*, 1986). The adenomas are probably precancerous for both types of carcinoma.

**Gross Morphology.** Adenomas are solitary or multiple growths in one or more glands and may measure as much as 4 cm in diameter. They are round or ovoid, well-circumscribed, encapsulated, and usually embedded in the mammary parenchyma. Papillary adenomas are occasionally found in the teat canal or larger ducts. Adenomas are usually firm, but sometimes soft, often cystic, lobulated in the solid areas, and gray, white, or tan.

**Histological Features.** Lobular adenoma occurs as proliferation of small, hyperchromatic, cuboidal or low columnar cells into the lumens of the alveoli and ducts (figs. 12.3A–D). The cells may enlarge later and when they fill the alveoli they show less dense staining. The basal location of nuclei presents a palisading (basiloid) appearance. The intraluminal growth occurs from budlike infoldings of alveolar lining epithelium or from solidly cellular intraluminal proliferations. It is not unusual to see expanded alveoli completely filled with epithelial cells. The epithelial cell growth may also fill the lobular ductules (fig. 12.3E). Lobular adenoma is probably precancerous for lobular carcinoma. The most valid histological feature used to distinguish the adenoma from early lobular carcinoma is absence of tumor cell infiltration of the intralobular stroma.

The papillary adenoma develops within the lobules, often from the intralobular duct system or from the interlobular ducts or teat sinus. Intraluminal papillae form in the dilated ducts or sinuses. The papillary extensions are sessile, stalked, or polypoid and have single or multiple points of attachment (figs. 12.4A and B). The duct of origin is dilated or cystic. The epithelium lining the duct is single or

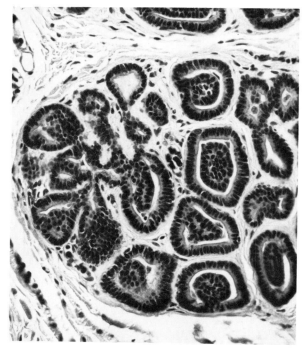

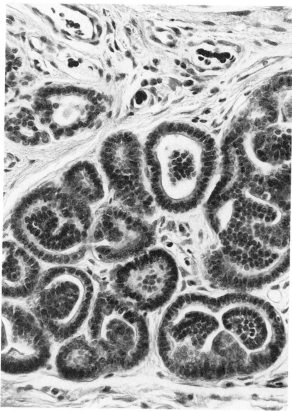

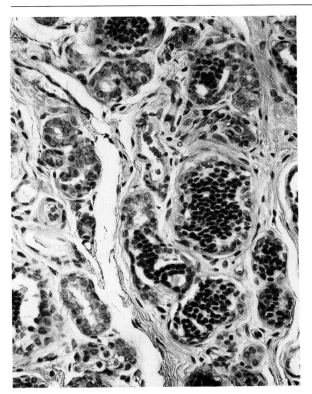

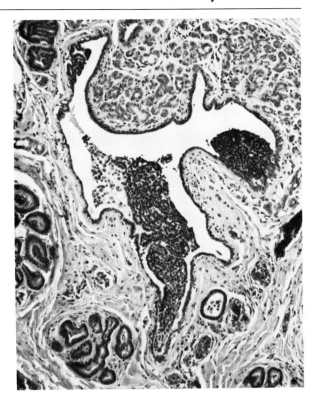

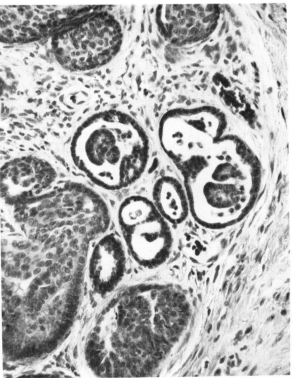

A | C | D
--- | --- | ---
B | E |

**FIGURE 12.3.** Lobular adenoma of the canine mammary gland. A and B. Lobular alveoli partly filled with neoplastic epithelial cells. Some alveoli show infolding of epithelium. Observe the basal location of the epithelial nuclei presenting a basiloid appearance. C. Dark staining cells almost fill the alveoli. D. Central lobular ductule partly filled with neoplastic cells. Alveoli in small peripheral lobules show beginning intraluminal growth (as in photographs A and B). E. Edge of a lobule showing alveoli with micropapillary growth of small, dark staining cells and alveoli filled with large, pale staining cells that suggest early carcinomatous change (carcinoma *in situ*).

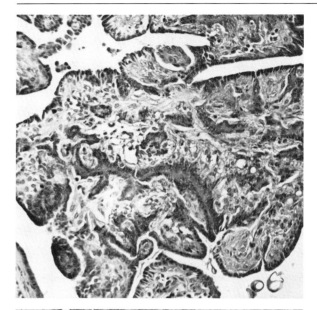

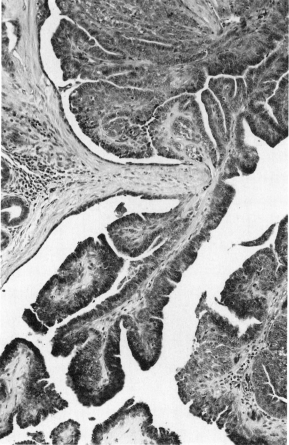

multilayered, sometimes flattened and atrophic, and simple cuboidal or columnar. The duct lumen usually contains a homogeneous acidophilic fluid and sometimes blood as well. The papillary growths are supported by narrow stalks of vascularized connective tissue and covered by epithelial cells varying from low cuboidal to tall columnar. Similar cells line glandular spaces within the body of the papillae.

When there is proliferation of myoepithelial cells in the papillary stalks, usually with formation of large, polypoid, blunted papillae, the neoplasm is placed in the mixed tumor category (see fig. 12.5C). In true papillary adenoma the stalk tissue consists of fibrous connective tissue and a small blood vessel for nourishment of the papillae.

The term *cystadenoma* means that the ducts or alveoli with intraluminal papillary growth are greatly dilated or cystic.

An uncommon form of mammary adenoma (that may be a hyperplastic change) occurs in male and female dogs and in cats and appears to arise from the ductule system. This neoplasm resembles the normal budding or rebuilding of the lobular ductule system during the change from the resting to the proliferative stage at the onset of estrus (the lobuloalveolar stage of mammary development). In the tumor, however, the epithelium is more active and irregularly piled up with more hyperchromatic nuclei than in the normal hyperplastic change. There is also marked proliferation of intralobular fibrous stroma. The overall histological picture may even suggest a carcinoma, but the growth remains restricted to the mammary lobules, never infiltrates surrounding tissue, and never metastasizes.

A
B
**FIGURE 12.4.** Papillary adenoma in the mammary gland of a bitch. This neoplasm formed from the intralobular ductules or interlobular ducts. A. Papillomatous growth in a dilated duct. B. Dilated duct showing intraluminal papillary growth.

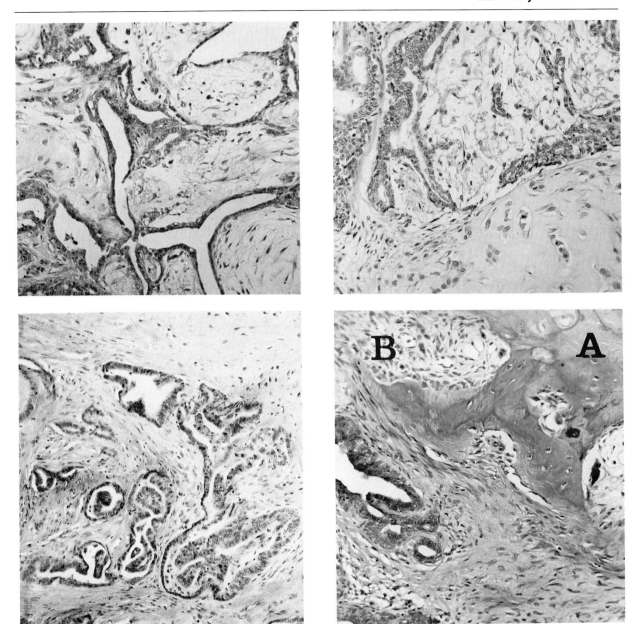

FIGURE 12.7. Mammary mixed tumor of the dog. A. Early formation of cartilage in myoepithelial cell stroma of intraductal papillae. B and C. Epithelial growth adjacent to hyaline cartilage. D. Bone (A) and myoepithelial tissue (B).

myxomatous and chondromatous parts of the neoplasm, where they are more separated, thicker, and straighter than in normal cells and much easier to discern. Other characteristic features of the neoplastic myoepithelial cells are an extensive Golgi apparatus, a large field of glycogen, and an ability of the cell to form basal membranelike structures (Bomhard and Sandersleben, 1974). As the myoepithelial cells proliferate and round-up and the tissue begins to resemble hyaline cartilage, the Golgi apparatus further enlarges and the cytoplasmic filaments decrease in number.

The cartilage that forms in mixed tumors appears in nodules or plates of variable size (figs. 12.7A–C). Osteoblasts participate actively in forming the bone, which appears as osteoid or well-mineralized osseous tissue (fig. 12.7D). Bone marrow with fat and hematopoietic cells is sometimes observed.

Fibrous connective tissue exists probably as a reaction to proliferation of epithelium in mixed tumor. The fibrous stroma often forms thick hyalinized collars around neoplastic glandular elements. When the fibrous tissue is densely cellular, it is difficult to distinguish from myoepithelial cell proliferation.

The epithelial components of mixed tumor show all degrees of proliferation from simple hyperplasia to disorderly papillomatous growth. The lobular architecture of the gland is poorly preserved. Ectatic ducts and cysts commonly contain papillary or polypoid growths of similar structure to those in papillary adenoma.

The glandular epithelium landlocked in chondromucinous stroma or hyaline cartilage of mixed tumor may appear as irregular cords and ducts of swollen, sometimes squamouslike, and occasionally degenerative cells suggestive of invasive carcinoma. This change makes it difficult to distinguish mixed tumor from invasive carcinoma unless attention is paid to the presence of myoepithelial cells and chondromucinous stroma.

Some large mixed tumors become infected through ulceration of the skin from trauma, and contain focal or diffuse collections of neutrophils and mononuclear cells. Foreign body giant cells are occasionally seen in areas of fat necrosis. Hemorrhage and necrosis are usually minimal. A few tumors exhibit cholesterol clefts in areas of necrosis, and hyalinization and calcification may be present, particularly in regions of cartilage and bone.

## Carcinoma

**Classification.** The classification of carcinomas is far from satisfactory; too many criteria have been proposed. Classification may be based on the type of cell involved (acinar, clear, spheroidal, mucous, or squamous cells), prominent tissue change (cribriform, solid, papillary, tubular or glandlike, or medullary), necrosis in solid ducts ("comedocarcinoma"), infiltration or lack of same, and stroma (fibrosing or scirrhous).

The presence or absence of infiltration in carcinoma is an important feature in diagnosis; it is far more important than determining the classification type. For this reason, in naming these carcinomas some pathologists designate them as infiltrating or noninfiltrating. The patterns of infiltrative growth are as follows: small or large solid epithelial cords, focal clusters of cells, single cells or ones invading single file, and tubular formation. In all forms of infiltration there is pronounced stromal fibrosis (scirrhous reaction). The very presence of fibrosis in the mammary gland should alert one to the possibility of invasive carcinoma. Fibrosis is also seen around lymphatic vessels carrying tumor emboli and in metastatic sites in the lymph nodes, lungs, etc. Care must be taken to not mistake myoepithelial proliferation for stromal fibrosis. Myoepithelial proliferation almost never occurs in carcinoma; it is only found in mixed tumor and myoepithelioma.

An ideal classification of carcinomas would be based on the origin of the carcinoma (histogenetic classification) and would allow designation according to whether the carcinoma was infiltrating or noninfiltrating. Unfortunately, the histological origin of carcinomas cannot always be determined. For example, the origin cannot be determined accurately when there is complete loss of lobular architecture or invasion of single cells or thin cords of cells in a diffuse fibrous stroma. Many are labeled duct carcinoma, although their ductal origin cannot be determined with certainty.

There are a variety of classification schemes proposed by pathologists. Cotchin (1958) subdivided these neoplasms into squamous cell carcinoma (arising from the lining of a teat canal or major duct or by metaplasia of glandular epithelium), duct carcinoma (including solid and papillary), adenocarcinoma, fibrosing (sclerosing or scirrhous) carcinoma, solid lobular carcinoma, and anaplastic carcinoma (no glandular pattern). Dobberstein and Matthias (1942) classified carcinomas as adenocarcinoma, spheroidal cell or solid carcinoma (including scirrhous and medullary), mucous carcinoma (tumor cells forming mucin), and squamous cell carcinoma. Jabara (1960*b*) used the classifications of adenocarcinoma, spheroidal cell (solid) carcinoma, and squamous cell carcinoma. Mulligan (1949) classified the carcinomas as duct carcinoma (papillary, solid, medullary, and fibrosing), lobular carcinoma, and mixed duct and lobular carcinoma. He stressed subdividing each type according to whether it was infiltrating or noninfiltrating. Willis' (1967) classification for canine mammary carcinomas included intraductal carcinoma (papillary, cribriform, lactiform, and solid), extraductal (adenocarcinoma, spheroidal, solid, and diffuse), and metaplastic (mucinous or colloid and squamous). He recognized transitions from epithelial hyperplasia to papilloma or carcinoma.

In the classification adopted by WHO (Hampe and Misdorp, 1974), carcinomas are subdivided into adenocarcinoma (simple and complex types of tubular, papillary, and papillary cystic types), solid carcinoma (simple and complex), spindle cell carcinoma (simple and complex), anaplastic carcinoma, squamous cell carcinoma, and mucinous carcinoma. In this classification, "simple" refers to pure carcinoma and "complex" refers to carcinoma with myoepithelial cell proliferation. This classification is unnecessarily complex and will not be used here. Its use, however, may be justified in the future, particularly if additional behavioral differences in the neoplasms can be related to histological types. A more recent classification proposed by Misdorp and Hart (1976) divides the malignant tumors into three main histological types, each type reflecting different biological behavior. The tumors are classified as simple carcinoma (one cell type, corresponding to adenocarcinoma), complex carcinoma (luminal epithelial plus myoepithelial cell proliferation), and carcinosarcoma (carcinomatous and/or sarcomatous parts). These workers also grade the carcinomas on the basis of differentiation (tubular formation) and cellular anaplasia (irregular cell size and shape, hyperchromatic nuclei, and high mitotic index).

If strict subdivision of carcinomas is necessary in veterinary medicine, the author recommends the following classification, which is based on anatomical site of tumor origin and the most prominent morphological feature. When more than one prominent feature is present, the tumor should be named on the basis of the one that predominates. All of these carcinomas may be infiltrating (invasive) or noninfiltrating (noninvasive). This classification (table 12.1) includes lobular carcinoma, papillary carcinoma, squamous cell carcinoma, and scirrhous (fibrosing) carcinoma. The term *adenocarcinoma,* which indicates glandular origin and/or glandular (tubular) histomorphology, has been discarded because all of these neoplasms have origin in a gland (the mammary gland), and most form tubular structures. *Anaplastic carcinoma, comedocarcinoma,* and *mucinous carcinoma* are subtypes of those listed above, and are not terms used here in naming the carcinomas. The term *solid carcinoma* usually refers to a lobular carcinoma where the mammary lobules have become greatly expanded and solidly (diffusely) infiltrated with neoplastic cells, and with little stromal fibrosis. The term *duct carcinoma* is still quite popular and indicates origin of the carcinoma from the mammary duct system. The author believes that this term should not be used unless there is clear histological evidence that the carcinoma has arisen in the ducts. For the most part, the carcinomas in dogs arise from the lobular alveoli and ductules (Moulton *et al.,* 1986). The one important exception is papillary carcinoma that may arise from interlobular ducts. The rare Paget's carcinoma of the nipple, reported in a bitch (Ajello, 1976), is described below as a distinct carcinoma type. The separation of mammary carcinomas, especially lobular type from scirrhous carcinoma type, may be artificial when there is extensive tumor cell infiltration and considerable stromal fibrosis. Usually in such carcinomas the histological site of origin cannot be determined and naming the tumor is largely guesswork. It is also important to realize that in lobular carcinoma there can be small epithelial infoldings (micropapillae) within the alveoli and intralobular ductules that may mimic early papillary carcinoma.

Lobular carcinoma comprises about 83% of these carcinomas, papillary type 7%, squamous type 4%, and scirrhous carcinoma 5% (Moulton *et al.,* 1986).

Since the terminology is sometimes confusing, we often diagnose these tumors simply as adenocarcinomas and indicate infiltration or noninfiltration and make no designation as to type. When histology can be better related to behavior, a classification will be adopted that reflects differences among types of carcinomas.

**Gross Morphology.** Carcinomas show rapid growth, often doubling in size in a few weeks. They invade locally, merging into surrounding normal tissue. Some seem encapsulated when compression of adjacent mammary tissue forms an interface that feels like a capsule on palpation. They often develop fibrous adhesions to the overlying skin and underlying fascia or musculature and cannot be moved freely. The skin may become thickened, dimpled, or ulcerated. Some have fibrous adhesions that pin the inner thigh region of the hindlimb to the flank (Owen, 1966). They often invade local lymphatics, the skin, or the adjacent gland on the same side. They may show retrograde growth within lymphatics.

The carcinomas vary greatly in size and appearance. The diameter averages 8 cm (ranging from 2 to 20 cm). The tumors are round, ovoid, discoid, fungiform, or of ill-defined shape. They usually occupy a large part of the mammary gland, but may affect several adjacent glands in continuity. The carcinomas are often poorly circumscribed, usually unencapsulated, and highly infiltrative. Many dogs have carcinoma and multilobular hyperplasia in the same or different mammary glands.

The lobular carcinomas are usually soft, and the cut surface displays diffuse or lobulated areas of homogeneous creamy white tissue. Approximately half of the papillary carcinomas are firm and half are soft and spongy. On section they are often lobulated and gray or white and often have multiple cysts, partly occluded by shaggy, irregular, papillary ingrowths and filled with slimy amber-colored fluid. The squamous cell carcinomas are firm, irregular in shape, lobulated, and gray or white with yellow mottling. Scirrhous carcinomas are irregular in shape, poorly circumscribed, and often show infiltration into adjacent mammary glands. They are hard, white, gray, or tan, and occasionally mottled brown or yellow. Many adhere to the skin or underlying musculature.

Misdorp and Hart (1979) have presented a useful method for clinical staging of the carcinomas based on gross appearance (table 12.2).

**TABLE 12.2. Clinical Stages of Canine Mammary Carcinomas**

| Stage | Size (cm) | Skin | Underlying tissues |
|---|---|---|---|
| I | <5 | Not involved | Not involved |
| II | 5 to 10 | Dimpled | Not involved |
| III | 11 to 15 | Infiltrated and ulcerated | Muscle fixation |
| IV | >15 or whole gland | | Chest or abdominal wall involved |

**Histological Features.** There is some evidence that carcinomas arise in the mammary lobules, possibly from alveoli that have undergone precancerous change (Moulton *et al.*, 1986). Carcinomas undoubtedly also arise *de novo* without precancerous change. The exact origin of many carcinomas in the canine mammary gland has not been established yet, probably because most of the available data come from histological examination of neoplasms removed surgically or obtained at necropsy; there have been few experimental studies on the histomorphology of carcinogenesis.

*Lobular Carcinoma*—This form of mammary carcinoma is composed of undifferentiated, often small and hyperchromatic cells, having an acinar or faintly tubular pattern (figs. 12.8A and B). Similar cells may fill the lobular ductule. The carcinoma first occurs within the lobule, possibly by cancerous change in adenoma (or in hyperplasia?). There are few distinct histological differences between adenoma and carcinoma in early stages of carcinoma development. One of the first changes indicative of carcinomatous change is filling of the lobular alveoli and ductules by proliferating tumor cells; this results in great expansion of these structures. As the alveoli and tubules become impacted by tumor cells there may be a change from small hyperchromatic cells to large, pale staining cells. The first unequivocal evidence of cancerous change is when the neoplastic cells infiltrate through the alveolar and ductular basement membranes and grow into the intralobular stroma (fig. 12.8C). This may or may not be attended by stromal fibrosis (figs. 12.8C and 12.9A). The infiltrative tumor cells may proliferate through-

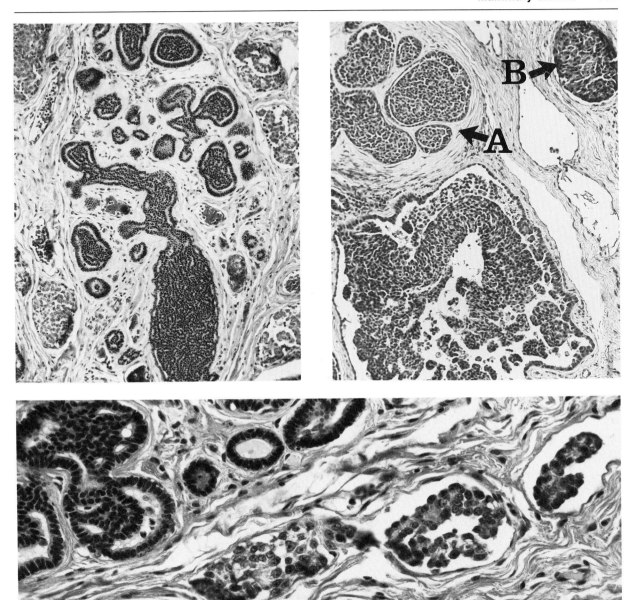

A|B
  C  **FIGURE 12.8.** Lobular carcinoma of the dog. A. Origin of carcinoma from lobular alveoli and ductules, some of which are occluded by tumor cells. B. Tumor tissue surrounded by fibrous tissue reaction (**arrow A**). Photograph also shows tumor embolus within interlobular lymphatic channel (**arrow B**). C. Higher magnification showing early carcinomatous change that is indistinguishable from lobular adenoma. Note the tumor emboli in the interlobular lymphatics. These may represent metastasis from carcinoma in another gland.

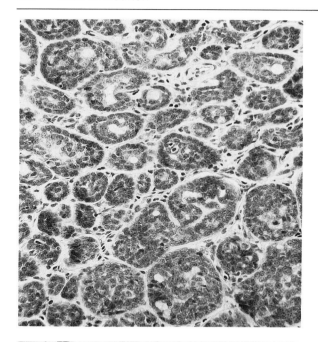

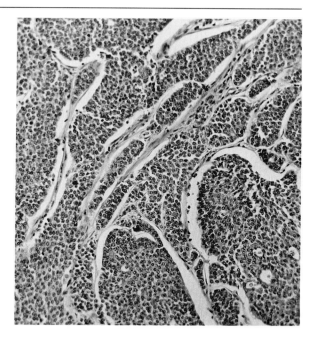

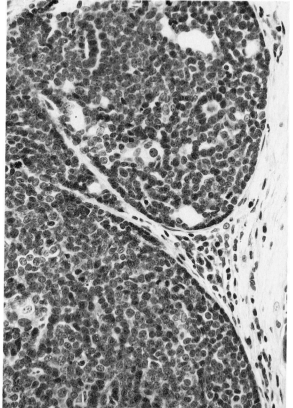

A|B
C|

**FIGURE 12.9.** Lobular carcinoma in mammary gland of the bitch. A. Lobular acini filled with tumor cells. B. Large diffuse masses of carcinoma cells, separated by thin stromal trabeculae. This is the so-called solid carcinoma variety of this tumor. C. Edge of solidly cellular mass.

out the entire lobule (figs. 12.9A and B), which becomes greatly enlarged. Solid lobular masses of tumor cells are often separated from one another by fibrous trabeculae (fig. 12.9C). At this stage the lobular carcinoma is indistinguishable from so-called solid carcinoma. The neoplastic cells are usually quite uniform in size and shape and have a high mitotic index. Occasionally, solid areas of tumor tissue become necrotic. In a few carcinomas (and also mammary carcinomas of other types) the neoplastic cells form cytoplasmic mucin vacuoles; mucin may also collect in dilated tubules. Depending on the extent of this change these tumors may be called mucinous carcinomas (figs. 12.10A and B). Most of the solid masses of tumor cells in lobular carcinoma display some evidence of tubular morphology (fig. 12.10C), but others show no tubular morphology. A few of the carcinomas have marked stromal fibrosis, especially if the tumor cells have infiltrated widely in the interlobular stroma.

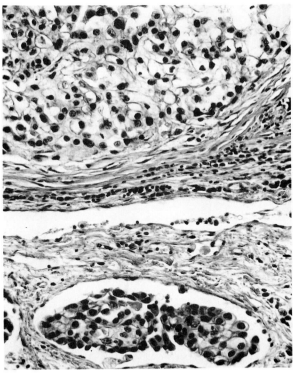

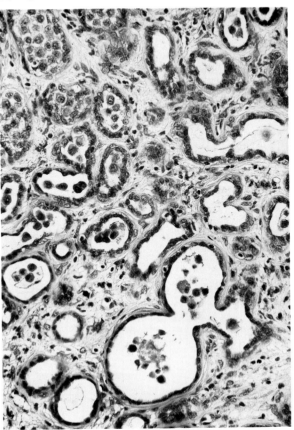

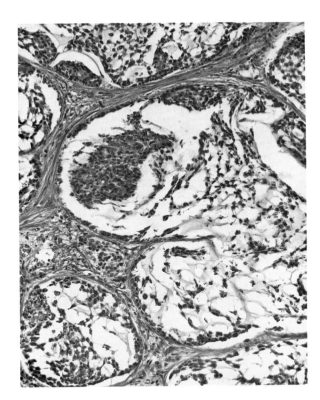

A | B
C |

**FIGURE 12.10.** Variations of lobular carcinoma of the bitch. A and B. Mucinous formation in the carcinoma. Mucin is secreted by the tumor cells and accumulates in the cell cytoplasm and also between the cells. C. Alveolar tubular formation and beginning stromal fibrosis. Observe irregular morphology of tubules, some that are filled with pale staining cells. (A and B, courtesy of Dr. W. Misdorp and *Vet. Path.*)

*Papillary Carcinoma*—Papillary carcinoma develops *de novo* or from malignant change in papillary adenoma. Papillary carcinoma may be multicentric in origin with simultaneous neoplastic change in separate, unrelated parts of the mammary gland. The carcinoma arises in three ways: (1) when an alveolus or alveolar ductule becomes dilated and forms intraluminal papillae; (2) when multiple alveolar ducts dilate and their thin intervening stromal septa rupture, converting the lobule into a cystic mass containing papillae; or (3) when interlobular ducts become papillomatous. The percentage of papillary carcinomas that develop from the mammary lobules or from the interlobular ducts is not known.

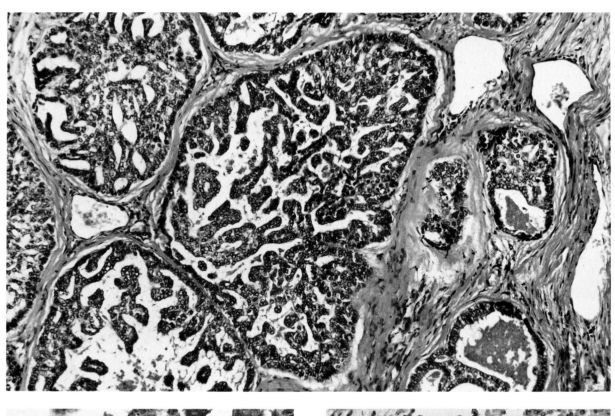

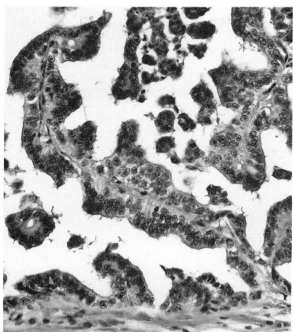
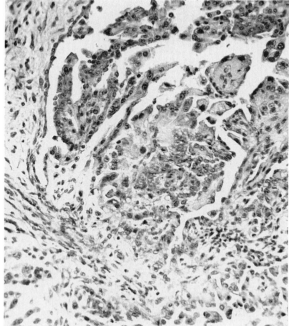

A
B | C
**FIGURE 12.11.** Papillary carcinoma of the bitch. A. The papillae are growing in the lumen of a duct. B. Higher magnification of papillae showing irregularity of covering epithelium and the fibrovascular stalk. C. Irregular papillary formation in more malignant carcinoma. (A, courtesy of *J. Small Anim. Pract.*; C, courtesy of *Cornell Vet.*)

Papillary carcinoma usually demonstrates multiple ductlike structures and is often cystic (papillary cystadenocarcinoma). The lumens are partly or completely filled with coalescing multibranched papillae (figs. 12.11A and B). The papillae may appear solidly epithelial or with delicate collagenous connective tissue stalks that have more than a single point of attachment. The papillae are often very irregular in formation and are covered by irregular stratifications of cells showing considerable loss of polarity (fig. 12.11C). When intraductal growth is complete, the papillae fuse and appear sievelike or are converted into solid cellular masses that may exhibit necrosis centrally, with only thin shells of viable tumor cells at the periphery. Intraductal papillae that form without connective tissue stalks often show necrosis. This form of the tumor within ducts is called *comedocarcinoma*.

The epithelial cells in papillary carcinoma are columnar or cuboidal and have large round or ovoid hyperchromatic nuclei and variable numbers of mitotic figures. The nucleoli are generally solitary and enlarged.

The separation of papillary carcinoma from papillary adenoma is often difficult. Several factors aid in making this distinction. The carcinoma has a piling up of the epithelial cells that cover the papillae, frequent mitotic figures, and cuboidal tumor cells with loss of polarity. The epithelial cells occasionally detach and accumulate in the gland lumens; seldom is there secretion in the lumens. The epithelial cells of papillary adenoma are cuboidal or columnar, usually single layered, have regular orientation, and rest on a basement membrane. Mitotic figures are uncommon. Proliferation of myoepithelial cells in the tumor almost always indicates a benign growth. Infiltration of tumor cells into the stalks or peripheral stroma aids in the diagnosis of carcinoma. Infiltration occurs in about 45% of papillary carcinomas.

*Squamous Cell Carcinoma*—Some carcinomas, mostly of duct origin, have squamous metaplasia of epithelium, and depending on the amount (a subjective decision) are called *squamous cell carcinomas*.

These carcinomas usually arise from the epithelium of the interlobular ducts or mammary cistern. They appear with solid cords (less often tubules) of invading cells that have undergone squamous metaplasia (figs. 12.12A and B). The carcinoma may have solid sheets of cells with central keratinization

and formation of keratin pearls. Suppuration and necrosis are often present.

*Scirrhous Carcinoma*—This carcinoma exhibits diffuse infiltration of neoplastic cells and productive fibrosis of the stroma (figs. 12.13A–E). There is close intermingling of fibrous stroma and carcinomatous elements. Scirrhous carcinoma usually shows a total breakdown of lobular structure, and the exact site of its origin (alveolar or ductal) usually cannot be determined. The infiltrating cells are arranged as small tubules, as solid tubules with or without necrotic centers, as thin cords of cells or cells infiltrating individually, and uncommonly as mucin-producing cells (mucinous carcinoma). The cells are cuboidal or irregular in shape and have a loss of polarity. Mitotic rate varies considerably between different tumors.

**Growth and Metastasis.** Data on the duration of growth of canine mammary carcinoma as reported by owners of dogs are usually incomplete. In general, however, the carcinomas are observed by owners over a few weeks to several years, usually for 2 to 6 months. The doubling time for carcinoma growth is 2.5 to 4 weeks. A frequent observation is rapid growth just prior to the dog's being brought to the veterinarian.

Misdorp and Hart (1976) summarized the different factors that influence survival of the dog with mammary carcinoma. These factors include the clinical state of the carcinoma (expansive, moderately infiltrative, or severely infiltrative growth), size and volume of the tumor, histological type, histological grade (based on undifferentiation of neoplastic cells and number of mitoses), and type of growth. They found that the size and volume of the tumors, even when corrected for clinical state, were associated with survival. The finding that infiltrative carcinoma was associated with invasion of lymphatics, a high histological grade, anaplasia, histological type of carcinoma, and involvement of regional lymph nodes demonstrated the relationship among different factors. They also observed that the localization of the carcinoma in the cephalad versus the caudal mammary glands did not seem to be an important characteristic in relationship to survival.

Owen (1966) stated that the course of survival averages 9 months after removal of most carcinomas, but only 3 months after removal of undifferentiated carcinomas. Most affected dogs die

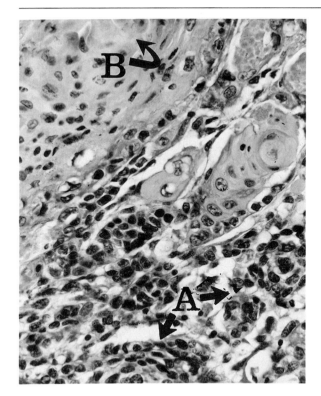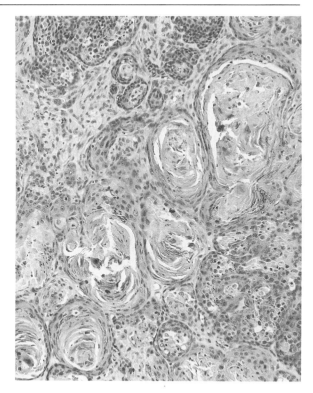

A | B    **FIGURE 12.12.** Mammary squamous cell carcinoma of the dog. A. Small, dark staining tumor cells (A) and large squamous cells (B), some of the latter cells showing keratinization. B. Extensive keratinization of neoplastic squamous cells. (A, courtesy of Dr. W. Misdorp and *Vet. Path.*)

from metastasis or recurrence of the growth, but many are euthanized. If lymphatic invasion is found in the primary carcinoma, it is usually associated with metastasis and short survival (Sandersleben, 1968). Survival after surgery is short (4 to 12 months) if there is lymphatic invasion in the primary neoplasm; survival is longer (1 to 2 years) if lymphatic invasion is absent.

Because of the invasiveness of carcinoma, surgical excision is often followed by recurrence. Recurrence occurs in more than 80% of mammary carcinomas within 6 months.

Misdorp and Hart (1979) stressed the importance of hematogenous as well as lymphogenous spread of carcinomas; in some highly malignant carcinomas both routes of metastasis occur.

If the mammary tumor is not removed surgically after diagnosis but is allowed to grow, the observed duration of growth before death of the dog is longer than generally reported. The carcinomas

may grow for 3 months to 6 years (average 2 to 4 years) (Moulton *et al.*, 1970).

The behavior of mammary carcinomas after diagnosis and treatment (surgery or other therapeutic measures) has been studied by Fowler *et al.* (1974) on 271 neoplasms from 154 bitches. Some interesting points were made in this study. The average duration of follow-up time after diagnosis for infiltrating papillary carcinoma was 5.6 months, less than for the other types. The average duration after diagnosis of infiltrating lobular carcinoma was 7.3 months. Scirrhous carcinoma had a longer follow-up time (9.7 months) than did nonfibrosing carcinoma. Most of the dogs with infiltrating papillary carcinomas died with metastatic disease. The behavior of scirrhous carcinoma resembled that of papillary carcinoma: seven of nine dogs that died or were killed had widespread metastases, recurrent neoplasms, or both. Two carcinomas were diagnosed as squamous type. One of these rapidly

## MAMMARY TUMORS OF THE CAT

### Carcinoma

**Incidence.** Aside from skin and the lymphoid and hematopoietic tissues, the most common site for neoplasia in the cat is the mammary gland. Carcinoma of the mammary gland is more common in the cat than in any other domestic species except the dog. The percentage of mammary tumors that are carcinomas is much higher (86%) in the cat than the dog (Cotchin, 1952, 1956; Nielsen, 1952). (Tumors of all types in the cat are frequently malignant.) The ratio of malignant to benign mammary tumors in the cat is 9 : 1. Adenoma is found occasionally, and myoepithelioma and mixed tumor are found rarely.

**Age, Breed, and Sex.** Carcinomas occur in older cats, mostly 8 to 12 years of age. Many feel that there is no known breed prevalence for feline mammary tumors, but according to Hayes *et al.* (1981), the Siamese breed has twice as much risk of developing mammary carcinoma as all other breeds combined. The age at diagnosis in the Siamese is younger than that in other breeds. Almost all (99%) mammary tumors appear in intact females. Evidence for the sparing effect of early ovariectomy is even stronger in the cat than in the bitch. Ovariectomized cats have only 0.6% of the risk of intact cats for carcinomas (Dorn *et al.*, 1968; Hayes *et al.*, 1981), but the optimal age when ovariectomy is prophylactic is not yet known. There are no data on the value of ovariectomy when the neoplasm is already present.

**Endocrine Influences.** There is limited and conflicting information regarding endocrine factors that may have an etiological bearing on feline mammary tumors. The sex of the cat, gonadal status, hormonal influence, genetic lineage, age, and possible viral infection may be implicated independently or in combination (Hayes *et al.*, 1981).

Estrogen receptors in feline mammary carcinoma are rare (Hamilton *et al.*, 1976) compared with human and canine mammary tumors. This rarity suggests a significant lack of estrogen dependency in this species. Nevertheless, the possibility remains that the tumors may be dependent on other hormones.

**Sites and Structures.** In most cats, only one mammary gland is involved, but no gland is spared.

According to Weijer *et al.* (1973), the tumors occur significantly less often in mammary glands 2 and 3. (The cat has two rows of four glands each which are numbered 1 to 4, cephalad to caudal.) These workers also observed that in 45 of 142 cats the tumors were in two or more adjacent glands and that in 42 cats the left as well as right mammary glands were involved. It is not known whether occurrence of tumors in multiple glands involves proliferation of a tumor from one gland to another or whether it is a simultaneous development of several tumors. The carcinoma types are adenocarcinoma, papillary, and scirrhous (Weijer *et al.*, 1972). Sarcomas rarely occur.

The carcinomas arise from both the duct and alveolar epithelium and are histologically similar to those in canines. On first examination the mammary tumor may appear benign, being a well-demarcated nodule within the gland. Nevertheless, carcinoma should always be suspected and dealt with accordingly (Anderson and Jarrett, 1966).

**Etiology.** It is not known if viruses play a role in the etiology of feline mammary tumors, but type-A and type-C virus particles have been detected in these neoplasms (Feldman and Gross, 1971; Weijer *et al.*, 1974).

**Growth and Metastasis.** Most carcinomas have highly infiltrative growth and 25% show invasion of lymphatics and blood vessels. Involvement of lymphatics is often seen as firm, thick cords in the skin. Most carcinomas grow rapidly and undergo necrosis.

In cats as in humans there is good correlation between histological grading of the carcinomas and prognosis of the patient. Factors of importance in grading these neoplasms are tumor volume, rapidity of growth, lymphatic or hematogenous invasion, and degree of cellular differentiation including mitotic rate. Cats with carcinomas have poor survival time after diagnosis of the neoplasm. Weijer *et al.* (1972) observed that 50% of cats with low-grade carcinomas survived 12 months, whereas only 10% of cats with high-grade carcinomas survived this long. Poor survival is related to the invasive nature of the neoplasm.

Death is due to a recurrence of the primary tumor, symptoms associated with metastasis, and intercurrent disease (Weijer *et al.*, 1973). The time between detection of the primary tumor and death is 12 months on the average. A significant correlation is found between the tumor volume and the 1-year survival. Most metastases are found in the lungs and regional axillary or inguinal lymph nodes (approximately 83% each). The pleura is involved in 42% of affected cats and the liver in 24%. Metastasis in the lungs is usually extensive. The intensity of pleuritic carcinoma is variable; accumulation of serohemorrhagic fluid is frequently encountered.

Metastasis to the abdominal organs and bones is also observed. Hattangady *et al.* (1963) reported a malignant mixed tumor in a cat in which the carcinomatous part metastasized.

## Fibroepithelial Hyperplasia

**Incidence.** This condition, also referred to as feline mammary hypertrophy, is rarely reported. A series of 11 such growths were described by Allen (1973), who also reviewed the literature on all benign mammary neoplasms in the cat. He reported that this condition was seen in about 12 of 500 biopsies done at the University of Pennsylvania. The condition is less common in studies by the author at the University of California.

**Age, Breed, and Sex.** Almost all cases of fibroepithelial hyperplasia occur in queens under 2 years of age and about half of these are in animals 1 year or less in age. Occasionally the lesion is found in older animals. There is no breed predilection and the condition has only been found in female cats. None of the females have been ovariectomized.

**Clinical Characteristics.** The female cats with this lesion are almost always nonpregnant, although the very rapid rate of growth (sometimes 2 to 3 weeks) of the mammary glands suggests enlargement with pregnancy. Allen (1973) had one affected cat in the early stages of pregnancy. He also reported a case with an ovarian corpus luteum and hyperplastic endometrial change. One of our cases was similar.

**Sites and Gross Morphology.** Usually all mammary glands are affected at the same time, although some glands may be larger than others. Often the right and left glands in the same location have a similar degree of enlargement. About half the time, one, two, or three pairs of glands (most often inguinal) are affected. The enlargements appear as firm, painless, dome-shaped masses that usually measure 2 to 5 cm or larger in greatest diameter. On cut section the lesion has a multinodular structure and is white to slightly pink.

**Histological Features.** The lesion is well-circumscribed but nonencapsulated and is located below normal mammary skin. It has a pattern of multilobulation, but distinct interlobular septa are usually not observed. A striking feature is the marked proliferation of the intralobular duct system. Interlobular duct proliferation is less evident. These ducts are identical in morphology to the proliferating ducts in the early stages of pregnancy before formation of alveoli. The branching ducts are lined by epithelial cells often three to four layers thick. These cells are hyperchromatic, and usually every cross-sectioned duct contains at least one mitotic figure. There is little or no tendency toward intraluminal papillary formation and no evidence of stromal invasion of epithelial cells.

The ducts proliferate in edematous, highly proliferative, intralobular, fibrous connective tissue that also commonly shows mitotic figures. The interlobular connective tissue is also hyperplastic, although less cellular and more collagenous than the intralobular connective tissue.

**Etiology.** Although the cause of feline fibroepithelial hyperplasia is unknown, it has a number of features that suggest a hormonal basis. It usually involves all or most of the mammary glands and often involves paired glands, unlike a neoplasm. Histologically, the gland has the appearance of mammary tissue in early pregnancy when it is first coming under the influence of progestogen.

## MAMMARY TUMORS OF OTHER DOMESTIC SPECIES

Mammary carcinoma has rarely been reported in the sow (Feldman, 1932; Rao *et al.*, 1976). Few mammary tumors have been found in the mare, although a series of 45 cases was cited by Feldman (1932).

The cow rarely has mammary tumors, although many dairy cows are allowed to survive to "cancer age" (Kenny, 1942). Mammary carcinomas are almost never found by the United States Department of Agriculture in the millions of udders examined every year. Povey and Osborne (1969) reported 21 bovine mammary tumors since 1902 and added one case of their own. They found reports of 9 carcinomas, with the rest being fibroma, fibrosarcoma, papillary adenoma, osteoma, and fibroadenoma. Primary carcinoma of the mammary gland has been reported rarely (Cleland, 1908; Elder *et al.,* 1954; Kenny, 1944; Misdorp, 1967; Sticker, 1902). These tumors involved the duct system and none arose from the alveolar epithelium. Metastasis was to the supramammary lymph nodes; also present in one case was metastasis to the lungs and liver. Squamous cell carcinoma involving the skin of the udder with invasion of the mammary gland is much more common than primary parenchymal carcinoma.

Papillomas of the teat canal and multiple polyps of the cistern have the highest incidence (Julian, 1948; Renk, 1955; Trotter, 1909), but still are not common. The cisternal polyps are multiple and appear as simple papillary outgrowths from the tunica propria. The polyps are fibrous lesions covered with one or several layers of epithelium. They show no evidence of neoplasia and probably represent proliferations of granulation tissue secondary to inflammation.

Papillomas and fibroadenomas of the mammary duct system have been reported in the water buffalo (*Bubalus bubalis*) in India (Bhowmik, 1979; Bhowmik and Iyer, 1978). The first case of carcinoma of the mammary gland of the water buffalo was reported by Mandal and Iyer (1969). This was diagnosed during the examination of 300 udders from female buffaloes in several abattoirs in India. All animals were 8 to 12 years of age. The neoplastic udder was shrunken and contained a solid mass 5 cm in diameter. Histologically, it appeared as an intraductal carcinoma, similar to the so-called comedocarcinoma of humans.

Mammary neoplasms are rarely found in goats: Singh and Iyer (1972) described 3 carcinomas, one with metastasis, among 220 goats and remarked on the rarity of mammary tumors in goats except when the animals are allowed to live to old age, as in India. While examining over 4,000 female goats for chronic lesions in the mammary glands, Singh and Iyer observed 10 mammary glands with fibrocystic disease (cystic hyperplasia) and 2 with intraductal carcinoma. All lesions appeared in adult female goats. Fibrocystic disease, a well-recognized

precancerous condition in women, was manifested by cystic dilation of the ducts with proliferation of epithelial lining cells. The carcinomas were multicentric in origin and primarily involved ducts, but affected some lobules completely. Most of the ducts showed intraluminal proliferation of cancerous epithelial cells with central necrosis. There was no mention of metastasis.

## REFERENCES

Ajello, A. (1976) Il cosiddetto morbo di Paget della mammella nella cagna. *Annali Fac. Med. Vet.* 13, 201–232.

Allen, A. C. (1940) So-Called Mixed Tumors of the Mammary Gland of Dog and Man. *Arch. Path.* 29, 589–624.

Allen, H. L. (1973) Feline Mammary Hypertrophy. *Vet. Path.* 10, 501–508.

Andersen, A. C. (1965) Parameters of Mammary Gland Tumours of Aging Beagles. *J. Amer. Vet. Med. Assoc.* 147, 1653–1654.

Andersen, A. C., and Rosenblatt, L. S. (1969) The Effect of Whole-Body X-Irradiation on the Median Lifespan of Female Dogs (Beagles). *Rad. Res.* 39, 177–200.

Anderson, L. J., and Jarrett, W. F. H. (1966) Clinico-Pathological Aspects of Mammary Tumours in the Dog and Cat. *J. Small Anim. Pract.* 7, 697–701.

Auler, H., and Wernicke, O. (1931) Über Tumoren des Hundes. *Z. Krebsforsch.* 35, 1–46.

Beckman, C. H. (1945) Sexual Hormones in Treatment of Mammary Tumors of Aged Bitches. *Vet. Med.* 40, 20–23.

Bhowmik, M. K. (1979) A Note on Mammary Fibroadenoma in a Buffalo (*Bubalus bubalis*). *Indian J. Anim. Sci.* 49, 147–149.

Bhowmik, M. K., and Iyer, P. K. R. (1978) Studies on the Pathology of Chronic Lesions in the Mammary Glands of Buffaloes (*Bubalus bubalis*). *Indian Vet. J.* 55, 418–419.

Biggs, R. (1947) The Myoepithelium in Certain Tumours of the Breast. *J. Path. Bact.* 49, 437–444.

Bloom, F. (1954) *Pathology of the Dog and Cat: The Genitourinary System with Clinical Considerations.* American Veterinary Publications (Evanston, Illinois), 418–424.

Bomhard, D., and Sandersleben, J. (1974) Über die Feinstruktur von Mammamischtumoren der Hündin. II. Das Vorkommen von Myoepithelzellen in chondroiden Arealen. *Virchows Arch.* 362, 157–167.

Briggs, M. H. (1980) Progestogens and Mammary Tumours in the Beagle Bitch. *Res. Vet. Sci.* 28, 199–202.

Brodey, R. S., Fidler, I. J., and Howson, A. E. (1966) The Relationship of Estrous Irregularity, Pseudopregnancy, and Pregnancy to the Development of Canine

Mammary Neoplasms. *J. Amer. Vet. Med. Assoc.* 149, 1047–1049.

Cameron, A. M., and Faulkin, L. J. (1971) Hyperplastic and Inflammatory Nodules in the Canine Mammary Gland. *J. Natl. Cancer Inst.* 47, 1277–1287.

Catellani, G. (1956) Sul comportamento della fosfatasi alcalina nelle displasie e nei tumori della cagna. *Acta Med. Vet.* 2, 131–152.

Cleland, J. B. (1908) Some Examples of Malignant Disease in Animals. *J. Comp. Path.* 21, 242–245.

Correll, N. O., and Langston, H. T. (1958) Pulmonary Lymphatic Drainage in the Dog. *Surg. Gynec. Obstr.* 107, 282–286.

Cotchin, E. (1952) Neoplasms in Cats. *Proc. R. Soc. Med.* 45, 671–674.

———. (1954) Further Observations on Neoplasms in Dogs, with Particular Reference to Site of Origin and Malignancy. I. Cutaneous, Female Genital and Alimentary Systems. II. Male Genital, Skeletal, Lymphatic and Other Systems. *Brit. Vet. J.* 110, 218–230, 274–286.

———. (1956) *Neoplasms of the Domesticated Mammals.* In: Review Series No. 4 of the Commonwealth Bureau of Animal Health. Commonwealth Agricultural Bureaus (Farnham Royal, Bucks, England).

———. (1958) Mammary Neoplasms of the Bitch. *J. Comp. Path.* 68, 1–22.

Dahme, E., and Weiss, E. (1958) Zur Systemetik der Mammatumoren des Hundes. *Dtsch. Tierärztl. Wschr.* 65, 458–461.

D'Arville, C. N., and Pierrepoint, C. G. (1979) Demonstration of Oestrogen, Androgen and Progestogen Receptors in the Cytosol Fraction of Canine Mammary Tumours. *Europ. J. Cancer* 15, 875–883.

Da Silva, R. A., Amorim, L. de M., and Cardoso, S. B. (1947) Estudos sobre a occorrencia de tumoures mammarios na cadela. *Veterinaria* (S. Paulo), 1, 49–54.

De Vitta, J. (1939) Mammary Adenofibroma of the Female Dog. *N. Amer. Vet.* 20, 53–55.

Dobberstein, J., and Matthias, D. (1942) Über das Mammacarcinom bei der Hündin. *Arch. Wiss. Prakt. Tierheilk.* 78, 18–31.

Dorn, C. R., Taylor, D. O. N., Frye, F. L., and Hibbard, H. H. (1968) Survey of Animal Neoplasms in Alameda and Contra Costa Counties, California. I. Methodology and Description of Cases. *J. Natl. Cancer Inst.* 40, 295–305.

Dozza, G., and Coluzzi, G. (1963) Dosaggio biologico degli estrogeni urinari in cagne affette da tumori della mammella. *Atti. Soc. Ital. Sci. Vet.* 17, 354–359.

Elder, C., Kintner, L. D., and Johnson, R. E. (1954) Bovine Mammary Gland Carcinoma. *J. Amer. Vet. Med. Assoc.* 124, 142–146.

El Etreby, M. F., and Wrobel, K. H. (1978) Effect of Cyporterone Acetate, d-Norgestrel and Progesterone on the Canine Mammary Gland. *Cell. Tiss. Res.* 194, 245–267.

Else, R. W., and Hannant, D. (1979) Some Epidemiological Aspects of Mammary Neoplasia in the Bitch. *Vet. Rec.* 104, 296–304.

Erichsen, S. (1955) A Histochemical Study of Mixed Tumours of the Canine Mammary Gland. *Acta Path. Microbiol. Scand.* 36, 490–502.

Evans, C. R., and Pierrepoint, C. G. (1975) Tissue–Steroid Interactions in Canine Hormone Dependent Tumors. *Vet. Rec.* 97, 464–467.

Feldman, D. G., and Gross, L. (1971) Electron Microscopic Study of Spontaneous Mammary Carcinomas in Cats and Dogs: Virus-like Particles in Cat Mammary Carcinomas. *Cancer Res.* 31, 1261–1267.

Feldman, W. H. (1932) *Neoplasms of Domesticated Animals.* W. B. Saunders (Philadelphia).

Fidler, I. J., and Brodey, R. S. (1967) A Necropsy Study of Canine Malignant Mammary Neoplasms. *J. Amer. Vet. Med. Assoc.* 151, 710–715.

Foreman, R. J. (1913) Metastatic Chondriomata in Dog. *Vet. J.* 69, 240–241.

Fowler, E. H., Wilson, G. P., and Koestner, A. (1974) Biologic Behavior of Canine Mammary Neoplasms Based on a Histogenetic Classification. *Vet. Path.* 11, 212–229.

Frye, F. L., Dorn, C. R., Taylor, D. O. N., Hibbard, H. H., and Klauber, M. R. (1967) Characteristics of Canine Mammary Gland Tumor Cases. *Anim. Hosp.* 3, 1–12.

Gardner, W. U. (1941) Inhibition of Mammary Growth by Large Amounts of Estrogen. *Endocrinology* 28, 53–61.

Hamilton, J. M. (1975) A Review of Recent Advances in the Study of the Aetiology of Canine Mammary Tumors. *Vet. Ann.* 15, 276–283.

Hamilton, J. M., Else, R. W., and Forshaw, P. (1976) Oestrogen Receptors in Feline Mammary Carcinomas. *Vet. Rec.* 99, 477–479.

———. (1977) Oestrogen Receptors in Canine Mammary Tumours. *Vet. Rec.* 101, 258–260.

Hampe, J. F., and Misdorp, W. (1974) Tumours and Dysplasias of the Mammary Gland. *Bull. Wld. Hlth. Org.* 50, 111–133.

Hattangady, S. R., Purohit, B. L., and Jamkhedkar, P. P. (1963) Adenocarcinoma of the Mammary Gland in a Cat. *Indian Vet. J.* 40, 53–55.

Hayes, H. M., Milne, K. L., and Mandell, C. P. (1981) Epidemiological Features of Feline Mammary Carcinoma. *Vet. Rec.* 108, 476–479.

Huggins, C., and Moulder, P. V. (1944) Studies on the Mammary Tumours of Dog. I. Lactation and the Influence of Ovariectomy and Suprarenalectomy Thereon. *J. Exp. Med.* 80, 441–454.

Hurley, J. V., and Jabara, A. G. (1964) Properties of "Cartilage" in Canine Mammary Tumours. *Arch. Path.* 77, 343–347.

Jabara, A. G. (1960a) Canine Mixed Tumours. *Aust. Vet. J.* 36, 212–221.

———. (1960b) Canine Mammary Carcinomata. *Aust. Vet. J.* 36, 389–398.

Julian, L. M. (1948) Multiple Cisternal Polyps of the Bovine Mammary Gland. *J. Amer. Vet. Med. Assoc.* 112, 238–240.

Kenny, J. E. (1942) Primary Adenocarcinoma of the Udder of a Milk Cow. *Vet. Rec.* 54, 240–241.

———. (1944) Some Observations on Bovine Neoplasia. *Vet. Rec.* 56, 69–71.

Kronberger, H. (1961) Kritische Sichtung des dem Institute in den Jahren 1917–1959 eingesandten Geschwulstmaterials von Häussaugetieren. *Mh. Vet. Med.* 16, 296–302.

Krook, L. (1954) A Statistical Investigation of Carcinoma in the Dog. *Acta Path. Microbiol. Scand.* 35, 407–422.

Kwapien, R. P., Giles, R. C., Geil, R. G., and Casey, H. W. (1980) Malignant Mammary Tumors in Beagle Dogs Dosed with Investigational Oral Contraceptive Steroids. *J. Natl. Cancer Inst.* 65, 137–142.

Lebeau, A. (1953) L'Age du Chien et Celui de l'Homme. Essai de Statistique sur la Mortalité Canine. *Bull. Acad. Vét. Fr.* 26, 229–232.

MacVean, D. W., Monlux, A. W., Anderson, P. S., Silberg, S. L., and Roszel, J. F. (1978) Frequency of Canine and Feline Tumors in a Defined Population. *Vet. Path.* 15, 700–715.

Mandal, P. C., and Iyer, P. K. R. (1969) Mammary Intraductal Carcinoma in a Buffalo (*Bubalus bubalis*). *Vet. Path.* 6, 534–537.

Meier, H. (1962) Some Aspects of Experimental and Spontaneous Tumorigenesis in Animals. *Adv. Vet. Sci.* 7, 43–86.

Misdorp, W. (1967) Tumours in Large Domestic Animals in the Netherlands. *J. Comp. Path.* 77, 211–216.

Misdorp, W., and den Herder, B. A. (1966) Bone Metastasis in Mammary Cancer: A Report of 10 Cases in the Female Dog and Some Comparison with Human Cases. *Brit. J. Cancer* 20, 496–503.

Misdorp, W. and Hart, A. A. M. (1976) Prognostic Factors in Canine Mammary Cancer. *J. Natl. Cancer Inst.* 56, 779–784.

———. (1979) Canine Mammary Cancer. I. Prognosis. II. Therapy and Causes of Death. *J. Small Anim. Pract.* 20, 385–404.

Misdorp, W., Cotchin, E., Hampe, J. F., Jabara, A. G., and Sandersleben, J. (1971) Canine Malignant Mammary Tumours. I. Sarcomas. *Vet. Path.* 8, 99–117.

———. (1972) Canine Malignant Mammary Tumours. II. Adenocarcinomas, Solid Carcinomas and Spindle Cell Carcinomas. *Vet. Path.* 9, 447–470.

———. (1973) Canine Malignant Mammary Tumours. III. Special Types of Carcinomas, Malignant Mixed Tumours. *Vet. Path.* 10, 241–256.

Monlux, A. W., Roszel, J. F., MacVean, D. W., and Palmer, T. W. (1977) Classification of Epithelial Mammary Tumors in a Defined Population. *Vet. Path.* 14, 194–217.

Moulton, J. E., Rosenblatt, L. S., and Goldman, M. (1986) Mammary Tumors in a Colony of Beagle Dogs. *Vet. Path.* 23, 741–749.

Moulton, J. E., Taylor, D. O. N., Dorn, C. R., and Andersen, A. C. (1970) Canine Mammary Tumors. *Path. Vet.* 7, 289–320.

Mulligan, R. M. (1944) Some Statistical Aspects of Canine Tumors. *Arch. Path.* 38, 115–120.

———. (1945) Some Endocrinologic Considerations of Canine Neoplastic Diseases. *Arch. Path.* 39, 162–171.

———. (1947) Some Effects of Chronic Doses of Stilbesterol in Female Dogs. *Exp. Med. Surg.* 5, 196–205.

———. (1949) *Neoplasms of the Dog.* Williams and Wilkins (Baltimore).

———. (1963) Comparative Pathology of Human and Canine Cancer. *Ann. N.Y. Acad. Sci.* 108, 642–690.

Nieberle, K. (1933) Zur Kenntnis der Sogenannten Mammamischgeschwulste des Hundes. *Z. Krebsforsch.* 39, 113–127.

Nielsen, S. W. (1952) The Malignancy of Mammary Tumors in Cats. *N. Amer. Vet.* 33, 245–252.

Owen, L. N. (1966) Prognosis and Treatment of Mammary Tumours in the Bitch. *J. Small Anim. Pract.* 7, 703–710.

Palmer, T. E., and Monlux, A. W. (1979) Acid Mucopolysaccharides in Mammary Tumors of Dogs. *Vet. Path.* 16, 493–509.

Poppensiek, G. C. (1961) *Neoplasms Studied in Selected Veterinary Diagnostic Laboratories in the United States and Canada.* New York State Veterinary College, Cornell University (Ithaca, New York).

Povey, R. C., and Osborne, A. D. (1969) Mammary Gland Neoplasia in the Cow: A Review of the Literature and Report of a Fibrosarcoma. *Path. Vet.* 6, 502–512.

Prier, J. E., and Brodey, R. S. (1963) Canine Neoplasia: A Prototype for Human Cancer Study. *Bull. Wld. Hlth. Org.* 29, 331–344.

Priester, W. A. (1979) Occurrence of Mammary Neoplasms in Bitches in Relation to Breed, Age, Tumour Type, and Geographical Region from Which Reported. *J. Small Anim. Pract.* 20, 1–11.

Pulley, L. T. (1973) Ultrastructural and Histochemical Demonstration of Myoepithelium in Mixed Tumors of the Canine Mammary Gland. *Amer. J. Vet. Res.* 34, 1513–1522.

Rao, A. T., Iyer, P. K. R., Chaudary, C., and Nayak, B. C. (1976) Mammary Intraductal Carcinoma in a Pig. *Indian Vet. J.* 53, 892.

Renk, W. (1955) Über chronisch-interstitielle Mastitis und Zystenbildung sowie über ein Adenom in Kuheuter. *Berl. Munch. Tierärztl. Wschr.* 68, 127–130.

Riser, W. H. (1947) Surgical Removal of the Mammary Gland of the Bitch. *J. Amer. Vet. Med. Assoc.* 110, 86–90.

Sandersleben, J. (1958) Beitrag zur Frage der Malignität der Mammatumoren des Hundes. *Mh. Tierheilk* 11, 191–198.

———. (1968) Die malignen Mammatumoren der Hündin unter Besonderer Berücksichtigung ihrer Prognose. *Zbl. Vet. Med.* 15, 111–115.

Schlotthauer, C. F., Hoskins, H. P., and Lacroix, J. V.

(1949) *Canine Surgery.* North American Veterinarian (Evanston, Illinois), 406–423.

Schmidt, I. (1933) Zur Frage des Entstehung der Mischgiwächse an Hand von zwei Fallen von Milchdrüsenmischgeschwulsten des Hundes. *Virchows Arch.* 291, 491–506.

Schneider, R., Dorn, R. C., Taylor, D. O. N. (1969) Factors Influencing Canine Mammary Cancer Development and Postsurgical Survival. *J. Natl. Cancer Inst.* 43, 1249–1261.

Sekhri, K. K., and Faulkin, L. J. (1970) The Mammary Gland. In: Andersen, A. C., ed., *The Beagle as an Experimental Dog.* Iowa State University Press (Ames, Iowa), 327–349.

Silver, I. A. (1966) The Anatomy of the Mammary Gland of the Dog and Cat. *J. Small Anim. Pract.* 7, 689–696.

Singh, B., and Iyer, P. K. R. (1972) Mammary Intraductal Carcinoma in Goats (*Capra hircus*) *Vet. Path.* 9, 441–446.

Sticker, A. (1902) Über den Krebs der Thiere. Insbesondere über die Empfänglichkeit der verschiedenen Hausthierarten und über die Unterschiede des Thierund Menschenkrebses. *Arch. Klin. Chir.* 65, 616–696, 1023–1087.

Tateyama, S., and Cotchin, E. (1977) Alkaline Phosphatase Reaction of Canine Mammary Mixed Tumours: A Light and Electron Microscopic Study. *Res. Vet. Sci.* 23, 356–364.

Taylor, G. N., Shabestari, L., Williams, J., Mays, C. W., Angus, W., and McFarland, S. (1976) Mammary Neoplasia in a Closed Beagle Colony. *Cancer Res.* 36, 2740–2743.

Trotter, A. M. (1909) Intracanalicular Papilliferous Fibroma of Mamma of Cow. *J. Comp. Path.* 22, 251–253.

Überreiter, O. (1960) Neubildungen bei Tieren. *Wien. Tierärztl. Mschr.* 47, 805–832.

Van Ooyen, P. G., and Misdorp, W. (1967) Metastasierte Mammatumoren beim Hund. I. Klinisch-pathologische Untersuchungen über Mammakarzinome. II. Klinisch-pathologische Untersuchungen über Sarkome und Karzinosarkome der Milchdrüse. *Zbl. Vet. Med.* A14, 315–327, 328–334.

Warner, M. R. (1976) Age Incidence and Site Distribution of Mammary Dysplasias in Young Beagle Bitches. *J. Natl. Cancer Inst.* 57, 57–61.

Weijer, K., Calafat, J., Daams, J. H., Hageman, P. C., and Misdorp, W. (1974) Feline Malignant Mammary Tumors. II. Immunologic and Electron Microscopic Investigations into a Possible Viral Etiology. *J. Natl. Cancer Inst.* 52, 673–679.

Weijer, K., Hampe, J. F., and Misdorp, W. (1973). Mammary Carcinoma in the Cat. A Model in Comparative Cancer Research? *Arch. Chiv. Neer.* 25, 413–425.

Weijer, K., Head, K. W., Misdorp, W., and Hampe, J. F. (1972) Feline Malignant Mammary Tumors. I. Morphology and Biology: Some Comparisons with Human and Canine Mammary Carcinomas. *J. Natl. Cancer Inst.* 49, 1697–1701.

Willis, R. A. (1967) *Pathology of Tumours.* 4th ed. Appleton-Century-Crofts (New York).

# 13

*Charles C. Capen*

# Tumors of the Endocrine Glands

## INTRODUCTION

Endocrine glands are collections of specialized cells that synthesize, store, and release their secretions directly into the bloodstream. Because they lack a duct system, they are often referred to as ductless glands of internal secretion. Secretory products of specialized endocrine cells are hormones that are released into the extracellular fluids and transported via the blood. They affect the rates of chemical reactions in target cells and other body tissues. Endocrine glands in concert with the nervous system are involved in integrating and coordinating a wide variety of activities concerned with the maintenance of homeostasis.

Endocrine glands are small in relation to other body organs, widely distributed in the body, and connected with one another only by the bloodstream. They are richly supplied with blood and there is a close anatomical relationship between endocrine cells and the capillary network. Peripheral cytoplasmic extensions of capillary endothelial cells have fenestrae covered by a single membrane that facilitate rapid transport of raw materials and secretory products between the bloodstream and endocrine cells.

Hormones secreted by mammals are divided chemically into three major groups, namely polypeptides (80%), steroids (15%), and tyrosine derivatives (5%). By knowing the chemical nature of a hormone, it is possible to predict much about its mechanism of action, receptors, solubility, half-life in blood, and binding characteristics to plasma proteins.

Polypeptide hormones share the following characteristics: (1) their primary site of action is the plasma membrane of target cells, (2) receptor proteins for the hormone are bound to the outer surface of the plasma membrane, (3) they are water soluble, (4) they have a short half-life in blood (usually measured in minutes), and (5) they lack specific plasma-binding proteins. There appears to be a single common intracellular pathway for many different polypeptide hormones. It begins with the activation of the enzyme adenylate cyclase in the plasma membrane of target cells, followed by intracellular formation of cyclic adenosine monophosphate from adenosinetriphosphate (ATP), and subsequent activation of cyclic adenosinemonophosphate- (AMP-) dependent protein kinases.

Steroid hormones account for approximately 15% of mammalian hormones and share the following characteristics: (1) their primary site of action is the nucleus of target cells, (2) their receptors are soluble proteins that bind the hormone in the cytoplasm of target cells, (3) they are lipid soluble, which facilitates their easy transport through the cell membrane, (4) they have a longer half-life in blood (typically measured in hours), and (5) they reversibly bind to high-affinity specific-binding proteins in plasma. After steroids are within target cells and bound to cytoplasmic receptors, the hormone−receptor complex is translocated to the nucleus where it binds to a receptor in the nuclear chromatin. The interaction of steroid hormones with the genetic information results in increased transcription of messenger ribonucleic acid (mRNA), which directs new protein synthesis by specific target cells.

The third chemical group of hormones are the tyrosine derivatives. They account for approximately 5% of mammalian hormones and include the catecholamines (epinephrine and norepinephrine) secreted by the adrenal medulla and the iodothyronines (thyroxine and triiodothyronine) produced by follicular cells of the thyroid gland. Catecholamines share a similar mechanism of action with polypeptide hormones, whereas iodothyronines more closely resemble steroid hormones.

There are certain morphological differences among endocrine cells that secrete polypeptide and steroid hormones. These structural differences that normally exist are also found in neoplastic cells derived from the different endocrine glands. Normal and neoplastic cells concerned with the synthesis of polypeptide hormone have a well-developed endoplasmic reticulum with many attached ribosomes for assembly of hormone. They also have a prominent Golgi apparatus for packaging hormone into granules for intracellular storage and transport.

Secretory granules are unique for cells that secrete polypeptide hormone (and catecholamine) and provide a mechanism for intracellular storage of preformed hormone. These membrane-limited granules represent macromolecular aggregations of active hormone, often in association with specific-binding protein. Upon receipt of an appropriate signal for hormone secretion, secretory granules are moved to the periphery of the endocrine cell where the limiting membrane of the granule fuses with the plasma membrane of the cell. The hormone-containing granule core is extruded into the extracellular perivascular space either by emiocytosis or exocytosis. Neoplasms derived from polypeptide hormone-secreting endocrine cells may release recently synthesized hormone on a continuous or episodic basis and may contain few characteristic secretory granules in their cytoplasm.

Neoplasms derived from polypeptide hormone-secreting endocrine cells usually consist of one predominant cell type and are associated with the secretion of one major polypeptide hormone. However, there is evidence accumulating from immunocytochemical and electron microscopic investigations to suggest that some endocrine tumors may be composed of more than one type of neoplastic cell and be capable of synthesizing multiple hormones.

Neoplasms derived from steroid hormone-secreting endocrine cells are characterized by having large lipid bodies in their cytoplasm that contain cholesterol and other precursor molecules for hormone synthesis. The lipid bodies are in close proximity to an extensive tubular network of smooth endoplasmic reticulum and large mitochondria that contain the hydroxylase and dehydrogenase enzyme systems concerned with attachment of the various side chains and radicals to the basic steroid nucleus. Steroid hormone-producing cells lack secretory granules and are unable to store significant amounts of preformed hormone. They are dependent on continued biosynthesis to maintain the normal secretory rate for a particular hormone.

The histopathological separation between nodular hyperplasia, adenoma, and carcinoma often is more difficult in endocrine glands than in most organs of the body. Criteria for their separation, however, should be established and applied in a uniform manner in the evaluation of proliferative lesions in endocrine glands. For many endocrine glands (especially thyroid C-cells, secretory cells of the adrenal medulla, and specific tropic hormone-secreting cells of the adenohypophysis) there appears to be a continuous spectrum of proliferative lesions between diffuse or focal hyperplasia and adenomas derived from a specific population of secretory cells.

It appears to be a common feature of endocrine glands that prolonged stimulation of a population of secretory cells predisposes to the subsequent development of a higher than expected incidence of tumors. Long-continued stimulation may lead to the development of clones of cells within the hyperplastic endocrine glands that grow more rapidly than the rest and are more susceptible to neoplastic transformation when exposed to the right combination of promoting carcinogens.

Focal ("nodular") hyperplasia usually appears as multiple small areas in one or both (for paired) endocrine gland(s) that are well-demarcated but not encapsulated from adjacent normal cells. Cells making up an area of focal hyperplasia closely resemble the cells of origin; however, the cytoplasmic area may be slightly enlarged and the nucleus more hyperchromatic than in the normal endocrine cell.

Generally, adenomas are solitary nodules in one endocrine gland (or occasionally in both for paired endocrine glands) that are larger than the multiple areas of focal hyperplasia. They are sharply demarcated from the adjacent normal glandular parenchyma by a thin, partial to complete, fibrous capsule. The adjacent parenchyma is compressed to varying degrees depending on the size of the adenoma. Cells composing an adenoma may closely resemble the cells of origin morphologically and in their architectural pattern of arrangement; however, there often are histological differences such as multiple layers of cells lining follicles and vascular trabeculae or solid clusters of secretory cells subdivided into packets by a fine fibrovascular stroma.

Carcinomas usually are larger than adenomas of an endocrine gland and result in a macroscopically detectable enlargement in one (or occasionally both, for paired) endocrine gland(s). The separation between adenoma and carcinoma of an endocrine gland often is more difficult than in other tissues of the body using only morphological criteria. Histopathological features that are suggestive of malignancy in an endocrine tumor include intraglandular invasion, invasion into and through the capsule of the gland with establishment of secondary foci of growth in the periglandular fibrous and adipose connective tissues, formation of tumor cell thrombi within vessels (especially muscular walled), and particularly the establishment of metastases at distant sites. The spread of neoplastic endocrine cells subendothelially in highly vascular benign tumors should not be mistaken for vascular invasion. Malignant endocrine cells often are more pleomorphic (including oval or spindle shaped) than normal, but nuclear pleomorphism is not a consistent criterion to distinguish adenoma from carcinoma. Mitotic figures may be frequent in malignant endocrine cells, but the significance of this criterion can vary considerably with the degree of background stimulation of the endocrine gland.

Many neoplasms derived from endocrine glands are functionally active, secrete an excessive amount of hormone either continuously or episodically, and result in dramatic clinical syndromes of hormone excess. Examples in animals that are described in

this chapter include the hypoglycemia of $\beta$-cell neoplasms of the pancreatic islets in dogs, hyperthyroidism of adenomas and carcinomas derived from thyroid follicular cells in cats and dogs, hypercalcitoninism in bulls and other animal species with thyroid C-cell tumors, and hyperadrenocorticism either associated with adrenocorticotropin- (ACTH-) secreting pituitary corticotroph adenomas or neoplasms derived from the adrenal cortex (zona fasciculata) in dogs, among other species.

Quantitation of hormone levels in serum of plasma in the basal or stimulated state and/or the measurement of hormonal metabolites in the urine over a 24-hour period of excretion is essential to confirm that an endocrine tumor is functional and releasing hormone at an abnormally elevated rate. Morphologically, an endocrine tumor often can be interpreted as endocrinologically active if the rim of normal tissue around the tumor, the opposite of paired endocrine glands, or the nontumorous endocrine glands undergo trophic atrophy due to negative feedback inhibition by the elevated hormone levels or an altered blood constituent. In response to the autonomous secretion of hormone by the tumor, these nonneoplastic secretory cells, especially in the cytoplasmic area, become smaller than normal, and eventually the number of cells is decreased. Functional pituitary neoplasms secreting an excess of a particular tropic hormone (e.g., ACTH) will be associated with striking hypertrophy and hyperplasia of target cells in the adrenal cortex (e.g., zonae fasciculata and reticularis) or follicular cells in the thyroid glands.

## TUMORS OF THE PITUITARY GLAND

### Functional Chromophobe ("Corticotroph") Adenoma in Pars Distalis

**Incidence.** Functional tumors arising in the pituitary gland are most commonly derived from corticotroph (ACTH-secreting) cells in the pars distalis or pars intermedia and associated with a clinical syndrome of cortisol excess (Cushing's-like disease) (Capen, 1983a). These neoplasms are encountered most frequently in dogs, infrequently in cats and horses, and rarely in other animal species. They develop in adult to aged dogs and have been reported in a number of breeds (Brodey and Prier, 1962; Brouwers and Tsiroyannis, 1957; Capen et al., 1967a; Clarkson et al., 1959; Coffin and Munson, 1953; Dahme and Schiefer, 1960; Diener and Langham, 1961; Hare, 1935; Jackson, 1960; Lesbouyries et al., 1942; Lucksch, 1923; Molinary and Mandelli, 1962; Mulligan, 1949; Palmer, 1960; Rijnberk et al., 1967, 1969; Streett and Herrero, 1966; Stunzi and Perlstein, 1958; Trapp et al., 1958; Verwer, 1959; White, 1938). Boxers and Boston terriers appear to be breeds having a high incidence of functional pituitary tumors. The spectrum of dramatic clinical manifestations and lesions that develop are primarily the result of a long-term overproduction of cortisol by hyperplastic adrenal cortices. These changes are the result of the combined gluconeogenic, lipolytic, protein catabolic, and antiinflammatory actions of glucocorticoid hormones on many organ systems of the body.

**Clinical Characteristics.** A number of distinctive clinical and functional alterations develop in dogs with corticotroph (ACTH-secreting) adenomas, resulting in the syndrome of hyperadrenocorticism (Capen et al., 1967a; Lubberink et al., 1971; Siegel et al., 1970). Peterson et al. (1982c) reported that 84% of dogs with pituitary-dependent hyperadrenocorticism had adenomas derived from cells either of the pars distalis or pars intermedia. Immunocytochemical staining of the tumor cells gave a positive reaction for ACTH, $\beta$-lipotrophin, and $\beta$-endorphin.

Centripetal redistribution of adipose tissue leads to prominent fat pads on the dorsal midline of the neck, giving the neck and shoulders a thick appearance. Appetite and intake of food may be increased or ravenous, either as a direct result of the hypercortisolism or involvement of hypothalamic appetite control centers by a large pituitary tumor. The muscles of the extremities and abdomen are weakened and atrophied. The loss of tone of abdominal muscles and muscles of the abaxial skeleton results in gradual abdominal enlargement ("pot belly"), lordosis, muscle trembling, and a straight legged skeletal-braced posture to support the body's weight. Profound atrophy of the temporal muscles may result in obvious concave indentations and readily palpable prominences of underlying skull bones. Hepatomegaly due to increased fat and gly-

cogen deposition and vacuolation of smooth endoplasmic reticulum in liver cells may contribute to the development of the distended, often pendulous abdomen.

Skin lesions occur in more than 90% of dogs with hyperadrenocorticism. The initial changes in the skin are over points of wear. The hair coat becomes thin, rough, and dry. Hair shafts can be easily broken and dislodged from their follicles. As the disease progresses these initial skin changes spread in a bilaterally symmetrical pattern to involve a significant portion of the body surface. The skin is of fine texture, coarsely wrinkled, and often paper thin. The basic lesion in the skin, caused by the excessive secretion of cortisol, is a loss of collagen and elastin fibers in the dermis and subcutis with severe atrophy of the epidermis and pilosebaceous apparatus. The majority of hair follicles are inactive and in the telogen phase of the growth cycle. The prominent comedones observed in the skin, particularly on the ventral abdomen, represent hair follicles distended with keratin and debris. The outer stratum corneum is thickened considerably from the accumulation of multiple layers of keratin on the surface. The accumulation of keratin often gives the skin surface a dry, roughened, scaly appearance.

Other distinctive skin changes in dogs with functional pituitary tumors include hyperpigmentation and mineralization. The accumulations of melanin pigment may be either focal or diffuse and consist of increased numbers of melanocytes in the basal epidermis, stratum corneum, and dermis. Cutaneous mineralization is a characteristic lesion in approximately 40% of dogs with hyperadrenocorticism. Numerous mineral crystals that are deposited along collagen and elastin fibers in the dermis may protrude through the atrophic and thinned epidermis. In less severe cases the epidermis remains intact and appears irregularly elevated by the opaque white deposits of mineral. Dermal vessels are prominent and readily visible through the thin skin. In an occasional dog with marked abdominal distension and loss of supporting dermal collagen and elastin fibers, the superficial vessels become severely stretched and dilated, forming striae similar to those described in human beings with Cushing's syndrome.

The syndrome of long-term cortisol excess is

often complicated by an increased susceptibility to infection with the development of bacterial or fungal infections in the skin, urinary tract, conjunctiva, and lung. Multifocal areas of suppurative folliculitis and dermatitis develop near the lip folds and footpads and elsewhere in the skin (Hall *et al.*, 1984). A frequent serious complication in dogs with hyperadrenocorticism is a suppurative bronchopneumonia that can be fatal if not detected early and treated appropriately.

Dogs with severe muscle asthenia and wasting have difficulty in supporting their body weight and may be recumbent for extended periods. They develop extensive pressure ulcerations of the skin that may be deep, exposing the underlying bony prominences. Until the hypercortisolism is corrected, lesions of this type heal slowly because of inhibition of fibroblastic proliferation by cortisol and the continued muscle weakness.

Several laboratory procedures are available to detect secondary derangements of function caused by an excessive secretion of adrenal cortical hormones. The blood levels of corticosteroids have consistent effects on the hematopoietic system. Lymphoid tissue involutes in response to the increased secretion of cortisol, resulting in a significant lymphopenia (approximately 6% of circulating leukocytes). Increased corticosteroid secretion also results in intravascular destruction of eosinophils or sequestration of circulating eosinophils, leading to eosinopenia. The total eosinophil count in dogs with hyperadrenocorticism often is reduced to below $100/mm^3$. The total white blood cell count is elevated (approximately $16,000/mm^3$), and the percentage of neutrophils is increased (approximately 90%). Dogs with hyperadrenocorticism infrequently develop significant alterations in the serum concentration of sodium, potassium, or chloride. This is in contrast to the frequent electrolyte imbalances in human patients with Cushing's syndrome.

Laboratory evaluation of adrenal cortical function became considerably more accurate with the development of satisfactory methods for measuring the concentration of corticosteroids in plasma. These methods permit adrenal cortical disease to be evaluated directly. The plasma levels in unstressed caged dogs range from 1.0 to 2.5 $\mu$g/100 ml in our laboratory by the competitive protein-binding method of Murphy (1967). Normal dogs not adapted to a veterinary hospital have higher concentrations, varying from 2.0 to 8.5 $\mu$g/100 ml (Martin *et al.*, 1971).

Adrenal function should be further evaluated by the response of the adrenal cortex to ACTH stimulation and dexamethasone suppression. The adrenal cortex of normal dogs responds to exogenous ACTH by increasing the plasma corticosteroid concentration to 7.5 to 18.0 $\mu$g/100 ml at 1 hour postinjection. The plasma concentration returns to preinjection levels, or nearly so, by 3 hours postinjection. Normal dogs respond to dexamethasone by a decrease in plasma corticosteroids to 0.2 to 0.8 $\mu$g/100 ml at 8 hours postinjection. The concentration of corticosteroids in the plasma of dogs with hyperadrenocorticism ranges from 3 to 10 $\mu$g/100 ml or higher. Most dogs with bilateral adrenal cortical hyperplasia (either idiopathic or caused by an ACTH-secreting pituitary tumor) respond to ACTH by an exaggerated increase in the plasma concentration of corticosteroids, ranging from 20 to 60 $\mu$g/100 ml at 1 hour postinjection. Some dogs respond with a lower but more prolonged elevation in corticosteroid concentration. The plasma corticosteroid level in dogs with hyperadrenocorticism usually will fall after the injection of dexamethasone only if the adrenal gland remains under the tropic control of hypophyseal ACTH (as with idiopathic cortical hyperplasia). If a dog has a corticotroph (ACTH-secreting) adenoma of the adenohypophysis or if the adrenal cortex is functioning independently of endogenous ACTH (e.g., carcinoma), the dexamethasone suppression test usually results in minimal or no significant decrease in plasma corticosteroid concentration.

Low doses of dexamethasone (15 $\mu$g/kg) suppress ACTH production and subsequently plasma cortisol levels in normal dogs, but do not suppress dogs with pituitary-dependent hyperadrenocorticism or adrenal cortical neoplasms. High doses of dexamethasone (1.0 mg/kg) usually suppress plasma cortisol levels in dogs with pituitary-dependent hyperadrenocorticism, but not significantly in dogs with adrenal cortical neoplasms (Peterson and Drucker, 1981).

The development of radioimmunoassays for plasma ACTH in the dog has demonstrated a mean concentration of 46 pg/ml (range 17 to 98 pg/ml)

(Feldman *et al.*, 1977). Assays for plasma ACTH are useful in differentiating between pituitary-dependent and other causes of adrenal cortical hyperplasia and the syndrome of cortisol excess. Dogs with functional adrenal cortical neoplasms have plasma ACTH concentrations two standard deviations or more below ($<20$ pg/ml) the mean value for normal dogs, whereas dogs with pituitary-dependent hyperadrenocorticism have plasma ACTH values of $>40$ pg/ml (Feldman, 1981, 1983). The differentiation between pituitary- and adrenal-dependent hyperadrenocorticism by laboratory methods has been reviewed by Peterson (1984*b*).

**Gross Morphology.** The pituitary gland is consistently enlarged in dogs with corticotroph adenomas and ranges in size from $0.7 \times 0.6 \times 0.5$ cm to $4.0 \times 2.5 \times 2.5$ cm. The occurrence or severity of functional disturbance, however, has no consistent direct relationship to the size of the neoplasm. Small chromophobe adenomas are as likely to be endocrinologically active as larger neoplasms. The larger adenomas are often firmly attached to the base of the sella turcica, but without evidence of erosion of the sphenoid bone. In the animal species most likely to develop pituitary neoplasms (dog and horse), the diaphragma sellae is incomplete. Therefore, the line of least resistance in the dog favors dorsal expansion of the gradually enlarging mass with resulting invagination into the infundibular cavity, dilatation of the infundibular recess and third ventricle, and eventual compression and replacement of the hypothalamus and thalamus. This differs from the situation in humans where the complete diaphragma sellae, which is a tough reflection of dura mater separating the hypophysis from the cranial cavity, favors ventrolateral growth of the neoplasm and erosion of the sphenoid bones that form the walls and base of the sella turcica. Dorsal expansion of the larger pituitary neoplasms results in either a broad-based indentation and compression of the overlying hypothalamus or extension into and replacement of the parenchyma of the hypothalamus and occasionally the thalamus (fig. 13.1A). Focal areas of hemorrhage, necrosis, mineralization, and liquefaction are frequently encountered in the larger neoplasms.

Dogs with functional corticotroph adenomas have bilateral enlargement of the adrenal glands (fig. 13.1A). This hyperplasia is often striking and is due entirely to an increased amount of cortical parenchyma, primarily in the zona fasciculata and to a lesser extent in the zona reticularis. Nodules of yellow-orange cortical tissue are often identified outside the capsule in the periadrenal fat as well as extending into the medulla. The corticomedullary junction is irregular, and the medulla is compressed.

**Histological Features.** Pituitary adenomas are composed of well-differentiated secretory cells supported by fine connective tissue septa. Chromophobe adenomas are subclassified into sinusoidal and diffuse types on the basis of the predominant pattern of cellular architecture. The tumor cells in the sinusoidal type are separated into compartments of varied sizes and shapes by delicate, often incomplete, connective tissue septa containing capillaries or small venules (fig. 13.1B). The sinusoidal type is more vascular than the diffuse type, and in some areas the blood sinusoids attain considerable size and appear to be lined by neoplastic cells. When the tumor cells palisade along the connective tissue septa or blood sinusoids, they are more elongated and have oval or spindle-shaped nuclei. The tumor cells in the diffuse type of chromophobe adenoma lack a characteristic architectural arrangement and appear as sheets or masses of large chromophobic cells (fig. 13.1C). Blood vessels are small and few in number. The connective tissue stroma is sparse.

Corticotroph adenomas are composed of either large or small chromophobic cells. Large chromophobes make up the majority of adenomas of this type. They are polyhedral and have large vesicular nuclei with one or two prominent nucleoli and an abundant eosinophilic cytoplasm with distinct cell boundaries. The cytoplasm is devoid of secretory granules detectable by the conventional histochemical procedures employed for pituitary cytology. Small chromophobic cells constitute the remaining pituitary adenomas of this type. They are roughly half the size of large chromophobes and have small dark nuclei with indistinct nucleoli and a small amount of cytoplasm. Mitotic figures are infrequent in both types of chromophobic cells.

Remnants of the pars distalis may be identified near the periphery of the chromophobe adenomas. Demarcation between the neoplasm and the pars distalis is not distinct. The separation is effected by an incomplete layer of condensed reticulum, and there is often not a complete capsule. Acidophils

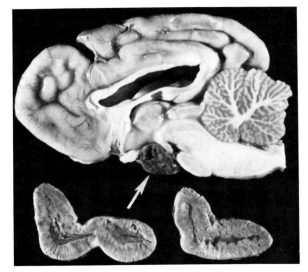

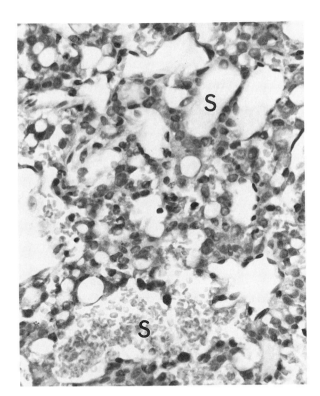

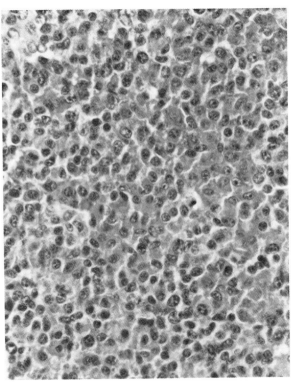

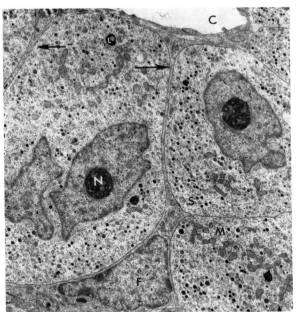

A|B
C|D

**FIGURE 13.1.** Functional chromophobe adenoma. A. Corticotroph adenoma (**arrow**) in the hypophysis with bilateral adrenal cortical hyperplasia in a dog. The hypothalamus is compressed by the dorsally expanding pituitary adenoma. B. Corticotroph adenoma, sinusoidal type. The neoplastic cells are separated into compartments by the numerous endothelial-lined vascular sinusoids (S). C. Corticotroph adenoma, diffuse type. The sheets of large chromophobic tumor cells lack a characteristic pattern of arrange-

ment. Capillaries are small, indistinct, and few in number. D. Neoplastic corticotrophs. The tumor cells have irregularly shaped nuclei and prominent nucleoli (N) and are supported by a reticular framework of follicular cells (F) that extend long cytoplasmic processes (**arrows**) to the perivascular spaces (C is capillary). The cytoplasm of the neoplastic cells contains numerous small secretory granules (S) of varying electron density, occasional dense lipid bodies (L), and scattered mitochondria (M).

and occasionally basophils are incorporated within the neoplasm near the margin. The pars distalis is either partly replaced by the neoplasm or severely compressed and composed principally of heavily granulated acidophils. The posterior lobe and infundibular stalk either are infiltrated and disrupted by tumor cells or completely incorporated within the larger neoplasms. The hypothalamus is severely compressed or invaded and replaced by the large, dorsally expanding corticotroph adenomas (fig. 13.1A). There are increased numbers of fibrous astrocytes and hemosiderin-laden macrophages, perivascular hemorrhages, a loss of neurons, and myelin degradation within the hypothalamus and occasionally in the thalamus around the expanding mass of neoplastic cells. Focal areas of hemorrhage, coagulation and liquefactive necrosis, mineralization, and cholesterol clefts occur within the larger corticotroph adenomas.

**Ultrastructural and Immunocytochemical Characteristics.** Cells constituting functional corticotroph adenomas in dogs have definite evidence of secretory activity (Capen and Koestner, 1967). Organelles concerned with protein synthesis (endoplasmic reticulum) and packaging of secretory products (Golgi apparatus) are well developed in tumor cells. The predominating neoplastic cells are large, relatively electron dense, and roughly polyhedral or cuboidal (fig. 13.1D). The outline of the neoplastic cells is irregular, and cytoplasmic projections tend to extend between neighboring cells or encompass them completely. The nucleus is usually centrally located and irregular in shape with deep indentations, and contains one or two dense nucleoli (fig. 13.1D).

The neoplastic cells are supported by a reticular framework of follicular cells (Capen and Koestner, 1967; Kagayama, 1965). These cells are stellate and have long cytoplasmic processes that extend between the neoplastic cells and terminate in the extracellular perivascular spaces (fig. 13.1D). The cytoplasmic matrix of the follicular cells is finely granular and comparatively electron dense because of the presence of numerous organelles.

Cells making up functional corticotroph adenomas contain mature secretory granules at the level of ultrastructure. This is in contrast to the absence of demonstrable secretory granules within the neoplastic cells as observed through light micros-

copy following the application of histochemical procedures. Secretory granules vary in number from cell to cell but are usually numerous (fig. 13.1D). The granules are roughly spherical and surrounded by a delicate limiting membrane. The space between the secretory granule and its covering membrane is relatively wide compared with the granules in other cells of the adenohypophysis of the dog. The secretory granules, particularly those in the vicinity of the Golgi apparatus, are small (mean diameter of 170 $\mu$m), extremely electron dense, and have a prominent submembranous space. Larger secretory granules may be admixed with the small secretory granules, particularly near the periphery of the neoplastic cells. They are uniformly less electron dense, finely granular, and limited by a definite membrane. Within the membranes of the Golgi apparatus are small prosecretory granules of variable size, presumably in the process of formation. Secretory granules are observed occasionally in the process of becoming detached from the Golgi membranes.

Immunocytochemical staining has demonstrated that ACTH- and melanocyte-stimulating hormone- (MSH-) staining cells—antisera to porcine ACTH, synthetic ACTH-$\beta$ (1–24) and ACTH-$\beta$ (17–39), and bovine-$\beta$-MSH—are polyhedral to round, sparsely granulated, and most numerous in the ventrocentral and cranial portions of the pars distalis in dogs where they occur in large groups (El Etreby and Dubois, 1980). They are less numerous in the dorsal and caudal regions of the pars distalis and throughout the pars tuberalis. In the pars intermedia of dogs most cells demonstrated immunoreactivity to either pACTH, $\alpha$-MSH, or $\beta$-MSH.

Pituitary adenomas arising in both the pars distalis and the pars intermedia, associated with the syndrome of cortisol excess in dogs, are composed of polyhedral cells that immunocytochemically stain selectively for ACTH and MSH (Attia, 1980; El Etreby et al., 1980). Focal areas of hyperplasia and microadenomas, composed of similar ACTH/MSH cells, are also present in both lobes of the adenohypophysis. Peterson et al. (1982c) reported that pituitary adenomas arising in both the pars distalis and pars intermedia had positive immunocytochemical staining for ACTH, $\beta$-lipotrophin, and $\beta$-endorphin.

Siperstein (1963), using high-resolution autoradiographic techniques with tritiated glycine in rats, has shown that the ACTH-producing cell in the hypophysis is a large chromophobic cell. Following adrenalectomy this chromophobic cell had the highest content of tritium and the fastest rate of both incorporation (hormone synthesis) and loss (hormone secretion) of tritium of all the hypophyseal cell types. The "adrenalectomy cell" is morphologically distinct from gonadectomy or thyroidectomy cells and from other cell types in the normal hypophysis. The cytoplasm is often compressed between or indented by the neighboring pituitary cells.

Cells constituting functional chromophobe adenomas in dogs share many histological and ultrastructural features with the corticotrophs or "adrenalectomy cell" reported in the hypophysis of rats (Kurosumi and Kobayashi, 1966; Kurosumi and Oota, 1966; Siperstein and Allison, 1965). They could be differentiated from acidophils and basophils of the canine hypophysis by the smaller size and lesser density of their secretory granules.

Chromophobe adenomas that possess secretory activity have been reported in humans and are associated with an increased secretion of adrenocorticotropin (Engel and Kahana, 1963; Nelson et al., 1958). Cushing's disease was described initially in association with basophil adenomas of the hypophysis.

## Nonfunctional Chromophobe Adenoma in Pars Distalis

**Incidence.** Nonfunctional (endocrinologically inactive) pituitary tumors are most common in dogs, cats, and parakeets and are rare in other species (Capen, 1983a; Capen et al., 1967a; Zaki and Liu, 1973). In contrast to the functional adenomas, there is no indication of any breed or sex predisposition. Although these chromophobe adenomas appear to be endocrinologically inactive, they may result in significant functional disturbances by virtue of compression atrophy of the pars nervosa and pars distalis or extension into the brain.

**Clinical Characteristics.** Animals with nonfunctional pituitary adenomas are usually presented with clinical disturbances related to dysfunction of the central nervous system or lack of secretion of pituitary tropic hormones and diminished end-organ function. The history often includes depression, incoordination and other disturbances of balance, weakness, collapse with exercise, and a marked change in personality. Animals may become unresponsive to people and develop a tendency to hide at the slightest provocation. In long-standing cases there may be evidence of blindness with dilated and fixed pupils (Heavner and Dice, 1977). Clinically, the body condition varies from a progressive loss of weight to obvious obesity. The animals appear to be dehydrated, as evidenced by a lusterless dry hair coat, and the owner may have noticed increased water consumption and frequent urination. Parakeets with chromophobe adenomas often develop exophthalmos due to extension of neoplastic cells along the optic nerve.

A consistent finding with both functional and nonfunctional pituitary tumors is the excretion of large volumes of dilute urine with a low specific gravity (approximately 1.007) (Capen et al., 1967a). Water intake is increased correspondingly and the owner often complains that the animal, previously housebroken, urinates frequently in the house. Disturbances of water balance are the result of either a direct diuretic effect exerted on the kidney by the elevated corticosteroid levels or an interference with the synthesis and release of antidiuretic hormone (ADH) (Koestner and Capen, 1967). The posterior lobe, infundibular stalk, and hypothalamus are often compressed or disrupted by neoplastic cells in dogs with pituitary tumors. This interrupts the nonmyelinated axons that transport ADH from the site of production in the hypothalamus to the site of release in the capillary plexus of the posterior lobe. Compression of neurosecretory neurons in the supraoptic nucleus of the hypothalamus by the tumor may result in decreased ADH synthesis.

Clinical signs in animals with nonfunctional pituitary adenomas and hypopituitarism are not highly specific and could be confused with other disorders of the central nervous system, such as brain tumors and encephalitis (e.g., toxoplasmosis), or chronic renal disease. Hypopituitarism caused by pituitary tumors should be included in the differential diagnosis of adult to older animals with signs of incoordination, depression, polyuria, blindness, and a sudden change in personality.

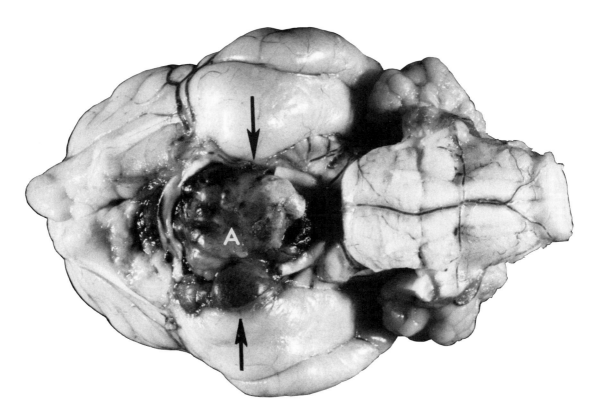

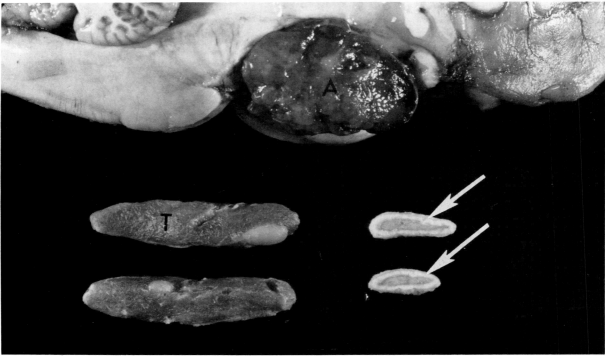

A
B
**FIGURE 13.2.** Nonfunctional chromophobe adenoma of the pituitary gland. A. Ventral view of the brain of a 4-year-old male Siamese cat illustrating a large chromophobe adenoma (A). The neoplasm has completely incorporated the pituitary, extended into the brain, and destroyed the optic nerves. Arrows mark the junction between the neoplastic tissue and brain parenchyma. B. Chromophobe adenoma (A) in a dog with expansion into the hypothalamus. There is severe trophic atrophy of the adrenal cortex (**arrows**), but the thyroid glands (T) are nearly normal size due to distention of follicles with colloid in the absence of thyrotropin.

acidophil. These hypertrophied acidophils are considered to be secretorily active cells. Cells with varying intergrades of organellar development and a number of mature secretory granules are observed between the extremes of storage and actively synthesizing acidophils.

The neoplastic acidophils often contain numerous mature secretory granules at the level of ultrastructure (fig. 13.7B). The granules are spherical to oval, uniformly electron dense, finely granular, and surrounded by a delicate limiting membrane. The submembranous space of the granule is narrow. Secretory granules are occasionally observed in the process of becoming detached from the Golgi membranes. The mean diameter of mature secretory granules in the neoplastic acidophils is 420 mμ (ranging from 320 to 600 mμ) (Capen *et al.,* 1967*b*).

Immunoreactive prolactin cells occur in small groups of large polygonal cells with prominent granules in the ventrocentral and cranial parts of the canine pars distalis (El Etreby and Fath El Bab, 1977). A diffuse increase in this population of cells occurs in female dogs near parturition (El Etreby *et al.,* 1980). Growth hormone-secreting cells are present singly along capillaries in the dorsal region of the pars distalis near the pars intermedia (El Etreby and Fath El Bab, 1977). They are small, round to oval, and have fine cytoplasmic granules. Somatotrophs frequently undergo diffuse hyperplasia and hypertrophy in old dogs, especially females with mammary dysplasia or neoplasia (El Etreby *et al.,* 1980).

## Pituitary Chromophobe Carcinoma

**Incidence.** Pituitary carcinomas are uncommon compared with pituitary adenomas, but have been seen in older dogs and cows (Powers and Winkler, 1977). They are usually endocrinologically inactive, but may result in significant functional disturbances by destruction of the pars distalis and neurohypophyseal system, leading to panhypopituitarism and diabetes insipidus.

**Gross Morphology and Histological Features.** Pituitary carcinomas are large and extensively invade the brain and sphenoid bone of the sella turcica (fig. 13.8A). Metastasis may occur to regional lymph nodes or to distant sites, such as the spleen or liver (fig. 13.8B).

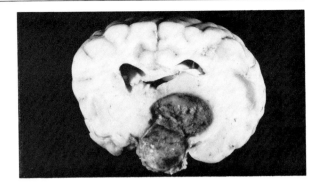
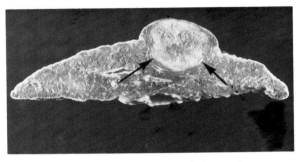

A    **FIGURE 13.8.** Pituitary chromophobe carcinoma.
B    A. Extensive dorsal invasion into the brain. B. Metastasis to the spleen (**arrows**).

Malignant tumors of pituitary chromophobes are highly cellular and often have large areas of hemorrhage and necrosis. Giant cells, nuclear pleomorphism, and mitotic figures are encountered more frequently than in chromophobe adenomas.

## Craniopharyngioma

**Incidence.** Craniopharyngioma is a benign tumor that is derived from epithelial remnants of the oropharyngeal ectoderm of the craniopharyngeal duct (Rathke's pouch). It occurs in animals younger than those with other types of pituitary neoplasms and is present either in a suprasellar or infrasellar location. It is one cause of panhypopituitarism and dwarfism in young dogs resulting from a subnormal secretion of somatotropin and other tropic hormones beginning at an early age, prior to closure of the growth plates (Eigenmann *et al.,* 1983).

**Clinical Features.** The clinical signs resulting from this type of pituitary tumor are usually a com-

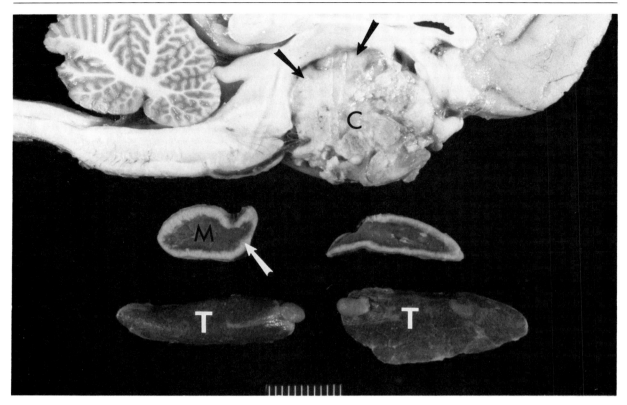

**FIGURE 13.9.** Craniopharyngioma (C) with dorsal extension and compression of the hypothalamus and thalamus (**black arrows**). The large neoplasm has incorporated the adenohypophysis and neurohypophysis, and resulted in severe trophic atrophy of the adrenal cortex (**white arrow**). The adrenal glands consist predominantly of medulla (M) surrounded by a thin rim of cortex (capsule plus zona glomerulosa). Although the thyroid follicular cells were flattened and atrophic, the overall gland (T) size was within normal limits due to distension of the follicles with colloid (scale is 1 cm).

bination of several factors. These include (1) lack of secretion of pituitary tropic hormones resulting in tropic atrophy and subnormal function of the adrenal cortex and thyroid (Neer and Reavis, 1983) (fig. 13.9), gonadal atrophy, and failure to attain somatic maturation due to a lack of growth hormone; (2) disturbances in water metabolism (polyuria, polydipsia, low urine specific gravity and osmolality) from interference in the release and synthesis of ADH by the large tumor (Saunders and Rickard, 1952); (3) deficits in cranial nerve function; and (4) central nervous system dysfunction due to extension into the overlying brain.

**Gross Morphology.** Craniopharyngiomas are often large and grow along the ventral aspect of the brain where they can incorporate several cranial nerves. In addition, they extend dorsally into the hypothalamus and thalamus (fig. 13.9).

**Histological Characteristics.** Craniopharyngiomas have alternating solid and cystic areas (White, 1938). The solid areas are composed of nests of epithelial cells (cuboidal, columnar, or squamous cells) with focal areas of mineralization. The cystic spaces are lined by either columnar or squamous cells and contain keratin debris and colloid. Ductlike structures may be formed that are lined by columnar cells.

## Basophil Adenoma of Pars Distalis

Tumors composed of granulated basophils are one of the most rare pituitary tumors in all animal species. Cushing's disease in humans was initially attributed to a hypersecretion of adrenocorticotropin by small basophilic adenomas in the pars distalis. Current evidence suggests they are a possible cause for a small percentage of patients with Cushing's disease (Daughaday, 1968). Several of the early reports on corticotropin-secreting pituitary tumors in dogs with hyperadrenocorticism reflected this concept and considered them to be basophil adenomas (Belmonte, 1934; Brandt, 1940; Coffin and Munson, 1953; Dämmrich, 1959; Diener and Langham, 1961; Lucksch, 1923; Spaar and Willie, 1959). Corticotroph (chromophobe) adenomas of the pars distalis and pars intermedia are responsible for the great majority of cases of Cushing's-like disease in dogs.

Basophil adenomas in humans may secrete thyrotropin (TSH) resulting in bilateral enlargement of both thyroid lobes ("goiter") (Yovos *et al.*, 1981). Serum thyroxine, triiodothyronine, and TSH are elevated and responsive to thyrotropin-releasing hormone. The neoplastic cells contain small secretory granules (diameter <150 nm) with prominent rough endoplasmic reticulum and Golgi apparatuses, characteristic of pituitary thyrotrophs.

Tsuchitani and Narama (1984) reported a well-circumscribed chromophobe adenoma in a male monkey (*Macaca fascicularis*). The round or polyhedral cells were arranged either into follicles or diffuse sheets. Although the neoplastic cells lacked basophilic or acidophilic granules, the small secretory granules (mean diameter 151 nm) and positive immunohistochemical staining for thyrotropin suggested that the tumor was derived from thyrotropic basophils in the pars distalis. The thyroid gland, however, did not show evidence of stimulation, but rather was composed of involuted follicles lined by atrophic follicular cells.

## Metastatic Tumors to the Pituitary Gland

The pituitary gland is occasionally either partially or completely destroyed by metastatic tumors from distant sites. Examples include malignant lym-

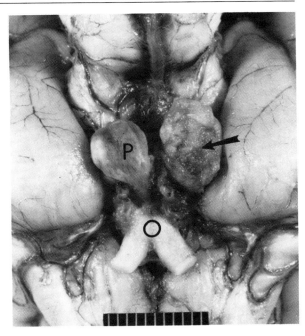

**FIGURE 13.10.** Meningioma (**arrow**) arising on ventral aspect of brain in a dog that exerted pressure on the hypothalamic–hypophyseal portal system and infundibular stalk. O, optic nerve; P, pituitary.

phoma of cattle and dogs, malignant melanoma of horses and dogs, transmissible venereal tumor (Spence *et al.*, 1978), and adenocarcinoma in the mammary gland of dogs. In addition, the pituitary may be destroyed by local infiltration or compression from an osteosarcoma of the sphenoid bone, ependymoma arising in the infundibular recess of the third ventricle, meningioma (fig. 13.10), and a glioma ("infundibuloma") of the infundibular stalk (Saunders *et al.*, 1951).

## NONNEOPLASTIC CYSTS OF THE PITUITARY GLAND

### Cysts of the Craniopharyngeal Duct

Cysts may develop from remnants of the distal craniopharyngeal duct, which normally disappears by birth in most animal species. The cysts are lined by ciliated, cuboidal to columnar epithelium and contain mucin (Rao and Bhat, 1971). In dogs, especially of the brachycephalic breeds, cysts from these remnants are frequently found at the periphery of the pars tuberalis and pars distalis. In one survey, cystic remnants of the craniopharyngeal duct were found in 53% of dogs of several breeds (Schiefer and Hänichen, 1967).

Craniopharyngeal duct cysts occasionally become large enough to exert pressure on the infundibular stalk and hypophyseal portal system, median eminence, or pars distalis. Structures adjacent to the cysts atrophy to varying degrees owing to compression and interference with the blood supply. Disruption of a large cyst with escape of the proteinic contents into adjacent tissues may incite an intense, local inflammation with subsequent fibrosis that interferes with pituitary function. Clinical signs may include visual difficulties due to pressure on the optic chiasma, diabetes insipidus, obesity, and hypofunction of the adenohypophysis (gonadal atrophy, decreased basal metabolic rate, and hypoglycemia).

## Cysts Derived from the Pharyngeal Hypophysis

The proximal portion of the adenohypophyseal anlage may persist in the dorsal aspect of the oral cavity in adults as undifferentiated remnants of cells along the craniopharyngeal canal or as differentiated cells similar to those of the definitive adenohypophysis. These remnants, called the *pharyngeal hypophysis*, have been described in dogs, cats, other animal species, and humans (McGrath, 1974). The pharyngeal hypophysis is physically separated from the sellar adenohypophysis in dogs, but in cats these structures may be continuous because of persistence of the craniopharyngeal canal.

The pharyngeal hypophysis is seen most frequently in brachycephalic breeds of dogs. It is a tubular structure lined by ciliated columnar epithelium, located on the midline of the nasopharynx, and is frequently continuous with a multilocular cyst that is lined by squamous, ciliated, cuboidal, or columnar epithelium. The cyst contains colloid material and cellular debris. A mass of differentiated

acidophilic, basophilic, and chromophobic cells similar to those of the sellar adenohypophysis usually extends from the cyst wall.

A cyst (as much as several centimeters in diameter) may be derived from the oropharyngeal end of the craniopharyngeal duct and project as a space-occupying mass into the nasopharynx in dogs. The predominant clinical sign may be related to respiratory distress due to ventral displacement of the soft palate and occlusion of the posterior nares (Slatter *et al.*, 1976). The cyst wall is hard on palpation because of the presence of partially mineralized woven bone. The contents of the cyst are often yellow-gray and caseous due to the accumulation of keratin and desquamated epithelial cells from the cyst lining. The squamous epithelial lining of the cyst appears to be derived from metaplasia of the remnants of the primitive oropharyngeal epithelium.

## Pituitary Dwarfism

Pituitary dwarfism in German shepherd dogs usually is associated with a failure of the oropharyngeal ectoderm of Rathke's pouch to differentiate into tropic hormone-secreting cells of the pars distalis. This results in a progressively enlarging, multiloculated cyst in the sella turcica and a partial to complete absence of the adenohypophysis (Alexander, 1962). The cyst is lined by pseudostratified, often ciliated, columnar epithelium with interspersed mucin-secreting goblet cells. The mucin-filled cysts eventually occupy the entire pituitary area in the sella turcica and severely compress the pars nervosa and infundibular stalk (fig. 13.11A). A few differentiated tropic hormone-secreting chromophils may be present in the pituitary region; these immunocytochemically stain for the specific tropic hormones. An occasional small nest or rosette of poorly differentiated epithelial cells is interspersed between multiloculated cysts, but the cell cytoplasm is usually devoid of hormone-containing secretory granules.

Cysts associated with pituitary dwarfism morphologically are distinct from the cysts that develop following the abnormal accumulation of colloid in the residual lumen of Rathke's pouch (fig. 13.11B). The normally developed pars distalis and pars nervosa are compressed to varying degrees by the abnormal accumulation of colloid in a cavity of the pituitary.

Pituitary dwarf pups appear normal or are indistinguishable from littermates at birth and until about 2 months of age. Subsequently, the slower growth rate than the littermates, retention of puppy hair coat, and lack of primary guard hairs gradually become evident in dwarf pups (fig. 13.11C). German shepherd dogs with pituitary dwarfism appear coyotelike or foxlike due to their diminutive size and soft woolly coat (Muller, 1979; Muller and Jones, 1973). A bilaterally symmetrical alopecia develops gradually and often progresses to complete alopecia except for the head and tufts of hair on the legs. There is progressive hyperpigmentation of the skin until it is uniformly brown-black over most of the body. Adult German shepherd dogs with panhypopituitarism vary in size from as tiny as 4 lb up to nearly half normal size, apparently depending on whether the failure of formation of the adenohypophysis is nearly complete or only partial.

Panhypopituitarism in German shepherd dogs often occurs in littermates and related litters, suggesting a simple autosomal recessive mode of inheritance (Andresen and Willeberg, 1976; Andresen *et al.*, 1974; Lund-Larsen and Grondalen, 1976; Nicholas, 1978; Willeberg *et al.*, 1975). The activity of somatomedin (a cartilage growth-promoting peptide whose production in the liver and plasma

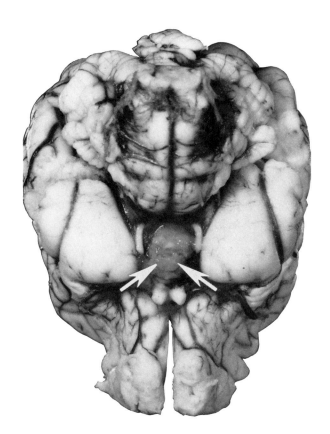

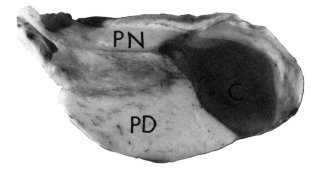

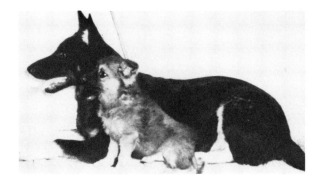

A
B
C

**FIGURE 13.11.** Pituitary cysts. A. Pituitary cysts resulting from a failure of the primitive oropharyngeal ectoderm of Rathke's pouch to differentiate into secretory cells of the adenohypophysis. The pituitary region is occupied by a large multiloculated cyst (**arrows**) that compressed adjacent structures. The dog developed panhypopituitary dwarfism due to a failure of secretion of growth hormone and other tropic hormones by the cystic pituitary gland. B. Cystic distention of residual hypophyseal lumen with colloid (C) compressing the pars distalis (PD) and pars nervosa (PN). Bovine hypophysis. C. Panhypopituitarism (pituitary dwarfism) in a 5-month-old German shepherd dog. An unaffected littermate weighed 60 lb and the dwarf pup 8.8 lb. Note the retention of the puppy haircoat on the dwarf. Courtesy of Dr. J. Alexander and *Can. Vet. J.* (1962).

activity are controlled by somatotropin) is low in dwarf dogs (Lund-Larsen and Grondalen, 1976). Intermediate somatomedin activity is present in the phenotypically normal ancestors suspected to be heterozygous carriers. Assays for somatomedin (a non-species-specific, somatotropin-dependent peptide) provide an indirect measurement of circulating growth hormone activity in dogs with suspected pituitary dwarfism (Van Wyk *et al.*, 1974; Willeberg *et al.*, 1975).

## TUMORS OF THE ADRENAL GLAND

### Tumors of the Adrenal Cortex

**Incidence.** Adenomas of the adrenal cortex are seen most frequently in old dogs (8 years and older) and sporadically in horses, cattle, goats, and sheep (László, 1942; Raethel, 1957; Richter, 1957, 1958; Sandison and Anderson, 1968; Schenke, 1934; Schofield, 1949; Sikora, 1953; Vince and Watson, 1982). Castrated male goats are reported to have a much higher incidence of cortical adenomas than intact males (Altman *et al.*, 1969).

Adrenal cortical carcinomas occur less frequently than adenomas. They have been reported most often in cattle (Tamaschke, 1951–1952; Wright and Conner, 1968), sporadically in old dogs (Chaistain *et al.*, 1978; Siegel *et al.*, 1967; Vince and Watson, 1982), and rarely in other species. Carcinomas develop in adult to older animals and there is no particular breed or sex prevalence.

**Clinical Characteristics.** Cortical adenomas that occur frequently in old dogs are usually incidental findings at necropsy. Occasionally, adenomas and carcinomas of the adrenal cortex in dogs are functional and secrete excessive amounts of cortisol. The clinical signs of cortisol excess in dogs produced by functional adrenal cortical tumors are essentially similar to those described previously for corticotroph (ACTH-secreting) adenomas of the pituitary. The clinical picture of adrenal cortical carcinoma may be complicated by compression of adjacent organs by the large tumor, invasion into the aorta or posterior vena cava leading to intraabdominal hemorrhage, and metastasis to distant sites. In horses, adrenal tumors have been reported to be associated with endocrine disturbances (Kral, 1951). The clinical signs of cortisol excess caused by a functional cortical adenoma or carcinoma usually cannot be reversed by the adrenalcytotoxic drug o,p'-DDD (Vince and Watson, 1982).

Peterson *et al.* (1982a) reported that the mean basal plasma cortisol was high (6.3 $\mu$g/dl) in dogs with functional adrenal cortical neoplasms compared to clinically normal control dogs (1.6 ± 1.0 $\mu$g/dl). In 59% of dogs with cortical adenomas (four dogs) and carcinomas (nine dogs), there was an exaggerated increase in plasma cortisol following administration of exogenous ACTH (20 units ACTH gel intramuscularly). The mean concentration of plasma cortisol was 37.9 $\mu$g/dl at 2 hours post-ACTH in dogs with adrenal cortical tumors. The plasma cortisol levels were approximately fourfold higher at 2 hours post-ACTH in dogs with functional carcinomas compared to those with cortical adenomas.

**Gross Morphology.** Cortical adenomas usually are well-demarcated single nodules in one adrenal gland, but they may be bilateral. Larger cortical adenomas are yellow to red, distort the external contour of the affected gland, and are partially or completely encapsulated. Adjacent cortical parenchyma is compressed and the tumor may extend into the medulla.

Smaller cortical adenomas are more yellow and similar in color to the normal adrenal cortex because of the high lipid content. They are surrounded on all sides by mildly compressed cortex with early attempts at encapsulation and may be difficult to distinguish from large areas of nodular cortical hyperplasia in old dogs. Usually, however, nodular hyperplasia consists of multiple foci of various sizes in both adrenals showing no evidence of encapsulation and is associated with extracapsular nodules of hyperplastic cortical tissue.

Adrenal cortical carcinomas are larger than adenomas and more likely to be bilateral (Davis *et al.*, 1933). In dogs they are composed of a variegated, yellow to brownish red, friable tissue that incorporates the affected adrenal gland. They are often fixed in location because of extensive invasion of surrounding tissues and the posterior vena cava, forming large tumor cell emboli. Carcinomas may attain considerable size in cattle (as much as 10 cm or more in diameter) and have multiple areas of mineralization or ossification (Montpellier, 1928).

Functional adrenal cortical adenomas and carcinomas are associated with profound cortical atro-

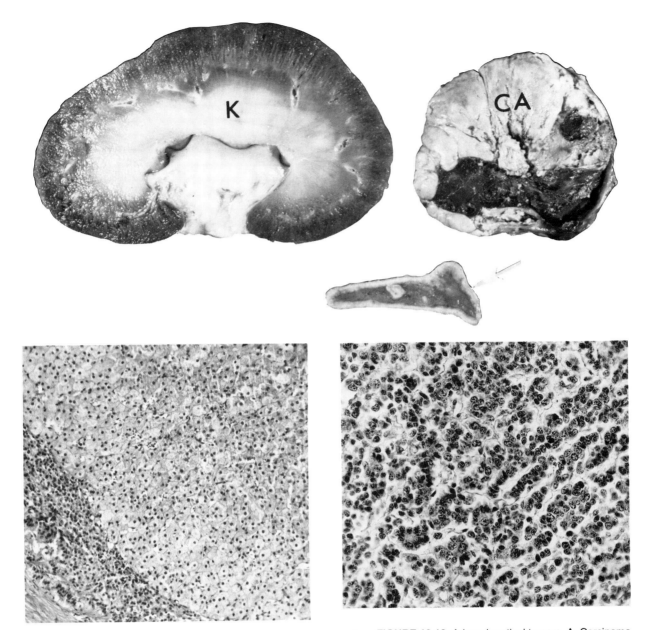

phy of the contralateral gland because of negative feedback inhibition of the pituitary corticotropin (ACTH) secretion by the elevated blood cortisol levels (fig. 13.12A) (Feldman, 1981). The atrophic cortex consists primarily of the adrenal capsule and zona glomerulosa, but few secretory cells remain in the zonae fasciculata and reticularis. A similar parenchymal atrophy may be present in the uncompressed cortex around functional adenomas. The adrenal medulla appears expanded and relatively more conspicuous because of the lack of cortical parenchyma.

A
B|C  **FIGURE 13.12.** Adrenal cortical tumors. A. Carcinoma (CA) from a dog with Cushing's-like syndrome of hyperadrenocorticism. The carcinoma was functional and secreted an excess of cortisol that resulted in prominent cortical atrophy (**white arrow**) of the contralateral adrenal gland. A longitudinal section of kidney (K) is at the left. B. Adenoma of the dog. Adenoma is composed of large lipid-laden cells with a vacuolated cytoplasm and small hyperchromatic nucleus. A rim of compressed adrenal cortex and adrenal capsule is seen at the upper left. C. Carcinoma of the cow. Cords of tumor cells with prominent hyperchromatic nuclei are separated by small vascular sinusoids.

**Histological Features.** Cortical adenomas are composed of well-differentiated cells that resemble secretory cells of the normal zona fasciculata or reticularis (fig. 13.12B). Tumor cells are arranged in broad trabeculae or nests separated by small vascular spaces. The abundant cytoplasmic area of tumor cells is lightly eosinophilic, often vacuolated, and filled with many lipid droplets. Adenomas are partially or completely surrounded by a fibrous connective tissue capsule of varying thickness and a rim of compressed cortical parenchyma. Focal areas of mineralization, hematopoiesis, and accumulations of fat cells may be found in cortical adenomas. Larger adenomas have areas of necrosis and hemorrhage near the center.

Adrenal cortical carcinomas are composed of more highly pleomorphic cells than adenomas that are subdivided into groups by a fibrovascular stroma of varying thickness. The architecture of the affected adrenal is completely obliterated by the carcinoma. The pattern of growth varies between individual tumors and within the same carcinoma and results in the formation of trabeculae, lobules, or nests of tumor cells (fig. 13.12C). Tumor cells are usually large and polyhedral and may have a vesicular nucleus with prominent nucleoli and a densely eosinophilic or vacuolated cytoplasm. Anaplastic carcinomas have some spindle-shaped cells with a smaller and more lightly eosinophilic cytoplasm (Monlux *et al.*, 1956). Areas of hemorrhage within the tumors are common because of rupture of thin-walled vessels (László, 1942). Invasion of tumor cells through the adrenal capsule into adjacent tissues and into vessels and lymphatics, forming emboli, is frequently detected in carcinomas of the adrenal cortex (Kelly *et al.*, 1971).

Nodular cortical hyperplasia and myelolipoma are two discrete cortical lesions that must be differentiated histologically from adrenal cortical adenomas. The presence of a partial or complete fibrous capsule surrounding one or two progressively expanding areas of proliferating cortical cells suggests an adenoma rather than nodular hyperplasia.

Myelolipoma is a benign lesion commonly encountered in the adrenal glands of cattle and nonhuman primates and infrequently in other ani-

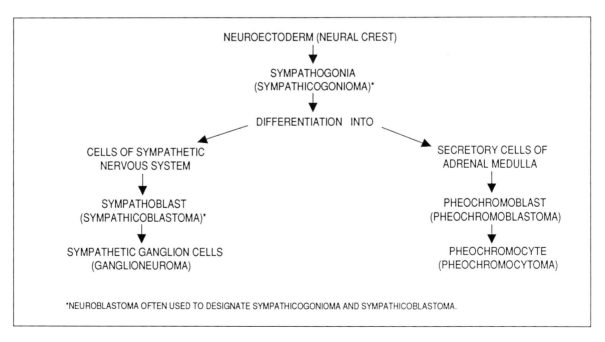

**FIGURE 13.13.** Histogenesis of tumors of the adrenal medulla.

mals. It is composed of accumulations of well-differentiated adipose cells and hematopoietic tissue, including both myeloid and lymphoid elements. Focal areas of mineralization or bone formation may occur in myelolipomas. Although the origin of these nodular aggregations of fat, bone, and myeloid cells is uncertain, they appear to develop by metaplastic transformation of cells in the adrenal cortex.

**Growth and Metastasis.** Adrenal cortical adenomas usually are slow-growing small tumors that are infrequently associated with a hypersecretion of cortisol or other steroid hormones. Carcinomas of the adrenal cortex are larger, locally invasive, and metastasize to distant sites (Kelly *et al.*, 1971). They often invade through the thin wall of the posterior vena cava, forming a large tumor cell thrombus, and into the adventitial layer of the abdominal aorta in dogs and cattle (Cohrs, 1927; Horne, 1905). Metastases are found primarily in the liver, kidney, and mesenteric lymph nodes (Cleland, 1908; Schlegel, 1908; Schofield, 1949).

## Tumors of the Adrenal Medulla

**Incidence and Classification.** Pheochromocytomas are the most common tumors in the adrenal medulla of animals, although other tumors may develop from the neuroectodermal cells, which differentiate into either secretory elements or sympathetic ganglion cells (fig. 13.13). Neuroblastomas arise from primitive neuroectodermal cells, often in younger animals, and form a large intraabdominal neoplasm that may metastasize to peritoneal surfaces. Ganglioneuromas are usually well-differentiated small tumors that have multipolar ganglion cells and neurofibrils.

Pheochromocytomas develop most often in cattle and dogs and infrequently in other domestic animals (Buckingham, 1970; Froscher and Power, 1982; László, 1941b; Tamaschke, 1955; West, 1975; White and Cheyne, 1977; Wright and Conner, 1968); they also occur frequently in certain strains of laboratory rats (DeLellis *et al.*, 1977). In bulls and humans pheochromocytomas often develop concurrently with calcitonin-secreting C-cell tumors of the thyroid gland (Black *et al.*, 1973b; Khairi *et al.*, 1975; Sipple, 1961; Sponenberg and

McEntee, 1983; Voelkel *et al.*, 1973). This appears to represent a neoplastic transformation of multiple types of endocrine cells of neuroectodermal origin in the same individual. Most affected animals are 6 years of age or more. Boxers appear to be the breed of dogs that are most predisposed to develop pheochromocytomas (Howard and Nielsen, 1965).

**Clinical Characteristics.** Functional pheochromocytomas have been reported infrequently in animals. Tachycardia, edema, and cardiac hypertrophy observed in several dogs and horses with pheochromocytomas were attributed to excessive catecholamine secretion (Dahme and Schlemmer, 1959; Howard and Nielsen, 1965). Ojemann (1941) reported arteriolar sclerosis and widespread medial hyperplasia of arterioles in dogs with pheochromocytomas that were associated with clinical signs suggestive of paroxysmal hypertension.

Norepinephrine is the principal catecholamine extracted from pheochromocytomas in dogs (Head and West, 1958; Müller *et al.*, 1955). This is similar to normal pups, where norepinephrine is the predominant catecholamine in the adrenal medulla, but is the reverse in adult dogs, where more epinephrine is present. Yarrington and Capen (1975, 1981) found that the catecholamine content in pheochromocytomas from bulls with concurrent C-cell tumors of the thyroid gland was higher than in the normal adrenal medulla. Urinary excretion of vanillylmandelic acid and free unconjugated catecholamines was elevated in bulls with pheochromocytomas.

Many of these tumors in animals are found as incidental findings at necropsy. They are often large and invade into the posterior vena cava forming an extensive tumor cell thrombus (fig. 13.14A). The vena cava is greatly distended and partially occluded by the thrombus leading to impaired venous return from the posterior extremities (fig. 13.14B). Large and vascular pheochromocytomas with invasion of the posterior vena cava may undergo extensive hemorrhage and form a blood-filled cyst near the kidney in horses (Yovich and Ducharme, 1983).

**Gross Morphology.** Pheochromocytomas are tumors of chromaffin cells and are almost always located in the adrenal gland of animals, although a few extraadrenal tumors have been found along the posterior aorta and vena cava in sites analogous with the organ of Zuckerkandl in humans (How-

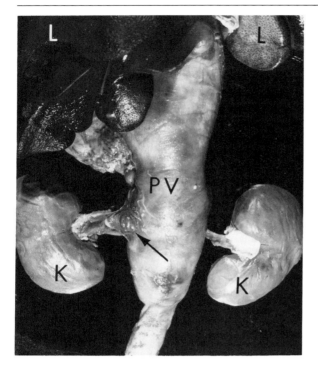

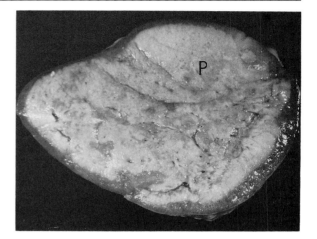

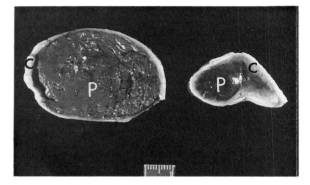

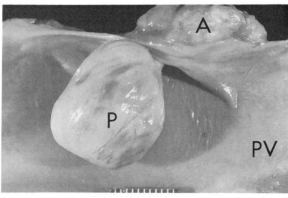

A|C
B|D
**FIGURE 13.14.** Pheochromocytoma. A Neoplasm in adrenal medulla (**arrow**) of a dog. The posterior vena cava (PV) is greatly distended due to invasion through the vessel wall and formation of a large tumor cell thrombus. Chronic passive congestion is evident in the liver (L) (K is kidney) (scale is 1 cm). B. Pheochromocytoma (P) extending from the region of the adrenal gland (A) to the wall of the posterior vena cava (PV) and forming a tumor cell thrombus in the lumen (scale is 1 cm). C. Pheochromocytoma (P) in adrenal medulla from a bull that also had a C-cell tumor of the thyroid. The surrounding adrenal cortex is thin and compressed by the expanding tumor in the medulla. D. Chromaffin positive reaction in bilateral pheochromocytomas (P) in the bovine adrenal gland. The surrounding cortex (C) is compressed to varying degrees (scale is 1 cm).

ard and Nielsen, 1965). They usually are unilateral and infrequently bilateral. Although size varies considerably, pheochromocytomas are often large (10 cm or more in diameter) and incorporate the majority of the affected adrenal. A small remnant of the adrenal gland usually can be found at one pole. Smaller tumors are completely surrounded by a thin compressed rim of adrenal cortex (fig. 13.14C).

Large pheochromocytomas are multilobular and variegated light brown to yellowish red due to areas of hemorrhage and necrosis. A valuable aid in macroscopic diagnosis of pheochromocytoma is the Henle chromoreaction with either potassium dichromate or iodate (fig. 13.14D). Application of Zenker's solution to the flat cut surface of a freshly sectioned tumor results in oxidation of catecholamines, forming a dark brown pigment within 5 to 20 minutes.

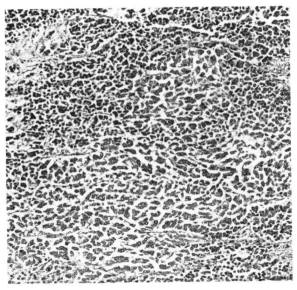

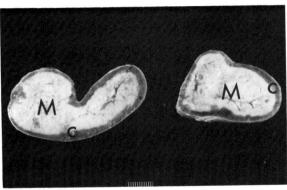

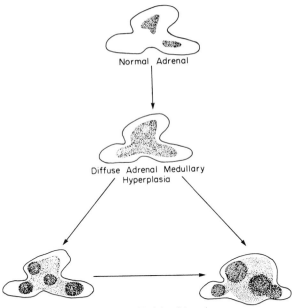

A|B
C| **FIGURE 13.15.** Adrenal medullary hyperplasia. A. Pheochromocytoma of a dog. Groups of small and large tumor cells are arranged along vascular sinusoids. The adrenal cortex (top) is compressed. B. Histogenesis of pheochromocytoma from diffuse and/or nodular adrenal medullary hyperplasia in humans with thyroid C-cell neoplasms. C. Bilateral diffuse hyperplasia of adrenal medulla in a bull with a concomitant C-cell carcinoma of the thyroid gland. The expanded adrenal medulla (M) compresses the surrounding adrenal cortex (C) (scale is 1 cm). (A, courtesy of DeLellis *et al.* [1976] and *Amer. J. Path.*; B, from Yarrington and Capen [1981] and courtesy of *Vet. Path.*)

Malignant pheochromocytomas have a thin fibrous capsule that is invaded at several points. They exert pressure on the posterior vena cava or infiltrate the vessel forming a tumor cell thrombus.

**Histological Features.** Tumor cells in pheochromocytomas vary from small cuboidal or polyhedral cells, similar to those in normal adrenal medulla, to large pleomorphic cells with multiple hyperchromatic nuclei. The cytoplasmic area is lightly eosinophilic, finely granular, and often indistinct because of early onset of autolysis in adrenal medullary tissue. Tumor cells are characteristically subdivided into small lobules by fine connective tissue septa and capillaries (fig. 13.15A). Vascular sinusoids may be lined directly by polyhedral to spindle-shaped tumor cells. Primary fixation with potassium dichromate (e.g., Zenker's solution) gives a positive chromaffin reaction and a brown granular

appearance to the cytoplasm of tumor cells. This chromaffin reaction is helpful in distinguishing anaplastic pheochromocytomas from adrenal cortical carcinomas.

The term *pheochromoblastoma* has been used to designate poorly differentiated anaplastic tumors of catecholamine-secreting cells in the adrenal medulla. *Malignant pheochromocytoma* often is used to designate medullary tumors that invade through the adrenal capsule and into adjacent structures (e.g., posterior vena cava and periadrenal fat) and/or metastasize to distant sites (e.g., liver, regional lymph nodes, or lungs). Multiple areas of coagulation necrosis and hemorrhage are often present in larger malignant pheochromocytomas. The neoplastic cells completely incorporate the medulla of the affected adrenal, invade most or all of the surrounding cortex, and often penetrate the adrenal capsule.

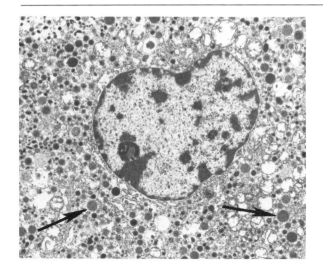 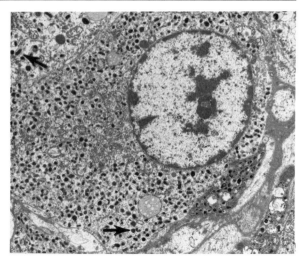

A|B  **FIGURE 13.16.** Ultrastructure of pheochromocytoma. A. Norepinephrine-secreting cell in pheochromocytoma from a bull in storage phase. Secretory granules have a wide space (**arrows**) between the core and limiting membrane. B. Epinephrine-secreting cell in storage phase from a pheochromocytoma of a bull. Secretion granules (**arrows**) are less dense and have a narrow submembranous space. Cytoplasmic organelles are poorly developed.

Evidence is common for invasion into adrenal sinusoids and lymphatics and the formation of distinct tumor cell emboli. The pattern of arrangement of neoplastic cells varies between different areas of the malignant pheochromocytoma, but includes small lobules, solid sheets, and palisading along blood sinusoids. Neoplastic cells tend to be larger and more pleomorphic (polyhedral and spindle shaped) and tend to have more frequent mitotic figures than those of more benign pheochromocytomas.

Diffuse or nodular adrenal medullary hyperplasia appears to precede the development of pheochromocytoma in bulls, laboratory rats, and humans with C-cell tumors of the thyroid gland (fig. 13.15B) (Carney *et al.*, 1975; DeLellis *et al.*, 1976; Yarrington and Capen, 1975, 1981). Medullary hyperplasia is detected by an increased total adrenal weight, a decrease in corticomedullary ratio (fig. 13.15C) due to an increase in the size and number of medullary cells, and the presence of frequent mitotic figures in the adrenal medulla.

Neuroblastomas are differentiated from pheochromocytomas by being composed of small tumor cells with a hyperchromatic nucleus and a scant amount of cytoplasm. They often resemble lymphocytes and tend to form pseudorosettes. Neurofibrils or unmyelinated nerve fibers can be demonstrated in neuroblastomas.

Ganglioneuromas are small benign tumors in the medulla composed of multipolar ganglion cells and neurofibrils with a prominent fibrous connective tissue stroma. Neoplastic cells in medullary tumors occasionally differentiate in two directions, resulting in adjacent pheochromocytomas and ganglioneuromas in the same adrenal gland.

**Ultrastructural Characteristics.** Pheochromocytomas are composed of either epinephrine-secreting cells, norepinephrine-secreting cells, or both (Lauper *et al.*, 1972; Yarrington and Capen, 1975, 1981). The principal distinguishing feature between these two populations of medullary cells is in the fine structure of their secretory granules. Pheochromocytomas from which norepinephrine is the principal catecholamine extracted are composed of cells of the type illustrated in figure 13.16A. The secretory granules have an eccentrically situated electron-dense core that is surrounded by a wide submembranous space. When

functional thyroid tumors have been described by Rijnberk (1971) and Rijnberk and der Kinderen (1969). Polyuria is the most consistent finding, but other common clinical signs are weight loss, polyphagia, weakness and fatigue, intolerance to heat, and nervousness. A dog described by Reid *et al.* (1963) with a functional thyroid adenocarcinoma had a mitral valve insufficiency that improved markedly following surgical excision of the tumor. Other dogs with bilateral thyroid carcinoma have destruction of both thyroid lobes leading to clinical evidence of hypothyroidism with hypercholesterolemia and corneal lipidosis (Harrington and Kelly, 1980).

### Gross Morphology

*Thyroid Adenoma*—Adenomas are usually white to tan, small, solid nodules that are well-demarcated from the adjacent thyroid parenchyma. The affected thyroid lobe is only moderately enlarged and distorted. A distinct, white, fibrous connective capsule of variable thickness separates the adenoma from the compressed parenchyma (fig. 13.18A). Only a single adenoma is usually present in a thyroid lobe.

Other thyroid adenomas are composed of thin-walled cysts filled with a yellow to red fluid (fig. 13.18B). The external surface is smooth and covered by an extensive network of blood vessels. Small masses of neoplastic tissue remain in the wall and form rugose projections into the cyst lumen. The thyroid parenchyma of the affected lobe may be completely obliterated.

*Thyroid Carcinoma*—Carcinomas are larger than adenomas, are coarsely multinodular, and often have large areas of hemorrhage and necrosis near their centers. Unilateral involvement by thyroid carcinoma is about twice as frequent in dogs as involvement of both thyroid lobes (fig. 13.18C) (Lindsay and MacLeod, 1910). Carcinomas are poorly encapsulated and invade locally into the wall of the trachea, cervical muscles, esophagus, larynx, nerves, and vessels (McClelland, 1941). Early invasion into branches of the cranial and caudal thyroid veins, with the formation of tumor cell thrombi (fig. 13.19), leads to multiple pulmonary metastases, often before involvement of the retropharyngeal and caudal cervical lymph nodes. White, gritty focal areas of mineralization or bone formation are scattered throughout a few thyroid carcinomas.

Although adenomas and carcinomas derived

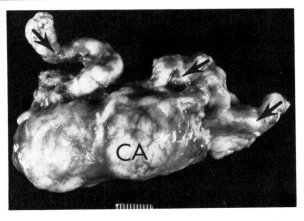

**FIGURE 13.19.** Prominent tumor cell thrombi distending thyroid veins (**arrows**) of a dog with an adenocarcinoma (CA) derived from thyroid follicular cells (scale is 1 cm).

from follicular cells usually arise in the neck from the thyroid lobes, they may develop from ectopic thyroid parenchyma in the mediastinum and must be included in the differential diagnosis of "heart base tumors" in dogs (Cheville, 1972; Walsh and Diters, 1984). Stephens *et al.* (1982) reported an ectopic thyroid carcinoma arising at the base of the heart in a dog that was invasive and metastasized to lung, pancreas, and kidney. The neoplastic cells ultrastructurally formed intra- or intercellular lumens with microvillar projections and contained large lysosomes and arrays of rough endoplasmic reticulum.

### Histological Features

*Thyroid Adenoma*—The adenomas are classified into follicular and papillary types. They are sharply demarcated and encapsulated from the adjacent compressed thyroid parenchyma by a fibrous capsule of varying thickness. Adenomas derived from follicular cells that retain the ability to form follicles, according to one of several patterns, are by far more common than papillary adenomas in animals (fig. 13.20A). Each follicular adenoma tends to have a consistent growth pattern within itself.

There are several different patterns of growth for follicles similar to those of the normal thyroid for the species involved. Microfollicular adenomas consist of tumor cells arranged in miniature follicles with small amounts of colloid or an absence of col-

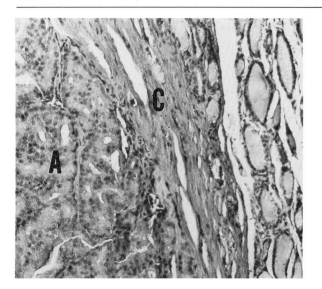

A
B

**FIGURE 13.20.** Thyroid adenoma. A. Follicular adenoma (A) from a horse with a prominent fibrous capsule (C) separating it from the adjacent compressed thyroid parenchyma (T). B. Functional adenoma of the cat. The neoplastic cells are arranged into a follicle with numerous long cytoplasmic processes (P) extending from the luminal surface to engulf colloid by endocytosis. There are many large lysosomal (L) bodies in follicular cells associated with colloid droplets (C) and long microvilli (**arrows**) on the surface bordering the colloid. Profiles of rough endoplasmic reticulum (E) often are dilated by a finely granular material (N is nucleus of follicular cell).

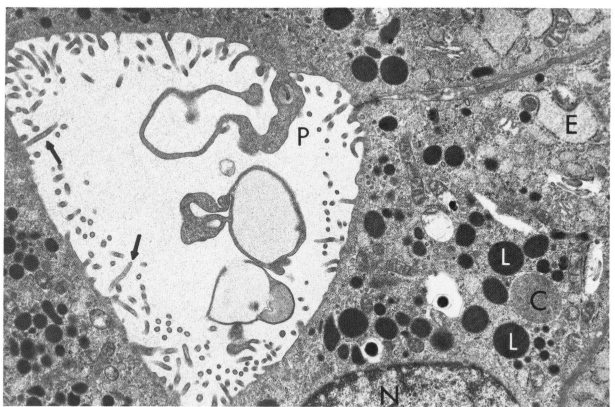

loid. Macrofollicular adenomas are formed by large, irregularly shaped follicles that are greatly distended with colloid and lined by flattened follicular cells. There may be extensive hemorrhage and desquamation of follicular cells into the lumens of the distended follicles.

Cystic adenomas consist of one or two large cavities filled with proteinic fluid, necrotic debris, and erythrocytes. Focal accumulations of tumor cells, forming either follicles or solid nests, are present in the capsule of dense fibrous connective tissue. These adenomas may develop by progressive cystic degeneration of one of the several types of follicular adenomas. Oxyphilic adenomas are composed predominantly or entirely of large cells with a densely eosinophilic granular cytoplasm arranged in indistinct follicles with little or no colloid formation. Oxyphilic (Hürthle) cells appear to be metabolically altered follicular cells that accumulate abnormally large numbers of mitochondria in their cytoplasm (Valenta *et al.*, 1974). Trabecular adenomas are the most poorly differentiated of the follicular type. The tumor cells are small and arranged in narrow columns separated by an edematous fibrous stroma. There is little evidence of follicle formation.

Papillary adenomas are recognized infrequently in most animal species. Columnar or cuboidal follicular cells are arranged in a single layer around a thin vascular connective tissue stalk. These papillary projections extend into the lumens of cystic spaces of various sizes. The cysts contain desquamated tumor cells, colloid, erythrocytes, and occasionally laminated foci of mineralization resembling psammoma bodies.

Thyroid adenomas in cats usually appear as solitary, soft nodules that enlarge and distort the contour of the affected lobe. A thin, fibrous connective tissue capsule separates the adenoma from the adjacent, often compressed, thyroid parenchyma. The neoplastic cells tend to form irregularly shaped follicles with occasional papillary infoldings of epithelium and variable amounts of colloid. Focal areas of necrosis, mineralization, and cystic degeneration are present in larger adenomas. Multiple sections of adenomas fail to reveal histological evidence of either vascular or capsular invasion by tumor cells.

Thyroid adenomas also must be differentiated from multinodular ("adenomatous") hyperplasia ("goiter") that occurs in old cats. These multiple areas of thyroid hyperplasia usually are microscopic and do not enlarge the affected lobe of thyroid. In contrast to adenomas, the areas of nodular hyperplasia are not encapsulated and adjacent thyroid parenchyma is not compressed. Histopathologically, the hyperplastic nodules are composed of irregularly shaped, colloid-filled follicles lined by cuboidal follicular cells.

Functional thyroid adenomas in cats associated with a clinical syndrome of hyperthyroidism are composed of cuboidal to columnar follicular cells that form follicles of varying sizes and shapes. The follicles usually are partially collapsed and contain little colloid because of the intense endocytotic activity of neoplastic follicular cells. Long cytoplasmic projections often extend from the follicular cells into the lumen to phagocytize colloid (fig. 13.20B). As a result of the marked endocytotic activity, numerous colloid droplets are present in the apical cytoplasm of follicular cells in close proximity to the many electron-dense lysosomal bodies.

Functional thyroid adenomas are partially or completely separated from remnants of the adjacent "normal" thyroid by a fine connective tissue capsule. Follicles in the rim of "normal" thyroid around a functional adenoma are enlarged and distended by an accumulation of colloid. The follicular cells are low cuboidal and atrophied, with little evidence of endocytotic activity in response to the elevated levels of thyroid hormones.

The opposite thyroid lobe should be carefully evaluated in cats with solitary adenomas for evidence of focal hyperplasia or "microadenomas." In the author's experience, the opposite thyroid lobe in cats with unilateral functional adenoma often has discrete, small areas of multinodular hyperplasia of follicular cells that cause recurrence of hyperthyroidism several months to a year or more after surgical removal of the tumor.

*Thyroid Carcinoma*—Malignant tumors of thyroid follicular cells are generally more highly cellular and have a greater degree of cellular pleomorphism than adenomas. Thompson *et al.* (1980) found a good correlation between fine needle aspiration cytology and histopathological evaluation of thyroid biopsies in the diagnosis of thyroid carcinomas in dogs. On the basis of the predominant histological pattern of growth, "differentiated" thyroid carcinomas are subdivided into follicu-

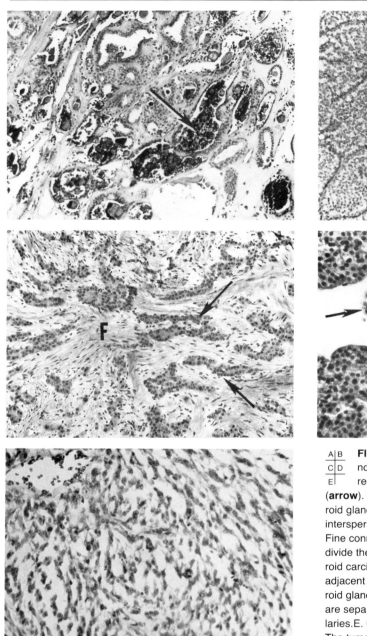

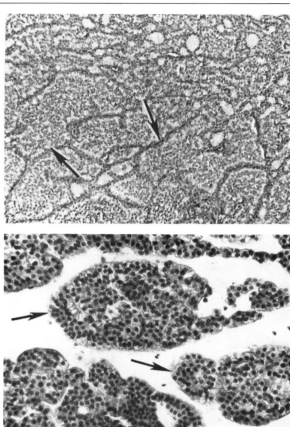

**FIGURE 13.21.** Thyroid carcinoma. A. Follicular adenocarcinoma in the thyroid gland of the dog. Many irregular follicules are filled with mineralized colloid (**arrow**). B. Follicular–compact-cellular carcinoma of the thyroid gland from a dog. Small colloid-containing follicles are interspersed between compact aggregations of tumor cells. Fine connective tissue septa with capillaries (**arrows**) subdivide the carcinoma into small lobules. C. Invasion of thyroid carcinoma (**arrows**) through the fibrous capsule (F) into adjacent tissues in a dog. D. Small cell carcinoma in the thyroid gland of a dog. Clusters of small tumor cells (**arrows**) are separated by an edematous fibrous stroma with capillaries. E. Giant cell carcinoma in the thyroid gland of a dog. The tumor cells are spindle shaped and there is a lack of follicle formation.

lar, papillary, and compact cellular (solid) types (Leav *et al.*, 1976; Meissner and Warren, 1969). In dogs, where thyroid carcinomas are seen most frequently, they often have both a follicular and compact-cellular growth pattern, whereas papillary carcinomas are rare. Papillary carcinoma is the most common type of thyroid carcinoma in humans (Meissner and Warren, 1969).

Follicular adenocarcinomas are diagnosed when the majority of tumor cells are arranged in a recognizable follicular pattern. It is possible to subdivide follicular carcinomas further on the basis of degree of follicle formation, as described for follicular adenomas, but that often is difficult because of the admixture of growth patterns present in any one tumor. Such subdivision is of little prognostic value. The tumor cells are tall cuboidal to columnar and form follicles of varying size, shape, and colloid content. Mitotic activity in the tumor cells is minimal. The colloid in follicular lumens occasionally is clumped and extensively mineralized (fig. 13.21A).

In compact-cellular carcinoma, tumor cells form compact aggregations or solid sheets of cells often separated by a fibrous stroma with little or no attempts at follicle formation and colloid secretion. The polyhedral cells are closely arranged and have an eosinophilic cytoplasm that is finely granulated or vacuolated. Immunocytochemical and ultrastructural studies (Leav *et al.*, 1976) have demonstrated that compact-cellular (solid) carcinomas are derived from follicular cells of the canine thyroid and not from C-cells as suggested by Williams *et al.* (1966). Moore *et al.* (1984) demonstrated thyroglobulin immunoreactivity by the peroxidase—antiperoxidase technique, but not calcitonin positive cells in compact-cellular thyroid tumors of dogs. The major patterns of thyroglobulin immunoreactivity included diffuse cytoplasmic staining, apical staining of the border of follicular lumens, intracytoplasmic droplets, and staining of colloid in the follicular lumens. The stroma has bands of fibrous connective tissue of varying thickness, but does not contain amyloid as reported in C-cell (medullary) carcinomas of the thyroid.

Schneider and Leav (1977) reported that compact-cellular carcinomas in the thyroid of dogs responded to thyrotropin (TSH) by increased phosphatide turnover, especially phosphatidic acid and phosphatidylinositol. The malignant tumor cells appeared to retain at least one complete control system from TSH receptors to the final metabolic product.

Follicular—compact-cellular carcinoma, which has approximately equal follicular and compact-cellular (solid) growth patterns, is the most common histological type of malignant thyroid tumor in dogs (fig. 13.21B). The follicles formed are often smaller and contain less colloid than in pure follicular carcinoma. The tumor cells arranged in compact nests appear to be morphologically and functionally less differentiated than those that form follicles and secrete colloid.

Papillary carcinomas, in which tumor cells form predominantly papillae extending into cystic spaces, are rare in animals in contrast to their frequent occurrence in humans. Single or multiple layers of cuboidal cells surround fibrovascular stalks that project into cystic spaces. Their nuclei are vesicular and pleomorphic, with prominent nucleoli. The nuclear vacuoles seen by light microscopy have been shown by electron microscopy to represent cytoplasmic evaginations into the nucleus (Gould *et al.*, 1972). Other areas of papillary thyroid tumors may form small follicles or solid sheets.

Infiltration of tumor cells through the fibrous connective tissue capsule (fig. 13.21C) and into adjacent tissues is frequent in thyroid carcinomas of dogs. The early formation of tumor cell emboli by invasion of thin-walled veins results in pulmonary metastasis in dogs prior to the development of secondary foci of growth in lymph nodes draining the affected thyroid lobe (Bartlett, 1914).

Undifferentiated thyroid carcinomas lack a characteristic architectural pattern of arrangement of tumor cells. They are an uncommon form of thyroid carcinoma in animals (Anderson and Capen, 1986).

Small cell carcinoma is one type of undifferentiated thyroid carcinoma. It is composed of highly malignant follicular cells with either a diffuse or compact pattern of growth. The small tumor cells are uniform in appearance and are closely packed together in clusters separated by a fibrous stroma (fig. 13.21D). The scant cytoplasm is eosinophilic and the oval nucleus is densely hyperchromatic. Mitotic figures are frequent.

Giant cell carcinoma is the second type of undifferentiated thyroid carcinoma. It is a highly malignant tumor and derived from poorly differentiated thyroid follicular cells. The anaplastic tumor cells are large, pleomorphic, and often spindle shaped, making a differentiation from fibrosarcoma difficult (fig. 13.21E) (Forman and Reed, 1917; Patnaik and Lieberman, 1979). Bustad *et al.* (1957) and Marks *et al.* (1957) reported a metastasizing fibrosarcoma in the thyroid gland of a sheep that had received 5 microcuries of radioactive iodine ($^{131}$I) for 53 months beginning at weaning. The demonstration of identifiable epithelial structures may require multiple sections from several areas of the tumor. Ultrastructural studies of giant cell carcinomas from humans have demonstrated microvilli, numerous dense bodies, and other nuclear and cytoplasmic characteristics similar to those of follicular cells (Fisher *et al.*, 1974; Graham and Daniel, 1974). Follicular remnants and transitional forms suggest that giant cell carcinomas are derived from thyroid follicular cells (Gaal *et al.*, 1975; Jao and Gould, 1975).

Malignant mixed thyroid tumors have been reported in the dog (Buergelt, 1968; Johnson and Patterson, 1981; Mason and Wells, 1929). The tumors contain both malignant thyroid follicular cells and malignant mesenchymal elements, usually osteogenic or cartilaginous (Clark and Meier, 1958; Ewald, 1915; Ruddick and Willis, 1938; Schlumberger, 1955).

An interesting case of bilateral thyroid neoplasms in a dog (follicular–compact-cellular on the left and malignant mixed tumor on the right) reported by Johnson and Patterson (1981) was accompanied by severe multifocal myxedema but a low normal serum thyroxine level. There was a marked accumulation of glycosaminoglycans, particularly hyaluronic acid leading to increased water-binding capacity in the dermis and subcutis over the head, footpads, elbows, and elsewhere.

Thyroid carcinomas occur less frequently in cats than either adenoma or multinodular hyperplasia of follicular cells. They often result in considerable enlargement of one or both thyroid lobes and may invade adjacent structures. Carcinomas are characterized by the invasion of vessels and the connective tissue capsule by neoplastic cells. Metastases to regional lymph nodes (retropharyngeal, mandibular, and deep cervical) and distant sites have been reported in less than 50% of thyroid carcinomas in cats (Leav *et al.*, 1976). The well-differentiated thyroid carcinomas are relatively solid and composed of a uniform pattern of small follicles containing little colloid and occasional compact cellular areas. Strands of dense connective tissue, with an abundant capillary network and foci of lymphocytes, subdivide the neoplastic cells into small lobules.

**Growth and Metastasis.** Thyroid adenomas grow slowly, only occasionally resulting in a palpable enlargement that is detected clinically in the anterior cervical region. Thyroid carcinomas are larger and more frequently produce a palpable enlargement and respiratory distress that is apparent clinically. Leav *et al.* (1976) reported that the probability of metastasis increases in proportion to the size and duration of the thyroid carcinoma. For example, metastases were found in only 14% of dogs with carcinoma when the tumor volume was less than 21 ml, but they were found in 78% when the tumor was larger than 21 ml. Therefore, it appears that early surgical removal of thyroid carcinomas before they attain a large size is critical for long-term survival. Pure follicular carcinomas in dogs appear to enlarge more rapidly than those with a compact cellular (solid) component. Radioisotope imaging has proven useful in determining the extent of local tissue involvement by a thyroid carcinoma (Branam *et al.*, 1982).

Carcinomas often grow rapidly, invade adjacent structures such as the trachea, esophagus, and larynx, and usually are fixed in position. Leav *et al.* (1976) reported metastasis in 38% of dogs with thyroid carcinomas, and other studies have found an even higher incidence (Brodey and Kelly, 1968). The earliest and most frequent site of metastasis is the lung because thyroid carcinomas tend to invade branches of the thyroid vein. Tumor cell emboli may be palpated in the thyroid or jugular veins in some dogs with thyroid carcinoma (fig. 13.19) (Brodey and Kelly, 1968). The retropharyngeal and caudal cervical lymph nodes are less frequent sites of tumor metastasis. Although metastasis of thyroid carcinoma to bone is rare in the dog, Krook *et al.* (1960) reported a case that spread to the skull bones, resulting in focal osteolysis and hypercalcemia that was clinically suggestive of a functional parathyroid tumor.

Thyroid carcinomas are less frequent in cats than in dogs. Metastases have been detected in approximately 40% of the cases studied (Clark and Meier, 1958; Holzworth *et al.*, 1955; Johnson and Osborne, 1970; Leav *et al.*, 1976; Lucke, 1964; Nielsen, 1964; Whitehead, 1967).

Canine thyroid carcinoma has been successfully transplanted to puppies treated with total body irradiation and nitrogen mustard (Allam *et al.*, 1954, 1957). Kasza (1964) established a thyroid carcinoma cell line of canine origin that had a regular growth pattern after 50 passages.

## Hyperplasia of Thyroid Follicular Cells

**Incidence.** Nonneoplastic and noninflammatory enlargement of the thyroid can develop in all domestic mammals, birds, and submammalian vertebrates from one of several pathogenic mechanisms. Certain forms of thyroid hyperplasia may present problems in differentiation from adenomas (Cubillos *et al.*, 1981). Iodine deficiency causing diffuse thyroid hyperplasia was common in certain enzootic goitrogenic areas throughout the world before the widespread addition of iodized salt to animal diets (Matthew and Thomas, 1935; Quinlan, 1928). Although iodine-deficient goiter still occurs worldwide in domestic animals, the outbreaks are sporadic and fewer animals are affected than prior to the widespread use of iodized salt. Young animals born to dams on iodine-deficient diets are more likely to develop severe thyroid hyperplasia and have clinical evidence of hypothyroidism. Offspring of iodine-deficient mothers may be stillborn or aborted late in pregnancy. Of the animals born alive, some are weak and partly hairless with subcutaneous edema of the head and neck.

Certain goitrogenic substances that interfere with thyroxinogenesis may precipitate the development of hyperplastic goiter in animals on a diet that is marginally iodine deficient. These substances include thiouracil, sulfonamides, anions of the Hofmeister series, and a number of plants from the genus *Brassica*. Isolated outbreaks of hyperplastic goiter develop in calves, lambs, kids, and pups as a consequence of an inability to synthesize thyroglobulin or an enzyme defect in the biosynthesis of the thyroxine by follicular cells (Falconer, 1966; Rac *et al.*, 1968; Theron and van Jaarsveld, 1972*a*, *b*; van Jaarsveld *et al.*, 1976).

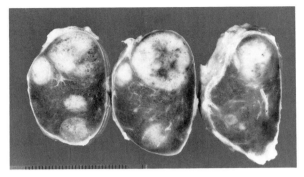

**FIGURE 13.22.** Multifocal hyperplasia of thyroid follicular cells ("nodular goiter") in an old horse. The light tan nodules of hyperplasia are not encapsulated and there is minimal compression of the adjacent thyroid parenchyma.

Although seemingly paradoxical, an excess of iodide in the diet can also result in thyroid hyperplasia in animals and humans. Foals of mares fed dry seaweed containing excessive iodide may develop thyroid hyperplasia and clinically evident goiter (Baker and Lindsey, 1968). The thyroid glands of the foal are exposed to higher blood iodide levels than the mare because of concentration of iodide first by the placenta and subsequently by the mammary gland. High blood iodide interferes with one or more steps of thyroxinogenesis (especially proteolytic cleavage of thyroid hormones from thyroglobulin), leading to lowered blood thyroxine levels and a compensatory increase in pituitary thyrotropin secretion (Wolff, 1969).

**Gross Morphology.** Nodular hyperplasia ("goiter") in thyroid glands of old horses appears as multiple white to tan nodules of varying size (fig. 13.22). The affected lobes are moderately enlarged and irregular in contour. In contrast to thyroid adenomas, the areas of nodular hyperplasia are not encapsulated and result in minimal compression of adjacent parenchyma.

Both lateral lobes and the isthmus of the thyroid in ruminants are uniformly enlarged in young animals with diffuse hyperplastic goiter associated with iodine deficiency. The enlargements may be extensive in severe cases and result in palpable swellings in the anterior cervical area. The affected lobes are firm and dark red because an extensive interfollicular capillary network develops under the influence of long-term thyrotropin stimulation.

Colloid goiter represents the involutionary phase of diffuse hyperplastic goiter in young adult to adult animals. Both thyroid lobes are diffusely enlarged but are more translucent. The differences in macroscopic appearance are the result of a lower degree of vascularity in colloid goiter and the development of macrofollicles due to involution and distention of follicles by colloid.

**Histological Features.** Nodular goiter consists of multiple foci of hyperplastic follicular cells that are sharply demarcated but not encapsulated from the adjacent thyroid. The microscopic appearance within a nodule is variable. Some hyperplastic cells form small follicles with little or no colloid. Other nodules are formed by larger irregularly shaped follicles lined by one or more layers of columnar cells that may form papillary projections into the lumen. Some of these follicles are involuted and filled with densely eosinophilic colloid. These changes appear to be the result of alternating periods of hyperplasia and colloid involution in the thyroid glands of old animals. The areas of nodular hyperplasia may be microscopic (as in old cats) or grossly visible causing asymmetrical enlargement of the thyroid (as in old horses).

The histological changes in diffuse hyperplastic and colloid goiters are more consistent throughout the diffusely enlarged thyroid lobes and essentially similar in all animal species (Marine and Lenhart, 1909; Schlumberger, 1955). The follicles are irregular in size and shape in hyperplastic goiter because of varying amounts of lightly eosinophilic and vacuolated colloid in the lumen. Some larger follicles are collapsed from lack of colloid. The lining epithelial cells are columnar with a deeply eosinophilic cytoplasm and small hyperchromatic nuclei that are often situated in the basilar part of the cell. The follicles are lined by single or multiple layers of hyperplastic follicular cells that in some follicles may form papillary projections into the lumen. Similar proliferative changes are present in ectopic thyroid parenchyma in the neck or mediastinum of certain species.

Colloid goiter represents the involutionary phase of diffuse thyroid hyperplasia, which may develop either after sufficient amounts of iodide have been added to the diet or after the requirements for thyroxine have diminished in an older animal (Marine,

1928). Blood thyroxine levels return to normal, and the secretion of thyrotropin by the pituitary gland is correspondingly decreased. Follicles are progressively distended with densely eosinophilic colloid because of diminished thyrotropin-induced endocytosis. The follicular cells lining the macrofollicles are flattened and atrophic. The interface between the colloid and luminal surface of follicular cells is smooth and lacks the characteristic endocytotic vacuoles of actively secreting cells. Interfollicular capillaries are less well-developed than with diffuse hyperplastic goiter.

## TUMORS OF THYROGLOSSAL DUCT REMNANTS

**Incidence.** Tumors arising in cystic remnants of the thyroglossal duct are rare in animals, but have been encountered in the dog (Harkema et al., 1984).

The canine thyroid originates as a thickened plate of epithelium in the floor of the pharynx. It is intimately related to the aortic sac in its development, and this association leads to the frequent occurrence of accessory thyroid parenchyma in the mediastinum of the adult dog, which may undergo neoplastic transformation (Cheville, 1972; Godwin, 1936; Kameda, 1972; Thake et al., 1971). Branched cell cords develop from the pharyngeal plate and migrate dorsolaterally, but remain attached to the pharyngeal area by the narrow thyroglossal duct. A portion of the thyroglossal duct may persist postnatally and form a cyst because of the accumulation of proteinic material secreted by the lining epithelium. Thyroglossal duct cysts are present in the ventral aspect of the anterior cervical region in dogs. Their lining epithelium may undergo neoplastic transformation and give rise to papillary carcinomas.

**Gross Morphology.** Tumors of thyroglossal duct remnants appear as well-circumscribed, fluctuant, movable enlargements (approximately 2 to 4 cm in diameter) on the ventral midline in the anterior cervical region. The clinical history usually indicates a slowly progressive expansion of the cervical mass. On cross section they have multilocular cystic areas containing a translucent proteinic fluid alternating with white solid areas (fig. 13.23A).

The thyroid glands appear to be normal in the

few cases studied in the dog. These tumors develop *de novo* from the epithelium of the thyroglossal duct and are not a cystic metastasis from a primary carcinoma in the thyroid gland.

**Histological Features, Growth, and Metastasis.** The tumors appear as well-differentiated papillary carcinomas. Multiple papillary outgrowths, covered by several layers of tall cuboidal to columnar epithelial cells, extend from the cyst wall into the lumen (fig. 13.23B) The lining of the cyst may undergo squamous metaplasia to form a keratinizing epithelium (Harkema *et al.*, 1984). The cyst wall is composed of dense fibrous connective tissue with focal areas of hemorrhage and cholesterol clefts. Aggregations of thyroidogenetic epithelium in the form of small follicles and cell cords are present within the fibrous capsule and in the surrounding connective tissue. These follicles are lined by a low cuboidal epithelium and contain variable amounts of colloid.

Carcinomas of thyroglossal duct remnants are well-differentiated and slow growing. They infrequently recur following complete surgical resection of the multilocular cyst and adjacent tissue.

## Thyroid C-Cell (Ultimobranchial) Tumors

**Incidence.** Tumors derived from C-cells (parafollicular cells) of the thyroid gland are encountered most frequently in adult to aged bulls (Capen and Black, 1974; Krook *et al.*, 1969), certain strains of laboratory rats (Boorman *et al.*, 1972; Lindsay *et al.*, 1968; Thompson and Hunt, 1963), adult to aged horses (Hillidge *et al.*, 1982; Turk *et al.*, 1983), but infrequently in other domestic species (Leav *et al.*, 1976; Wadsworth *et al.*, 1981). Jubb and McEntee (1959) reported that approximately 30% of aged bulls had C-cell neoplasms and an additional 15 to 20% had hyperplasia of C-cells and ultimobranchial derivatives. These frequently occurring hyperplastic and neoplastic changes in C-cells have been observed often in bulls and rarely in cows. McEntee *et al.* (1980) reported a progressive increase in the incidence of thyroid C-cell tumors with advancing age in bulls. This coincided with an increase in the development of vertebral osteophytes (table 13.1).

The high incidence of C-cell tumors in bulls differs from the situation in humans in which medul-

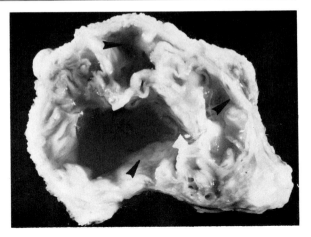

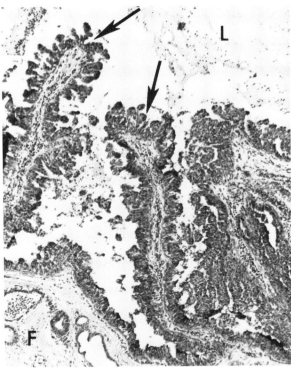

A
—
B

**FIGURE 13.23.** Tumors of thyroglossal duct remnants. A. Carcinoma in the thyroglossal duct remnants of a dog. The multicystic tumor (**arrowheads**) was removed from the ventral midline of the anterior cervical region. B. Papillary carcinoma of thyroglossal duct remnants from a dog. Papillary outgrowths covered with multiple layers of tall cuboidal to columnar cells (**arrows**) project from the fibrous capsule (F) into the cyst lumen (L).

**TABLE 13.1. Vertebral Osteophytosis and C-Cell Tumors Related to Age**[a]

| Age (years) | No. of bulls | C-cell tumors | Osteophytosis | Vertebral fractures |
|---|---|---|---|---|
| 5 to 8 | 469 | 52 (11.1%)[b] | 100 (21.3%)[b] | 2 (0.4%)[b] |
| 8 to 11 | 162 | 48 (29.6%) | 79 (48.8%) | 11 (6.7%) |
| 11 to 14 | 119 | 52 (43.7%) | 62 (52.1%) | 6 (5.0%) |
| 14 to 18 | 32 | 21 (65.6%) | 22 (68.8%) | 4 (12.5%) |
| TOTAL | 782 | 173 (22.1%) | 263 (33.6%) | 23 (2.9%) |

[a] From McEntee *et al.* (1980).
[b] Percentages of total number of bulls in each age group with that particular malady.

lary carcinoma accounts for only 6 to 10% of all thyroid tumors (Hill *et al.*, 1973). The development of C-cell tumors in both humans and bulls is preceded by a multifocal C-cell hyperplasia (Wolfe *et al.*, 1973). Medullary carcinoma in humans is the only type of thyroid tumor known to have a genetic basis, and it appears to be transmitted as an autosomal dominant trait in certain families (Melvin *et al.*, 1972).

The syndrome of C-cell tumors in bulls shares many similarities with medullary thyroid carcinoma in humans (Capen and Black, 1974; Melvin *et al.*, 1972). Multiple endocrine tumors, especially bilateral pheochromocytomas and occasionally pituitary adenomas, are coincidentally detected in bulls with C-cell tumors (Black *et al.*, 1973b; Wilkie and Krook, 1970). This may represent a simultaneous neoplastic transformation of multiple endocrine cell populations of neural crest origin in the same individual (Weichert, 1970). Sponenberg and McEntee (1983) reported a high frequency of thyroid C-cell tumors and pheochromocytomas in a family of Guernsey bulls that suggested an autosomal dominant pattern of inheritance. A diffuse or focal ("nodular") hyperplasia of secretory cells in the adrenal medulla appears to precede the development of pheochromocytoma (Carney *et al.*, 1975).

Peterson *et al.* (1982d) reported a thyroid C-cell carcinoma in a dog that also had a pheochromocytoma and parathyroid hyperplasia. Immunoreactive calcitonin levels were elevated approximately 10-fold, but the dog was hypercalcemic (12.9 mg/dl) because of primary parathyroid hyperplasia and moderate elevations of immunoreactive parathyroid hormone.

**Clinical Characteristics.** Thyroid C-cell adenomas in bulls may result in a slight palpable enlargement of the anterioventral cervical region. C-cell carcinomas often attain considerable size and cause extensive multinodular enlargements along the ventral aspect of the neck because of the primary tumor in the thyroid and metastasis in anterior cervical lymph nodes (fig. 13.24A).

Severe vertebral osteosclerosis with ankylosing spondylosis deformans and degenerative osteoarthrosis, resulting in clinical lameness, often is detected in bulls with thyroid C-cell neoplasms. Skeletal lesions of this type have been reported to occur frequently in adult bulls, but are rare in cows of the same age and breed (Thomson, 1969). The relationship of excess calcitonin secretion by C-cell hyperplasia or neoplasia to the pathogenesis of skeletal lesions in bulls is currently uncertain and requires additional investigation. Prominent bone lesions have not been reported in human patients with medullary thyroid carcinoma despite the secretion of excessive calcitonin by the tumor (Fletcher, 1970; Melvin *et al.*, 1971; Meyer and Abdel-Bari, 1968; Steiner *et al.*, 1968).

The blood calcium level is usually in the normal or low normal range in animals with C-cell tumors. A bilateral medullary (C-cell) carcinoma in the thyroid of a dog reported by Patnaik *et al.* (1978) was associated with hypocalcemia (5 to 6 mg/dl) that returned to slightly above normal (12.8 mg/dl) following surgical excision of the tumor. The hypocalcemia recurred with regrowth of the C-cell carcinoma in regional lymph nodes.

**Gross Morphology.** C-cell adenomas appear as discrete, single or multiple, gray to tan nodules in one or both thyroid lobes (fig. 13.24B). Adenomas are smaller (approximately 1 to 3 cm in diameter) than carcinomas and are separated from the thyroid parenchyma by a thin fibrous connective tissue capsule. The adjacent thyroid is compressed but not invaded by neoplastic C-cells.

Thyroid C-cell carcinomas result in extensive multinodular enlargements of one or both thyroid lobes (fig. 13.24C). The entire thyroid gland may be incorporated by the proliferating neoplastic tissue. Multiple metastases in anterior cervical lymph nodes are usually large and have areas of necrosis and hemorrhage. Pulmonary metastases are present infrequently and appear as discrete tan nodules throughout all lobes of the lung.

**Histological Features.** Focal and/or diffuse hyperplasia of C-cells often precedes the development of C-cell neoplasms in animals and humans (Burek, 1978; DeLellis *et al.*, 1977; Kakudo *et al.*, 1984) (fig. 13.25). C-cells appear normal with an abundant, lightly eosinophilic, granular cytoplasm. Nodular hyperplasia of C-cells consists of focal accumulations less than the size of colloid-filled follicles. Calcitonin immunoreactivity has been localized to the cytoplasm of the hyperplastic C-cells (Deftos *et al.*, 1980).

The neoplastic cells in C-cell adenoma are divided into small groups or nests by coarse fibrous connective tissue septa that originate from the capsule. Other cells are columnar or tall cuboidal and form small acinar or ductal structures that contain a colloidlike material. The formation of follicles and secretion of thyroglobulin have also been reported in medullary thyroid carcinoma in humans (Ljunggren *et al.*, 1973). The neoplastic C-cells are well-

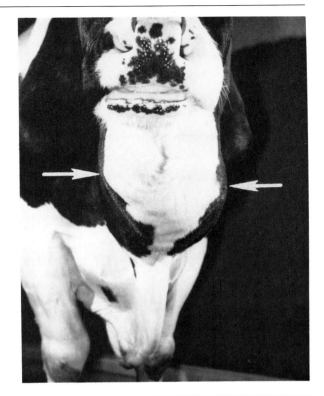

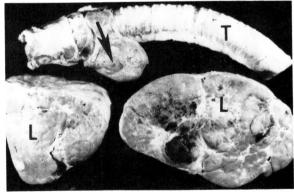

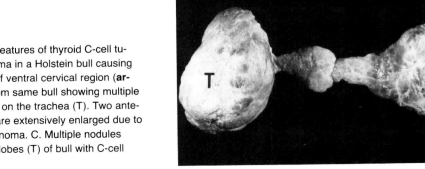

| A |
|---|
| B |
| C |

**FIGURE 13.24.** Gross features of thyroid C-cell tumors. A. C-cell carcinoma in a Holstein bull causing massive enlargement of ventral cervical region (**arrows**). B. C-cell carcinoma from same bull showing multiple nodules in the thyroid (**arrow**) on the trachea (T). Two anterior cervical lymph nodes (L) are extensively enlarged due to metastases of the C-cell carcinoma. C. Multiple nodules (**arrowheads**) in both thyroid lobes (T) of bull with C-cell carcinoma.

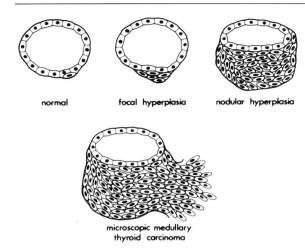

**FIGURE 13.25.** Focal and/or nodular hyperplasia of C-cells preceding the development of C-cell neoplasms. (Courtesy of Dr. J. D. Burek and CRC Press.)

differentiated and have an abundant cytoplasmic area that is lightly eosinophilic or clear on sections stained with hematoxylin and eosin (fig. 13.26A). The nucleus has one or more nucleoli and evenly distributed chromatin.

C-cell adenoma presents a discrete, expansive mass of cells greater in size than a colloid-distended follicle. They are well-circumscribed or partially encapsulated from adjacent follicles that are compressed to varying degrees. C-cell adenomas may be subdivided into packets of cells by fine connective tissue septa and capillaries.

C-cell carcinomas are more highly cellular and the tumor cells are more pleomorphic than with C-cell adenomas. They often have evidence of intrathyroidal and/or extracapsular invasion, occasionally with metastasis to distant sites. The neoplastic cells are polyhedral to spindle shaped with a lightly eosinophilic, finely granular, indistinct cytoplasmic area. The vesicular nuclei are oval or elongate and have more frequent mitotic figures than in adenomas. C-cells are often subdivided into small groups by fine connective tissue septa that contain small capillaries (fig. 13.26B). Only occasional ducts and acini are present in C-cell carcinomas. A similar histological pattern is also present in the metastatic lesions in cervical lymph nodes and lung.

Ultimobranchial tumors in the thyroid glands of bulls often have a more complex histological structure than the typical C-cell (medullary) carcinoma in humans and certain strains of laboratory rats. Areas in the tumor composed of differentiated C-cells consist of focal accumulations of neoplastic cells with an abundant lightly eosinophilic cytoplasm in the wall of thyroid and ultimobranchial follicles or they consist of larger nodules with a solid histological structure. This often is accompanied by a multifocal hyperplasia of C-cells in other parts of the thyroid lobes and hilus. The neoplastic C-cells are often embedded in an increased amount of hyalinized stroma that may contain amyloid. Parts of this thyroid neoplasm in bulls that appear to be derived from less differentiated ultimobranchial remnants consist of folliclelike structures, cysts, and tubules composed of immature small basophilic cells. These tumors in bulls and other species closely resemble undifferentiated or stem cells of the normal ultimobranchial body that develop into both C-cells and follicular cells. Thyroid follicles and cribriform structures with colloidlike material formed by cells resembling differentiated follicular cells are often present in the neoplasms in close association with these more primitive ultimobranchial-derived structures. The heterogeneous histological structure of ultimobranchial neoplasms

A | B
C | D
E

**FIGURE 13.26.** Microscopic features of thyroid C-cell tumors. A. C-cell adenoma of a bull. Neoplastic cells are subdivided into small groups by prominent connective tissue septa (**arrowhead**) arising from the capsule (C). There are scattered colloid-containing follicles (F) in the adenoma. B. C-cell carcinoma of a bull. The neoplastic C-cells are spindle shaped or polyhedral and subdivided into discrete groups by a fine connective tissue septa with capillaries (**arrows**). C. Extensive network of microfilaments (**arrows**) in a C-cell carcinoma of a bull. Membrane-limited secretory granules (S) are scattered in the network of microfilaments. The nucleus is indented by the microfilaments and profiles of rough endoplasmic reticulum (E) are distended. D. Poorly differentiated C-cells in an ultimobranchial carcinoma from a bull. There are numerous clusters of free ribosomes (**arrow**) and a prominent Golgi apparatus (G) with small vesicles but few secretory granules in the cytoplasm. E. C-cell tumor from a bull illustrating large aggregations of fine amyloid fibrils (A) interspersed in the stroma between bundles of collagen fibers (C).

ture fibrous connective tissue. The bone lesion of fibrous osteodystrophy is generalized throughout the skeleton, but is accentuated in local areas.

**Incidence.** Adenomas of parathyroid glands are encountered infrequently in older dogs (Capen *et al.*, 1975; Goulden and MacKenzie, 1968; Krook, 1957; Renk, 1962; Stavrou, 1968; Wilson *et al.*, 1974), laboratory rats (Burek, 1978), and mice (Lewis and Cherry, 1982). Inadequate numbers of cases have been studied to determine any breed or sex predisposition. Tumors of parathyroid chief cells do not appear to be a sequela of long-standing secondary hyperparathyroidism of renal or nutritional origin. Parathyroid carcinoma is rare in animals, but has been diagnosed in older dogs and cats. It is the parathyroid lesion responsible for approximately 4% of the cases of primary hyperparathyroidism in humans (Roth and Capen, 1974).

**Clinical Characteristics.** The clinical disturbances observed with functional parathyroid tumors are the result of a weakening of bones by excessive resorption. Lameness due to fractures of long bones may occur after relatively minor physical trauma. Compression fractures of vertebral bodies exert pressure on the spinal cord and nerves, resulting in motor or sensory dysfunction or both. Facial hyperostosis with partial obliteration of the nasal cavity and loosening or loss of teeth from alveolar sockets have been observed in dogs with primary hyperparathyroidism. Hypercalcemia results in anorexia, vomiting, constipation, depression, polyuria, polydipsia, and generalized muscular weakness due to decreased neuromuscular excitability.

Primary hyperparathyroidism should be considered in older dogs and cats if they have a history of multiple fractures associated with severe generalized skeletal demineralization and normal renal function. Radiographic evaluation reveals areas of subperiosteal cortical resorption, loss of lamina dura around the teeth, soft tissue mineralization, bone cysts, and a generalized decrease in bone density with multiple fractures in advanced cases.

The most important and practical laboratory test to aid in establishing the diagnosis of primary hyperparathyroidism is quantitation of total blood calcium. Although other laboratory findings may be variable, hypercalcemia is a consistent finding and is the result of accelerated release of calcium from bone. Calcium values consistently above 12

mg/100 ml in an adult animal should be considered to be in the hypercalcemic range. Dogs evaluated with primary hyperparathyroidism have had a greatly elevated (13 to 20 mg/100 ml or higher) blood calcium level.

The blood phosphorus level is low (4 mg/100 ml) or in the low to normal range because of inhibition of renal tubular resorption of phosphorus by excess parathyroid hormone. Alkaline phosphatase activity may be elevated in the serum of animals with overt bone disease. The increased activity of this enzyme is thought to result from a compensatory increase in osteoblastic activity along trabeculae as a response to mechanical stress in bones weakened by excessive resorption. The urinary excretion of calcium and phosphorus is increased and may predispose to the development of nephrocalcinosis and urolithiasis. Accelerated bone matrix catabolism is reflected by an increased excretion of hydroxyproline in the urine. The detection of elevated circulating levels of parathyroid hormone by radioimmunoassay in humans and animals has greatly facilitated early diagnosis of hyperparathyroidism (Aurbach *et al.*, 1973; Feldman and Krutzik, 1981; Meuten *et al.*, 1983*b*).

Other causes of hypercalcemia that must be considered in differential diagnosis of functional parathyroid tumors are vitamin D intoxication, malignant neoplasms with osseous metastases, and PTH-like humoral substances or other bone-resorbing factors, such as osteoclast-activating factor, prostaglandins, or transforming growth factor, produced by malignant neoplasms of nonparathyroid origin without metastasis of bone.

**Gross Morphology.** Chief cell adenomas usually result in considerable enlargement of a single parathyroid gland. They are light brown to red and are located either in the cervical region near the thyroids or infrequently within the thoracic cavity near the base of the heart (Cheville, 1972; Krook, 1957). Parathyroid neoplasms in the precardial mediastinum are derived from ectopic parathyroid tissue displaced into the thorax along with the expanding thymus during embryonic development. The adenomas are sharply demarcated and encapsulated from the adjacent thyroid gland (fig. 13.28A). Multiple white foci may be seen in the thyroids of dogs with functional parathyroid tumors. These represent areas of C-cell hyperplasia in response to

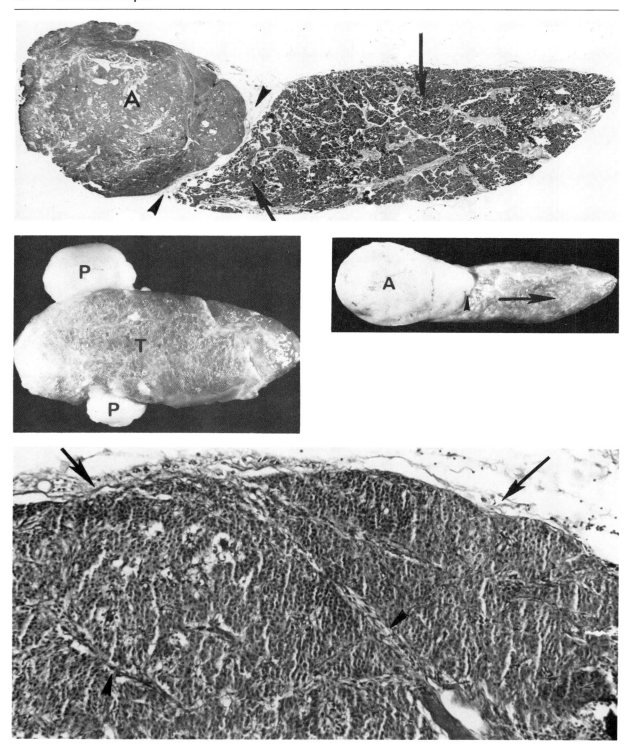

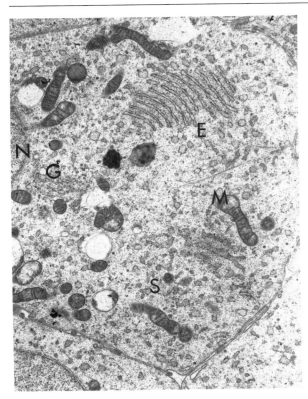

A E

B C

D

**FIGURE 13.28.** Tumors of the parathyroid gland. A. Chief cell adenoma (A) in the external parathyroid gland of a dog with primary hyperparathyroidism. The adenoma is sharply demarcated and encapsulated (**arrowheads**) from the adjacent thyroid gland. The cranial pole of the thyroid is compressed and there are multifocal areas of C-cell hyperplasia (**arrows**). B. Moderate enlargement of the internal and external parathyroids (P) in a dog with secondary chief cell hyperplasia associated with chronic renal failure (T is thyroid gland; scale is 1 cm). C. Parathyroid adenoma (A) causing extensive enlargement of one parathyroid gland. The tumor is encapsulated (**arrowhead**) and there are multicentric areas of C-cell hyperplasia in the thyroid (**arrow**) as a response to the long-term hypercalcemia. D. Parathyroid adenoma illustrating closely packed chief cells subdivided into small groups by fine fibrous septa and capillaries (**arrowheads**). A thin capsule of fibrous connective tissue (**arrows**) surrounds the tumor. E. Active chief cell in a functional parathyroid adenoma from a dog with primary hyperparathyroidism. There are large lamellar arrays of rough endoplasmic reticulum (E), a prominent Golgi apparatus (G), large mitochondria (M), but few secretory granules (S) in the abundant cytoplasmic area (N is nucleus).

the long-term hypercalcemia (figs. 13.28A and C).

Hyperparathyroidism due to chief cell hyperplasia is common in animals as part of the compensatory reaction to chronic renal disease and nutritional imbalances. Chief cells undergo organellar hypertrophy initially and cellular hyperplasia later to increase parathyroid hormone synthesis and secretion in response to a hypocalcemic stimulus. In secondary chief cell hyperplasia, all four parathyroids are enlarged two to five times their normal size (fig. 13.28B). A parathyroid adenoma enlarges a single gland to a much greater degree (fig. 13.28C), while the remaining parathyroids will be atrophic and smaller than normal. Histopathological demonstration of a compressed rim of parathyroid parenchyma and a fibrous capsule in an enlarged gland points to the diagnosis of adenoma rather than chief cell hyperplasia.

Primary parathyroid hyperplasia has been described in German shepherd pups associated with hypercalcemia, hypophosphatemia, increased immunoreactive parathyroid hormone, and increased fractional clearance of inorganic phosphate in the urine (Thompson *et al.*, 1984). Clinical signs include stunted growth, muscular weakness, polyuria, polydipsia, and a diffuse reduction in bone density. Intravenous infusion of calcium fails to suppress the autonomous secretion of parathyroid hormone by the diffuse hyperplasia of chief cells in all parathyroids. Lesions include nodular hyperplasia of thyroid C-cells and widespread mineralization of the lungs, kidney, and gastric mucosa. The disease is inherited as an autosomal recessive.

Hypercalcemia and hypophosphatemia develop in certain dogs affected with malignant lymphoma or apocrine gland carcinoma of the anal sac and in humans affected with several different types of malignant neoplasms (e.g., carcinomas of the kidney, lung, or ovary) in the absence of bone metastasis and functional lesions in the parathyroid glands (Omenn, 1973). A syndrome of pseudohyperparathyroidism has been reported in dogs and cats with disseminated malignant lymphoma (Chew *et al.*, 1975; Osborne and Stevens, 1973). Antemortem differentiation between primary hyperparathyroidism and pseudohyperparathyroidism is difficult, especially if there are no overt clinical signs of lymphoma, since both have hypercalcemia, hypophosphatemia, and often increased alkaline phosphatase.

The degree of skeletal demineralization is usually less severe with pseudohyperparathyroidism.

**Histological Features.** Parathyroid adenomas are composed of closely packed chief cells subdivided into small groups by fine connective tissue septa with many capillaries (fig. 13.28D). The chief cells are cuboidal or polyhedral, and the cytoplasm stains lightly eosinophilic. Occasional oxyphil cells, water-clear cells, and transitional forms may be distributed throughout the adenoma. Fat cells and mast cells are often present in the stroma of the tumor. Adenomas are surrounded by a fine connective tissue capsule and may compress the adjacent thyroid gland (fig. 13.28A). A rim of compressed parathyroid parenchyma is usually present outside the capsule of small adenomas. These atrophic chief cells are small, irregular in shape, and densely eosinophilic.

**Ultrastructural Characteristics.** Chief cells constituting functional parathyroid adenomas are usually in the actively synthesizing stage of the secretory cycle (fig. 13.28E) (Capen *et al.*, 1975). Multiple large lamellar arrays of rough endoplasmic reticulum and clusters of free ribosomes are present in the cytoplasm. Few mature secretory ("storage") granules are seen, however, suggesting that parathyroid hormone is secreted at a faster rate than synthesis and storage in autonomous chief cells (fig. 13.28E). Large mitochondria and prominent Golgi apparatuses are present in neoplastic chief cells. The annulate lamellae that occur frequently in parathyroid adenomas have not been reported in normal chief cells (Roth and Capen, 1974).

Parathyroid adenoma may contain secretory granules as well as mature oxyphil cells and transitional forms with well-developed organelles that control hormonal synthesis and packaging. This is in marked contrast to the oxyphil cell of normal parathyroid glands, which has a cytoplasm filled with tightly packed mitochondria but a poorly developed endoplasmic reticulum and Golgi apparatus (Roth and Capen, 1974).

Parathyroid carcinoma is composed of chief cells with a highly variable development of cytoplasmic organelles. Alterations of the nuclear morphology have been described in malignant chief cells (Roth and Capen, 1974).

**Growth and Metastasis.** Parathyroid adenomas are usually slow growing and compress the adjacent thyroid. They are well-encapsulated and can be sur-gically excised without difficulty. Successful removal of a functional parathyroid adenoma results in a rapid decrease in circulating parathyroid hormone levels because the half-life of the hormone in plasma is only about 20 min. It should be kept in mind that plasma calcium levels in humans with overt bone disease may decrease rapidly and be subnormal within 12 to 24 hours, resulting in hypocalcemic tetany. Postoperative hypocalcemia is the result of depressed secretory activity in the remaining parathyroid tissue resulting from long-term suppression by the chronic hypercalcemia and decreased bone resorption combined with accelerated mineralization of organic matrix formed by the hyperplastic osteoblasts along bone surfaces. Infusion of calcium gluconate, high calcium diets, and supplemental vitamin D therapy in pharmacological doses will correct this postoperative complication.

Parathyroid carcinomas are larger than adenomas, invade the capsule and adjacent structures (e.g., thyroid glands and cervical muscles), and may metastasize to regional lymph nodes and the lung.

## Nonneoplastic Parathyroid Cysts

Small cysts occur within the parenchyma of the parathyroid or in the immediate vicinity of the gland and are observed frequently in dogs and occasionally in other animal species (fig. 13.29A). Parathyroid cysts are usually mutiloculated, lined by a cuboidal to columnar (often ciliated) epithelium, and contain a densely eosinophilic proteinic material. The lining epithelial cells have an electron-dense cytoplasm and numerous microvilli projecting into the lumen of the cyst, but poorly developed synthetic and secretory organelles (fig. 13.29B). Chief cells adjacent to larger cysts may be moderately compressed.

Parathyroid cysts (Kürsteiner's cyst) appear to develop from a persistence and dilatation of remnants of the duct that connects the parathyroid and thymic primordia during embryonic development. Similar cysts may be present in the anterior mediastinum when remnants of the embryonic duct are displaced with the caudal migration of the thymus (fig. 13.29C). They are lined by pseudostratified columnar epithelium and contain a proteinic material.

Parathyroid cysts are distinct from midline cysts

diameter) nodules visible from the serosal surface. They are of similar consistency to or slightly firmer than the surrounding pancreatic parenchyma. Functional adenomas occur singly or as multiple nodules occasionally (Botha and Irvine-Smith, 1978) in the same or different lobes of the pancreas. A thin layer of fibrous connective tissue completely encapsulates adenomas from the adjacent parenchyma (fig. 13.37A).

A review of our cases and those reported in the literature revealed that carcinomas of the pancreatic islets are more common in dogs than adenomas (Capen and Martin, 1969; Njoku *et al.*, 1972). This differs from the situation in humans, where adenomas are encountered much more often (as much as 90% of all pancreatic islet tumors) than islet cell carcinoma. Clinicopathological evidence suggesting hyperinsulinism has been reported more frequently with β-cell carcinoma than with adenoma in dogs. The duodenal (right) lobe of the pancreas appears to be a site of more frequent involvement with islet cell tumors in dogs than the splenic (left) part of the pancreas, although the numbers of islets per given area are greater in the splenic lobe.

Carcinomas of the pancreatic islets can be differentiated from adenomas by their larger size, multilobular appearance, extensive invasion into adjacent parenchyma (fig. 13.37B) and lymphatics, and establishment of metastases in extrapancreatic sites. Important anatomical sites that must be examined for metastasis are the regional lymph nodes, liver, mesentery, and omentum. Larger neoplasms fre-

quently have focal areas of necrosis, hemorrhage, and liquefaction. Carcinomas in the pancreatic angle may result in parenchymal atrophy of distal portions of the duodenal and splenic branches of the pancreas (fig. 13.37B).

**Histological Features.** Islet cell adenomas are sharply delineated from the adjacent parenchyma and surrounded by a complete, thin capsule of fibrous connective tissue. Small nests of acinar epithelial cells may be present throughout the neoplasm, but particularly near the periphery. Numerous connective tissue septa containing small capillaries radiate from the capsule into the neoplasm and subdivide the cells into small lobules or packets. The neoplastic cells are well-differentiated, varying from cuboidal to columnar, and have a lightly eosinophilic and finely granular cytoplasm with indistinct cell membranes. The cellular structure and tinctorial properties of both adenoma and carcinoma are retained best in tissues fixed immediately in Bouin's fluid. Autolysis of neoplastic cells progresses rapidly if the interval between death and fixation is prolonged. The cytoplasm of the neoplastic cells is blue on sections stained with chromium hematoxylin–phloxine after fixing or mordanting in Bouin's fluid. Scattered dark blue granules are observed in some cells but are not numerous. Islets in the surrounding pancreatic tissue appear normal or slightly reduced in size.

Irregularly shaped ducts are observed frequently within islet cell adenomas. The cuboidal to columnar lining epithelium has basal nuclei and eosinophilic cytoplasm. The ducts are intimately associated with the neoplastic cells, occur in greater numbers than would be expected for preexisting pancreatic ducts, and are considered to be part of the neoplasm.

Islet cell carcinomas are consistently larger than adenomas, are multilobular, and invade the adjacent pancreatic parenchyma. Although there is a peripheral condensation of connective tissue in some areas, neoplastic cells invade into and through the fibrous capsule (fig. 13.37C). The dense bands of fibrous tissue that course through the neoplasm give rise to fine connective tissue septa (with capillaries) that subdivide the cells into small cords or lobules (fig. 13.37D). The well-differentiated neoplastic cells in islet cell carcinomas are closely packed and may be less uniform in size and shape

**FIGURE 13.37.** Tumors of the pancreatic islets. A. β-Cell adenoma (A) of pancreatic islets in a dog. The neoplasm is well-delineated from the exocrine pancreas by a fibrous capsule (**arrow**). B. Functional β-cell carcinoma of pancreatic islets (B) with invasion into the adjacent pancreas. The distal portion (A) of the pancreatic lobe is atrophic (scale is 1 cm). C. Functional β-cell carcinoma of pancreatic islets invading through the fibrous connective tissue capsule (**arrow**) into adjacent exocrine pancreas (E). D. β-Cell carcinoma illustrating characteristic pattern of arrangement of cells that resembles the structure of normal pancreatic islets. The closely packed neoplastic beta cells are subdivided into small groups by fine connective tissue septa with capillaries (**arrows**).

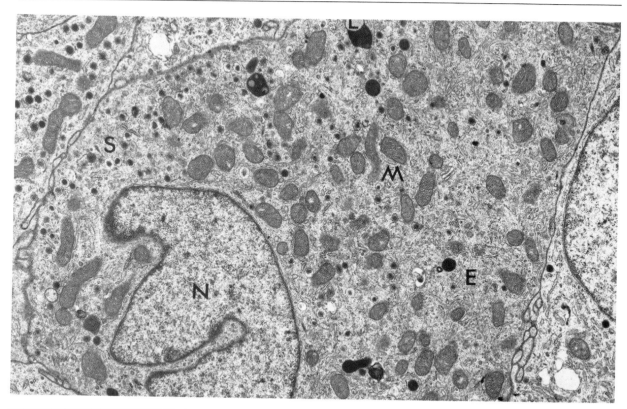

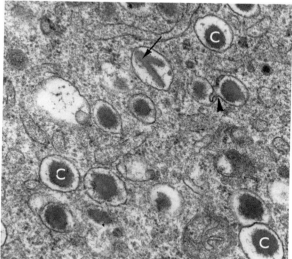

**FIGURE 13.38.** β-Cell carcinomas of pancreatic islets. A. Functional β-cell carcinoma. The neoplastic cells are polyhedral and have indented nuclei (N). The plasma membranes of adjacent cells are straight with uncomplicated interdigitations. The cytoplasm contains flat profiles of rough endoplasmic reticulum (E), scattered secretory granules (S), numerous mitochondria (M), and lipofuscin (L). B. Mature secretory granules in functional β-cell carcinoma. The internal cores (C) are circular or V-shaped (**arrow**), surrounded by a wide halo, and often situated eccentrically within the granule. Fine fibrils extend outward from the indistinct margins of internal cores. The limiting membranes of adjacent granules appear fused or interdigitated (**arrowhead**).

than the cells composing adenomas. They are either cuboidal or polyhedral and have a granular eosinophilic cytoplasm. Mitotic figures are seen infrequently. Ductules are present within $\beta$-cell carcinomas, and there may be evidence of a transition of ductal epithelium into neoplastic $\beta$-cells.

Pathologists evaluating biopsies of islet cell tumors should be aware that even small neoplasms composed of well-differentiated $\beta$-cells may have already invaded lymphatics and vessels and metastasized to the liver and regional lymph nodes. Multiple sections often are necessary to demonstrate clear-cut evidence of lymphatic and vascular invasion and the formation of tumor cell emboli.

**Ultrastructural and Immunocytochemical Characteristics.** Cells composing functional islet cell neoplasms in dogs have ultrastructural, histochemical, and immunocytochemical characteristics of $\beta$-cells. The neoplastic $\beta$-cells are irregularly cuboidal or polyhedral, closely packed, and contain numerous electron-dense cytoplasmic organelles (Capen and Martin, 1969) (fig. 13.38A). The cytoplasmic area is usually abundant compared with the area of the nucleus. Insulin reactivity can be demonstrated over the cytoplasmic area of neoplastic $\beta$-cells by peroxidase–antiperoxidase immunocytochemical techniques (Stromberg *et al.*, 1983). Nuclei of neoplastic cells are irregularly indented and have peripheral condensations of nuclear chromatin. The plasma membranes of adjacent cells have uncomplicated interdigitations, and desmosomal attachments join adjacent cells.

$\beta$-Cells in different stages of secretory activity are observed in functional islet cell neoplasms. Sparsely granulated $\beta$-cells are considered to be in the "actively synthesizing phase" of their secretory cycle because of the extensive network of rough endoplasmic reticulum, large cytoplasmic area, numerous free ribosomes, and large mitochondria. Densely granulated $\beta$-cells are interpreted to be in the "storage phase" of their secretory cycle since they have less endoplasmic reticulum and fewer ribosomes. Cells are observed with fine structural characteristics intermediate between these two extremes of organellar development and granulation.

Secretory granules are readily visible throughout the cytoplasm of neoplastic $\beta$-cells. The granules vary in shape, size, and electron density. The smallest granules are spherical in outline, uniformly electron dense, and have a narrow electron-lucent space subjacent to the continuous limiting membrane. The mean diameter of this type of granule is approximately 200 m$\mu$. The larger oval or spherical granules, with a wide submembranous space and bar-shaped internal cores, are considered to represent mature secretory granules since they are the most common type reported in $\beta$-cells of normal dogs (Lacy, 1957, 1967, 1968; Munger *et al.*, 1965; Sato *et al.*, 1966). They are encountered less frequently in neoplastic $\beta$-cells and are surrounded by a continuous agranular limiting membrane (fig. 13.38B). The mature granules appear to develop from the uniformly electron-dense, small, secretory granules by a central condensation of their contents. The finely granular internal core of the mature secretory granule is circular, bar- or V-shaped, and frequently situated eccentrically within the granule. A wide electron-lucent space ("halo") separates the internal core from the outer limiting membrane. The margins of the internal cores are indistinct, and fine fibrils extend into the wide submembranous space. Limiting membranes of adjacent granules are sometimes fused together so that two internal cores are surrounded by a continuous membrane (fig. 13.38B). The membranes of other adjacent granules are deeply interdigitated. Mature secretory granules of $\beta$-cells have a mean diameter of 340 m$\mu$ and internal cores measuring about 210 m$\mu$. Bar-shaped or rectangular internal cores measure 280 m$\mu$ in greatest length by 82 m$\mu$ in width and have a fibrillar or laminated substructure.

There is no consistent polarity of secretory granules within the neoplastic $\beta$-cells, although large numbers of granules are often in the portion of cytoplasm bordering the perivascular space. Secretory granules are frequently aligned immediately subjacent to the plasma membrane of the cell. A portion of the limiting membrane of the secretory granule often fuses with the plasma membrane, and a hiatus is formed for extrusion of the granule contents into the extracellular space. This process of secretion is termed *emiocytosis*.

The neoplastic $\beta$-cells can be differentiated readily from $\alpha$-cells of the pancreatic islets in dogs by the unique rectangular or crystalloid internal cores and wide submembranous space of the mature secretory granules. $\alpha$-Cells have round secretory granules with a closely applied limiting membrane in normal dogs (Munger *et al.*, 1965). The neoplastic $\beta$-cells can also be differentiated from the other cell types (F- and D-cells) normally found in the pancreatic islets by the ultrastructure of their secretory granules (Lacy, 1957; Legg, 1967; Sato *et al.*, 1966).

**Growth and Metastasis.** Adenomas of $\beta$-cells usually grow slowly and compress adjacent pancreatic parenchyma. Their sharp delineation and complete encapsulation permit successful surgical excision. Although $\beta$-cell adenomas are usually single in the dog, the entire pancreas should be examined for the presence of multiple tumors. Complete surgical removal of islet cell adenomas dramatically ameliorates the hypoglycemia and associated neurological signs unless there have been irreversible changes in the central nervous system (Wilson and Hulse, 1974).

Occasional small insulin-secreting $\beta$-cell neoplasms may appear as well-delineated single nodules closely resembling an adenoma. However, tumor cells will have already invaded through the fibrous capsule into lymphatics and vessels, and established multiple metastases in the liver. Islet cell carcinomas are usually considerably larger than adenomas and invade adjacent pancreatic parenchyma. Multiple metastases develop early in the liver and draining lymph nodes (duodenal, hepatic, splenic, and mesenteric). Chemotherapy with $\beta$-cell cytotoxins (e.g., streptozotocin) has not proven useful in the long-term management of carcinoma because of the development of nephrotoxicity (Meyer, 1976).

## Non-$\beta$-cell (Gastrin-secreting) Tumors

**Incidence.** Gastrin-secreting, non-$\beta$ islet cell tumors of the pancreas have been reported in humans, dogs (Jones *et al.*, 1976; Happé *et al.*, 1980), and a cat (Middleton *et al.*, 1983). The hypersecretion of gastrin in humans results in the well-documented Zollinger–Ellison syndrome consisting of hypersecretion of gastric acid and recurrent peptic ulceration in the gastrointestinal tract. The non-$\beta$ islet cell tumors derived from ectopic amine precursor uptake decarboxylase (APUD) cells in the pancreas produce an excess of the hormone gastrin, which normally is secreted by gastrin-secreting cells of the antral and duodenal mucosa. The incidence of gastrin-secreting pancreatic tumors in dogs and cats is uncertain, but it appears to be uncommon compared to insulin-secreting $\beta$-cell neoplasms.

**Clinical Characteristics.** The few cases studied in the dog and cat have been presented with clinical signs of anorexia, vomiting of blood-tinged material, intermittent diarrhea, progressive weight loss, and dehydration. The prominent functional disturbances appear to be the result of the multiple ulcerations of the gastrointestinal mucosa that develop from the gastrin hypersecretion.

**Gross Morphology.** Animals with Zollinger–Ellison-like syndrome have single or multiple tumors of varying size in the pancreas (Happé *et al.*, 1980; Jones *et al.*, 1976; Middleton *et al.*, 1983). They are often firm on palpation because of an increase of fibrous connective tissue in the stroma. There were attempts at encapsulation, but the tumor usually extended into the surrounding pancreatic parenchyma.

**Histological Features.** The basic histological pattern of pancreatic islet cell tumors in animals is similar whether they are secreting insulin or gastrin. Happé *et al.* (1980) recognized three histological patterns in non-$\beta$ islet cell tumors in dogs: (1) a ribbon or trabecular arrangement of neoplastic cells with occasional pseudorosettes and an intimate relationship to capillaries; (2) solid nests of cells with a delicate, highly vascularized stroma; and (3) an acinar pattern with arrangement of cuboidal neoplastic cells around a central lumen. The stroma may be prominent and hyalinized in some dogs with gastrin-secreting tumors.

**Ultrastructural and Immunocytochemical Characteristics.** The abundant cytoplasmic area of gastrin-secreting neoplastic cells contains scattered small secretory granules (100 to 150 nm in diameter) (Happé *et al.*, 1980). They are surrounded by a closely applied limiting membrane and have a round internal core. The internal core of the secretory granule in gastrin-secreting cells is different than that in the insulin-secreting $\beta$-cell in the dog, which often is bar- or V-shaped with a wide submembranous space. Specific immunocytochemical reaction has localized gastrin immunoreactivity to the cytoplasm of the neoplastic cells.

The cat with a non-$\beta$ islet cell carcinoma had elevated serum gastrin levels (1,000 pg/ml) compared to clinically normal cats (mean 87.6 pg/ml). Neoplastic cells stained by the unlabeled immunoperoxidase method were positive for gastrin and glucagon (Middleton *et al.*, 1983).

**Laboratory Data.** Extracts of the pancreatic tumor contained 1.72 and 0.03 $\mu$g gastrin equivalents per gram of wet tissue in dogs reported by Happé *et al.* (1980). Gastrin component III was the prominent molecular form in the tumor in one dog, whereas in a second case gastrin components II and III were present in equimolar amounts.

Serum gastrin levels have been evaluated in a limited number of dogs with non-$\beta$ islet cell tumors of the pancreas. Happé *et al.* (1980) reported that gastrin levels in one dog with a Zollinger–Ellison-like syndrome varied from 155 to 2,780 pg/ml, whereas the mean serum gastrin in clinically normal control dogs ($n = 17$) was $70.9 \pm 5.1$ pg/ml. The dog studied by Jones *et al.* (1976) had a plasma immunoreactive gastrin level of 360 pg/ml.

**Growth and Metastasis.** The gastrin-secreting tumors of the pancreas that have been studied in dogs appear to invade locally into the adjacent parenchyma and often metastasize to regional lymph nodes and liver. The dogs have either single or multiple ulcerations in the gastrin and/or duodenal mucosa associated with free blood in the lumen.

## TUMORS OF THE CHEMORECEPTOR ORGANS

**Introduction.** The chemoreceptor organs are sensitive barometers of changes in the blood carbon dioxide content, pH, and oxygen tension and aid in the regulation of respiration and circulation. Carotid and aortic bodies can initiate an increase in the depth, minute volume, and rate of respiration by way of parasympathetic nerves, which results in an increased heart rate and elevated arterial blood pressure by way of the sympathetic nervous system. They are normally composed of parenchymal (chemoreceptor and glomus) cells and stellate-shaped sustentacular cells (Höglund, 1967; Kobayashi, 1968). Nerve endings with synaptic vesicles and nerve fibers are seen in close association with the chemoreceptor cells. Although the embryological origin of chemoreceptor organs is not precisely known, there is considerable evidence to suggest that they arise from perivascular mesodermal cells that are invaded by cells of neuroectodermal origin (Pryse-Davis *et al.*, 1964).

Chemoreceptor tissue is present at several sites in the animal including the carotid body, aortic bodies, nodose ganglion of the vagus nerve, ciliary ganglion in the orbit, pancreas, bodies on the internal jugular vein below the middle ear, and glomus jugulare along the recurrent branch of the glossopharyngeal nerve (LeCompte, 1951). Nonidez (1937) demonstrated that normal aortic bodies of dogs consist of clusters of cells embedded in adventitia at multiple sites including the innominate artery immediately below the origin of the right subclavian artery, on the anterior surface of the aortic arch, beneath the arch between the aorta and pulmonary artery, between the ascending aorta and pulmonary artery near the left coronary artery, and scattered in the wall of the pulmonary artery.

**Incidence.** Although chemoreceptor tissue is widely distributed in the body, tumors develop principally in the aortic and carotid bodies.

Aortic body tumors are encountered more frequently than neoplasms of the carotid body in animals (Dean and Strafuss, 1975), but the reverse is true for humans (LeCompte, 1951; Scotti, 1958). *Chemodectoma* and *nonchromaffin paraganglioma* are synonyms that are frequently used to designate neoplasms arising in chemoreceptor organs (Jubb and Kennedy, 1957). These tumors develop primarily in dogs (Bloom, 1943; Johnson, 1968; Kast, 1958; Misdorp and Elders, 1965; Parodi and Lekkas, 1970; Tisseur and Parodi, 1963) and rarely in cats (Buergelt and Das, 1968) and cattle (Nordstoga, 1966). Brachycephalic breeds of dogs such as the boxer and Boston terrier are highly predisposed to develop tumors of the aortic and carotid bodies (S. P. Bishop, 1975, personal communication; Howard and Nielsen, 1965; Jubb and Kennedy, 1957; Nilsson, 1955). The majority of dogs with chemodectomas are 8 years of age or older. Male dogs appear to have a greater frequency of chemodectomas than females (Dean and Strafuss, 1975; Hayes, 1975a; Howard and Nielsen, 1965; Johnson, 1968).

**Clinical Characteristics.** Tumors of the aortic and carotid bodies in animals are not functional (i.e., they do not secrete excess hormone into the circulation), but as space-occupying lesions may result in a variety of clinical signs. Clinical signs associated with larger aortic body adenomas and carcinomas usually are manifestations of cardiac decompensation due to pressure on the atria, vena cava, or both (Johnson, 1968; Riser and Bailey, 1949). There may be evidence of dyspnea, coughing, vomiting, cyanosis, hydrothorax, hydropericardium, ascites, edema of the subcutaneous tissue of the head, neck, and forelimbs, and passive congestion of the liver. The accumulation of serous, often blood-tinged, fluid in the pericardial sac results from the invasion of tumor cells into lymphatics at the base of the heart or the compression of small pericardial veins.

Dogs with carotid body tumors are usually presented with a palpable, slowly enlarging mass in the anterolateral cervical region near the angle of the mandible. Larger neoplasms interfere with swallowing because of pressure on the esophagus and result in circulatory disturbances from compression of the larger veins in the neck. Other clinical signs may be related to the presence of an aortic body tumor in the same animal. Dyspnea and coughing have been observed in dogs with malignant carotid body tumors that have multiple pulmonary metastases (Sander and Whitenack, 1970).

**Etiology.** Although the etiology of chemodectomas is unknown, Hayes (1975*a*) suggested that a genetic predisposition aggravated by chronic hypoxia may account for the higher risk of certain brachycephalic breeds such as the boxer and Boston terrier to develop aortic and carotid body tumors. Carotid bodies of several mammalian species, including dogs, have been shown to undergo hyperplasia when subjected to chronic hypoxia by living in a high altitude environment (Edwards *et al.*, 1971). Saldana *et al.* (1973) demonstrated that humans living at high altitudes have 10 times the frequency of chemodectomas as those living at sea level.

**Gross Morphology.** Aortic body tumors appear most frequently as single masses or occasionally as multiple nodules within the pericardial sac near the base of the heart (Johnson, 1968). They vary considerably in size from 0.5 to 12.5 cm, and carcinomas are generally larger than adenomas. Solitary small adenomas are either attached to the adventitia of the pulmonary artery and ascending aorta or em-

bedded in the adipose connective tissue between these major vascular trunks. They have a smooth external surface, and on cross section are white and mottled with red to brown areas. Larger adenomas may indent the atria or displace the trachea. Their surface is more coarsely nodular, and large areas of hemorrhage or necrosis are present in the tumor. The larger aortic body adenomas are multilobular and partially surround the major arterial trunks at the base of the heart. Although the vessels may be completely surrounded by neoplastic tissue, there is little evidence of vascular constriction.

Malignant aortic body tumors occur less frequently in dogs than adenomas. Carcinomas may infiltrate the wall of the pulmonary artery to form papillary projections into the lumen or invade through the wall into the lumens of the atria (fig. 13.39A). A large mural thrombus is occasionally attached to the neoplastic tissue extending into the atrium. Although tumor cells often invade blood vessels, metastasis to the lung and liver occurs infrequently in dogs with aortic body tumors (Johnson, 1968; Nillson, 1956). However, local invasion of the pericardium, epicardium, myocardium, and walls of great vessels at the base of the heart by aortic body tumors occurs frequently (S. P. Bishop, 1975, personal communication).

Carotid body tumors arise near the bifurcation of the common carotid artery in the cranial cervical area (Comroe and Schmidt, 1938). They usually appear as a unilateral slow-growing mass (Dean and Strafuss, 1975), and only rarely develop on both sides in the same animal (Jubb and Kennedy, 1957). Adenomas vary from approximately 1 to 4 cm in diameter, are well-encapsulated, and have a smooth external surface. The bifurcation of the carotid artery is incorporated in the mass, and tumor cells firmly adhere to the tunica adventitia. A branch of the glossopharyngeal nerve may be traced into the capsule of the tumor by careful dissection. Adenomas are firm and white with scattered areas of hemorrhage and are extremely vascular. Biopsy and complete surgical excision are often difficult because of the high degree of vascularity and intimate relationship of the tumor with major arterial trunks in the neck.

Malignant carotid body tumors are larger (as much as 12 cm in diameter) and more coarsely multinodular than adenomas. Multiple areas of hemorrhage and cystic degeneration are present within

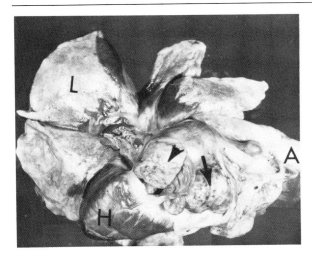
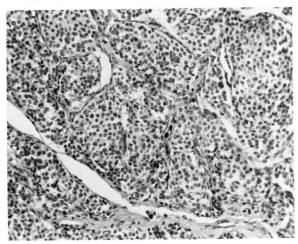
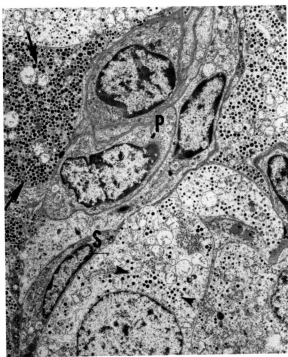
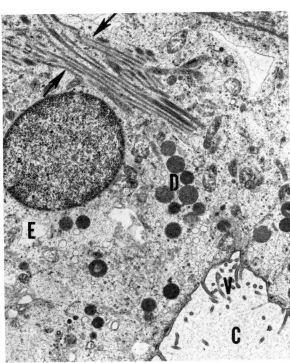

$\dfrac{A|B}{C|D}$  **FIGURE 13.39.** Tumors of the chemoreceptors. A. Aortic body carcinoma of a dog with multiple nodules (**arrow**) at the base of the heart (H) and extension into the adjacent atrium (**arrowhead**) (L is diaphragmatic lobe of lung, A is aorta). B. Characteristic histological pattern of arrangement of neoplastic cells in a chemoreceptor tumor (carotid body tumor from a dog). Tumor cells are subdivided into groups or lobules by fine connective tissue septa with many capillaries. C. Carotid body adenoma from a dog illustrating lightly (**arrowheads**) and densely (**arrows**) granulated tumor cells. The small secretory granules have a closely applied limiting membrane. A sustentacular cell (S) extends processes toward several perivascular cells (P). D. A follicular adenoma derived from ectopic thyroid tissue located at the base of the heart. The thyroid follicular cells contain dense bodies (D), endoplasmic reticulum (E), and numerous microvilli (V) projecting into the colloid (C) of the follicular lumen, but lack the small secretory granules found in aortic and carotid body tumors. Long dense tubules are present within the cisternae of endoplasmic reticulum in the tumor cells (**arrows**). (B, courtesy of Dr. P. C. Kennedy and *Cancer;* C and D, courtesy of Dr. N. F. Cheville and *Vet. Path.*)

the tumor. Although carcinomas appear to be encapsulated, tumor cells invade the capsule and the walls of adjacent vessels and lymphatics. The external jugular vein and several cranial nerves, in addition to the carotid bifurcation, may be incorporated by the neoplasm. Larger tumors result in extensive dorsolateral deviation of the trachea. Dean and Strafuss (1975), in a review of 22 carotid body tumors reported in the dog, found that approximately 30% of those with adequate descriptions of lesions had evidence of metastasis. Metastasis of carotid body tumors has been found in the lung, bronchial and mediastinal lymph nodes, liver, pancreas, and kidney (Dean and Strafuss, 1975; Jubb and Kennedy, 1957; Sander and Whitenack, 1970). Occasionally the metastases to parenchymal organs, such as the kidney, may be extensive and nearly obliterate the affected organ.

Multicentric neoplastic transformation of chemoreceptor tissue occurs frequently in brachycephalic breeds of dogs. Approximately 65% of the reported carotid body tumors (i.e., those cases with adequate descriptions of lesions) also have aortic body tumors (Dean and Strafuss, 1975; Hubben *et al.*, 1960; Kurtz and Finco, 1969).

**Histological Features.** The histological characteristics of chemoreceptor tumors are similar whether they are derived from the carotid or the aortic body. The neoplastic chemoreceptor cells are subdivided into lobules by prominent branching trabeculae of connective tissue that originate from the fibrous capsule (Jubb and Kennedy, 1957). They are further subdivided into small compartments by fine septa that contain collagen and reticulum fibers plus small capillaries (fig. 13.39B). Tumor cells are commonly aligned along and around the small capillaries in chemodectomas. Focal accumulations of lymphocytes and hemosiderin-laden macrophages are frequently present in the capsule and major connective tissue trabeculae.

The tumor cells of chemodectomas are discrete, cuboidal to polyhedral, and closely packed (fig. 13.39B). The cytoplasm is lightly eosinophilic, finely granular, and often vacuolated. Cells forming chemodectomas rapidly undergo autolysis. Cell boundaries become indistinct, and the cytoplasm appears clear if the postmortem interval is prolonged. Chromaffin granules cannot be demonstrated in the cytoplasm of cells forming chemodectomas as in pheochromocytomas of the adrenal

medulla. The nuclei are round to oval and usually placed centrally in the cell. There is a finely granular chromatin pattern and mitotic figures are infrequent (Nilsson, 1955).

In larger aortic body adenomas or in carcinomas, there are scattered areas where the tumor cells are larger and more pleomorphic. Mononuclear tumor giant cells with bizarre-shaped, multilobed, densely basophilic nuclei are intermingled with the cuboidal tumor cells. Although tumor giant cells are more consistently detected in carcinomas, they are by no means an unequivocal criterion of malignancy. Small, well-differentiated chemodectomas occasionally have a considerable number of tumor giant cells.

Aortic and carotid body tumors are very vascular and have numerous muscular arterioles, large thin-walled veins, and an abundant network of capillaries in the connective tissue septa (Johnson, 1968). Focal areas of hemorrhage from disruption of thin-walled vessels and areas of coagulation necrosis are a consistent finding in chemodectomas (Nilsson, 1955). Cholesterol clefts and foci of mineralization often are present in the areas of necrosis. Several layers of tumor cells may radiate along fine connective tissue septa from the thin-walled vessels. Tumor cells frequently invade blood vessels and lymphatics with the formation of emboli. Carcinomas have evidence of tumor cell invasion through the capsule and into the walls of large muscular arteries and adjacent structures (e.g., wall of the atrium, bifurcation of the trachea, and the pericardium). The invading tumor cells are pleomorphic, hyperchromatic with frequent mitotic figures, and arranged in broad sheets with little tendency to form distinctive packets of cells.

Adenomas and carcinomas derived from ectopic thyroid tissue account for approximately 5 to 10% of "heart base" tumors in dogs (S. P. Bishop, 1975, personal communication; Stünzi and Teuscher, 1953). They often compress or invade structures in the anterior mediastinum near the base of the heart.

Areas of ectopic thyroid tumors with a compact cellular (solid) pattern of arrangement are difficult to distinguish histologically from aortic body tumors. In general, cells of ectopic thyroid tumors are smaller than in aortic body tumors and have more hyperchromatic nuclei and eosinophilic cytoplasm. The neoplastic follicular cells are not consistently subdivided into small packets by fine strands of *tron Microscopy Society of America.* Claitor's Publishing (Baton Rouge), 44–45.

Young, D. M., Capen, C. C., and Black, H. E. (1971) Calcitonin Activity in Ultimobranchial Neoplasms from Bulls. *Vet. Path.* 8, 19–27.

Yovich, J. V., and Ducharme, N. G. (1983) Ruptured Pheochromocytoma in a Mare with Colic. *J. Amer. Vet. Med. Assoc.* 183, 452–464.

Yovos, J. G., Falko, J. M., O'Dorisio, T. M., Malarkey, W. B., Cataland, S., and Capen, C. C. (1981) Thyrotoxicosis and a Thyrotropin-Secreting Pituitary Tumor Causing Unilateral Exophthalmos. *J. Clin. Endocrinol. Metabol.* 52, 338–343.

Zaki, F. A., and Liu, S. K. (1973) Pituitary Chromophobe Adenoma in a Cat. *Vet. Path.* 10, 232–237.

Zenoble, R. D., and Rowland, G. N. (1979) Hypercalcemia and Proliferative, Myelosclerotic Bone Reaction Associated with Feline Leukovirus Infection in a Cat. *J. Amer. Vet. Med. Assoc.* 175, 591–595.

# 14

*Donald R. Cordy*
# Tumors of the Nervous System and Eye

## TUMORS OF THE NERVOUS SYSTEM

**General Considerations.** Primary neoplasms of the nervous system, once regarded as rare, have a frequency in animals probably approaching that in humans; this is certainly the case for dogs. Substantial numbers are also reported in other species.

Except for an unusual incidence of meningioma in cats and of neuroblastoma and nerve sheath tumors in cattle, no species differences are apparent. Glioma is distinctly more common among brachycephalic breeds of dogs, especially boxers, but this seems to be the only example of breed predilection in any species.

Except for the few primitive neoplasms seen in younger animals, most affected animals are middle-aged or older. In a large series, Luginbühl (1963) noted that 83% of dogs with nervous system neoplasms were 5 years of age or more, and 50% were 9 years or more. No significant differences between sexes were found.

Too few cases of the less common neoplasms are reported for any significant host incidence to be established. Consequently, the occurrence or non-occurrence of scattered cases by host is not given here.

**Classification.** Modern classification schemes spring largely from the early attempt of Bailey and Cushing (1926) to relate specific neoplasms to postulated embryonic cell types, some of which have proved illusory (Boulder Committee, 1970). Except for the infrequent primitive tumors of young animals, neoplasms are currently regarded as arising by transformation, with varying degrees of anaplasia, from adult cell types.

The classification of nervous system neoplasms used here generally follows that of Russell and Rubinstein (1971), Rubinstein (1972a), and Harkin and Reed (1969) for human tumors. The present author has presumed to drop some historical terms in favor of names more accurately identifying the cell of origin, and has generally not, in view of meager information in animals, subdivided types as extensively. Many single neoplasms vary from one part to another, whether the result of variable differentiation, real admixture, or the influence of host tissue structure on tumor growth pattern (Scherer, 1938). Multiple sections are often useful in defining this range of variability.

The animal tumor classifications of Luginbühl *et al.* (1968) and Fankhauser *et al.* (1974) are very useful, but because they are based on Zulch's (1965) scheme for humans, they reflect terminology not fully accepted by many British and American pathologists.

Malignancy is not a useful concept for tumors of the central nervous system because all of these neoplasms are space occupying and most are eventually harmful. While local spread through the cerebrospinal fluid spaces occurs with several rapidly growing, friable tumors, almost none metastasize extraneurally without surgical intervention having occurred. Probably rapidity of growth and invasiveness are the best correlates of malignancy.

## Ependymoma

Derived from ependymal cells, ependymoma grows into the ventricular system and often compresses adjacent parenchyma. Rapidly growing varieties can invade the brain or cord and metastasize by the cerebrospinal fluid pathways. The neoplasm arises anywhere in the ventricle system, but most frequently is found associated with the lateral ventricles and the central canal of the spinal cord. Macroscopically, the tumor is soft, grayish pink, and fairly well defined (fig. 14.4A). Microscopically, there are sheets and broad bands of cells with variable numbers of true rosettes (figs. 14.4B and C). In the rosettes the cells surround an empty lumen and usually contain blepharoplasts and sometimes cilia. Some perivascular pseudorosettes are also seen in which cell processes form a nucleus-free zone around the vessel. A well-vascularized but scanty glial stroma supports the neoplasm. The tumor is highly cellular, and the component cells are polygonal to pyriform with round hyperchromatic nuclei. Cell outlines are indistinct. The number of mitotic figures is variable. Malignant ependymoma is characterized by anaplastic changes, invasiveness, and frequent mitoses. Differentiation can be made from choroid plexus tumors and neuroblastomas, both of which lack true rosettes with cells containing blepharoplasts and cilia.

## Mixed Gliomas

Composite glial tumors have extensive areas of astrocytic, oligodendroglial, or ependymal differentiation and are not rare in animals. It seems more appropriate to call these neoplasms mixed gliomas than to submerge their varied differentiation in a category indicating only one line of differentiation. Hart *et al.* (1974) suggested that when populations of two cell types are about equally mixed in a tumor or when different cell types appear in separate areas of a tumor, such neoplasms be called mixed gliomas.

## Microglioma

The present author agrees with Vandevelde *et al.* (1981) that there is a distinctive group of rare neoplasms that can be called microglioma. Since resting microglia are not part of the mononuclear phagocyte system (Oehmichen *et al.*, 1979; Wood *et al.*, 1979) and are probably glial (Fujita *et al.*, 1981), the tumors should be placed with other gliomas and entirely dissociated from lymphomas and other tumors.

We would include only those neoplasms forming streams or drifts of cells with elongated, twisted nuclei and meager, ill-defined cytoplasm. Immunoperoxidase methods fail to demonstrate immunoglobulins. The mode of growth is diffusely infiltrative and not particularly perivascular. Reticulum formation is not evident. As with other gliomas, boxer dogs are especially prone to these neoplasms.

## Choroid Plexus Papilloma and Carcinoma

Neoplasms derived from choroid plexus epithelium are commonly designated as papillomas and carcinomas. They are usually benign. Most occur in the dog, where they are not a rare neoplasm and probably are relatively more frequent than in humans. About three-fourths of affected dogs are 4 years of age or more. There is no predilection for brachycephalic breeds. Males are affected about twice as often as females. Arising from any of the choroid plexi, more than half develop from the lateral part of the plexus of the fourth ventricle. Here they often occupy the cerebellopontine angle with a preference for the left side. Besides compressing brain structures, these neoplasms may cause hydrocephalus by obstruction or excessive production of cerebrospinal fluid.

Plexus papillomas are macroscopically well-defined, grayish white to red, granular or cauliflower-like masses growing into the ventricle or out into the cerebellopontine angle. Microscopically, the papillomas show a branching arboriform pattern with a single layer of cuboidal or columnar cells covering a modest vascular stroma of leptomeningeal derivation (fig. 14.4D). A few acinuslike rings of somewhat paler cells are often seen in the basal areas of the larger fronds. Edema, hemorrhage, necrosis, and mineralization are not infrequent and probably reflect pressure effects rather than malignancy. Mitosis is uncommon.

Choroid plexus carcinoma is rare, and probably many reported cases are actually papillomas. Malig-

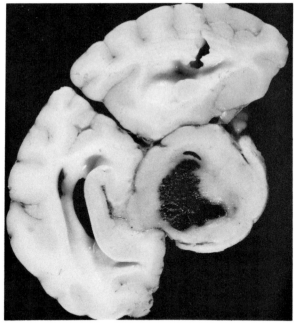

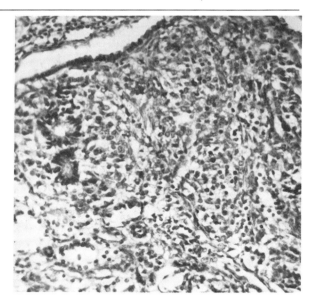

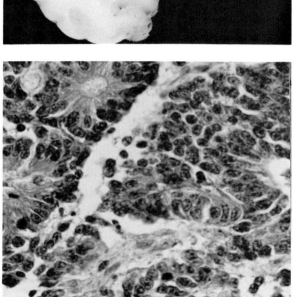

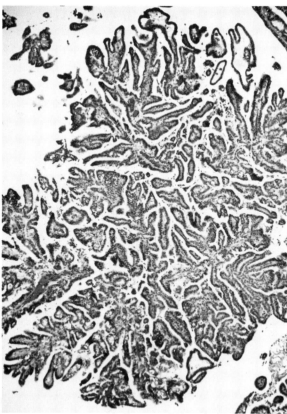

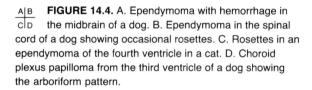 **FIGURE 14.4.** A. Ependymoma with hemorrhage in the midbrain of a dog. B. Ependymoma in the spinal cord of a dog showing occasional rosettes. C. Rosettes in an ependymoma of the fourth ventricle in a cat. D. Choroid plexus papilloma from the third ventricle of a dog showing the arboriform pattern.

nancy is marked by anaplasia, frequent mitosis, true invasiveness, and some replacement of the papillary pattern by solid areas. Spreading through the cerebrospinal fluid to meningeal sites does not constitute real metastasis since it is also seen with benign papillomas. Perhaps the position of the tumor in the flow of fluid facilitates cerebrospinal fluid spread that is usually characteristic of malignant examples of other types of neoplasms.

One must be very critical in determining invasiveness. Choroid plexus neoplasms are firm tumors, and when located outside the brain in the cerebellopontine angle, their growth causes some of the papillae to deeply indent the adjacent brainstem or to enter perivascular spaces simulating invasion. In many of these the glial basement membrane is probably still intact and true invasion has not occurred. One must also be wary of mistaking hyperplastic vessels subjacent to such contact surfaces for tumor cells.

Choroid plexus tumors may be differentiated from ependymoma by having a collagen-containing stroma and by having neither cilia nor basal bodies except in some young subjects (Patnaik *et al.*, 1980).

## Cholesterol Granuloma of the Choroid Plexus

Often called cholesteatomas, these nonneoplastic masses are usually seen in the choroid plexi of the lateral ventricles of older horses. They may be unilateral or, more commonly, bilateral. Many are clinically silent. Others enlarge to distend the ventricle and compress the brain tissue. Occasionally they occlude the interventricular foramen causing hydrocephalus. In their early stages they are small, soft, and grayish yellow. Microscopically, at this stage one sees only distended foamy cells infiltrating the choroid stroma (fig. 14.5). Older lesions are usually discrete, yellowish brown, firm, and granular. At this later stage the bulk of the lesion is composed of cholesterol clefts that reflect extracellular accumulation of cholesterol crystals. These are surrounded by a limited amount of granulomatous tissue, including macrophages containing hemosiderin. The identity of the initial foamy storage cell (whether macrophage, leptomeningeal cell, or ependymal cell) is undetermined, as is the mechanism of cholesterol accumulation (Shuangshoti and

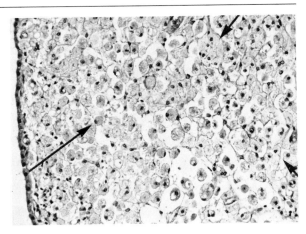

**FIGURE 14.5.** Cholesterol granuloma ("cholesteatoma") in the horse in early stage with cholesterol-filled foam cells (**arrows**) in the stroma of the choroid plexus.

Netsky, 1966). The presence of hemosiderin has suggested that prolonged stromal extravasation of erythrocytes may be the source of the cholesterol.

## Neuroblastoma and Ganglioneuroma

**Classification.** Neuroblastoma and ganglioneuroma are rare neoplasms that make up a group presumably derived from surviving primitive neuroepithelial cells, not from dedifferentiation of mature cells. They show varying degrees of differentiation toward postmitotic neuroblasts (neuroblastoma) or neurons (ganglioneuroma). Intermediate mixtures, perhaps the most frequent type, are called ganglioneuroblastoma.

*Peripheral Neuroblastoma*—This neoplasm, a derivative of neural crest cells, is seen most often in humans as a malignant tumor of childhood. Tiny *in situ* neuroblastomas are frequent in the adrenals in humans up to 3 months of age (Beckwith and Perrin, 1963; Turkel and Itabashi, 1974). It is suggested that most of these regress spontaneously or lie dormant, but that a few proliferate and differentiate to various levels of the neuroblastoma–ganglioneuroma series.

Peripheral neuroblastoma is most often reported in animals as an incidental finding in adult slaughter cattle (Monlux *et al.*, 1956; Monlux and Monlux, 1972; Wright and Conner, 1968). Such

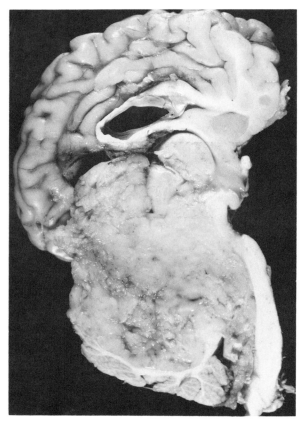

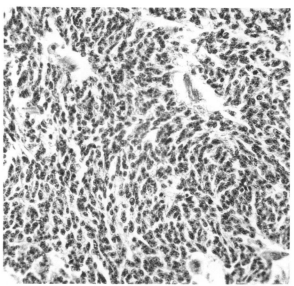

A
B

**FIGURE 14.6.** Cerebellar neuroblastoma ("medulloblastoma"). A. Involving cerebellum, medulla, and midbrain in a 2-month-old calf. B. From the region of the fourth ventricle in a steer showing small, uniform, pyriform, hyperchromatic cells around vessels. (B, courtesy of *Cornell Vet.*)

lesions are usually small and rarely metastasize. These may be analogous to the *in situ* neuroblastomas of humans.

Malignant neuroblastomas are reported in premature and stillborn calves and in dogs of all ages. Rapid growth, invasiveness, and frequent metastasis are characteristic. Usual sites of the tumor are adrenal medulla or sympathetic ganglia, although the primary site is often difficult to discern in these rapidly spreading neoplasms. Rare olfactory neuroblastomas occur in the nasal cavity.

These tumors are soft and gray, although sometimes varicolored due to hemorrhage and necrosis. Metastasis is initially to local lymph nodes or liver, but is often widespread.

These neoplasms are composed of sheets of small, poorly defined cells with dark round or elongated nuclei. Typically there are pseudorosettes of cells arranged around a tangle of processes representing primitive axons.

*Cerebellar Neuroblastoma (Medulloblastoma)* — Probably derived from primitive cells of the external granular layer (Rubinstein, 1972*b*), cerebellar neuroblastoma is seen chiefly in calves and puppies. Cases occur in the cerebellum of adult dogs where, as in humans, the usual site is hemispheric rather than vermal as in young animals. Local extension to the fourth ventricle, meninges, or adjacent brain stem may occur. Extensive dissemination can occur through cerebrospinal fluid pathways.

These neoplasms are soft, friable, gray to pink, and fairly well-defined (fig. 14.6A). Hemorrhage, cysts, and necrosis are infrequent. Microscopically, the neoplasm is composed of uniform, closely packed cells with hyperchromatic, round to elongated nuclei, and ill-defined, round to pyriform cell outlines. The cells are arranged in sheets and broad bands, sometimes radiating around small vessels (fig. 14.6B). The hallmark of neuroblastic differentiation is the appearance of pseudorosettes in which the cells are arranged around a tangle of their unipolar processes. Mitosis is frequent and growth rapid. There is a scanty vascular stroma.

Most of the few cerebral neuroblastomas reported in animals are too inadequately described to permit detailed comment, but this neoplasm, as in humans (Horten and Rubinstein, 1976), occurs occasionally in the cerebrum.

*Ganglioneuroma* — These are rare neoplasms containing neoplastic neurons of some recognizable degree of differentiation. They occur in various species and are found in neuraxis, cranial nerve ganglia, autonomic ganglia, and adrenal medulla. Growth is slow and the neoplasm benign. They are gray or white, firm, lobulated, and fibrillar. The neurons occur in groups or are scattered singly among the axon bundles. The cells are ovoid, pyramidal, or irregular in shape. The nuclei are large and often eccentric. Nissl substance, often meager, must be demonstrated in some of the neoplastic neurons. Most tumors of animals contain areas of small undifferentiated cells and are actually ganglioneuroblastomas. Often considerable stroma is present, showing glial cells centrally and Schwann cells and collagen peripherally.

One must distinguish neoplastic neurons from normal neurons entrapped in other types of neoplasms, from ectopic neurons, and from giant mononuclear cells in undifferentiated astrocytoma.

## Vascular Tumors

While most vascular masses in the central nervous system are either metastatic hemangiosarcomas or hamartomas (capillary telangiectasis, cavernous angioma, or arterovenous malformations), a few true primary hemangiomas do occur (Cordy, 1979a). These latter are discrete, pinkish to dark red masses composed microscopically of tangles of endothelium-lined channels that may contain blood. There is a variable amount of stroma. Often there is central sclerosis with more stroma and fewer channels. The nature of the stromal cells is debated; some may be neoplastic endothelium, others are trapped astrocytes. In differentiating any vascular mass, one should also keep in mind the possibility of exceptionally well vascularized meningiomas and gliomas.

## Teratoid Lesions

Included here are a variety of rare nonneuroectodermal tumors of maldevelopmental character. Some are true neoplasms, some are developmental defects, and some are entities of uncertain nature.

Rarely, germ cell neoplasms, identical to those of the gonads, occur intracranially in midline sites involving pineal, hypothalamic, or suprasellar areas.

Teratomas, germinomas, and teratomas with areas of other types have been reported.

Craniopharyngioma (described with endocrine neoplasms) has been reported a few times in dogs where it has a suprasellar site and, by pressure, may lead to the adiposogenital syndrome and diabetes insipidus.

Dorsal midline meningeal lesions overlying brain or spinal cord and composed chiefly of adipose tissue are occasionally reported. Some are associated with meningocele or other defects. It is uncertain whether these represent neoplasms or developmental anomalies.

Epidermal and dermoid cysts, the former associated most often with the choroid plexus of the fourth ventricle, are occasionally seen.

## Lymphoma

**General Considerations.** General information on lymphoma in animals is provided in chapter 6 of this volume, but a few remarks on involvement of the nervous system seem appropriate. Only recently have immunohistological methods been used on animal lymphomas of the nervous system (Vandevelde *et al.*, 1981). Judging from studies in humans (Houthoff *et al.*, 1978), probably all morphological types seen extraneurally also occur in the neuraxis. As in humans, most animal lymphomas have been found to be of B-cell origin showing maturation arrest at various stages (Holmberg *et al.*, 1976).

### Primary Histiocytic Lymphoma

Probably the most common primary neuraxial lymphoma and the type causing the most diagnostic confusion is the large cell or "histiocytic" lymphoma, once called reticulum cell sarcoma. This category probably includes most cases of so-called primary neoplastic reticulosis (Fankhauser *et al.*, 1972; Russo, 1979), which remain after one has eliminated cases of canine granulomatous meningoencephalomyelitis (Braund *et al.*, 1978; Cordy, 1979b).

These neoplasms are usually found in the cerebrum or diencephalon. Some tumors show fairly well-defined outlines, but most appear only as a vague increase in volume of the affected part of the brain. The cut surface may appear granular and occasionally mottled by necrosis. Some neoplasms are multicentric.

The typical neoplastic cell has a large, pleomorphic, vesicular nucleus with a distinct nuclear membrane and prominent nucleoli. There is appreciable acidophilic cytoplasm with poorly defined margins and angular in outline where apparent. Mitosis is frequent and growth rapid. Occasionally mononucleate or multinucleate giant cells suggestive of Sternberg–Reed cells are seen. Lymphocyte and plasma cell admixtures are common. The degree of tumor cell pleomorphism and cell admixture is variable across a broad spectrum. Reticulum may be prominent in a lamellar pattern around vessels, but is only occasionally seen among tumor cells at a distance. Its inconsistent appearance suggests that it is actually part of the stromal response and not produced by tumor cells.

These neoplasms are highly cellular. Solid sheets of tumor cells characterize the center of the mass with more evident predilection for perivascular spaces at the margins. Parenchyma intervening between ensheathed vessels may be nearly normal, somewhat edematous, or frankly necrotic. Diffusely scattered neoplastic cells appear well beyond the limits of the tumor proper.

### Secondary Lymphoma

About 5% of generalized lymphomas in dogs and cats have secondary metastases in the nervous system (Meincke *et al.*, 1972; Squire *et al.*, 1973). The most common way that these affect the nervous system (although actually extraneural) is through occurrence of epidural infiltrates compressing the spinal cord, especially in the thoracolumbar area (Zaki and Hurvitz, 1976; Zaki *et al.*, 1975). Inboard to the dura the most frequent site is the leptomeninges, including adjacent perivascular spaces and choroid plexi. Craniospinal roots, ganglia and nerves, the pituitary area, dura mater, and the neuraxial parenchyma itself are sometimes involved.

### Other Secondary Neoplasms

A number of neoplasms affect the central nervous system by extension from adjacent cranial and vertebral sites or by growing through foramina or through bone itself to impinge on nervous tissue. Bony and cartilaginous neoplasms and spinal epidural lymphoma are probably the most frequent. Also reported are malignant melanoma, plasmacytoma, and carcinoma of nasal mucosa, olfactory glands, skin, or conjunctiva.

More frequent are the hematogenous metastases of neoplasms to brain and cord from extraneural primary sites. Mammary carcinomas are most frequent, but other adenocarcinomas, hemangiosarcoma, malignant melanoma, canine venereal tumor, and fibrosarcoma also occur. Such metastases are usually discrete, spherical, and located in gray substance or at the gray–white junction.

## Meningioma

**Classification.** Meningiomas, among the most frequent intracranial neoplasms of animals, are derived from leptomeningocytes. These cells are not conventional fibroblasts, but are derived from neural crest cells or are mesenchymal derivatives induced by contact with neural crest cells. Ultrastructurally, the normal and neoplastic cells are characterized by the ability to form collagen, by desmosomes and cytoplasmic fibrils, and by their complex interdigitating pattern of elongated processes (Tedeschi *et al.*, 1981).

**Sites in Cats.** Meningiomas are especially frequent in older cats, where they may be multiple and clinically silent (Andrews, 1973; Luginbühl, 1961; McGrath, 1962; Nafe, 1979; Zaki and Hurvitz, 1976). Most cat tumors are supratentorial, where they are most frequent about the falx and in the transverse fissure under the fornix of the hippocampus. These latter tumors sometimes protrude into the lateral or third ventricles.

**Sites in Dogs.** Basal locations are the most common sites in dogs, although the neoplasm also occurs over the cerebral and cerebellar convexities, around the falx and tentorium, and in the pontocerebellar angle. Tumors also occur over the spinal cord, where they are most frequent around nerve roots of cervical segments. Retrobulbar meningiomas are occasionally seen, either as extensions of perichiasmal tumors or as primary meningiomas of the distal part of the meningeal sheath of the optic nerve. Rarely, extraneural meningiomas of typical ultrastructural appearance are reported in epidural

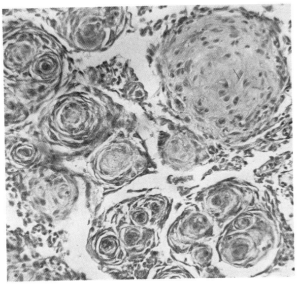

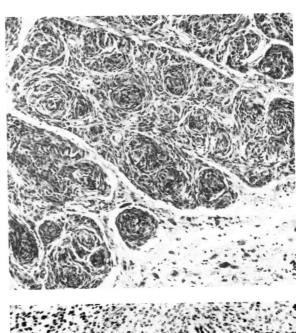

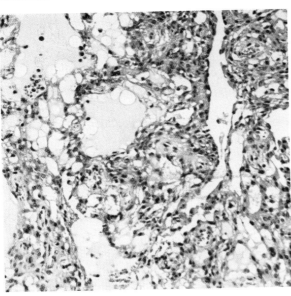

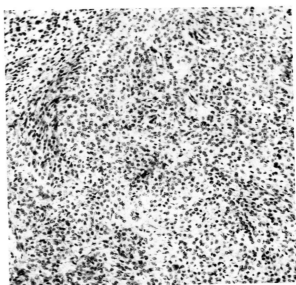

|A|B|
|C|D|

**FIGURE 14.7.** Meningioma. A. Meningioma over the right frontal lobe of a dog showing whorls of flattened cells. B. Meningioma overlying the cerebellum of a dog with lobules containing tight whorls of cells. C. Highly vascular meningioma of a dog. D. Meningioma composed of sheets of cells with vague cell outlines. Whorls are not seen. (B and D, courtesy of Dr. A. C. Palmer and *Res. Vet. Sci.*)

sites (Fagerland and Greve, 1980) or subcutaneous sites (Herrera and Mendoza, 1981; Vuletin *et al.*, 1978).

**Gross Morphology.** Meningiomas may be spheroid, lobate, lenticular, or plaquelike. Usually solitary in most species, they are often multiple in cats. The tumors are well-defined, firm, white, and thinly encapsulated. The cut surface may be lobulated and fibrillar. Some meningiomas become secondarily attached to the dura. Growth is usually expansive, and the mass is often bedded in an atrophic depression in the brain substance. Extension into cranial marrow spaces may lead to reactive hyperostosis.

**Histological Features.** Meningiomas have been divided into several subtypes depending on their microscopic pattern (figs. 14.7A–D). Because many of these neoplasms show two or more subtypes within the same tumor and because all are ultrastructurally composed of the same cell, it is not particularly useful to subdivide the group.

The most common microscopic pattern is one of laminated whorls of elongated crescentric cell profiles. These whorls may range from two to many cells in diameter and may show central calcified material (psammoma bodies). There is not usually a central blood vessel. Other patterns include streams and crescents of similar cells or lobulated islands of polygonal cells. The cells, whether flattened or not, have open nuclei and vague cell outlines. There is a variable and sometimes substantial amount of reticulum and collagen. Rarely, bone or cartilage islands are found.

**Growth and Metastasis.** Malignancy is rare and characterized by infiltrative growth, anaplasia, and increased mitosis. One should be careful of ascribing malignancy to the occasional blunt tongues of tumor that may indent the brain substance without intimate infiltration. There may be benign extensions into perivascular spaces where leptomeningeal cells are normally present. Meningioma is one intracranial neoplasm occasionally reported to develop extracranial metastases, especially to the lungs.

## Sarcoma

Occasionally diagnosed but poorly defined are the "sarcomas" of the central nervous system (Luginbühl *et al.*, 1968). Some are probably malignant meningiomas, undifferentiated astrocytomas, cerebellar neuroblastomas, or "histiocytic" lymphomas. A few may be fibrosarcomas of dural origin. The origin of others is unknown.

These tumors are macroscopically focal or diffuse and usually involve the meninges, but are also reported within the brain or cord. They are composed of fusiform or polygonal cells, with occasional multinucleate giant cells. Reticulum fibers may be demonstrated. Much more study needs to be made of this strangely assorted group before more definitive statements can be made.

## Schwannoma

**Classification.** Schwannomas (neurolemmomas) are neoplasms arising from Schwann cells, and perhaps the related perineurial cells, of the peripheral nerve sheaths (Canfield, 1978a,b). These cells are distinguished from fibroblasts by possessing a basal lamina. They are also facultative collagen formers.

A complication in classification of these tumors in humans has been their confusing association with von Recklinghausen's neurofibromatosis, a hereditary syndrome. This author does not believe that the multiple Schwannomas of cattle are analogous to von Recklinghausen's disease. There are certain rare cutaneous neoplasms of calves associated with nerves (Slanina *et al.*, 1976) that may be analogous, although these appear to be fibroblastic in origin since the tumor cells have no basal lamina.

The terms *neurofibroma* and *perineurial fibroblastoma* would well be abandoned since they suggest a fibroblastic origin and imply relationship to von Recklinghausen's disease. This is not to deny the possible rare occurrence of conventional fibromas arising from endoneurial fibroblasts (Vandevelde *et al.*, 1977).

**Incidence.** Schwannomas occur most frequently in cattle, where they are usually benign and often multiple (Canfield, 1978a; Monlux and Davis, 1953; Monlux and Monlux, 1972; Monlux *et al.*, 1956). Canfield and Doughty (1980) described viruslike particles in the tumor cells, perhaps explaining the unusually high incidence in cattle. Cattle are affected at all ages, but chiefly at maturity. If one is properly skeptical of suspicious skin Schwannomas in dogs, occurrences in species other than cattle are not common.

**Sites.** Schwannomas may occur nearly anywhere in the peripheral nervous system. In cattle, granted the limitations of meat inspection examination, the most common sites are the brachial plexus, intercostal nerves, and cardiac nerves. Less frequent are occurrences in other retroserosal sites in the thorax and abdomen, in nerves to skeletal muscles (especially the tongue), and in roots and ganglia of cervical spinal nerves. Schwannomas of the acoustic nerve are usually solitary in cattle. Cutaneous tumors are rare.

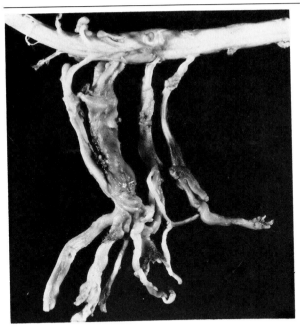

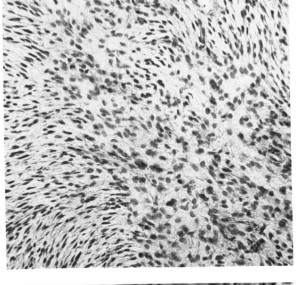

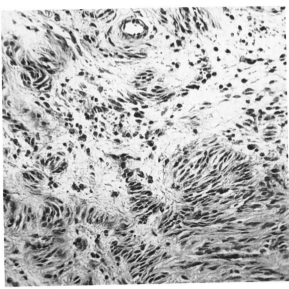

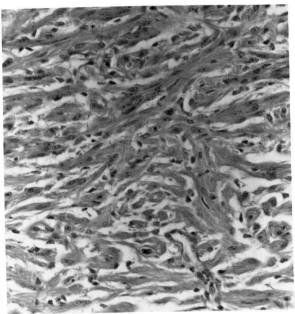

<table>
<tr><td>A</td><td>B</td></tr>
<tr><td>C</td><td>D</td></tr>
</table>

**FIGURE 14.8.** Schwannoma. A. Schwannoma of a dog showing cylindrical thickening of the eighth cervical nerve of the brachial plexus. B. Antoni type-A and type-B tissue patterns in Schwannoma of the ox. C. Palisading or regimentation of nuclei in Schwannoma of a dog. D. Schwannoma of the ox. Unusual cordlike pattern of Schwann cells with much intervening space. (A, courtesy of Dr. P.C. Kennedy and *Cancer*.)

In the dog, Schwannomas have been reported most often on cranial nerve roots (especially the fifth), on spinal nerve roots (especially at the caudal cervical level), and in the brachial plexus. Suspicious nodular lesions in the skin of dogs provide a difficult diagnostic problem. An association with a nerve should be shown to permit a diagnosis of Schwannoma. Many of these lesions are probably fibromas or hemangiopericytomas (see chap. 2). Ultrastructural studies should help clarify the problem.

**Gross Morphology and Histological Features.** Schwannomas are seen either as nodular masses or as varicose thickenings of large nerve trunks (fig. 14.8A). They vary from firm to gelatinous and are white or gray, shiny, and fairly well-circumscribed. Dumbbell-shaped tumors may be seen where a nerve root neoplasm has grown through the foramen and expanded.

Neoplastic Schwann cells are usually arranged in interwoven bundles or whorls of closely approximated, elongated, fusiform cells with a modest amount of intervening reticulum or collagen (Antoni type-A pattern) (figs. 14.8B and C). Often the nuclei of the bundled cells are parallel with each other in a regimented or palisaded pattern (fig. 14.8C). Other areas may show a looser texture with irregularly arranged cells of plumper fusiform or stellate outline with more intervening extracellular space (Antoni type-B pattern). Sometimes one sees a pattern of cordlike outgrowths of tumor cells with abundant extracellular space containing collagen and mucoid material (fig. 14.8D). The latter should not be confused with the Renaut bodies of normal nerves (Asbury, 1973).

It is uncertain how much of the lesion may be a nonneoplastic reaction to nerve trunk damage. This may account for much of the fibrosis seen, especially in the diffusely thickened parts of the nerve. The onion bulb-like structures (Canfield, 1978a,b) may also reflect reaction rather than neoplasia.

Usually the nerve of origin is located eccentrically, but some neoplasms show nerve fibers coursing through the tumor mass. Encapsulation is variable in extent or even absent.

Differential diagnosis is often difficult, especially with solitary cutaneous tumors. Whorling may also be seen in nerve root meningiomas and in hemangiopericytomas. Streaming bundles of elongated cells also characterize leiomyomas, equine sarcoids, and some fibromas. Even nuclear palisading is not specific for Schwannoma, being seen occasionally in other neoplasms with compact parallel arrangements of elongated dividing cells.

**Growth and Metastasis.** Malignant Schwannomas are infrequent and are characterized by mitosis, high cellularity, anaplasia, and rare metastasis to lymph nodes or lungs. Local benign involvement of nerves in parenchymal organs should be distinguished from actual metastasis.

## Granular Cell Tumors

Sometimes called myoblastomas, these rare tumors are often regarded as deriving from Schwann cells of small nerves (see chaps. 3 and 7). In dogs the tongue is the most common site, in horses the lung (Misdorp and Nauta-van Gelder, 1968; Parker et al., 1978). Rarely they arise in the central nervous system or skin.

The neoplasm appears as a dense, white, discrete mass. It is composed of lobules or rows of pale granular cells of variable size, some very large. Nuclei are oval and vesicular. Ultrastructurally, the cells are clad by basal laminae and contain granules and vesicles of probable lysosomal origin. The granules stain positively with periodic acid–Schiff and Sudan black B, sometimes regarded as evidence of myelin constituents.

## TUMORS OF THE EYE

This section deals with ocular squamous cell carcinoma and intraocular neoplasms. Except for the former, neoplasms of the lids and extraocular orbital sites are covered in chapter 2. Classification generally follows that of Kircher et al. (1974) and Reese (1963). Eye tumors are also reviewed by Gelatt (1972), Morgan (1969), Saunders (1971), and Saunders and Rubin (1975).

## Ocular Squamous Carcinoma of Cattle

**Incidence.** Ocular squamous carcinoma of cattle, a very common neoplasm, is of great economic importance. Between 1950 and 1954 the Meat Inspection Division of the United States Department of Agriculture recorded a 0.2% incidence of this tumor in cattle. The animals with the tumor accounted for 82% of all cattle condemned for neoplasia (Russell *et al.*, 1956). In some regions of the United States the incidence of ocular carcinoma in cattle is nearly 5% (Woodward and Knapp, 1950). The incidence in living animals is probably greater than that in slaughtered animals because many tumors are removed by veterinarians before the cattle reach the abattoir. In addition, the animals that die of the tumor are not accounted for in these statistics, nor are those killed in nonfederal abattoirs.

**Geographic Distribution.** "Cancer eye" in cattle has also been reported in Europe, South America, Africa, Asia, the United Kingdom, and Australia. In the United States the majority of cases are in the southwest, perhaps because of a greater exposure to ultraviolet radiation there (Anderson and Skinner, 1961; Guilbert *et al.*, 1948).

**Age, Breed, and Sex.** The average age of cattle with ocular squamous carcinoma is 8 years. The tumors are not common in animals younger than 5 years old and are rare in animals less than 1 year of age (Russell *et al.*, 1956). All breeds are affected, but the Hereford breed is thought to be the most susceptible. A lack of pigmentation around the eyes in this breed has been suggested (Anderson *et al.*, 1957a) as a predisposing factor, but that should affect only the incidence of the eyelid tumors. Most other reports agree that the Hereford has the highest incidence, but many of the incriminating statistics might be challenged on the basis that Herefords in the United States outnumber all other breeds of range cattle combined.

There is probably no sex difference in the incidence of cancer eye, although a falsely higher incidence is established since more males than females are sent to the abattoir before the age of peak incidence.

**Sites.** Russell *et al.* (1956) and Monlux *et al.* (1957) reported the sites of a combined total of more than 1,000 ocular carcinomas and benign precursor lesions. Approximately 75% were on the bulbar conjunctiva and cornea. Of these, 90% were at the limbus and 10% on the cornea proper. The majority of the lesions of the limbus appeared in the lateral and medial sides; fewer lesions were in the superior and inferior areas. Russell *et al.* (1956)

found more lesions at the lateral limbus than at the medial limbus, whereas Monlux *et al.* (1957) noted an equal distribution. It is of interest that the lateral or medial limbus, being at the point of palpebral closure, is more subject to irritation from foreign matter and ultraviolet radiation than are other areas of the eye. The remaining 25% of the lesions were found about equally distributed in the conjunctiva of the eyelids and membrana nictitans and the skin of the eyelids.

**Gross Morphology and Histological Features.** The various lesions and their incidence may be listed as follows: plaques, 11%; papillomas, 7%; noninvasive carcinoma, 3%; and invasive carcinoma, 79%. These lesions have been described in detail by Russell *et al.* (1956) and Monlux *et al.* (1957). In addition to having the plaque, papilloma, and carcinoma, the skin of the eyelid may exhibit hyperkeratosis, particularly near the mucocutaneous junction at or near the hairline. Extensive keratosis in this area usually appears as a cutaneous horn. The keratotic lesions become moistened by tears, collect debris, and become dirty brown and may be easily pulled off, leaving a bleeding surface. Carcinomas occasionally develop from these hyperkeratotic lesions.

*Plaque*—This is a small area of hyperplastic epithelium, and most of the conjunctival lesions can be traced to this lesion. The plaques are single or multiple in the eye. They are slightly raised and are circular, oblong, or irregular in shape (fig. 14.9A). The surface is smooth or irregular and moderately firm or hard from keratinization. At the limbus, where plaques are usually found, the shape is often curvilinear, following the arc of the junction of the cornea and sclera. The plaque is opaque and grayish white.

Microscopically, a plaque represents an area of hyperplastic conjunctival epithelium (fig. 14.9B). It involves any or all layers of the epithelium, but the cells of the stratum spinosum are principally involved. Varying degrees of hyperkeratosis appear, and rarely, extreme keratosis forms a horny growth. As the epithelial cell hyperplasia develops, the underlying connective tissue proliferates and becomes vascularized. It forms tortuous projections into the overlying epithelium, and at this stage the plaque becomes a papilloma.

*Papilloma*—This has multiple, hard, spinelike

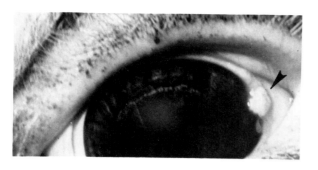

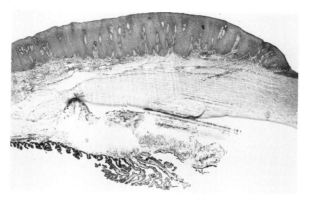

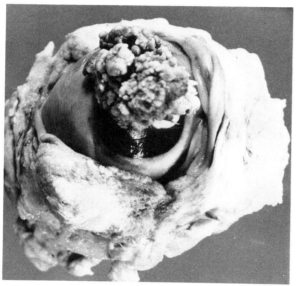

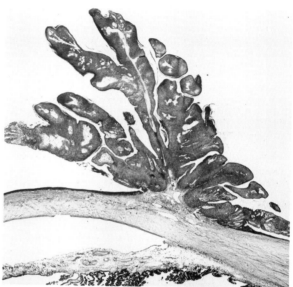

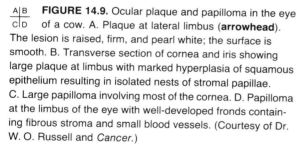

A|B
---
C|D

**FIGURE 14.9.** Ocular plaque and papilloma in the eye of a cow. A. Plaque at lateral limbus (**arrowhead**). The lesion is raised, firm, and pearl white; the surface is smooth. B. Transverse section of cornea and iris showing large plaque at limbus with marked hyperplasia of squamous epithelium resulting in isolated nests of stromal papillae. C. Large papilloma involving most of the cornea. D. Papilloma at the limbus of the eye with well-developed fronds containing fibrous stroma and small blood vessels. (Courtesy of Dr. W. O. Russell and *Cancer.*)

projections of variable size and a connective tissue core. It has a small base or multiple rounded protuberances with a large confluent base. A few papillomas are mushroom shaped with narrow stalks (fig. 14.9C).

When fully developed the papilloma consists microscopically of multiple papillary projections covered by proliferative epithelium and supported by vascular connective tissue stalks (fig. 14.9D). The covering epithelium shows all degrees of hyperkeratosis.

*Noninvasive Carcinoma*—This lesion follows the plaque-to-papilloma sequence or arises directly from the plaque. It grossly resembles papilloma and exhibits no invasion.

Microscopically, this form of the neoplasm shows malignant transformation of the epithelial cells in the basilar layer or, less commonly, in the stratum spinosum (figs. 14.10A–D). These cells display hyperchromatic nuclei, increased numbers of mitotic figures, pleomorphism, and loss of polarity. The

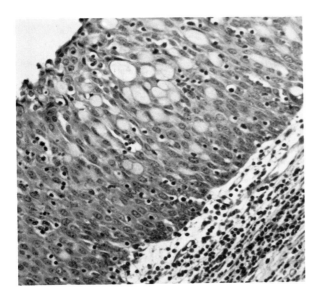

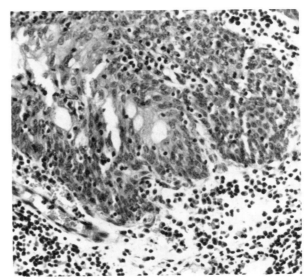

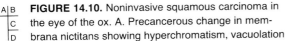

A | B
C
D

**FIGURE 14.10.** Noninvasive squamous carcinoma in the eye of the ox. A. Precancerous change in membrana nictitans showing hyperchromatism, vacuolation of epithelium, and infiltration of lymphocytes and plasma cells in the stroma below. B. Noninvasive carcinoma on bulbar conjunctiva showing loss of polarity in cells of basal layer, hyperchromatism, vacuolation of epithelium, variation in size of nuclei, and inflammation of stroma. C. Noninvasive carcinoma of the membrana nictitans. D. Early invasive carcinoma of bulbar conjunctiva showing infiltrating cords of large, hyperchromatic cells which have loss of polarity. Observe infiltration of mononuclear cells below. (B, courtesy of Dr. W. O. Russell and *Cancer.*)

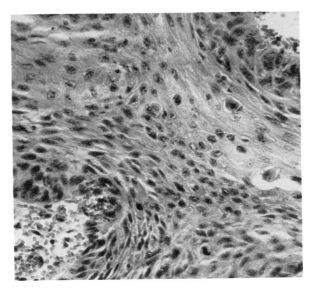

neoplasm may show beginning downward penetration, and subepithelial infiltrations of mononuclear cells are common at such sites.

*Invasive Carcinoma*—This carcinoma is generally large and protrudes through the palpebral fissure where it causes open fixation of the eyelids. The carcinoma can invade the anterior or posterior chambers of the eye and replace the entire eye (figs. 14.11A and B). Carcinoma arising from the conjunctiva of the membrana nictitans commonly replaces this structure but seldom invades the cartilage. When carcinoma arises strictly in the cornea, there is less downward invasion because of the resistance of the substantia propria and the membranes of Bowman and Descemet. The carcinoma also shows minimal invasion of the sclera, because of the resistance of this dense tissue. Secondary changes such as necrosis, ulceration, hemorrhage, and inflammatory cell infiltration appear in more than 40% of invasive carcinomas.

Microscopically, invasive carcinoma is well-dif-

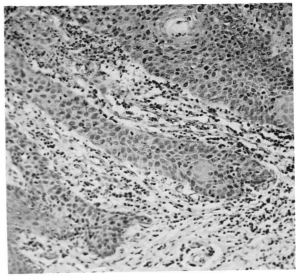

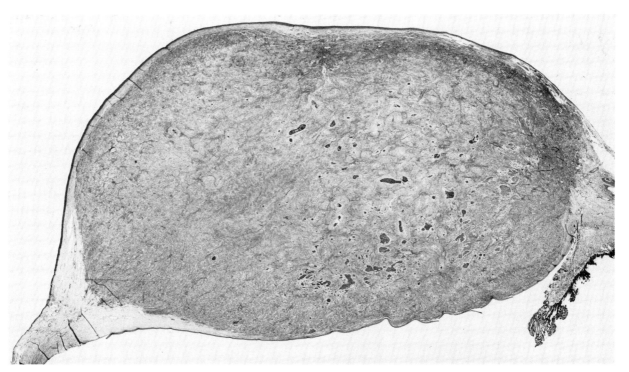

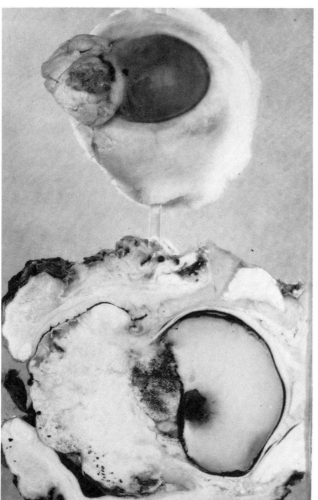

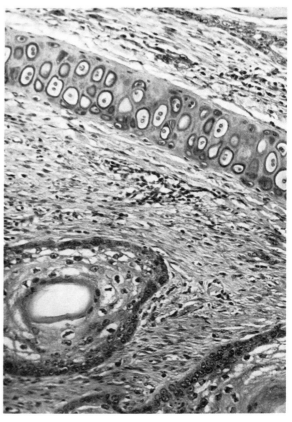

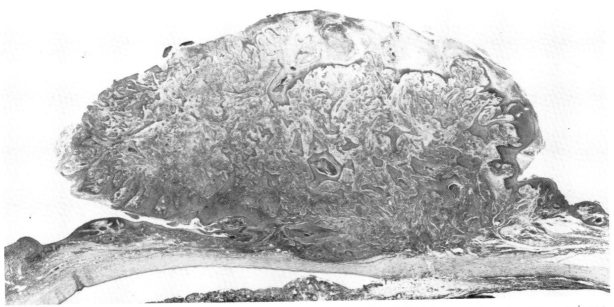

A / B

**FIGURE 14.12.** Invasive ocular squamous carcinoma of the ox. A. Carcinoma growing outward from the limbus with infiltrating cords of cells, keratinization, and abundant fibrous stroma. Note absence of invasion of the sclera. B. Infiltrating cords of cells in squamous carcinoma of the limbus. (A, courtesy of Dr. W. O. Russell and *Cancer*.)

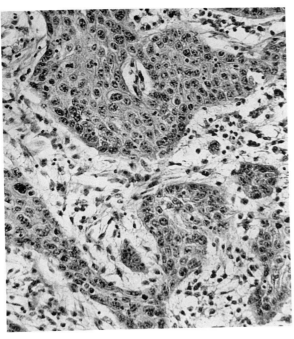

← 

**FIGURE 14.11.** Invasive ocular squamous carcinoma of the ox. A. Poorly differentiated squamous carcinoma filling anterior chamber; Descemet's membrane is intact. Note displaced ciliary body, reflected downward on the right. B. Top: carcinoma at the medial limbus of the eye. Bottom: meridinal section of the eye showing infiltrative squamous carcinoma obliterating cornea and involving anterior chamber. C. Invasive cords of squamous carcinoma adjacent to cartilage of the membrana nictitans. (A, courtesy of Dr. W. O. Russell and *Cancer*.)

ferentiated and exhibits keratin pearl formation or is highly anaplastic and consists of small, hyperchromatic cells that have no keratinization (figs. 14.11C and 14.12A and B). The tumor invades the tissues of the eye and its own connective tissue stroma.

**Etiology.** Ocular squamous carcinoma is not associated with trauma, irritation from dust or pollen, or photosensitization. That a transmissible agent causes this condition is suspected but not proved. Such an agent, perhaps a virus, would be compatible with the high incidence of the neoplasm in multiple and bilateral forms and with the progress of the tumor from hyperplasia to papilloma to carcinoma.

Taylor and Hanks (1969) reported an interesting association of infectious bovine rhinotracheitis virus (a herpes virus) with ocular carcinoma, but a cause and effect relationship is unlikely. A number of other herpes viruses have been demonstrated to be oncogenic in various species (Klein, 1972). Viral transformation has also been shown to be enhanced by ultraviolet light (Lytle *et al.*, 1970), a possible explanation of the roles of pigmentation and sunshine. Tumor cells do not exhibit the usual type of viral inclusion bodies, but they do contain viruslike particles as shown by electron microscopy (Hod and Perk, 1973).

Predisposition to cancer eye in cattle is probably inherited as a recessive character (Blackwell *et al.*, 1956; Woodward and Knapp, 1950). Anderson and Chambers (1957) found the tumor in 44.4% of the progeny of two affected parents, in 23.7 to 26.7% of the progeny of one affected and one un-affected parent, and in 8.8% of the progeny of two unaffected parents.

A predisposing factor of some importance in cancer eye is lack of pigmentation of the eyelids. A decreased pigmentation in the eyelids has been re-lated to development of this tumor in the skin of the lids (Anderson *et al.*, 1957b; Guilbert *et al.*, 1948). The characteristics of eyelid pigmentation are inherited in about 45% of Hereford cattle (An-derson *et al.*, 1957a); thus incidence of the tumor could be reduced by breeding for heavier eyelid pigmentation. The effect on the overall incidence of cancer eye would be minor, however, because the eyelids are the sites for only about 10% of these tumors.

**Growth and Metastasis.** Some carcinomas in-vade the orbital bones, maxilla, and orbital part of the frontal bones. The anterior chamber of the eye was invaded in 67 of 471 carcinomas in the series reported by Monlux *et al.* (1957). The posterior chamber was affected less often, and invasion there generally occurred around the lens rather than through the dense scleral tissue.

Metastasis probably develops late in these tu-mors. Metastatic cells from the eye tumor pass through a chain of lymph nodes in the head and neck before reaching the thoracic duct and venous circulation. Metastatic secondaries are found in the parotid lymph nodes in 5 to 15% of cases (Monlux *et al.*, 1957; Russell *et al.*, 1956). They are also found in the atlantal, retropharyngeal, submaxil-lary, mandibular, and cervical lymph nodes. Some metastases have been observed in the lungs, heart, pleura, liver, kidneys, and the bronchial and medi-astinal lymph nodes.

## Ocular Squamous Carcinoma of Other Species

**Incidence.** Ocular squamous carcinoma is rela-tively uncommon in animals other than cattle. The neoplasm has been reported in the horse, sheep, dog, and cat (in approximate order of decreasing frequency). The average age of affected horses is 8 years. The tumors are found in other animals of adult or old age. There is no breed or sex predilec-tion in any of these species.

**Sites and Structure.** Squamous cell carcinoma in the horse usually arises from the conjunctiva of the membrana nictitans, but also involves the eye-lids, limbus, and cornea. No favored site has been noted in other species.

These tumors are structurally similar to those in cattle, and both cornifying and noncornifying types exist.

**Metastasis.** A small percentage of the reported cases have included metastasis. Mainly involved were the mandibular, submaxillary, anterior cer-vical, and pharyngeal lymph nodes. No metastasis to the lungs was found.

## Ocular Dermoid

**Incidence.** Ocular dermoid is not a true tumor but rather a developmental defect in which a piece of skin, usually with hair, is situated on some part of the cornea or conjunctiva. Since this lesion is congenital, its presence in newborn or very young animals is not surprising. Smythe (1958) claimed that the condition is inherited and is very common in some strains of German shepherd (Alsatian) dogs.

**Site and Structure.** This lesion appears as a plaque of pigmented skin, usually with hair, often at the limbus but also on the conjunctiva and cor-nea. It is usually unilateral but may be bilateral. A crop of fairly stiff hairs from the surface of the growth is common and may attain considerable length. These hairs in the horse and ox are often luxuriant. Histologically, the lesion has practically the same structure as normal skin, consisting of an epidermis, dermis, sebaceous and sweat glands, hair follicles, and sometimes muscle fibers. The glands are occasionally cystic and filled with secretion. This lesion seldom grows very large and never shows malignant change, but it may cause irritation and become infected.

## Intraocular Melanocytic Tumors

**Classification.** Melanocytic tumors are the most common primary intraocular neoplasms of animals. Although most have been regarded as malignant, the dearth of follow-up studies makes the correlation of tumor morphology and clinical behavior uncertain (Diters *et al.*, 1983; Kircher *et al.*, 1974).

A subdivided classification is used for humans that does correlate well with clinical behavior (Wilder and Paul, 1951). It is based on cell type (spindle type-A, spindle type-B, epithelioid, and mixed types) and on the amount of pigment and reticulum present. Spindle type-A is the least malignant. Similar cell types occur in animals.

**Incidence and Sites.** Most cases have been found in dogs (Saunders and Barron, 1958) and cats (Bellhorn and Henkind, 1970). Despite the frequency of cutaneous melanocytic tumors in horses, intraocular tumors are rare in that species. Malignant melanomas arise most often in the anterior uveal tract, especially in the iris, and are infrequent in the choroid. A benign epibulbar form has been reported in or on the sclera at the limbus (Diters *et al.*, 1983).

**Structure and Growth.** These neoplasms are white, gray, or black. Except for necrotic areas they are firm. They may diffusely enlarge the affected part of the eye or appear as discrete masses, often occupying much of the interior of the eye.

Tumor cells vary (as described above) from spindle shaped to round or polygonal. Many of the latter type are large cells with abundant pale cytoplasm. Spindle cells may be in whorled or interwoven patterns, but sheets of cells are most common. Mitosis and pigmentation are highly variable, but necrosis is frequent. Neoplastic cells may be found growing along scleral vessels, occasionally reaching extraocular orbital sites. Hematogenous metastasis is not rare.

## Neoplasms of Iridociliary Epithelium

**Classification and Incidence.** A number of well-described adenomas and adenocarcinomas of pigmented or nonpigmented iridociliary epithelium in dogs have been reported (Bellhorn, 1971; Saunders and Barron, 1958) as primary tumors (fig. 14.13). They are second in frequency only to uveal melanocytic tumors among dogs.

**Structure and Behavior.** These neoplasms are of variable form, from tiny nodules to masses filling the bulb. Usually white, they may be partly gray or black depending on the inclusion of pigmented cells.

Adenomas are well-differentiated, with cuboidal to columnar cells in papillary, tubular, or solid patterns. Some mimic the ciliary processes, and their appearance varies with the plane of section, with cross-cut tubules suggesting rosettes or cordlike networks. Mitosis is infrequent.

Adenocarcinomas are characterized by pleomorphic columnar, fusiform, or polygonal cells with frequent mitoses. Tissue patterns are like those of adenomas but more irregular. The neoplasms are locally invasive and may reach episcleral sites. Hematogenous metastasis is rare and usually occurs to the lungs.

## Other Primary Intraocular Neoplasms

Intraocular primary mesenchymal neoplasms are rare in animals. Barron and Saunders (1959) described hemangioma of the iris and leiomyosarcoma of iris and ciliary body in dogs and chondrosarcoma of the uveal tract in a cat.

Neuroepithelial neoplasms are also rare. Well-differentiated astrocytoma and Schwannoma have been reported. Several medulloepitheliomas, which are primitive neoplasms arising from the inner layer of the optic cup epithelium, have been described in dogs and horses (Bistner, 1974; Eagle *et al.*, 1978; Lahav *et al.*, 1976; Langloss *et al.*, 1976). Nonteratoid medulloepitheliomas are composed of folded sheets and tubules of polarized columnar cells mimicking the embryonal retina. Teratoid types also show areas of nervous tissue, cartilage, skeletal muscle, or primitive mesenchyme. Usually arising in the pars ciliaris retinae, the tumors may be found wherever the primitive ventricular layer has existed, such as in the retina or optic nerve (Bistner *et al.*, 1983).

A few purported retinoblastomas have been described, but none were thought to be true retinoblastomas by Kircher *et al.* (1974) or Saunders and Rubin (1975). Possibly the case of Saliba and Alvarenga (1966) may qualify. These neoplasms, most

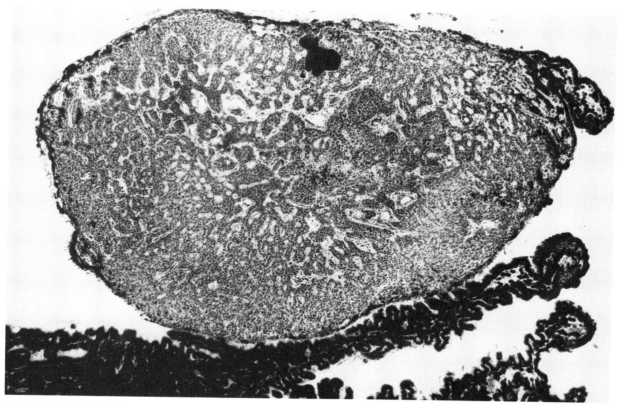

**FIGURE 14.13.** Small adenoma of the ciliary body attached to one of the ciliary processes in an aged dog. (Courtesy of Dr. L. Z. Saunders and *Cancer Res.*)

common in young children, are very similar to neuroblastoma of the nervous system. They are composed of small, densely packed, undifferentiated cells with dark nuclei and scanty, ill-defined cytoplasm. True rosettes are seen in some of the more differentiated tumors.

## Secondary Tumors of the Eye

### Spread by Local Extension

Two neoplasms account for most of the invasions of the bulb by extension from nearby primary sites. Squamous cell carcinoma, chiefly bovine, may invade from corneoconjunctival sites through the limbus to reach the iris and anterior chamber. Monlux *et al.* (1957) found that 20% of bovine squamous cell carcinomas of the eyeball behaved in this manner. Meningiomas, arising in the perichiasmal region and extending along the optic nerve or arising independently in the distal meningeal sheath of the optic nerve, may form large retrobulbar masses. Although they often surround and compress the optic nerve, they rarely invade it. Limited invasion of sclera, choroid, or retina may occasionally occur near the optic papilla. In some species, e.g. the dog and horse, carcinoma of the nasal cavity or sinuses can invade around the optic nerve and into the ocular orbit.

### Spread by Hematogenous Metastasis

Generalized lymphomas of various types not uncommonly metastasize late to intraocular sites in dogs and cats. The most frequent spread is to iris and ciliary body, but choroid and other parts are occasionally involved (Cello and Hutcherson, 1962; Meincke, 1966; Saunders and Barron, 1958). Anterior chamber hemorrhage and secondary glaucoma are often observed, and spread through the limbus may produce corneal opacity. Exophthalmos, which is prominent in orbital lymphoma in cattle, is not common in dogs and cats, in which most of the tumor is intraocular.

A small number of carcinomas, sarcomas, and malignant melanomas have been described as metastasizing to uveal sites (Barron *et al.,* 1963a; Bellhorn, 1972). Barron *et al.* (1963b) reported several cases of transmissible venereal tumors in dogs that metastasized to the uveal tract, an unusual affinity in neoplasms that rarely metastasize.

# REFERENCES

Anderson, D. E., and Chambers, D. (1957) Genetic Aspects of Cancer Eye in Cattle. In: *Oklahoma Agricultural Experiment Station Miscellaneous Publication MP-48*, 28–33.

Anderson, D. E., and Skinner, P. E. (1961) Studies on Bovine Ocular Squamous Carcinoma ("Cancer Eye"). XI. Effects of Sunlight. *J. Anim. Sci.* 20, 474–477.

Anderson, D. E., Chambers, D., and Lush, J. L. (1957a) Studies on Bovine Ocular Squamous Carcinoma ("Cancer Eye"). III. Inheritance of Eyelid Pigmentation. *J. Anim. Sci.* 16, 1007–1016.

Anderson, D. E., Lush, J. L., and Chambers, D. (1957b) Studies on Bovine Ocular Squamous Carcinoma ("Cancer Eye"). II. Relationship between Eyelid Pigmentation and Occurrence of Cancer Eye Lesions. *J. Anim. Sci.* 16, 739–746.

Andrews, E. J. (1973) Clinicopathologic Characteristics of Meningiomas in Dogs. *J. Amer. Vet. Med. Assoc.* 163, 151–157.

Asbury, A. K. (1973) Renaut Bodies. A Forgotten Endoneurial Structure. *J. Neuropath. Exp. Neurol.* 32, 334–343.

Bailey, P., and Cushing, H. A. (1926) *A Classification of the Tumors of the Glioma Group on a Histogenetic Basis with a Correlated Study of Prognosis.* J. B. Lippincott (Philadelphia).

Barron, C. N., and Saunders, L. Z. (1959) Intraocular Tumors in Animals. II. Primary Nonpigmented Intraocular Tumors. *Cancer Res.* 19, 1171–1174.

Barron, C. N., Saunders, L. Z., and Jubb, K. V. (1963a) Intraocular Tumors in Animals. III. Secondary Intraocular Tumors. *Amer. J. Vet. Res.* 24, 835–853.

Barron, C. N., Saunders, L. Z., Seibold, H. R., and Heath, M. K. (1963b) Intraocular Tumors in Animals. V. Transmissible Venereal Tumor of Dogs. *Amer. J. Vet. Res.* 24, 1263–1269.

Beckwith, J. B., and Perrin, E. V. (1963) *In Situ* Neuroblastomas: A Contribution to the Natural History of Neural Crest Tumors. *Amer. J. Path.* 43, 1089–1104.

Bellhorn, R. W. (1971) Ciliary Body Adenocarcinoma in the Dog. *J. Amer. Vet. Med. Assoc.* 159, 1124–1128.

———. (1972) Secondary Ocular Adenocarcinoma in Three Dogs and a Cat. *J. Amer. Vet. Med. Assoc.* 160, 302–307.

Bellhorn, R. W., and Henkind, P. (1970) Intraocular Malignant Melanoma in Domestic Cats. *J. Small Anim. Pract.* 10, 631–637.

Bistner, S. I. (1974) Medullo-Epithelioma of the Iris and Ciliary Body in a Horse. *Cornell Vet.* 64, 588–595.

Bistner, S., Campbell, R. J., Shaw, D., Leininger, J. R., and Gholbrial, H. K. (1983) Neuroepithelial Tumor of the Optic Nerve in a Horse. *Cornell Vet.* 73, 30–40.

Blackwell, R. L., Anderson, D. E., and Knox, J. H. (1956) Age Incidence and Heritability of Cancer Eye in Hereford Cattle. *J. Anim. Sci.* 15, 943–951.

Boulder Committee. (1970) Embryonic Vertebrate Central Nervous System: Revised Terminology. *Anat. Rec.* 166, 257–261.

Braund, K. G., Vandevelde, M., Walker, T. L., and Redding, R. W. (1978) Granulomatous Meningoencephalomyelitis in Six Dogs. *J. Amer. Vet. Med. Assoc.* 172, 1195–1200.

Canfield, P. (1978a) A Light Microscopic Study of Bovine Peripheral Nerve Sheath Tumours. *Vet. Path.* 15, 283–291.

———. (1978b) The Ultrastructure of Bovine Peripheral Nerve Sheath Tumours. *Vet. Path.* 15, 292–300.

Canfield, P. J., and Doughty, F. R. (1980) A Study of Virus-like Particles Present in Bovine Nerve Sheath Tumours. *Aust. Vet. J.* 56, 257–261.

Cello, R. M., and Hutcherson, B. (1962) Ocular Changes in Malignant Lymphoma of Dogs. *Cornell Vet.* 52, 492–523.

Cordy, D. R. (1979a) Vascular Malformations and Hemangiomas of the Canine Spinal Cord. *Vet. Path.* 16, 275–282.

———. (1979b) Canine Granulomatous Meningoencephalomyelitis. *Vet. Path.* 16, 325–333.

Diters, R. W., Dubielzig, R. R., Aguirre, G. D., and Acland, G. M. (1983) Primary Ocular Melanoma in Dogs. *Vet. Path.* 20, 379–395.

Eagle, R. C., Jr., Font, R. L., and Swerczek, T. W. (1978) Malignant Medulloepithelioma of the Optic Nerve in a Horse. *Vet. Path.* 15, 488–494.

Fagerland, J. A., and Greve, J. H. (1980) Unusual Psammoma Bodies in an Extracranial Syncytial Meningioma from a Dog. *Vet. Path.* 17, 45–52.

Fankhauser, R., Fatzer, R., Luginbühl, H., and McGrath, J. T. (1972) Reticulosis of the Central Nervous System (CNS) in Dogs. *Adv. Vet. Sci.* 16, 35–71.

Fankhauser, R., Luginbühl, H., and McGrath, J. T. (1974) Tumours of the Nervous System. *Bull. Wld. Hlth. Org.* 50, 53–69.

Fujita, S., Tsuchihashi, Y., and Kitamura, T. 1981. *Eleventh International Congress of Anatomy.* Alan R. Liss (New York), 141–169.

Gelatt, K. N. (1972) Recent Advances in Veterinary and Comparative Ophthalmology. *Adv. Vet. Sci.* 16, 1–33.

Guilbert, H. R., Wahid, A., Wagnon, K. A., and Gregory, P. W. (1948) Observations on Pigmentation of

Eyelids of Hereford Cattle in Relation to Occurrence of Ocular Epitheliomas. *J. Anim. Sci.* 7, 426–429.

Harkin, J. C., and Reed, R. J. (1969) Tumors of the Peripheral Nervous System. In: *Atlas of Tumor Pathology.* 2d series, fascicle 3. Armed Forces Institute of Pathology (Washington, D.C.).

Hart, M. N., Petito, C. K., and Earle, K. M. (1974) Mixed Gliomas. *Cancer* 33, 134–140.

Herrera, G. A., and Mendoza, A. (1981) Primary Canine Cutaneous Meningioma. *Vet. Path.* 18, 127–130.

Hod, I., and Perk, K. (1973) Intranuclear Microspherules in Bovine Ocular Squamous Cell Carcinoma. *Ref. Vet.* 30, 41–44.

Holmberg, C. A., Manning, J. S., and Osburn, B. I. (1976) Canine Malignant Lymphomas: Comparison of Morphologic and Immunologic Parameters. *J. Natl. Cancer Inst.* 56, 125–135.

Horten, B. C., and Rubinstein, L. J. (1976) Primary Cerebral Neuroblastoma. A Clinicopathological Study of 35 Cases. *Brain* 99, 735–756.

Houthoff, J., Poppema, S., Ebels, E. J., and Elema, J. D. (1978) Intracranial Malignant Lymphomas. Morphologic and Immunocytologic Study of Twenty Cases. *Acta Neuropath.* 44, 203–210.

Kircher, C. H., Garner, F. M., and Robinson, F. R. (1974) Tumours of the Eye and Adnexa. *Bull. Wld. Hlth. Org.* 50, 135–142.

Klein, G. (1972) Herpesviruses and Oncogenesis. In: *Proceedings of the National Academy of Sciences of the U.S.A.* 69, 1056–1064.

Lahav, M., Albert, D. M., Kircher, C. H., and Percy, D. H. (1976) Malignant Teratoid Medulloepithelioma in a Dog. *Vet. Path.* 13, 11–16.

Langloss, J. M., Zimmerman, L. E., and Krehbiel, J. D. (1976) Malignant Intraocular Teratoid Medulloepithelioma in Three Dogs. *Vet. Path.* 13, 343–352.

Luginbühl, H. (1961) Studies on Meningiomas in Cats. *Amer. J. Vet. Res.* 22, 1030–1040.

———. (1963) Comparative Aspects of Tumors of the Nervous System. *Ann. N.Y. Acad. Sci.* 108, 702–721.

Luginbühl, H., Fankhauser, R., and McGrath, J. T. (1968) Spontaneous Neoplasms of the Nervous System in Animals. *Prog. Neurol. Surg.* 2, 85–164.

Luse, S. A. (1960) Electron Microscopic Studies of Brain Tumors. *Neurol.* 10, 881–905.

Lytle, C. D., Hellman, K. B., and Telles, N. C. (1970) Enhancement of Viral Transformation by Ultraviolet Light. *Intl. J. Rad. Biol.* 18, 297–300.

McGrath, J. T. (1960) *Neurologic Examination of the Dog.* Lea and Febiger (Philadelphia).

———. (1962) Meningiomas in Animals. *J. Neuropath. Exp. Neurol.* 21, 327–328.

Meincke, J. E. (1966) Reticuloendothelial Malignancies with Intraocular Involvement in the Cat. *J. Amer. Vet. Med. Assoc.* 148, 157–161.

Meincke, J. E., Hobbie, W. V., and Hardy, W. D., Jr. (1972) Lymphoreticular Malignancies in the Cat: Clinical Findings. *J. Amer. Vet. Med. Assoc.* 160, 1093–1099.

Misdorp, W., and Nauta-van Gelder, H. L. (1968) "Granular-Cell Myoblastoma" in the Horse. A Report of 4 Cases. *Path. Vet.* 5, 385–394.

Monlux, A. W., and Davis, C. L. (1953) Multiple Schwannomas of Cattle (Nerve Sheath Tumors; Multiple Neurilemmomas; Neurofibromatosis). *Amer. J. Vet. Res.* 14, 499–509.

Monlux, A. W., Anderson, W. A., and Davis, C. L. (1956) A Survey of Tumors Occurring in Cattle, Sheep, and Swine. *Amer. J. Vet. Res.* 17, 646–677.

———. (1957) The Diagnosis of Squamous Cell Carcinoma of the Eye (Cancer Eye) in Cattle. *Amer. J. Vet. Res.* 18, 5–34.

Monlux, W. S., and Monlux, A. W. (1972) *Atlas of Meat Inspection Pathology.* Agriculture Handbook No. 367, U.S. Department of Agriculture (Washington, D.C.).

Morgan, G. (1969) Ocular Tumours in Animals. *J. Small Anim. Pract.* 10, 563–570.

Nafe, L. A. (1979) Meningiomas in Cats: A Retrospective Clinical Study of 36 Cases. *J. Amer. Vet. Med. Assoc.* 174, 1224–1227.

Oehmichen, M., Wietholter, H., and Greaves, M. F. (1979) Immunological Analysis of Human Microglia: Lack of Monocytic and Lymphoid Membrane Differentiation Markers. *J. Neuropath. Exp. Neurol.* 38, 99–103.

Parker, G. A., Botha, W., Van Dellen, A., and Casey, H. W. (1978) Cerebral Granular Cell Tumor (Myoblastoma) in a Dog: Case Report and Literature Review. *Cornell Vet.* 68, 506–520.

Patnaik, A. K., Erlandson, R. A., Lieberman, P. H., Fenner, W. R., and Prata, R. G. (1980) Choroid Plexus Carcinoma with Meningeal Carcinomatosis in a Dog. *Vet. Path.* 17, 381–385.

Reese, A. B. (1963) *Tumors of the Eye.* 2d ed. Hoeber (New York).

Rubinstein, L. J. (1972a) Tumors of the Central Nervous System. In: *Atlas of Tumor Pathology.* 2d series, fascicle 6. Armed Forces Institute of Pathology (Washington, D.C.).

———. (1972b) Cytogenesis and Differentiation of Primitive Central Neuroepithelial Tumors. *J. Neuropath. Exp. Neurol.* 31, 7–26.

Russell, D. S., and Rubinstein, L. J. (1971) *Pathology of Tumours of the Nervous System.* 3d ed. Williams and Wilkins (Baltimore).

Russell, W. O., Wynne, E. S., and Loquvam, G. S. (1956) Studies on Bovine Ocular Squamous Carcinoma ("Cancer Eye"). I. Pathological Anatomy and Historical Review. *Cancer* 9, 1–52.

Russo, M. E. (1979) Primary Reticulosis of the Central Nervous System in Dogs. *J. Amer. Vet. Med. Assoc.* 174, 492–500.

Saliba, A. M., and Alvarenga, J. (1966) Neuroepithelioma da retina em cao. *Arquivos da Escola Veterinaria* (Minas Gerais, Brazil) 18, 91–94.

Saunders, L. Z. (1971) *Pathology of the Eye of Domestic Animals.* Verlag P. Parey (Berlin).

Saunders, L. Z., and Barron, C. N. (1958) Primary Pigmented Intraocular Tumors in Animals. *Cancer Res.* 18, 234–244.

Saunders, L. Z., and Rubin, L. F. (1975) *Ophthalmic Pathology of Animals.* S. Karger (Basel).

Scherer, H. J. (1938) Structural Development in Gliomas. *Amer. J. Cancer* 34, 333–351.

Shein, H. M. (1970) Neoplastic Transformation of Hamster Astrocytes and Choroid Plexus Cells in Culture by Polyoma Virus. *J. Neuropath. Exp. Neurol.* 29, 70–88.

Shuangshoti, S., and Netsky, M. G. (1966) Xanthogranuloma (Xanthoma) of Choroid Plexus. *Amer. J. Path.* 48, 503–533.

Slanina, L., Konrad, V., Vajda, V., Lojda, L., Zibrin, M., Skarda, R., Bajova, V., Lehocky, J., Sokol, J., and Madar, J. (1976) Hromadný výskyt kongenitálnej kožnej neurofibromatózy u teliat. [Mass outbreak of congenital cutaneous neurofibromatosis in calves]. *Veterinárstvi* 26, 245–249.

Smythe, R. H. (1958) *Veterinary Ophthalmology.* Bailliere, Tindall and Cox (London).

Squire, R. A., Bush, M., Melby, E. C., Neeley, L. M., and Yarbrough, B. (1973) Clinical and Pathologic Study of Canine Lymphoma: Clinical Staging, Cell Classification and Therapy. *J. Natl. Cancer Inst.* 51, 565–574.

Taylor, R. L., and Hanks, M. A. (1969) Viral Isolations from Bovine Eye Tumors. *Amer. J. Vet. Res.* 30, 1885–1886.

Tedeschi, F., Brizzi, R., Trabattoni, G., Ferrari, C., and Tagliavini, F. (1981) Meningiomas. A Light and Electron Microscopy Study. *Acta Neuropath.* suppl. VII, 122–125.

Turkel, S. B., and Itabashi, H. H. (1974) The Natural History of Neuroblastic Cells in the Fetal Adrenal Gland. *Am. J. Path.* 76, 225–244.

Vandevelde, M., Braund, K. G., and Hoff, E. J. (1977) Central Neurofibromas in Two Dogs. *Vet. Path.* 14, 470–478.

Vandevelde, M., Fatzer, R., and Fankhauser, R. (1981) Immunohistological Studies on Primary Reticulosis of the Canine Brain. *Vet. Path.* 18, 577–588.

Vuletin, J. C., Friedman, H., and Gordon, W. (1978) Extraneuraxial Canine Meningioma. *Vet. Path.* 15, 481–487.

Wilder, H. C., and Paul, E. V. (1951) Malignant Melanoma of the Choroid and Ciliary Body: A Study of 2535 Cases. *Milit. Surg.* 109, 370–378.

Wood, G. W., Goolahon, K. A., Tibzer, S. A., Vats, T., and Marantz, R. A. (1979) The Failure of Microglia in Normal Brain to Exhibit Mononuclear Phagocyte Markers. *J. Neuropath. Exp. Neurol.* 38, 369–376.

Woodward, R. R., and Knapp, B., Jr. (1950) The Hereditary Aspect of Eye Cancer in Hereford Cattle. *J. Anim. Sci.* 9, 578–581.

Wright, B. J., and Conner, G. H. (1968) Adrenal Neoplasms in Slaughtered Cattle. *Cancer Res.* 28, 251–263.

Zaki, F. A., and Hurvitz, A. I. (1976) Spontaneous Neoplasms of the Central Nervous System of the Cat. *J. Small Anim. Pract.* 17, 773–782.

Zaki, F. A., Prata, R. G., Hurvitz, A. I., and Kay, W. J. (1975) Primary Tumors of the Spinal Cord and Meninges in Six Dogs. *J. Amer. Vet. Med. Assoc.* 166, 511–517.

Zulch, K. J. (1964) On the Definition of the Polymorphous Oligodendroglioma. *Acta Neurochir.* suppl. X, 166–172.

———. (1965) Brain Tumors: Their Biology and Pathology. 2d American ed. Springer Publishing (New York).

# Index